BOARD BUSTER

STEP 1

BOARD BUSTER

STEP 1

Stanley Zaslau, MD, MBA, FACS

Associate Professor
Division of Urology
West Virginia University
Morgantown, West Virginia

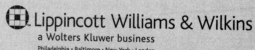 Lippincott Williams & Wilkins
a Wolters Kluwer business
Philadelphia · Baltimore · New York · London
Buenos Aires · Hong Kong · Sydney · Tokyo

Acquisitions Editor: Donna M. Balado
Managing Editor: Selene Steneck
Marketing Manager: Emilie Linkins
Production Editor: Sirkka E. H. Bertling
Design Coordinator: Holly Reid McLaughlin
Interior Designer: Leslie Haimes
Compositor: Circle Graphics, Inc.
Printer: Victor Graphics, Inc.

351 West Camden Street
Baltimore, MD 21201
530 Walnut Street
Philadelphia, PA 19106

Library of Congress Cataloging-in-Publication Data

Zaslau, Stanley.
   Board buster step 1 / Stanley Zaslau.
        p. ; cm.
   Includes index.
   ISBN 1-4051-0469-4
   1. Medicine—Examinations, questions, etc. 2. Physicians—Licenses—United States—Examinations—Study guides. I. Title. II. Title: Board buster step one.
   [DNLM: 1. Medicine—Case Reports. 2. Medicine—Examination Questions. W 18.2 Z38b 2006]
R834.5.Z36 2006
610.76—dc22

                                                    2005033108

To purchase additional copies of this book, call our customer service department at **(800) 638-3030** or fax orders to **(301) 223-2320**. International customers should call **(301) 223-2300**.

Visit Lippincott Williams & Wilkins on the Internet: http://www.LWW.com. Lippincott Williams & Wilkins customer service representatives are available from 8:30 am to 6:00 pm, EST.

06 07 08 09
1 2 3 4 5 6 7 8 9 10

Preface

One of the most challenging events in medical school is passage of the United States Medical Licensing Examination (USMLE). This three-step examination is not only required for licensure to practice medicine in the United States but is also used by some residency programs to select applicants for interviews. Thus, demonstration of high scores on this examination can have major importance for students.

Question-and-answer study guides form an important framework to study for licensure examinations. These simulated clinical vignettes place students in nearly "real-life" and examination-like situations. Students using question-and-answer books will effectively learn not only the correct answer for each vignette but also other pertinent information about why distracter choices (which are also possible answers but not the best ones) are incorrect. Use of these question-and-answer books will also prepare students for situations they will face on their clinical rotations. Patient presentations are the real-life form of the clinical vignettes in question-and-answer books.

The best question-and-answer books are written by students who have experienced these types of examinations first hand. It is with these premises in mind that the *Board Buster* series has been created. All of the questions in this book were written by medical students at West Virginia University School of Medicine. The questions are arranged according to body system. This allows students to use this book to review for classroom examinations. Questions are also arranged into a practice examination. This will give students the opportunity to simulate an actual licensure examination.

These questions were reviewed by ten other medical students, interns, and residents from programs throughout North America for level of difficulty, format, and accuracy. Additionally, the final, revised questions were given a final review by faculty.

We hope that you will find *Board Buster Step 1* to be both beneficial to your studies for your examination and a useful adjunct to your clinical rotations. We believe that this book of new vignettes will truly "bust the boards" for each user.

Stanley Zaslau, MD, MBA, FACS
Morgantown, WV

Contributors

Melany Atkins
West Virginia University School of Medicine, Class of 2006
Melany is a medical student at WVU School of Medicine, graduating in May 2006. She graduated summa cum laude from WVU with a bachelor's degree in chemistry in 2002. She is from Morgantown, West Virginia, and is the daughter of Billy and Carolyn Atkins.

Tania Babar
West Virginia University School of Medicine, Class of 2006
Born in New York City, Tania grew up in Holland and then moved to West Virginia. She did her undergraduate study at the University of Charleston in West Virginia, where she majored in both biology and psychology. She will receive her medical degree in 2006 from WVU School of Medicine. During her free time, Tania enjoys rowing, skiing, and traveling.

Gary Breetz
West Virginia University School of Medicine, Class of 2006
Gary is a medical student at WVU, class of 2006. His interest is in emergency medicine. Gary received a chemical engineering degree at the University of Louisville and worked as an engineer for 3 years before entering medical school. He enjoys kayaking, snowboarding, and mountain biking, including statewide racing. Past activities include a 1-week race in the French Pyrenees and a 3-month backpacking trip in Australia. He has been happily married to Karen Breetz, M.D., since December 2002; their daughter, Rachel Elizabeth Breetz, was born April 2, 2005.

Hyland Cronin
West Virginia University School of Medicine, Class of 2006
Hyland attended the University of Notre Dame for undergraduate study; she majored in science preprofessional and graduated summa cum laude. She is currently attending medical school at the WVU School of Medicine. In her free time, Hyland enjoys dancing, running, and skiing.

Courtney D. Cuppett
West Virginia University School of Medicine, Class of 2005
Courtney was born and raised in Uniontown, Pennsylvania. She attended Duquesne University for undergraduate study, majoring in biology with a focus on cellular and molecular studies. After graduating from Duquesne, Courtney entered WVU School of Medicine. She graduated in 2005 with her medical degree and is currently an ob/gyn resident at WVU. In her free time, Courtney enjoys running and spending time with her Weimaraner, Sammy.

Matthew Evans
West Virginia University School of Medicine, Class of 2006
Matthew is currently in his senior year at WVU School of Medicine. He anticipates training in internal medicine at Walter Reed Medical Center in Washington, DC, and has a particular interest in the care of adults with congenital heart disease.

Philip Granchi
West Virginia University School of Medicine, Class of 2005
Phil Granchi holds both a BS and MS in geology from Purdue University. After working for a few years in the petroleum and environmental fields, he pursued some of his creative interests through multimedia design and production.

Justin Harris
West Virginia University School of Medicine, Class of 2006
Justin was born and raised in Charleston, West Virginia. He attended WVU for undergraduate study and received a BA in biology. He will receive his medical degree in 2006 from WVU School of Medicine. Whenever he has free time, Justin enjoys digital photography, pinball, and weight lifting.

Noel DeSantos Ibanez
West Virginia University School of Medicine, Class of 2007
Noel was born in Charlestown, West Virginia, and raised in Huntington, West Virginia. He attended WVU for undergraduate study, where he majored in biology and graduated summa cum laude. He will receive his medical degree from WVU School of Medicine.

Collin John
West Virginia University School of Medicine, Class of 2007
Collin grew up in the historic town of Gettysburg, Pennsylvania. After attending Penn State University and obtaining a BA in premedicine, he enrolled in the MD/MPh program at WVU. He expects to obtain these degrees in 2007. For fun, Collin enjoys racquetball, white-water rafting, and scuba diving.

John Lynam
Intern, Maimonides Medical Center, Brooklyn, NY
John was born and raised on Long Island, NY. For his undergraduate study, he attended the State University of New York at Stony Brook, where he double majored in psychology and sociology and double minored in women's studies and human sexual/gender development. He attended the University of Miami for his postbaccalaureate work and recently received his medical degree from Western University of the Health Sciences/COMP in Southern California. He is currently completing his internship at Maimonides Medical Center in Brooklyn, New York, and applying for a residency in urological surgery.

Rocco A. Morabito, Jr.
West Virginia University School of Medicine, Class of 2006
Rocco is currently in his fourth year at WVU School of Medicine. He is most interested in urology, hoping to attain a residency and fulfill his ultimate goal in life: to work beside his father in his rapidly expanding practice, Huntington Urological Association, in Huntington, West Virginia. He values hard work and dedication and has great leadership qualities. He loves spending time with friends and family. In his spare time he enjoys traveling, cooking, weight training, and attending church.

Matthew Oliverio
West Virginia University School of Medicine, Class of 2006
Matt is currently a medical student at WVU School of Medicine and will graduate in 2006. As an undergraduate at WVU he majored in animal science.

Christopher Osborne
West Virginia University School of Medicine, Class of 2006
Chris is currently attending WVU School of Medicine. When he is not extrapolating a seemingly endless differential diagnosis, he can be found composing music or words. Currently, he aspires to be a pediatric hematologist/oncologist.

Haynes Ralsten
West Virginia University School of Medicine, Class of 2006
After completing a BA in French and an MA in linguistics, Haynes moved to Japan, where she taught English, studied Japanese, and learned to samba. She returned home to attend medical school and will receive her degree in 2006. After work, her dogs Samba and Gil take Haynes hiking on nearby trails.

Zeshan Rana
West Virginia University School of Medicine, Class of 2005
Zeshan received his M.D. degree in May 2005 from WVU School of Medicine. He will be completing a preliminary year in internal medicine at Christiana Care in Wilmington, Delaware. In his spare time he enjoys being with friends and family, playing sports, being outdoors, and traveling. He aspires to be a great physician, like the many before him.

Nasira Roidad
West Virginia University School of Medicine, Class of 2006
Nasira was born and raised in Fairmont, West Virginia. She attended WVU for her undergraduate study, majoring in biology. She will graduate from the WVU School of Medicine in May 2006. In her free time, she enjoys reading novels and spending time with family and friends.

Julie Balch Samora
West Virginia University School of Medicine, Class of 2009
Julie holds BFA degrees in biological sciences and bassoon performance from Carnegie Mellon University and an MA in music from Yale University. She began the MD/PhD program at WVU in 2001 and is currently in her third year of research in microvascular physiology. During her first year of research, she obtained an MPh degree; she will complete an MA in public administration with a specialization in health care administration in December 2005. Julie and her husband Quincy just celebrated the birth of their first child, Ethan Christopher Samora.

Stacey N. Shreve
West Virginia University School of Medicine, Class of 2006
Stacey, currently attending WVU School of Medicine, attended WVU for undergraduate study and received a BS in biology. In her free time, she enjoys traveling, skiing, and hiking with her black lab, Merlin.

Melanie E. Watkins
West Virginia University School of Medicine, Class of 2006

Melanie, currently a student at WVU School of Medicine, graduated from Emory University in 1999, where she earned a BS in biology. After graduation, Melanie moved to Boston, where she conducted research in gene therapy at Harvard Medical School. Melanie plans to enter the field of ob/gyn and complete her residency in the Northeast. During her free time, she enjoys running road races with her father.

Jeffrey M. Williams
West Virginia University School of Medicine, Class of 2006

Jeff was born in Morgantown, West Virginia, but mainly grew up in Bozeman, Montana. He graduated from Montana State University, having majored in chemical engineering, and worked as an engineer for 10 years in Houston before returning to medical school. Whenever he finds free time, Jeff enjoys playing tennis, fly fishing, and mountain biking.

Joel Yednock
West Virginia University School of Medicine, Class of 2006

Joel was born and raised in the small town of Point Marion, Pennsylvania. He attended North Carolina Wesleyan College as an undergrad and was a member of the NCAA Division III National Champion baseball team. Joel plans to remain at WVU and complete a residency in internal medicine.

Amy Schneid Yester
West Virginia University School of Medicine, Class of 2006

Amy was born in Wheeling, West Virginia. She attended Wheeling Central Catholic High School and WVU. She graduated cum laude in 2002 with a BS in biology. Currently Amy is completing her fourth year of medical school at WVU. She aspires to become an ob/gyn. In her free time she enjoys being with her husband, Marc Yester; they were married in June 2005.

Marc Yester
West Virginia University School of Medicine, Class of 2006

Marc is a lifelong resident of Morgantown, West Virginia. He attended WVU as an under-graduate, majoring in chemistry. He looks forward to entering a pediatric residency and a career in international health. By the time this book is printed, he will be married to Amy Schneid, another contributor to this book. In his free time, Marc enjoys movies, Playstation, and golfing.

Reviewers

Bob Armin
Class of 2006
David Geffen School of Medicine
Los Angeles, California

Jessica M. Ghaferi
Class of 2006
The Johns Hopkins School of Medicine
Baltimore, Maryland

Alexander Ho
Class of 2006
Washington University School of Medicine
St. Louis, Missouri

Sarah Katel
Class of 2006
Drexel University College of Medicine

Susan Knowles
Class of 2006
University of Nevada School of Medicine
Las Vegas, Nevada

Andrea Musel
Class of 2006
University of Minnesota Medical School
Minneapolis, Minnesota

Tejas N. Patel
Class of 2006
Temple University School of Medicine
Philadelphia, Pennsylvania

Luwam Semere
Class of 2006
Harvard Medical School
Boston, Massachusetts

Acknowledgments

The success of *Board Buster Step 2* and the enthusiasm of my West Virginia University medical students have infused energy to the creation of *Board Buster Step 1*. Completion of this seemingly monumental task would not have been possible without Beverly Copland, whose positive support and encouragement were timely. Selene Steneck has done another outstanding job as editor. Special thanks to my WVU medical students for their excellent work on a challenging project. Finally, a heartfelt thanks to my wife, April, and son, Darren, for always being there for me.

Contents

Figure Credits

Diagnostic Test

Figure 1: Used with permission from the Department of Imaging, Cedars-Sinai Medical Center, Los Angeles, California.

Figure 2: Used with permission from Axford J, O'Callaghan C. Medicine. 2nd ed. Oxford, UK: Blackwell Science Ltd., 2004, p. 1067.

Figure 3: Used with permission from Taylor GJ. 150 Practice ECGs: Interpretation and Review. 2nd ed. Malden, MA: Blackwell Publishing, Inc., 2002, p. 47.

Figure 4: Used with permission from Axford J, O'Callaghan C. Medicine. 2nd ed. Oxford, UK: Blackwell Science Ltd., 2004, p. 892.

Figure 5: Used with permission from Axford J, O'Callaghan C. Medicine. 2nd ed. Oxford, UK: Blackwell Science Ltd., 2004, p. 1105.

Figure 6: Used with permission from Axford J, O'Callaghan C. Medicine. 2nd ed. Oxford, UK: Blackwell Science Ltd., 2004, p. 258.

Figure 7(a, b, and c): Used with permission from Axford J, O'Callaghan C. Medicine. 2nd ed. Oxford, UK: Blackwell Science Ltd., 2004, p. 735.

Figure 8: Used with permission from Armstrong P, Wastie M, Rockall A. Diagnostic Imaging. 5th ed. Oxford, UK: Blackwell Science Ltd., 2004, p. 18.

Figure 9: Used with permission from Axford J, O'Callaghan C. Medicine. 2nd ed. Oxford, UK: Blackwell Science Ltd., 2004, p. 243.

Figure 10(a and b): Used with permission from Axford J, O'Callaghan C. Medicine. 2nd ed. Oxford, UK: Blackwell Science Ltd., 2004, p. 480.

Figure 11: Used with permission from Axford J, O'Callaghan C. Medicine. 2nd ed. Oxford, UK: Blackwell Science Ltd., 2004, p. 740.

Figure 12(a, b, and c): Used with permission from Axford J, O'Callaghan C. Medicine. 2nd ed. Oxford, UK: Blackwell Science Ltd., 2004, p. 518.

Figure 13: Used with permission from Axford J, O'Callaghan C. Medicine. 2nd ed. Oxford, UK: Blackwell Science Ltd., 2004, p. 854.

Figure 15: Used with permission from Burns T, Breathnach S, Cox N, Griffiths C. Rook's Textbook of Dermatology. 7th ed. Oxford, UK: Blackwell Science, Ltd., 2005.

Figure 16: Used with permission from Axford J, O'Callaghan C. Medicine. 2nd ed. Oxford, UK: Blackwell Science Ltd., 2004, p. 1035.

Figure 17: Used with permission from Axford J, O'Callaghan C. Medicine. 2nd ed. Oxford, UK: Blackwell Science Ltd., 2004, p. 1147.

Figure 18: Used with permission from Seaton A, Leitch AG, Seaton D. Crofton and Douglas's Respiratory Diseases. 5th ed. Oxford, UK: Blackwell Science Ltd., 2000.

Figure 19: Used with permission from Axford J, O'Callaghan C. Medicine. 2nd ed. Oxford, UK: Blackwell Science Ltd., 2004, p. 169.

Figure 20: Used with permission from Axford J, O'Callaghan C. Medicine. 2nd ed. Oxford, UK: Blackwell Science Ltd., 2004, p. 852.

Figure 21: Used with permission from the Department of Imaging, Cedars-Sinai Medical Center, Los Angeles, California.

Figure 22: Used with permission from the Department of Imaging, Cedars-Sinai Medical Center, Los Angeles, California.

Figure 23: Used with permission from Axford J, O'Callaghan C. Medicine. 2nd ed. Oxford, UK: Blackwell Science Ltd., 2004, p. 887.

Figure 24: Used with permission from Axford J, O'Callaghan C. Medicine. 2nd ed. Oxford, UK: Blackwell Science Ltd., 2004, p. 1163.

Figure 25: Used with permission from Axford J, O'Callaghan C. Medicine. 2nd ed. Oxford, UK: Blackwell Science Ltd., 2004, p. 266.

Figure 26: Used with permission from Axford J, O'Callaghan C. Medicine. 2nd ed. Oxford, UK: Blackwell Science Ltd., 2004, p. 317.

Figure 27: Used with permission from Axford J, O'Callaghan C. Medicine. 2nd ed. Oxford, UK: Blackwell Science Ltd., 2004, p. 465.

Figure 28(a and b): Used with permission from Kincaid-Smith P, Whitworth JA. The Kidney: A Clinico-Pathological Study. 2nd ed. Oxford, UK: Blackwell Scientific Publications, 1987.

Figure 29: Used with permission from Patel PR. Lecture Notes Radiology. 2nd ed. Oxford, UK: Blackwell Science, Ltd., 2005, p. 204.

Figure 30: Used with permission from Axford J, O'Callaghan C. Medicine. 2nd ed. Oxford, UK: Blackwell Science Ltd., 2004, p. 1140.

Figure 31: Used with permission from Axford J, O'Callaghan C. Medicine. 2nd ed. Oxford, UK: Blackwell Science Ltd., 2004, p. 892.

Figure 32: Used with permission from Axford J, O'Callaghan C. Medicine. 2nd ed. Oxford, UK: Blackwell Science Ltd., 2004, p. 215.

Chapter 1

Figure 1-1: Used with permission from the Department of Imaging, Cedars-Sinai Medical Center, Los Angeles, California.

Figure 1-2: Used with permission from the Department of Imaging, Cedars-Sinai Medical Center, Los Angeles, California.

Figure 1-3: Used with permission from the Department of Imaging, Cedars-Sinai Medical Center, Los Angeles, California.

Figure 1-4: Used with permission from the Department of Imaging, Cedars-Sinai Medical Center, Los Angeles, California.

Figure 1-5: Used with permission from the Department of Imaging, Cedars-Sinai Medical Center, Los Angeles, California.

Figure 1-6: Used with permission from the Department of Imaging, Cedars-Sinai Medical Center, Los Angeles, California.

Figure 1-7: Used with permission from the Department of Imaging, Cedars-Sinai Medical Center, Los Angeles, California.

Chapter 2

Figure 2-1: Used with permission from the Department of Imaging, Cedars-Sinai Medical Center, Los Angeles, California.

Figure 2-3: Used with permission from Patel PR. Lecture Notes Radiology. 2nd ed. Oxford, UK: Blackwell Science, Ltd., 2005, p. 272.

Figure 2-4: Used with permission from the Department of Imaging, Cedars-Sinai Medical Center, Los Angeles, California.

Chapter 3

Figure 3-1: Used with permission from Axford J, O'Callaghan C. Medicine. 2nd ed. Oxford, UK: Blackwell Science Ltd., 2004, p. 498.

Figure 3-2(a and b): Used with permission from Axford J, O'Callaghan C. Medicine. 2nd ed. Oxford, UK: Blackwell Science Ltd., 2004, p. 500.

Figure 3-3: Used with permission from the Department of Imaging, Cedars-Sinai Medical Center, Los Angeles, California.

Figure 3-4: Used with permission from Armstrong P, Wastie M, Rockall A. Diagnostic Imaging. 5th ed. Oxford, UK: Blackwell Science Ltd., 2004, p. 297.

Figure 3-5: Used with permission from the Department of Imaging, Cedars-Sinai Medical Center, Los Angeles, California.

Figure 3-6: Used with permission from the Department of Imaging, Cedars-Sinai Medical Center, Los Angeles, California.

Figure 3-7: Used with permission from Axford J, O'Callaghan C. Medicine. 2nd ed. Oxford, UK: Blackwell Science Ltd., 2004, p. 473.

Figure 3-8: Used with permission from Axford J, O'Callaghan C. Medicine. 2nd ed. Oxford, UK: Blackwell Science Ltd., 2004, p. 460.

Figure 3-9: Used with permission from Axford J, O'Callaghan C. Medicine. 2nd ed. Oxford, UK: Blackwell Science Ltd., 2004, p. 467.

Figure 3-10: Used with permission from Axford J, O'Callaghan C. Medicine. 2nd ed. Oxford, UK: Blackwell Science Ltd., 2004, p. 387.

Chapter 4

Figure 4-1(a and b): Used with permission from Axford J, O'Callaghan C. Medicine. 2nd ed. Oxford, UK: Blackwell Science Ltd., 2004, p. 918.

Figure 4-2: Used with permission from Armstrong P, Wastie M, Rockall A. Diagnostic Imaging. 5th ed. Oxford, UK: Blackwell Science Ltd., 2004, p. 297.

Figure 4-3: Used with permission from Axford J, O'Callaghan C. Medicine. 2nd ed. Oxford, UK: Blackwell Science Ltd., 2004, p. 888.

Figure 4-4: Used with permission from Axford J, O'Callaghan C. Medicine. 2nd ed. Oxford, UK: Blackwell Science Ltd., 2004, p. 923.

Figure 4-5: Used with permission from Axford J, O'Callaghan C. Medicine. 2nd ed. Oxford, UK: Blackwell Science Ltd., 2004, p. 934.

Figure 4-6: Used with permission from Axford J, O'Callaghan C. Medicine. 2nd ed. Oxford, UK: Blackwell Science Ltd., 2004, p. 935.

Figure 4-7: Used with permission from Axford J, O'Callaghan C. Medicine. 2nd ed. Oxford, UK: Blackwell Science Ltd., 2004, p. 935.

Chapter 5

Figure 5-1: Used with permission from Axford J, O'Callaghan C. Medicine. 2nd ed. Oxford, UK: Blackwell Science Ltd., 2004, p. 857.

Figure 5-2: Used with permission from the Department of Imaging, Cedars-Sinai Medical Center, Los Angeles, California.

Figure 5-3: Used with permission from Axford J, O'Callaghan C. Medicine. 2nd ed. Oxford, UK: Blackwell Science Ltd., 2004, p. 854.

Figure 5-4: Used with permission from Patel PR. Lecture Notes Radiology. 2nd ed. Oxford, UK: Blackwell Science, Ltd., 2005, p. 266.

Figure 5-5: Used with permission from Axford J, O'Callaghan C. Medicine. 2nd ed. Oxford, UK: Blackwell Science Ltd., 2004, p. 838.

Chapter 6

Figure 6-1: Used with permission from Kelsen DP, Daly JM, Kern SE, Levin B, Tepper JE. Gastrointestinal Oncology: Principles and Practice. Philadelphia: Lippincott Williams & Wilkins, 2002.

Figure 6-3: Used with permission from Cotton P, Williams C. Practical Gastrointestinal Endoscopy: The Fundamentals. 5th ed. Oxford, UK: Blackwell Science Ltd., 2003.

Figure 6-4: Used with permission from the Department of Imaging, Cedars-Sinai Medical Center, Los Angeles, California.

Figure 6-5: Used with permission from Forbes A, Misiewicz JJ Compton CC, Levine MS, Rubesin SE, Thuluvath P, Quraishy MS. Atlas of Clinical Gastroenterology. 3rd ed. London: Elsevier Science, 2004.

Chapter 7

Figure 7-1: Used with permission from Axford J, O'Callaghan C. Medicine. 2nd ed. Oxford, UK: Blackwell Science Ltd., 2004, p. 1063.

Figure 7-2: Used with permission from Axford J, O'Callaghan C. Medicine. 2nd ed. Oxford, UK: Blackwell Science Ltd., 2004, p. 1043.

Figure 7-3: Used with permission from Axford J, O'Callaghan C. Medicine. 2nd ed. Oxford, UK: Blackwell Science Ltd., 2004, p. 1066.

Figure 7-4: Used with permission from Axford J, O'Callaghan C. Medicine. 2nd ed. Oxford, UK: Blackwell Science Ltd., 2004, p. 1042.

Figure 7-5: Used with permission from Axford J, O'Callaghan C. Medicine. 2nd ed. Oxford, UK: Blackwell Science Ltd., 2004, p. 1054.

Figure 7-6: Used with permission from Patel PR. Lecture Notes Radiology. 2nd ed. Oxford, UK: Blackwell Science, Ltd., 2005, p. 204.

Figure 7-7: Used with permission from Axford J, O'Callaghan C. Medicine. 2nd ed. Oxford, UK: Blackwell Science Ltd., 2004, p. 1066.

Chapter 8

Figure 8-1: Used with permission from the Department of Imaging, Cedars-Sinai Medical Center, Los Angeles, California.

Figure 8-2: Used with permission from Axford J, O'Callaghan C. Medicine. 2nd ed. Oxford, UK: Blackwell Science Ltd., 2004, p. 290.

Figure 8-3: Used with permission from Axford J, O'Callaghan C. Medicine. 2nd ed. Oxford, UK: Blackwell Science Ltd., 2004, p. 243.

Figure 8-4: Used with permission from Axford J, O'Callaghan C. Medicine. 2nd ed. Oxford, UK: Blackwell Science Ltd., 2004, p. 223.

Figure 8-5: Used with permission from Axford J, O'Callaghan C. Medicine. 2nd ed. Oxford, UK: Blackwell Science Ltd., 2004, p. 258.

Figure 8-6: Used with permission from Axford J, O'Callaghan C. Medicine. 2nd ed. Oxford, UK: Blackwell Science Ltd., 2004, p. 230.

Chapter 9

Figure 9-1: Used with permission from Axford J, O'Callaghan C. Medicine. 2nd ed. Oxford, UK: Blackwell Science Ltd., 2004, p. 528.

Figure 9-2: Used with permission from Axford J, O'Callaghan C. Medicine. 2nd ed. Oxford, UK: Blackwell Science Ltd., 2004, p. 533.

Figure 9-3: Used with permission from the Department of Imaging, Cedars-Sinai Medical Center, Los Angeles, California.

Figure 9-4: Used with permission from Axford J, O'Callaghan C. Medicine. 2nd ed. Oxford, UK: Blackwell Science Ltd., 2004, p. 545.

Figure 9-5: Used with permission from Axford J, O'Callaghan C. Medicine. 2nd ed. Oxford, UK: Blackwell Science Ltd., 2004, p. 517.

Figure 9-6: Used with permission from Becker GJ, Whitworth JA, Kincaid-Smith P. Clinical Nephrology in Medical Practice. Oxford, UK: Blackwell Scientific Publications, 1992.

Figure 9-7: Used with permission from the Department of Imaging, Cedars-Sinai Medical Center, Los Angeles, California.

Figure 9-8: Used with permission from Axford J, O'Callaghan C. Medicine. 2nd ed. Oxford, UK: Blackwell Science Ltd., 2004, p. 533.

Chapter 10

Figure 10-1: Used with permission from Axford J, O'Callaghan C. Medicine. 2nd ed. Oxford, UK: Blackwell Science Ltd., 2004, p. 164.

Figure 10-2: Used with permission from Patel PR. Lecture Notes Radiology. 2nd ed. Oxford, UK: Blackwell Science, Ltd., 2005, p. 248.

Figure 10-3: Used with permission from the Department of Imaging, Cedars-Sinai Medical Center, Los Angeles, California.

Figure 10-4: Used with permission from Axford J, O'Callaghan C. Medicine. 2nd ed. Oxford, UK: Blackwell Science Ltd., 2004, p. 161.

Figure 10-5: Used with permission from the Department of Imaging, Cedars-Sinai Medical Center, Los Angeles, California.

Figure 10-6: Used with permission from Axford J, O'Callaghan C. Medicine. 2nd ed. Oxford, UK: Blackwell Science Ltd., 2004, p. 167.

Chapter 11

Figure 11-1: Used with permission from Bannister B, et al. Infectious Disease. 2nd ed. Oxford, UK: Blackwell Science Ltd., 2000.

Figure 11-2: Used with permission from Patel PR. Lecture Notes Radiology. 2nd ed. Oxford, UK: Blackwell Science, Ltd., 2005, p. 36.

Figure 11-3: Used with permission from Patel PR. Lecture Notes Radiology. 2nd ed. Oxford, UK: Blackwell Science, Ltd., 2005, p. 50.

Figure 11-4: Used with permission from the Department of Imaging, Cedars-Sinai Medical Center, Los Angeles, California.

Figure 11-5: Used with permission from the Department of Imaging, Cedars-Sinai Medical Center, Los Angeles, California.

Figure 11-6: Used with permission from Armstrong P, Wastie M, Rockall A. Diagnostic Imaging. 5th ed. Oxford, UK: Blackwell Science Ltd., 2004, p. 75

Figure 11-7: Used with permission from Armstrong P, Wastie M, Rockall A. Diagnostic Imaging. 5th ed. Oxford, UK: Blackwell Science Ltd., 2004.

Figure 11-8: Used with permission from the Department of Imaging, Cedars-Sinai Medical Center, Los Angeles, California.

Chapter 12

Figure 12-1: Used with permission from Axford J, O'Callaghan C. Medicine. 2nd ed. Oxford, UK: Blackwell Science Ltd., 2004, p. 1144.

Figure 12-2: Used with permission from Axford J, O'Callaghan C. Medicine. 2nd ed. Oxford, UK: Blackwell Science Ltd., 2004, p. 1150.

Figure 12-3: Used with permission from Axford J, O'Callaghan C. Medicine. 2nd ed. Oxford, UK: Blackwell Science Ltd., 2004, p. 1102.

Figure 12-4: Used with permission from Axford J, O'Callaghan C. Medicine. 2nd ed. Oxford, UK: Blackwell Science Ltd., 2004, p. 1147.

Figure 12-5: Used with permission from Burns T, Breathnach S, Cox N, Griffiths C. Rook's Textbook of Dermatology. 7th ed. Oxford, UK: Blackwell Science, Ltd., 2005.

Figure 12-6: Used with permission from Axford J, O'Callaghan C. Medicine. 2nd ed. Oxford, UK: Blackwell Science Ltd., 2004, p. 1125.

Figure 12-7: Used with permission from Axford J, O'Callaghan C. Medicine. 2nd ed. Oxford, UK: Blackwell Science Ltd., 2004, p. 1124.

Chapter 13

Figure 13-1: Used with permission from Axford J, O'Callaghan C. Medicine. 2nd ed. Oxford, UK: Blackwell Science Ltd., 2004, p. 1107.

Figure 13-2: Used with permission from Axford J, O'Callaghan C. Medicine. 2nd ed. Oxford, UK: Blackwell Science Ltd., 2004, p. 1144.

Figure 13-3: Used with permission from Axford J, O'Callaghan C. Medicine. 2nd ed. Oxford, UK: Blackwell Science Ltd., 2004, p. 421.

Figure 13-4: Used with permission from Axford J, O'Callaghan C. Medicine. 2nd ed. Oxford, UK: Blackwell Science Ltd., 2004, p. 743.

Figure 13-5: Used with permission from Axford J, O'Callaghan C. Medicine. 2nd ed. Oxford, UK: Blackwell Science Ltd., 2004, p. 717.

Normal Laboratory Values

Blood, Plasma, Serum

Alanine aminotransferase (ALT, GPT at 30°C)	8–20 U/L
Alpha-fetoprotein (AFP)	0–10 ng/mL
Amylase, serum	25–125 U/L
Aspartate aminotransferase (AST, GOT at 30°C)	8–20 U/L
Bilirubin, serum (adult) Total/Direct	0.1–1.0 mg/dL/0.0–0.3 mg/dL
Calcium, serum (Ca^{2+})	8.4–10.2 mg/dL
Cholesterol, serum	Recommend: < 200 mg/dL
Cortisol, serum	0800h: 5–23 ng/dL/1600h: 3–15ng/dL/ 2000h: ≤ 50% of 0800h
Creatine kinase, serum	Male: 25–90 U/L Female: 10–70 U/L
Creatinine, serum	0.6–1.2 mg/dL
Electrolytes, serum	
Sodium (Na^+)	136–145 mEq/L
Chloride (Cl^-)	95–105 mEq/L
Potassium (K^+)	3.5–5.0 mEq/L
Bicarbonate (HCO_3^-)	22–28 mEq/L
Magnesium (Mg^{2+})	1.5–2.0 mEq/L
Ferritin, serum	Male: 15–200 ng/mL Female: 12–150 ng/mL

Follicle-stimulating hormone, serum/plasma	Male: 4–25 mIU/mL
	Female: premenopause 4–30 mIU/mL
	      midcycle peak 10–90 mIU/mL
	      postmenopause 40–250 mIU/mL

Gases, arterial blood (room air)	
PH	7.35–7.45
PCO_2	33–45 mm Hg
PO_2	75–105 mm Hg
Glucose, serum	Fasting: 70–110 mg/dL 2-h postprandial: < 120 mg/dL
Growth hormone-arginine stimulation	Fasting: < 5 ng/mL Provocative stimuli: > 7 ng/mL
Human chorionic gonadotropin (hCG)	< 5 mIU/mL
Iron	50–70 ug/dL
Lactate dehydrogenase, serum	45–90 U/L

Luteinizing hormone, serum/plasma	Male: 6–23 mIU/mL
	Female: follicular phase 5–30 mIU/mL
	      midcycle 75–150 mIU/mL
	      postmenopause 30–200 mIU/mL

Osmolality, serum	275–295 mOsmo/kg
Parathyroid hormone, serum, N-terminal	230–630 pg/mL
Phosphate (alkaline), serum (p-NPP at 30°C)	20–70 u/L
Phosphorus (inorganic), serum	3.0–4.5 mg/dL

Prolactin, serum (hPRL)	< 20 ng/mL
Proteins, serum	
Total, recumbent	6.0–7.8 g/dL
Albumin	3.5–5.5 g/dL
Globulin	2.3–3.5 g/dL
Prostate specific antigen	0–4 ng/mL
Testosterone, serum	300–1000 ng/dL
Thyroid-stimulating hormone, serum or plasma	0.5–5.0 nU/mL
Thyroidal iodine (^{123}I) uptake	8–30% of administered dose/24 h
Thyroxine (T_4), serum	5–12 ng/dL
Triglycerides, serum	35–160 mg/dL
Triiodothyronine (T_3), serum (RIA)	115–190 ng/dL
Triiodothyronine (T_9), resin uptake	25–35%
Urea nitrogen, serum (BUN)	7–18 mg/dL
Uric acid, serum	3.0–8.2 mg/dL

Hematologic

Bleeding time (template)	2–7 minutes
Erythrocyte count	Male: 4.3–5.9 million/mm³
	Female: 3.5–5.5 million/mm³
Erythrocyte sedimentation rate (Westergren)	Male: 0–15 mm/h
	Female: 0–20 mm/h
Hematocrit	Male: 41–53%
	Female: 36–46%
Hemoglobin A1C	≤ 6%
Hemoglobin, blood	Male: 13.5–17.5 g/dL
	Female: 12.0–16.0 g/dL
Leukocyte count and differential	
Leukocyte count	4,500–11,000/mm³
Segmented neutrophils	54–62%
Bands	3–5%
Eosinophils	1–3%
Basophils	0–0.75%
Lymphocytes	25–33%
Monocytes	3–7%
Mean corpuscular hemoglobin	25.4–34.6 pg/cell
Mean corpuscular hemoglobin concentration	31–36% Hb/cell
Mean corpuscular volume	80–100 nm³
Partial thromboplastin time (activated)	25–40 seconds
Platelet count	150,000–400,000/mm³
Prothrombin time	11–15 seconds
Reticulocyte count	0.5–1.5% of red cells
Thrombin time	< 2 seconds deviation from control
Volume	
Plasma	Male: 25–43 mL/kg
	Female: 28–45 mL/kg
Red cell	Male: 20–36 mL/kg
	Female: 19–31 mL/kg

Urine

Calcium	100–300 mg/24 h
Chloride	varies with intake
Creatine clearance	Male: 97–137 mL/min
	Female: 88–128 mL/min
Osmolality	50–1,400 mOsmol/kg
Oxalate	8–40 ng/mL
Potassium	varies with diet
Proteins, total	< 150 mg/24 h
Sodium	40–220 mEq/24 h
Uric acid	210–750 mg/24 h

Urinalysis

Color	clear
Odor	none
Glucose	none
Ketones	none
Protein	< 150 mg/24 h
pH	4.5–8.0
Specific gravity	1.001–1.035
Red cells	0–3/HPF
White cells	0–3/HPF
Bacteria	negative
Crystals	negative
Epithelial cells	not significant

Seminal Fluid Analysis

Appearance	Opaque, gray-white, highly viscid
Volume	2–5 mL
Liquefaction	complete within 30 minutes
pH	7.2–8.0
Leukocytes	occasional or absent
Count	20–250 million/mL
Motility	50–80% with progressive active motility
Morphology	50–90% with normal forms

STEP 1

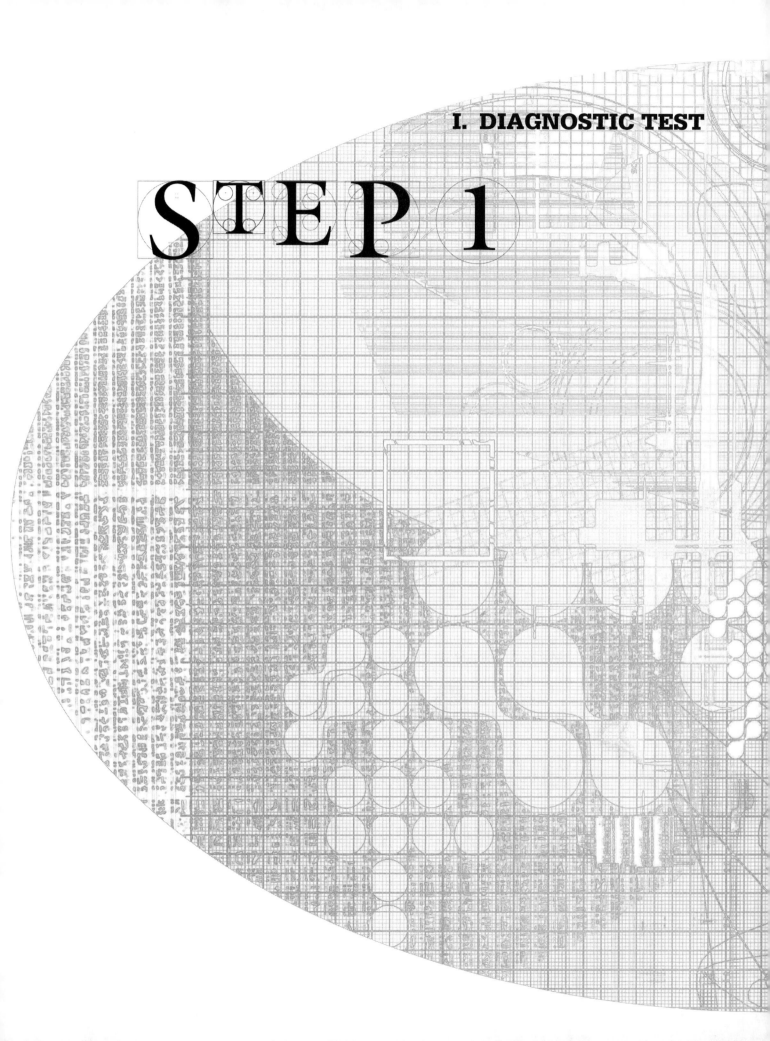

Diagnostic Test

Block 1

1. A medical student is involved in a summer research project to determine the effects of molecular size and charge on movement through the plasma membrane. The project will use ion electrophoresis. The ultimate goal is to determine the effect of cholesterol on membrane transport. It is likely that cholesterol in the plasma membrane:

   A. Acts as a carrier molecule
   B. Acts as a signaling molecule
   C. Decreases fluidity
   D. Disrupts the structural integrity
   E. Serves as an attachment site

2. A 38-year-old man presents to his primary care physician with severe headaches, which he has now had for 2 days. He states that the pain is located behind the left eye only and does not radiate. The episodes are reported as intermittent throughout the day without aggravating factors. He also says that during each occurrence, he has tearing eyes and runny nose. What is the most likely diagnosis?

   A. Cluster headache
   B. Giant cell arteritis
   C. Migraine with aura
   D. Migraine without aura
   E. Tension headache

3. What epidermal cell located in the stratum spinosum is similar in structure and function to dendritic cells in the thymus, spleen, and lymph nodes and is responsible for the initiation of the cutaneous contact hypersensitivity reactions?

   A. Adipocyte
   B. Keratinocyte
   C. Langerhans cell
   D. Melanocyte
   E. Merkel cell

4. A hiker from a town near sea level is climbing to an altitude of 12,000 ft. He has a prior medical history of recurrent otitis media and pharyngeal infections. Which of the following adaptations will have occurred to compensate for his increase in altitude?

   A. Decrease in 2,3 DPG concentration
   B. Decrease in pulmonary vascular resistance
   C. Increase in alveolar P_{O_2}
   D. Increase in arterial P_{O_2}
   E. Increase in ventilation rate

5. The arms and legs are part of the appendicular skeleton. As the limb buds of the musculoskeletal system form, muscles around the bones separate into either dorsal or ventral components. The upper limb rotates such that the extensor muscles are _____, and the lower limb rotates such that the extensor muscles are _____, respectively.

   A. anterior, posterior
   B. posterior, anterior
   C. anterior, anterior
   D. posterior, posterior
   E. transverse, posterior

6. On presentation to the emergency department, a 43-year-old man is unresponsive. His electrocardiogram (ECG) reveals ventricular tachycardia and atrial fibrillation. Which of the following antiarrhythmics is best suited for this condition?

   A. Adenosine
   B. Amiodarone
   C. Flecainide
   D. Lidocaine
   E. Quinidine

7. A 29-year-old man has taken an overdose of sleeping pills. He is awake, alert, and oriented enough to realize the need to seek help. He calls the local poison control center and is told to self-administer syrup of ipecac. This agent has a mechanism of action that involves which of the following?

   A. Stimulating the gag reflex
   B. Stimulating the trigger zone of chemotaxis
   C. Suppressing gastric outlet pressures
   D. Suppressing the gag reflex
   E. Suppressing the motor cortex

8. A 28-year-old woman presents to her primary care physician because of malaise, generalized edema, and hematuria. Physical examination also reveals a facial rash. Urinalysis reveals hematuria and proteinuria. A 24-hr urine reveals > 6 g proteinuria/day. Serum total cholesterol is 300 mg/dL. Renal biopsy is performed. Light microscopy reveals glomerular scarring and subendothelial immune complex deposition. What is the most likely diagnosis?

   A. Berger's disease
   B. Diabetic nephropathy
   C. Lupus nephropathy
   D. Renal amyloidosis
   E. Renal artery stenosis

9. A 10-year-old girl presents to the county health clinic requesting oral contraceptives. She mentions no prior medical or surgical history. Physical examination of the heart, lungs, and abdomen is within normal limits. In all but a few states, which of the following criteria must she meet in order to be treated without signed parental consent?

   A. No one under the age of 18 can be given contraceptives without parental or guardian consent.

   B. She must be at least 15 years of age before she can be assessed for emancipated minor status.

   C. She must be married, in the military, financially independent, or living away from home.

   D. She must first undergo screening for sexually transmitted diseases, and, if positive, undergo treatment.

   E. She need not meet any criteria as long as she can give informed consent.

10. A 60-year-old woman with a history of uncontrolled hypertension decides to visit her family physician for the first time in 20 years. A chest x-ray is obtained (Figure 1). An echocardiogram of this patient's heart would most likely reveal what pathological change?

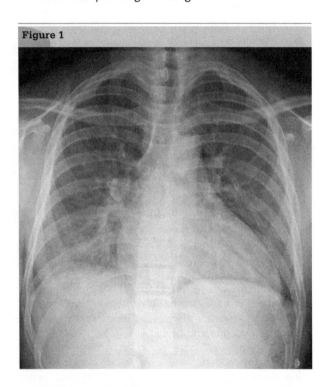

Figure 1

   A. Left ventricular concentric hypertrophy
   B. Left ventricular eccentric hypertrophy
   C. Left ventricular hyperplasia
   D. Left ventricular metaplasia

11. A 52-year-old man presents for a renal biopsy. He has a history of rheumatoid arthritis and has chronic edema and proteinuria. Renal biopsy is performed. Results include positive birefringence under polarized light as well as reactivity with Congo red and thioflavin T. A criss-cross pattern of fibrillary deposits is found by electron microscopy. What is the most likely diagnosis?

   A. IgA nephropathy
   B. Lupus nephropathy
   C. Renal amyloidosis
   D. Renal artery stenosis
   E. Rheumatoid-associated (RA) nephropathy

12. A 48-year-old man is brought to the emergency department by paramedics after complaining of blurry vision and weakness and then beginning to have a new-onset seizure. Past medical history is significant only for a 20-lb weight gain over the past 6 months, and his wife points out that he has been snacking more frequently. He takes no medications. The patient is unconscious on arrival. Physical examination reveals an overweight man with a body-mass index (BMI) of 29 whose vital signs are within normal limits. His ECG shows no abnormalities. The first set of cardiac enzymes is within normal limits. Serum glucose value is 35 mg/dL, while serum insulin and C-peptide levels are markedly elevated. Electrolytes and complete blood count are within normal limits. The most likely explanation for this man's symptoms is:

   A. Cerebrovascular accident
   B. Dehydration
   C. Insulinoma
   D. Myocardial infarction
   E. Self-administration of exogenous insulin

13. A mother brings her young child in for a routine well-child visit. This child has been developmentally normal so far. In reviewing the developmental milestones, the mom states the child has recently mastered the following; coos, smiles, laughs, raises body on hands, rolls over front to back, grasps a rattle, and can control its head well. Based on these milestones, which of the following would you also expect this child to have mastered?

   A. Cruises and takes steps alone
   B. Drinks from cup
   C. May be cutting first tooth
   D. Pulls to stand
   E. Reaches for objects and bats them

14. A 65-year-old man presents to his primary care physician with fever and chills. Two hours later, the patient's blood pressure drops precipitously and he is brought to the emergency department. He is admitted to the intensive care unit. Blood cultures reveal methicillin-resistant *Staphylococcus aureus*. The patient is begun on an intravenous antibiotic. About 30 min later, the patient develops severe flushing of the skin. What is the most likely explanation for this finding?

   A. Ampicillin
   B. Cefotaxime
   C. Chloramphenicol
   D. Trimethoprim-sulfamethoxazole
   E. Vancomycin

15. A 56-year-old man complains to his primary care physician of no longer having enough energy to do anything and attributes his weakness to just getting old. His symptoms have increased significantly over the past week, and his appetite is diminished. His speech is slow and he often seems to be confused during the interview. Laboratory values include a serum sodium level of 110 mEq/L, potassium level of 4.0 mEq/L, chloride of 84 mEq/L, and bicarbonate level of 20 mEq/L. What is the most likely diagnosis?

A. Clear cell carcinoma of the kidney

B. Pheochromocytoma

C. Renal cell carcinoma

D. Small cell carcinoma of the lung

E. Squamous cell carcinoma of the lung

16. A 52-year-old man with a 30-pack-year smoking history presents to his primary care physician for a yearly physical examination. He was diagnosed with emphysema at the age of 47 and continues to smoke without modification. Chest x-ray reveals lung hyperinflation. He is at much higher risk for which of the following?

A. Bacterial endocarditis

B. Cor pulmonale

C. Deep venous thrombosis

D. Mitral valve prolapse

E. Pulmonary embolus

17. A 43-year-old woman with a family history of renal disease presents for evaluation. She also has a history of hypertension and microhematuria. Renal ultrasound reveals enlarged kidneys bilaterally with at least five cystic lesions per kidney. The cysts are of varying sizes. Which of the following situations is most problematic for this patient?

A. Berry aneurysm

B. Diabetes mellitus

C. Renal stones

D. Recurrent urinary tract infections

E. Tuberculous orchitis

18. A 25-year-old previously healthy woman with no past medical history presents to her primary care physician with a lump in her left breast. She states that she noticed the lump a couple of days ago after performing a self-examination of her breast. She denies any pain or discharge from the nipple. She has been afebrile the entire time. Physical examination reveals that the breast lump is firm, mobile, round, and well circumscribed. The right breast is without lumps or nodules. Cardiac, pulmonary, and abdominal examinations are noncontributory. What is the most likely diagnosis?

A. Cystosarcoma phyllodes

B. Fibroadenoma

C. Fibrocystic disease

D. Intraductal papilloma

E. Mammary duct ectasia

19. A 19-year-old college student is brought to the emergency department by his friends after a party. His behavior is found to be impulsive and belligerent. He has no prior medical history. Physical examination reveals horizontal and vertical nystagmus. During the examination he also claims to see things on the wall that are actually not there. What substance did this student most likely abuse?

A. Cocaine

B. LSD (lysergic acid diethylamide)

C. Marijuana

D. Opioids

E. PCP (phencyclidine)

20. A medical student is attending a lecture on the female reproductive tract. The professor is discussing the different pathological diseases associated with the system. From what site are most ovarian cancers most likely derived?

A. Epithelial tissue

B. Germ cells

C. Metastasis

D. Sex cord tissue

E. Stromal tissue

21. A 25-year-old man complains of unilateral headaches with increased drainage from his nose and tearing of the right eye. His headaches are precipitated by alcohol. He experiences multiple episodes a day. What is the most likely diagnosis?

A. Cluster headache

B. Migraine

C. Sinusitis

D. Tension headache

E. Tuberculosis

22. A 15-year-old girl presents to her primary care physician with a pruritic rash localized to the wrist. Papules and vesicles are noted to appear in a bandlike fashion. What is the most likely etiology?

A. Contact dermatitis

B. Herpes simplex virus

C. Seborrheic dermatitis

D. Shingles

E. Normal skin

23. A 2-year-old boy is brought into the emergency department by his mother, who has noted blood in the stools and abdominal distension. The child's laboratory tests are all within limits. A barium enema is done, revealing a sausage-shaped structure near the ileum. What is the most likely explanation of these findings?

A. Colonic volvulus

B. Intussusception

C. Meckel's diverticulum

D. Rotavirus infection

E. Normal variant

24. A 7-year-old boy is brought to his primary care physician with limb weakness and difficulty walking. He has to use both his hands to push himself up in order to stand. His mother has noticed that his calves seem to be larger than those of other boys his age. Physical examination of the heart, lungs, and abdomen is within normal limits. His gastrointestinal examination reveals no guarding, rebound tenderness, or peritoneal signs. Genitourinary examination reveals a circumcised penis with bilateral descended testicles. This boy most likely has a defect in which protein?

   A. Collagen
   B. Dystrophin
   C. Fibrillin
   D. Myelin
   E. Spectrin

25. A 67-year-old man presents to his primary care physician with fatigue, mucosal bleeding, and bruising. The patient also mentions a recent upper respiratory infection and poor appetite, with weight loss of 15 lb over 2 months. This patient's medical history is significant for a 40-pack-year history of cigarette smoking, diabetes mellitus, and hypercholesterolemia. Physical examination reveals bruising of the skin and petechiae throughout. Laboratory studies reveal a hematocrit of 29%, mean corpuscular volume (MCV) 86, platelet count 11,0000/mm^3, prothrombin time 11 sec, activated partial thromboplastin time (aPTT) 34 sec, leukocyte count 2,800, blood urea nitrogen (BUN) 34, creatinine 2.9, serum protein 9.6, serum albumin 2.9, serum calcium 11, serum protein electrophoresis IgG lambda monoclonal spike. Bone marrow aspirate is shown below (Figure 2). What is the most likely cause of the patient's bleeding and bruising?

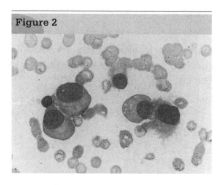

Figure 2

   A. Acquired factor VIII deficiency
   B. Acquired platelet function defect
   C. Disseminated intravascular coagulopathy
   D. Renal insufficiency
   E. Thrombocytopenia
   F. Vitamin K deficiency secondary to decreased appetite

26. A 45-year-old man presents to his primary care physician with multiple tan- to brown-colored, coin-shaped plaques with a granular surface. These are located on his trunk, head, neck, and extremities and have a "stuck on" appearance. Microscopic examination of a punch biopsy of one of these lesions reveals keratin-filled epidermal pseudocysts. What is the most likely diagnosis?

   A. Acanthosis nigracans
   B. Actinic keratosis
   C. Basal cell carcinoma
   D. Histiocytosis X
   E. Malignant melanoma
   F. Psoriasis
   G. Squamous cell carcinoma

27. Control of the muscles in standing and moving is not something that we are able to do from birth. What is the order of muscles (from the first skill to the last skill) that babies learn to coordinate and control?

   A. Muscles of the body, muscles of the neck, muscles of the shoulders and arms
   B. Muscles of the neck, muscles of the shoulders and arms, muscles of the body
   C. Muscles of the shoulders and arms, muscles of the body, muscles of the neck
   D. Muscles of the neck, muscles of the body, muscles of the shoulders and arms

28. A patient suspected of having a brain lesion experiences symptoms of a motor aphasia in which he cannot formulate words; however, he appears to possess functional comprehension when spoken to. Which of the following areas of the brain will produce this disorder?

   A. Arcuate fasciculus
   B. Amygdala
   C. Basal ganglia
   D. Broca's area in the frontal lobe
   E. Wernicke's area in the temporal lobe

29. A 14-year-old boy complains of polyuria, fatigue, dizziness, headaches, and blurred vision. Physical examination of the heart, lungs, and abdomen is normal. Urinalysis reveals glucosuria and ketonuria. Serum glucose is 450 mg/dL. The ketoacidosis associated with this condition is a consequence of

   A. accelerated fat breakdown
   B. decreased insulin and increased glucagon
   C. hepatic failure
   D. hyperglycemia
   E. renal failure

30. A 33-year-old man presents to his physician for an annual examination. A medical student who is learning how to examine patients is shadowing the physician. The student is attempting to palpate the left kidney. What is the location of the kidneys with respect to the vertebrae?

   A. C1–C8
   B. T1–T4
   C. L1–L4
   D. S2–S4
   E. S4

31. A 38-year-old woman presents to her primary care physician with a bloody discharge from her right breast. She explains that for the last several months her right breast has felt tender, especially in the region of the nipple, which itself became swollen. Biopsy reveals an invasive ductal carcinoma with marked nuclear atypia in the nipple. To which of the following lymph nodes would the metastatic cells first spread?

A. Apical axillary node

B. Central axillary node

C. Parasternal node

D. Pectoral node

E. Subscapular node

32. A 59-year-old obese man with a history of unstable angina presents to the emergency department with an episode of chest pain. To monitor any changes in cardiac function and electrical signal transmission throughout the myocardium, an ECG is ordered (Figure 3). Which of the following corresponds to the passage of the electric signal from the atria to the ventricle via the AV node?

A. P wave

B. PR interval

C. QRS wave

D. QT interval

E. T wave

33. A 13-year-old girl who had just come back from a camping trip in the northeastern part of the country comes to clinic with a fever, headache, runny nose, and a general feeling of malaise. She developed a lesion described as a bull's-eye rash with central clearing. She does not recall being bitten by an insect but is unsure. She is diagnosed with Lyme disease and started on tetracycline. What is the mechanism of action of this agent?

A. Blocks the translocation step in protein synthesis

B. Blocks transpeptidase cross-linking of the cell wall

C. Inhibits 50S ribosome peptidyl transferase

D. Inhibits formation of the initiation complex causing misreading of mRNA

E. Prevents attachment of aminoacyl-tRNA to 30S ribosome

34. One of your young male patients comes to the office for his yearly well-child visit. Genital examination reveals the growth of dark, coarse, and curly hair spreading sparsely over the pubic symphysis. The hair is darker and curlier than it was the previous year. The penis has also grown larger, especially in length. The glans penis has yet to develop fully and penis has not grown in width. The testes have also grown over the past year. What is the most likely Tanner stage for this patient?

A. Tanner 1

B. Tanner 2

C. Tanner 3

D. Tanner 4

E. Tanner 5

35. A 63-year-old woman is brought to the emergency department with severe back pain. She also has a history of easy bruising and has cutaneous striae over the lower abdomen. Magnetic resonance imaging (MRI) of the spine reveals a compression fracture of L1. During her hospital course, she ultimately expired owing to septic shock. Autopsy revealed adrenal atrophy. Which of the following explains these findings?

A. Corticosteroid therapy

B. Cretinism

C. Cushing's disease

D. Diabetes

E. Osteoporosis

36. During a difficult hysterectomy in a 42-year-old woman, the left ureter is accidentally ligated. It is then repaired by ureteroureterostomy. The ureter is accompanied in its course by which of the following structures?

A. Mesometrium

B. Mesosalpinx

C. Rectouterine ligaments

D. Sacrocervical ligaments

E. Uterine artery

37. A 72-year-old man presents to his primary care physician accompanied by his wife. He has severe motor deficits. He was fine when he went to bed the night before, but on waking this morning he had total motor paralysis on the left side of his body. He is showing no sensory deficits. An MRI is obtained (Figure 4). Where would be the most probable location for the lesion that would explain these findings?

A. Caudate

B. External capsule

C. Internal capsule

D. Putamen

E. Thalamus

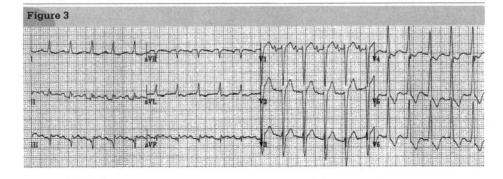

Figure 3

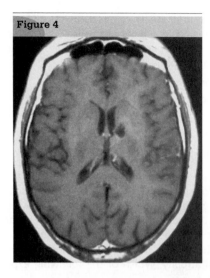

Figure 4

38. The parents of a 3-year-old girl are concerned because she is overweight compared to the other children her age. She has a raging appetite and she steals and hoards food. This behavior came as a shock to her parents because until she reached 1 year of age, she was hypotonic and feeding poorly. What is the most likely explanation of these findings?

A. Deletion in chromosome 5

B. Deletion in chromosome 22

C. Loss of maternal imprinting

D. Loss of paternal imprinting

E. Missense mutation

39. A 29-year-old woman presents to her primary care physician complaining of generalized malaise and intermittent itchiness. Her family history is positive for blood disorders, particularly hemolytic anemia. Physical examination reveals scleral icterus, and her skin appears jaundiced. Cardiac and pulmonary examinations are within normal limits. The spleen tip is palpable. Laboratory studies are obtained and reveal a total bilirubin of 6 and an indirect bilirubin of 4.9. Hematocrit is 28%. What is the most appropriate treatment for this patient?

A. Phenobarbital

B. Dialysis

C. Liver transplant

D. Splenectomy

E. Quinidine

40. A 7-year-old boy is brought to the pediatrician with a 5-day history of cough, runny nose, and a rash, which began as individual lesions on his head, neck, and shoulders. These lesions are now beginning to coalesce and spread downward toward his torso. Physical examination reveals gray-white macules noted on the buccal mucosa. What is the most likely explanation for these findings?

A. Human herpesvirus 6

B. Measles

C. Group A beta-hemolytic streptococcus

D. Parvovirus B19

E. *Staphylococcus epidermidis*

41. A 35-year-old man presents to his primary care physician for his yearly physical examination. He has a history of recurrent sinus infections and bronchiectasis. He mentions that he has been married for 10 years. He and his wife have been unsuccessfully trying to have children for several years now. Physical examination reveals that the heart sounds are on the right and that there is a mass on the left side of the abdomen. What will most likely be found in this patient?

A. C-ANCA

B. Extra X chromosome

C. Extra Y chromosome

D. Immotile cilia

E. P-ANCA

F. Trisomy 21

42. A 45-year-old bridge maintenance worker presents to his primary care physician with numbness and pain in his ring finger and the middle finger on his right hand. His sleep at night has been disrupted. He has experienced this constellation of symptoms for 3 months. He has tried using wrist splints and anti-inflammatory medications, neither of which has helped. He is asked to hold his forearms upright by pointing his fingers down and pressing the backs of his hands together for a minute and almost immediately complains of pain. What is the most likely diagnosis?

A. Acute arthritis

B. Carpal tunnel syndrome

C. Medial epicondylitis

D. Lateral epicondylitis

E. Tenosynovitis

43. A 47-year-old man is brought to the emergency department with a 1-hr onset of crushing chest pain radiating down the left arm, followed by diaphoresis and nausea. The patient has a history of a previous MI 2 years earlier. His ECG shows ST-segment elevation in the anterior leads. What is the most appropriate treatment?

A. Aspirin

B. Heparin

C. Streptokinase

D. Ticlopidine

E. Warfarin

44. A 41-year-old woman, while drunk, is stabbed by a male friend. She is brought to the emergency department for evaluation. She is alert, awake, and oriented. Her vital signs are stable. Physical examination reveals multiple stab wounds in the right axilla and a large wound that leaves the pelvis above the piriformis muscle. Which of the following structures can be damaged by this large stab wound?

A. Inferior gluteal artery

B. Internal pudendal artery

C. Posterior femoral cutaneous nerve

D. Sciatic nerve

E. Superior gluteal nerve

45. A 14-year-old boy is hospitalized because of blurred vision, polyuria, and polydipsia. He is 61 in tall and weighs 240 lb. His family history is positive for diabetes mellitus (grandfather). His temperature is 38.2° C (100.7°F), blood pressure 136/80 mm Hg, heart rate 90 bpm, and respiratory rate of 22/min. Acanthosis nigricans is noted on his neck. He has a serum glucose of 264 mg/dL; serum ketones are negative. What is the most likely explanation for this patient's hyperglycemia?

A. Hyperthyroidism

B. Maturity diabetes of youth

C. Type I diabetes

D. Type II diabetes

E. Secondary diabetes

46. A mother brings her 17-year-old daughter to the family physician because she has never had a menstrual period. Urine β-hCG is negative. On physical examination, the patient is noted to be 5 ft 11 in tall, with breasts at Tanner Stage 5. No axillary or pubic hair is noted. Her physical and cognitive development has been unremarkable. What is most likely etiology of her gonadal abnormality?

A. Anorchia

B. Complete androgen insensitivity

C. Cryptorchidism

D. Kallman's syndrome

E. Klinefelter's syndrome

47. A 62-year-old man with a long-standing history of chronic tophaceous gout was recently started on a new uricosuric agent that works by blocking the active reabsorption of uric acid in the proximal tubules. Which medication is this patient taking?

A. Allopurinol

B. Colchicine

C. Indomethacin

D. Oxypurinol

E. Phenylbutazone

F. Probenecid

48. A 19-year-old African American woman presents to her primary care physician for a general checkup. She has several discrete depigmented white patches on her skin throughout her body. A picture of her hands is shown in Figure 5. She states she has had these patches since she was 12 years old. If the depigmented areas of skin are caused by loss of melanocytes in those areas, what is the most likely diagnosis?

A. Bullous pemphigoid

B. Cicatricial pemphigoid

C. Erythema multiforme

D. Psoriasis

E. Vitiligo

49. A 35-year-old man presents to his primary care physician with a combination of symptoms including recurrent diarrhea, cutaneous flushing, and asthmatic wheezing. An increased level of 5-hydroxyindoleacetic acid (5-HIAA) is found on urinalysis. What is the most likely site of this patient's tumor?

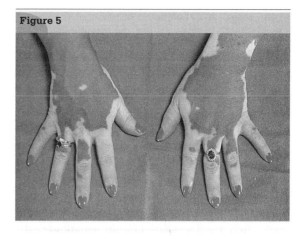

Figure 5

A. Appendix

B. Esophagus

C. Jejunum

D. Rectum

E. Transverse colon

F. Sigmoid colon

G. Stomach

50. A 60-year-old woman is brought to the emergency department for evaluation of three episodes of extreme lethargy over the past several days. She cannot even stay awake long enough to answer all of your questions. You find out that she has recently been talking to someone about feeling sad and lonely since her children moved away. She has also lost interest in activities she used to share with her friends. You manage to find out that she has started taking a new medication. What medication is she most likely taking?

A. Amitriptyline

B. Lithium

C. Paroxetine

D. St. John's wort

E. Thioridazine

Block 2

51. A 19-year-old woman presents to her primary care physician with the complaint of amenorrhea for the previous 4 months. She denies any weight loss or change in appetite. She is currently not on any medications and has had no fevers. She also states that she has had a discharge from both nipples for a month. There is no history of breast cancer in the family but the patient is worried about this possibility. She has never been sexually active. Physical examination reveals engorged breasts bilaterally without the presence of mass lesions or lymphadenopathy. Elevation of which of the following hormones would explain these findings?

A. β-hCG

B. FSH

C. LH

D. Prolactin

E. TSH

52. A 36-year-old man complains of having had erectile dysfunction for 4 months. He has just recently undergone an emotionally painful divorce. He now wants a prescription for sildenafil (Viagra). Prior to giving such a prescription, it would be important to ascertain information regarding his baseline erectile function. In general, penile erection occurs in which stage of sleep?

- **A.** Rapid eye movement
- **B.** Stage 1
- **C.** Stage 2
- **D.** Stage 3
- **E.** Stage 4

53. A 50-year-old man has been having increased difficulty urinating for 2 months. He has difficulty initiating the stream and has increased frequency, urgency, and nocturia. His prostate is 40 g in size and without nodules. His testes are descended bilaterally and are without masses. Urinalysis reveals four red blood cells per high-power field. What is the most likely diagnosis?

- **A.** Benign prostatic hyperplasia
- **B.** Bladder tumor
- **C.** Urethral stricture
- **D.** Urinary tract infection
- **E.** Pyelonephritis

54. An 18-year-old girl, a high school soccer player, is in excellent health except for the absence of menses. On examination she is Tanner stage 5 with respect to breasts and pubic hair. Her cervical examination is normal, as is her bimanual exam. What is the most likely etiology of her primary amenorrhea?

- **A.** Anorexia nervosa
- **B.** Gonadal agenesis
- **C.** Hypogonadotropic hypogonadism
- **D.** Testicular feminization
- **E.** Imperforate hymen

55. A 2-month-old is brought to the primary care physician for a checkup. He has no prior medical history and was born to a mother who received prenatal care; he was delivered by spontaneous vaginal delivery. Physical examination reveals a continuous murmur in all areas of auscultation. The murmur is of a vibratory type. What is the most likely diagnosis?

- **A.** Patent ductus arteriosus
- **B.** Peripheral pulmonic stenosis
- **C.** Still's murmur
- **D.** Venous hum
- **E.** Uremic pericarditis

56. A 19-year-old male has already been seen in the clinic for urethral discharge. He is given an injection of ceftriaxone, but the discharge has not resolved. Physical examination of the heart, lungs, and abdomen is within normal limits. The culture is returned as "no growth." What is the most likely explanation for these findings?

- **A.** *Chlamydia psittaci*
- **B.** *Chlamydia trachomatis*

- **C.** Herpes simplex virus
- **D.** *Neisseria gonorrhoeae*
- **E.** *Treponema pallidum*

57. A 22-year-old man is brought to the emergency department by his roommate after being found on the floor with labored breathing and vomiting. Physical examination reveals that the patient is disoriented and has pinpoint pupils. Cardiac examination reveals a grade I systolic ejection murmur heard best at the apex. Pulmonary examination is unremarkable. Abdominal examination reveals no evidence of guarding or rebound tenderness. There is some significant bruising along his forearms. What is the most appropriate treatment for this patient?

- **A.** Atropine
- **B.** Ethyl alcohol
- **C.** Flumazenil
- **D.** *N*-acetylcysteine
- **E.** Naloxone

58. A 16-year-old boy has excessive bleeding whenever he cuts himself shaving. He states that neither of his parents has the propensity to bleed but that both of his grandfathers had a similar problem. Physical examination is unremarkable. Laboratory studies are normal. An extensive hematological workup with electrophoresis reveals lack of platelet glycoprotein Ib. What is the most likely explanation for these findings?

- **A.** Bernard Soulier disease
- **B.** Glanzmann's thrombasthenia
- **C.** Idiopathic thrombocytopenic purpura
- **D.** Thrombotic thrombocytopenic purpura
- **E.** Thrombocytopenia

59. A 1-month-old girl is brought to the emergency department because she suddenly developed a high fever, cough, and runny nose. Physical examination reveals palpebral edema, bulging fontanelle, and injected pharynx. Her laboratory values reveal marked leukopenia. She is admitted to the hospital for observation overnight. The next day she wakes up with no fever, feeling and acting better, but with a rash on her neck and trunk which is described as 2- to 5-mm maculopapules with a white halo. What is the most likely diagnosis?

- **A.** Human herpesvirus 6
- **B.** Morbillivirus
- **C.** Group A beta-hemolytic streptococcus
- **D.** Parvovirus B19
- **E.** *Staphylococcus aureus*

60. A 60-year-old farmer (BMI 37) is experiencing dermatomal pain to the medial side of the knee that worsens the more time he spends outside. Hand x-rays are obtained (Figure 6). This disease is best characterized by which of the following?

- **A.** Calcium oxalate crystals in the joint
- **B.** Decreased proteoglycan and cartilage synthesis
- **C.** Inflammation of the tendon resulting in hyperextension and flexion joints in the hands
- **D.** Most common in wrist and ankle

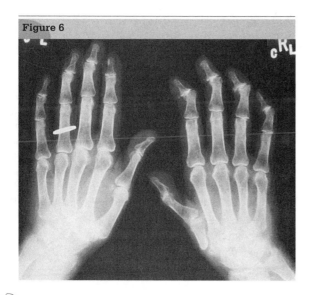

Figure 6

61. A patient presents with findings consistent with encephalitis. Pathologic findings are giant cells with eosinophilic inclusions involving both the nucleus and cytoplasm. What other finding in the patient's history would be consistent with the diagnosis?

A. Acquired immunodeficiency syndrome

B. Childhood polio infection

C. Ritual ingestion of the brains of deceased tribesmen in New Guinea, his place of birth

D. Ingestion of beef from an area where mad cow disease is endemic

E. Recent bite by a raccoon

62. A 40-year-old smoker presents to his primary care physician with a productive cough. He states that he has had the cough for several weeks and had a similar cough the previous year. Physical examination reveals wheezes and crackles in both lung fields. What further finding would be expected in this patient?

A. Bronchial hyperresponsiveness

B. Diffuse pulmonary interstitial fibrosis with ferruginous bodies

C. FEV_1/FVC ratio > 80%

D. Hereditary alpha$_1$-antitrypsin deficiency

E. Hypertrophy of the mucus-secreting cells of the bronchioles

63. A 31-year-old HIV-positive man presents to his primary care physician with severe diarrhea, which he has had for 3 weeks. He does not remember having eaten anything different from his usual diet, and he has not traveled in the last year. A stool sample reveals acid-fast cysts. The most likely cause of his diarrhea is:

A. *Clostridium difficile*

B. *Cryptosporidium parvum*

C. *Giardia lamblia*

D. *Vibrio cholerae*

E. *Yersinia enterocolitica*

64. A 48-year-old woman with a long history of hypertension is currently taking furosemide, isosorbide dinitrate, triamterene, and atenolol. Her blood pressure is 128/86 mm Hg. Physical examination of the heart, lungs, and abdomen is unremarkable. Her recent laboratory studies are shown below:

Electrolytes, serum

Sodium	43 mEq/L
Chloride	99 mEq/L
Potassium	3.3 mEq/L
Bicarbonate	24 mEq/L
Magnesium	2.0 mEq/L
Creatinine	1.1 mg/dL

Leukocyte count and differential

Leukocyte count	12,000/mm^3
Segmented neutrophils	55%
Bands	5%
Eosinophils	3%
Basophils	1%
Lymphocytes	23%
Monocytes	4%

Blood, plasma, serum

Alanine aminotransferase (ALT)	12 U/L
Amylase	55 U/L
Aspartate aminotransferase (AST)	11 U/L
Calcium	9 mg/dL
Glucose	106 mg/dL
Hematocrit	39%
Urea nitrogen, serum (BUN)	10 mg/dL

Urinalysis

Urine pH	6.0
Red cells	2/HPF
White cells	2/HPF
Nitrates	Negative
Bacteria	Negative

What is the site of action of furosemide?

A. Collecting duct

B. Distal convoluted tubule

C. Proximal convoluted tubule

D. Thick ascending limb of loop of Henle

E. Thin descending limb of loop of Henle

65. The end product of G-protein activation is cAMP. What is the next piece of intracellular machinery that cAMP stimulates in the peptide hormone activation cascade?

A. Nuclear transcription factor β

B. Phosphodiesterase

C. Protein kinase A

D. Protein kinase G

E. Xylene D

66. A teenager complains to his parents that he isn't feeling well and doesn't think he will be able to go to school. When his mom leaves his room to call the doctor for an expert opinion, the boy proceeds to place the thermometer near his bedside lamp and dumps water on his nightshirt to give the appearance of "sweats." Finally, he uses makeup to make his face appear paler and to give himself dark circles under his eyes. What is the most likely diagnosis?

    A. Bipolar disorder type 1
    B. Body dysmorphic disorder
    C. Factitious disorder
    D. Major depressive disorder
    E. Malingering

67. A young couple wants to start a family. They want information regarding the most fertile period of the menstrual cycle. The number of fertile hours during a normal menstrual cycle is which of the following?

    A. 20
    B. 60
    C. 100
    D. 120
    E. 200

68. A 23-year-old female presents to her primary care physician with a 4-month history of low-volume bloody diarrhea along with some lower abdominal pain. She has had a recent weight loss of 15 lb. She also reports a prolonged fever. She claims that she had been diagnosed with hemorrhoids before, but they have never lasted this long. Digital rectal examination reveals fecal occult blood. The patient has never had a sigmoidoscopy or colonoscopy. Labs show mild leukocytosis and an elevated sedimentation rate. Sigmoidoscopy is performed and biopsies taken. The results are shown in Figure 7. What is the most likely diagnosis?

    A. Bacterial colitis
    B. Crohn's disease
    C. Irritable bowel syndrome
    D. Diverticulitis
    E. Ulcerative colitis

69. A 46-year-old Caucasian man presents to his primary care physician with a 3-month history of tuberculosis treated by isoniazid, rifampin, ethambutol, and pyrazinamide. He is also taking trimethoprim-sulfamethoxazole for an infection with *Pneumocystis carinii*. The patient thinks he has been having gross hematuria and that his contact lenses have become slightly tinted with a red-orange color. What is the most likely explanation for these findings?

    A. Ethambutol
    B. Isoniazid
    C. Pyrazinamide
    D. Rifampin
    E. Trimethoprim-sulfamethoxazole

70. An 8-year-old boy is brought in to his family physician because he had a fever of 101°F (38.3°C) and has been extremely lethargic for 3 days. Physical examination reveals a palpable spleen below the left costal margin. The heterophil antibody test is positive. If blood were to be drawn from this patient, there would be atypical cells of what type?

    A. B cells
    B. Eosinophils
    C. Macrophages
    D. Polymorphonuclear leukocytes
    E. T cells

71. A 26-year-old presents with a circular, erythematous lesion on her arm with an area of central clearing. The dermatologist scrapes the skin from her lesion and places the scrapings under a microscope with 10% potassium chloride solution. This slide shows hyphae. What is the cause of this lesion?

Figure 7

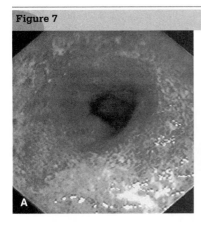
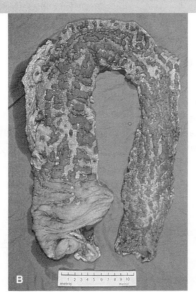
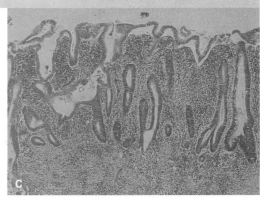

A. *Borrelia burgdorferi*

B. *Candida albicans*

C. *Plasmodium falciparum*

D. *Sporothrix schenkii*

E. *Tinea corporis*

72. A 33-year-old man presents for an employment history and physical examination. He denies any prior medical history of significance. Cardiac, pulmonary, and abdominal examinations are within normal limits. Figure 8 shows a chest x-ray from this individual. Which of the following statements is correct regarding this patient?

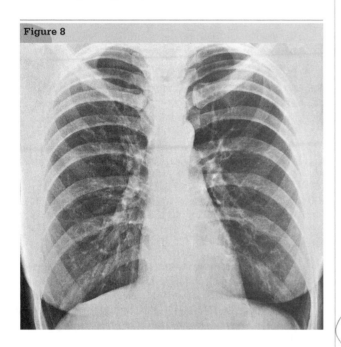

Figure 8

A. He probably has a history of coarctation of the aorta

B. He probably has a history of congestive heart failure

C. He probably has a history of neurofibromatosis

D. His cardiothoracic ratio is measured from the AP projection

E. The left lateral film may confirm the cardiac appearance

73. A 23-year-old man presents to his primary care physician with a 1-week history of numbness and tingling in his toes. A few days after these symptoms developed, he began having increased difficulty walking. Physical examination reveals deep tendon reflexes bilaterally throughout the lower extremities. Lumbar puncture is performed and testing of the cerebrospinal fluid (CSF) reveals significant elevations in protein concentration with only a slight increase in cell count. What event most likely preceded this patient's symptoms?

A. Preceding viral upper respiratory infection

B. Recent fall resulting in trauma to parietal region

C. Recurrent history of the described symptoms, with each episode progressively worse than the previous

D. Several mutations in the APP gene of chromosome 21

E. Ten-year history of alcoholism

74. A 55-year-old man presents to his primary care physician because of hoarseness. He has a 30-pack-year history of smoking. He is found to have a neoplasm on his true vocal cords. If dysplasia is found, one should fear progression to which of the following?

A. Adenocarcinoma

B. Laryngeal polyp

C. Laryngotracheobronchitis

D. Mucoepidermoid carcinoma

E. Squamous cell carcinoma

75. A mother presents to the emergency department with her 14-month-old son. She is concerned because earlier in the day the infant fell down two steps onto a tiled floor. Since the fall, the infant has not been walking and seems agitated. The mother is concerned that the child may have broken a bone. To date, the child has been fairly healthy and has had regular checkups. He is up to date with his immunizations and on schedule with his developmental milestones. On examination, his heart, lung, and abdominal exams are all within normal limits. It is noted that the child's sclerae have a bluish hue. Some mild bruising is obvious on his left lower extremity and he cries when the area is palpated. He is sent for radiographic evaluation, which reveals a fracture of the distal tibia. It also shows decreased bone density in the x-rayed area. What is the most likely diagnosis?

A. Child abuse

B. Osteogenesis imperfecta

C. Osteopetrosis

D. Osteosarcoma

E. Scurvy

76. A 33-year-old man who weighs 170 lb has begun an athletic diet to maximize his muscle weight in preparation for running a half-marathon. He consumes 50 g of carbohydrate, 10 g of protein, and 20 g of fat per day. This individual consumes approximately which of the following estimates of calories per day?

A. 1000

B. 800

C. 600

D. 400

E. 200

77. A 25-year-old woman who has just given birth to a healthy infant suddenly develops dyspnea, cyanosis, and shock. She later develops seizures. What is the most likely explanation for these findings?

A. Air emboli

B. Amniotic fluid emboli

C. Bacterial emboli

D. Fat emboli

E. Thrombus

F. Tumor emboli

78. A 29-year-old sexually active monogamous African American woman presents to her primary care physician complaining of menorrhagia and dysmenorrhea, which she has had for several months. Her symptoms are caused by the most common uterine tumor. Which of the following is true of this tumor?

A. Her racial background decreases her risk of developing recurrent uterine tumors.

B. It often decreases in size during pregnancy.

C. It may increase in size during menopause.

D. It is a benign neoplasm that has a malignant transformation rate of 15%.

E. It usually occurs at multiple separate foci simultaneously.

79. A 43-year-old man presents for evaluation of a 6-month history of weight loss, generalized weakness, and nausea/vomiting after meals. He also reports feeling that he is "tanning" without being in the sun and is getting progressively darker. He complains of dizziness. Blood pressure is 100/60 mm Hg, pulse is 80 bpm. Physical examination reveals tanning throughout the trunk. What is the most likely diagnosis?

A. Addison's disease

B. Conn's syndrome

C. Hemochromatosis

D. Pineal gland tumor

E. Wermer's syndrome

80. A 68-year-old man presents to the clinic with new-onset hip pain bilaterally and proximal muscle weakness that has gotten progressively worse over the previous month. The patient states that the pain has become so bad that it has affected his gait, in that he feels he is waddling. The patient has a history of chronic renal failure secondary to diabetes mellitus type II, for which he receives dialysis. Physical examination of the heart, lungs, and abdomen is normal. The musculoskeletal examination reveals proximal muscle weakness of the lower limb girdle along with an unsteady, waddling gait. Neurological examination is normal. Upon further evaluation, it is determined that this patient is suffering from osteomalacia secondary to chronic renal failure. Given this diagnosis, what laboratory values are most likely to have been found?

A. Elevated levels of $1,25(OH)_2D$

B. Hyperphosphatemia, hypocalcemia, and low levels of $1,25(OH)_2D$

C. Hypophosphatemia, normocalcemia, and low levels of $25(OH)D$ levels

D. Low serum $25(OH)D$ only

E. Normal serum calcium levels and hypophosphatemia

81. A 37-year-old man presents to his dermatologist complaining of the development of an itchy rash that has recently developed. When asked about other medical problems, the patient notes that his doctor has advised him to avoid bread and wheat products, as they cause him severe diarrhea. Physical examination reveals a series of urticarial plaques and vesicles that occur in groups. Which of the following would most likely be seen upon further workup of the patient?

A. A netlike pattern of intercellular IgG deposits

B. Extensive parakeratosis

C. Granular deposits of IgA in the tips of the dermal papillae

D. HLA-B27 positivity

E. Linear deposition of immunoglobulin along the basement membrane

82. A newborn started to gag and turn blue after his first feeding. The mother states that his abdomen seems to swell after he cries. Cardiac examination reveals tachycardia and a systolic ejection murmur. Pulmonary auscultation reveals mild wheezes bilaterally. What is the most likely diagnosis?

A. Barrett's esophagus

B. Pulmonary hypoplasia

C. Pyloric stenosis

D. Respiratory distress syndrome

E. Tracheoesophageal fistula

83. A 63-year-old African American woman with a history of arrhythmia fails rate control with a beta-blocker; thus rhythm control is attempted. A few weeks after beginning therapy, she develops petechiae, purpura lab values, and smear consistent with immune thrombocytopenic purpura. What is the most likely explanation for these findings?

A. Amiodarone

B. Bretylium

C. Lidocaine

D. Mexiletine

E. Quinidine

84. A 35-year-old woman presents to her primary care physician because of vaginal itching, which she has had for 3 months. She has been treated in the past with oral fluconazole, which decreased the symptoms; however, they eventually returned. She has a family history of breast cancer. Which of the following is most associated with possible vulvar cancer in this patient?

A. Breast cancer

B. Cervical cancer

C. Colon cancer

D. Endometrial cancer

E. Ovarian cancer

85. A 48-year-old man presents to clinic complaining of severe pain in his left big toe. He was awakened during the previous night by a sharp, burning sensation localized to the first metatarsophalangeal joint. His history is significant only for hyperlipidemia, which is well controlled with atorvastatin (Lipitor), and intermittent alcohol abuse. The patient admits to recently having been on a drinking binge, consuming, on average, a case of beer per day for a week. Physical examination reveals the joint to be erythematous, warm, and extremely painful to touch. The affected toe is pictured in Figure 9. The rest of the physical examination is normal. What is the most appropriate next step in the management of this patient?

A. Aspiration of fluid from the affected joint

B. Empiric treatment with allopurinol

C. Empiric treatment with corticosteroids

D. Examination of the affected joint via x-ray

E. Measurement of serum urate concentration

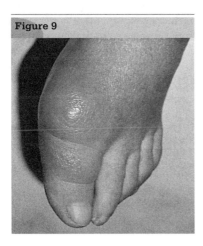

Figure 9

86. A 3-year-old girl is seen in the pediatrics clinic with her parents for follow-up in her care for hypophosphatemic rickets, a rare X-linked dominant condition. Her father suffers from the same condition but her mother does not. Her mother is pregnant and, as they are leaving, the mother casually asks whether there is a chance that her next child will suffer from the same condition. She informs you that the child's sex has been confirmed and that it is a boy. What is the most appropriate statement to make to the mother?

   A. She does not need to worry. Since she is having a boy, there is no risk.

   B. She should worry, as there is a 100% chance that her son will have the condition.

   C. She should worry, as there is a 50% chance that her son will have the condition.

   D. She should worry, as there is a 25% chance that her son will have condition.

   E. You will not know until the baby is born and can be tested.

87. A 60-year-old woman is hospitalized for chest pain. Cardiac catheterization reveals a severe stenosis of the right coronary artery. The vessel is stented and she was begun on nitrates, atenolol, ticlopidine, and verapamil. Four weeks later she returns with a low-grade temperature, and her platelet count is now 25,000/mm³. Schistocytes are seen on peripheral smear. Which of the following is the next step in management?

   A. Stop atenolol

   B. Stop nitrates

   C. Stop ticlopidine

   D. Give antibiotics

   E. Give platelets

88. A medical student is undertaking a research project that involves the passage of two substances through a membrane. Substance A is a charged molecule with a long fatty-acid chain while substance B is an aromatic hydrocarbon that is protonated. If the reflection coefficient of solute A is 1, this implies which of the following?

   A. The solute generates an osmotic effect

   B. The solute is completely permeable

   C. The solute will cause water flow

   D. The solute is probably similar in size to urea

89. After running a marathon on a hot, sunny, 85°F day, what would you expect the runner's volume and concentration status to be before any fluid replacement?

	ECF Volume	ICF Volume	ECF Osmolarity
A	Increase	No change	No change
B	Decrease	No change	No change
C	Increase	Decrease	Increase
D	Decrease	Decrease	Increase
E	Increase	Increase	Decrease
F	Decrease	Increase	Decrease

90. A 29-year-old woman presents to the emergency department with a 6-hr history of fever and general malaise. Her family is concerned because her condition has rapidly deteriorated. Physical examination reveals a new murmur. Ophthalmoscopic evaluation reveals bilateral round white spots on the retina. Two-dimensional echocardiography is obtained and shown in Figure 10. What organism is most likely to be responsible for this condition?

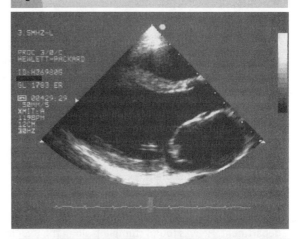

Figure 10

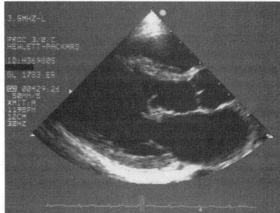

   A. *Staphylococcus aureus*

   B. *Streptococcus pneumoniae*

   C. *Streptococcus pyogenes*

   D. *Treponema pallidum*

   E. *Streptococcus viridans*

91. A 24-year-old sexually active woman presents to her primary care physician complaining of an inability to become pregnant, although she has tried for the past 2 years. Upon further history and clinical examination, the physician finds that she has significant abdominal obesity and increased hair growth on her face and back. In addition, she has been experiencing amenorrhea for several months. The most likely diagnosis of this patient is:

A. Chocolate cyst

B. Corpus luteum cyst

C. Follicular cyst

D. Polycystic ovary syndrome

E. Theca-lutein cyst

92. A 35-year-old woman presents to her primary care physician with numerous complaints. All of her symptoms—gastrointestinal, genitourinary, and cardiopulmonary problems—are vague and include multiple organ systems. Physical examination of the heart, lungs, and abdomen is within normal limits. What is the most likely diagnosis?

A. Obsessive-compulsive disorder

B. Schizotypal personality disorder

C. Schizophreniform disorder

D. Schizophrenia

E. Somatization disorder

93. Progestational hormones, adrenal hormones, and sex hormones all have the same first step in their synthesis from a common precursor molecule. The initial step in their synthesis involves which of the following?

A. Androstenedione

B. Dehydroepiandrosterone (DHEA)

C. Pregnenolone

D. 17-hydroxypregnenolone

E. 17-hydroxyprogesterone

94. A 45-year-old homeless man is brought to the emergency department. He was found stumbling along the middle of a busy downtown street in a severely confused state. When you try to speak to him, it appears that his extraocular muscle movements are not intact. In addition, you remember that this man has presented to the emergency department numerous times before for alcohol-related incidents. What is the etiology of disease from which this individual is suffering?

A. Degeneration of the lateral corticospinal tracts

B. Depigmentation of the substantia nigra and locus ceruleus

C. Increased numbers of CAG repeats in the short arm of chromosome 4

D. Marked cortical atrophy, especially in the frontal and temporal lobe regions

E. Marked demyelination of the cerebral cortex, pons, cerebellar vermis, and mamillary bodies

95. A woman in her eighth month of pregnancy recently moved from Denver, Colorado, to Los Angeles, California. Thinking about possible issues with this particular pregnancy, which of the following involves an increased risk secondary to her prior place of residence?

A. Atrial septal defect

B. Down's syndrome

C. Mitral valve prolapse

D. Patent ductus arteriosis

E. Trisomy 18

96. A new pharmacologic agent is found to decrease nausea in patients who are undergoing chemotherapy. This agent might have a mechanism of action at which of the following receptors?

A. 5HT1

B. 5HT2

C. 5HT3

D. Dopamine

E. Norepinephrine

97. A 40-year-old woman complains of a recently developed beard and mustache. She presents to her primary care physician for evaluation. She mentions that she developed pubic and axillary hair at the age of 8 years. She is 5 ft 6 in tall and weighs 120 lb. Blood tests reveal decreased levels of cortisol and aldosterone as well as increased ACTH. An increased renin level is also found. What is the most likely diagnosis?

A. Meig's syndrome

B. Polycystic ovary syndrome

C. Virilization

D. 17 alpha-hydroxylase deficiency

E. 21 beta-hydroxylase deficiency

98. A 53-year-old woman presents to her primary care physician for her annual visit. She has a long-standing history of hypertension, rheumatoid arthritis, and type II diabetes mellitus. She is 5 ft 4 in tall and weighs 180 lb. She does not smoke but drinks alcohol on occasion. She is married and has three children. She is on several medications including insulin, metformin, lisinopril, metoprolol, Lasix, indomethacin, sulfasalazine, Prempro, and an over-the-counter multivitamin. She is currently trying to lose weight and exercises three times a week. She has no new complaints; to date, her previously diagnosed medical conditions seem to be fairly well controlled. Physical examination of the heart, lungs, and abdomen is within normal limits. Her pelvic exam was deferred, since she has annual visits with a gynecologist. She has some evidence of wrist swelling and pain bilaterally, but this is normal for her. She has no obvious lower extremity edema and 2+ pulses bilaterally. Based on this patient's history, which medication listed is considered to be a disease-modifying antirheumatic drug?

A. Indomethacin

B. Lisinopril

C. Metformin

D. Premarin

E. Sulfasalazine

99. A 25-year-old woman presents to clinic with complaints of weight loss, malaise, and vague joint pain and stiffness. The joint pain is more prominent in the mornings and subsides after a few hours of movement. The patient's mother and grandmother both suffer from a similar condition. What is the most likely explanation of these findings?

A. Ankle sprain

B. Ankylosing spondylitis

C. Osteoarthritis

D. Reiter's syndrome

E. Rheumatoid arthritis

100. You acquire a karyotype of a patient you suspect of having a chromosomal rearrangement. The pathology report comes back stating that there is a rearrangement involving two breaks in a single chromosome with inverted reincorporation of the segment. The inversion involves only one arm of the chromosome. What type of chromosomal mutation is this?

A. Deletion

B. Insertion

C. Isochromosome

D. Paracentric inversion

E. Pericentric inversion

F. Ring chromosome

Block 3

101. A 26-year-old woman presents with a 1-year history of intermittent diarrhea and abdominal pain that occurs every few weeks. Usually the diarrhea lasts for a few days or even a week. She has noticed that she occasionally has a fever during these episodes. A colonoscopy is performed; a representative picture of the ascending colon is shown in Figure 11. What is a possible extraintestinal manifestation of this disease that this patient may develop?

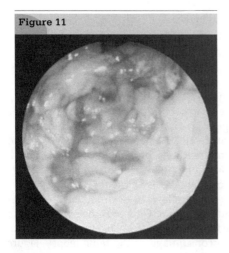

Figure 11

A. Erythema nodosum

B. Infection

C. Megaloblastic anemia

D. Pseudopolyps

E. Sarcoidosis

102. A 20-year-old woman in her first pregnancy presents for her initial prenatal visit at 6 weeks' gestation. She is concerned because she had used cocaine and heroin about 1 month before her pregnancy. She smokes a pack of cigarettes per day. In addition, she drinks one or two beers each day. Physical examination reveals tachycardia without murmurs or gallops. Pulmonary and abdominal examinations are unremarkable. Which of the following has the highest correlation with congenital anomalies for her fetus?

A. Alcohol

B. Caffeine

C. Cocaine

D. Opiates

E. Tobacco

103. A 24-year-old woman presents to the emergency department with the complaint of numbness and weakness in her lower extremities, which has existed for the past week. She informs the physician that she and her husband have been going through tough times and were planning to get a divorce. Physical examination of the heart, lungs, and abdomen is unremarkable. What is the most likely diagnosis?

A. Adjustment disorder

B. Conversion disorder

C. Hypochondriasis

D. Posttraumatic stress disorder (PTSD)

E. Somatization disorder

104. A 30-year-old woman (G1P1) presents to her primary care physician with the complaint of severe cramps with her menses. The pain has been so excruciating that it has caused her to miss many days at work. Her past medical history is insignificant. Physical examination of the heart, lungs, and abdomen is unremarkable. Pelvic examination reveals suprapubic tenderness and a uterus palpable above the pelvis. What is the most likely cause of her symptoms?

A. Adenomyositis

B. Asherman's syndrome

C. Pregnancy

D. Uterine carcinoma

E. Urinary tract infection

105. A 60-year-old man has developed gnawing epigastric pain that is worse after he eats. He recently increased his daily dose of an osteoarthritic medication because he heard that it had cardioprotective properties. Physical examination of the heart reveals no evidence of rubs, murmurs, or gallops. Pulmonary auscultation reveals no evidence of wheezes, rhonchi, or rales. Abdominal examination reveals no evidence of guarding or rebound tenderness. There is mild midepigastric tenderness to deep palpation. Upper gastrointestinal endoscopy reveals mild gastritis with punctate hemorrhages. Biopsies are taken. What is the most likely explanation for these findings?

A. Aspirin

B. Chloroquine

C. Ibuprofen

D. Indomethacin

E. Methotrexate

106. A brother and a sister both have a disease that has left them blind because of rapid optic nerve death. The brother, Sam, has six children (three boys and three girls), who are all completely normal. The sister, Susan, also has six children, all of whom have the disease. Susan's husband is completely normal. What is the most likely mode of inheritance for this disease?

A. Autosomal dominant

B. Autosomal recessive

C. Maternal inheritance of a mitochondrial mutation

D. X-linked dominant

E. X-linked inheritance

107. A 41-year-old woman presents to her primary care physician complaining of easy bruisability, which started about 2 weeks earlier. She mentions that after she bumps into anything, large bruises appear. She denies any other symptoms and takes no medications. She denies use of tobacco or alcohol. Physical examination is significant for numerous bruises and petechiae on her shins. On the basis of the laboratory studies shown below, what is the most likely diagnosis?

Hgb: 12.8 g/dL

WBC, 7,600: neutrophils, 70%; lymphocytes, 24%; eosinophils, 1%; monocytes, 4%

Platelets, 21,000

PT, normal

PTT, normal

Chemistries, normal

LFT, normal

A. Acute myelogenous leukemia

B. Disseminated intravascular coagulation

C. Idiopathic thrombocytopenic purpura

D. Thrombotic thrombocytopenic purpura

E. Pseudothrombocytopenia

108. A researcher studying neurological pathways is able to selectively stimulate a structure in a healthy female subject. Normally, this structure is naturally stimulated by which of the following stimuli?

A. Electromagnetic radiation

B. Fine touch

C. Hot temperature

D. Pressure

E. Sound

109. Physical examination of a newborn boy is unremarkable except for dimpling noticed in the lower lumbar region. Palpation of the underlying area is negative for a protruding mass. What prenatal precautions could the mother have taken to prevent this congenital defect in her child?

A. Abstaining from alcohol use

B. Amniocentesis testing

C. Folic acid supplementation

D. Measles, mumps, rubella (MMR) vaccination

E. Monitoring hypertension with appropriate treatment

110. A 22-month-old boy is brought into the clinic because his mother has noticed a decline in his appetite over the preceding 2 weeks. On examination he is found to have a cleft lip as well as an abnormal facial appearance. Cardiac, pulmonary, and abdominal examinations are within normal limits. Routine labs reveal a serum calcium of 6.5 mg/dL. What is the most likely cause of this child's symptoms?

A. Failure of pharyngeal pouches 3 and 4 to develop

B. Failure of the maxillary prominence to fuse with the medial nasal prominence

C. Failure of the palatine shelves to fuse with each other or the primary palate

D. Premature closure of sutures in the skull

E. Failure of the tongue to be freed from the floor of the mouth

111. A 19-year-old Wisconsin dairy farmer who drinks well water developed a painful, hard, enlarging mass at the upper end of his tibia. X-ray study reveals a shadow between the cortex and the periosteum. Labs show elevated alkaline phosphatase. What is the most likely explanation for these findings?

A. Ewing's sarcoma

B. Failure of differentiation into mature structures

C. Proliferation of growth-plate cartilage

D. Radium in the water

E. *Staphylococcus aureus* infection

112. A 3-year-old child presents for a general checkup with his pediatrician. At this time the physician notes a 2/6 holosystolic murmur but decides to watch its progression rather than act on it. By the time the child is 18 years old, the murmur is no longer detectable. What is the most appropriate explanation for these findings?

A. Aortic stenosis

B. Atrial septal defect

C. Patent ductus arteriosus

D. Situs inversus

E. Tetralogy of Fallot

F. Transposition of the great vessels

G. Ventricular septal defect

113. A 17-year-old young woman who is hepatitis B–positive presents to her primary care physician with weakness and fatigue. Physical examination of the heart, lungs, and abdomen is unremarkable. Laboratory studies reveal a serum creatinine of 2.9 mg/dL and serum blood urea nitrogen of 35 mg/dL. Renal biopsy is performed. Light microscopy reveals thickened capillary walls and basement membrane, with electron-dense immune complexes in subepithelium. Figure 12A below shows a silver stain from this patient's adrenal biopsy. Figure 12B is an electron-microscopic image of the renal biopsy. Figure 12C is an image of the renal biopsy with fluorescence microscopy. What is the most likely diagnosis?

A. Diabetic nephropathy

B. Lupus nephropathy

C. Membranous glomerulonephritis

Figure 12

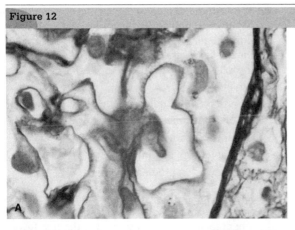

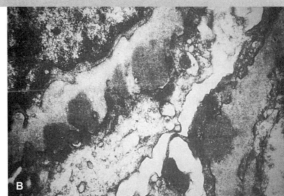

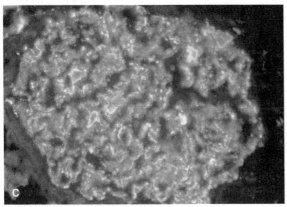

D. Minimal change disease

E. Renal amyloidosis

F. Renal artery stenosis

G. Renal vein thrombosis

H. Ureterolithiasis

114. A 26-year-old man presents to the emergency department complaining of recurrent, colicky midabdominal pain. His father had a colon polyp removed several years ago. Physical examination reveals a palpable abdominal mass and several areas of increased pigmentation on this patient's lips, palms, and soles. What is the most likely diagnosis?

A. Familial polyposis coli

B. Gardner's syndrome

C. Intussusception

D. Peutz-Jeghers syndrome with intussusception

E. Ulcerative colitis

115. An otherwise healthy 24-year-old sexually active woman presents to her primary care physician with a history of four unprotected sexual encounters in the past month. Clinical examination of the labia reveals a soft, painful ulcerated lesion. Which of the following organisms is most likely responsible for her symptoms?

A. *Calymmatobacterium granulomatis*

B. *Chlamydia trachomatis* L1, L2, or L3

C. *Haemophilus ducreyi*

D. Herpes simplex virus type 2

E. *Neisseria gonorrhoeae*

116. A 7-year-old Muskrat Scout returns from a five-night camping adventure in the Rocky Mountains with well-demarcated areas of redness on his face, neck, arms, and lower legs that correspond to zones not covered by his regulation shirt and shorts. He returned from the trip with leaves and grass of nine different species of plant in his hair, an excoriated and erythematous insect bite in his left axillary region, and a weathered piece of antler that his troop leader has identified as once belonging to a member of *Cervus canadensis*. After 3 days of supportive care provided by his parents, he recovers fully and returns to his normal summer routine. Nine days later, the boy develops malaise, fever, nausea, oliguria, and some swelling around his eyes. Later in the day, at the local emergency department, a nurse notes that the boy's urine has a grayish color. What causative findings for the boy's condition are likely to be discovered on further investigation?

A. Appearance of flagellated organisms with an eye-like appearance on urine culture

B. Contiguous segments of immunofluorescence of glomerular basement membrane

C. Intracellular Gram-negative bacteria in the endothelial cells of renal capillaries

D. Intracellular Gram-negative bacteria in macrophages

E. Granular deposits of immunoglobulin and C3 in the mesangium and basement membrane

117. A 22-year-old woman who was recently married presents to the clinic requesting help to conceive. She states that she has not been able to smell since birth and that her mother also has this problem and also had much difficulty trying to conceive. She is prescribed clomiphene. Which of the following conditions was present in the patient?

A. Polycystic ovary syndrome

B. Kallman's syndrome

C. Klinefelter's syndrome

D. Turner's syndrome

E. XYY syndrome

118. In which of the following cases would it be necessary to waive someone's right to confidentiality:

A. A famous person has been admitted to the hospital and the local newspaper has called for a statement.

B. You see one of your neighbors in the lobby and he asks what is going on with Mr. Smith (your patient).

C. A young mother brings her child to you and you notice hand-shaped bruises on the child's back.

D. A father calls in demanding to know whether his 18-year-old daughter (your patient) is on birth control.

119. A 58-year-old man with a long-standing history of gout and kidney stones presents for a follow-up examination. Physical examination of the heart, lungs, and abdomen is within normal limits. What would be used as first-line therapy in the chronic treatment of his gout?

A. Allopurinol

B. Colchicine

C. Indomethacin

D. Phenylbutazone

E. Probenecid

120. A 32-year-old woman presents to her primary care physician for her first prenatal visit. She has a history of two single births at 39 and 40 weeks, a set of twins born at 28 weeks, and two miscarriages. All four children are currently living and are well. Physical examination reveals a midline thyroid mass. Cardiac examination reveals a systolic ejection murmur grade I and an S_3 heart sound. Pulmonary auscultation reveals no wheezes, rhonchi, or rales. Which of the following is the most accurate description of her gravida and parity status?

A. G5P2004

B. G5P3224

C. G6P3014

D. G6P2124

E. G6P2224

121. Which of the following cell types has a surface marker that recognizes CD4+ T cells?

A. Hepatocytes

B. B cells

C. Primary spermatogonia

D. Enteric neurons

E. Mast cells

122. A 18-year-old college freshman presents to the emergency department with fever, headache, and a stiff neck. To confirm your diagnosis, lumbar puncture is performed between the L3 and L4 vertebrae slightly off of the midline. Which of the following structures will the needle pass through during this procedure?

A. Anterior longitudinal ligament

B. Conus medullaris

C. Dentate ligament

D. Ligamentum flavum

E. Posterior longitudinal ligament

123. A 9-year-old girl becomes infected with the chickenpox virus. She has not had any previous exposure to this virus. If her blood serum is measured in the first few days after infection, what antibody will be present in the highest amount?

A. IgA

B. IgD

C. IgE

D. IgG

E. IgM

124. A 45-year-old man presents to his primary care physician with a previous wrist fracture and current pain in the left hip, which he attributes to his work. Ultrasound assessment shows low bone density. Further studies show erosion of the femoral head, which required a surgical prosthetic replacement. What is his most likely occupation?

A. Body builder

B. Car salesman

C. Durable goods factory worker

D. Elementary school teacher

E. Loan officer

125. A 32-year-old female presents to the ambulatory care clinic complaining of recent abdominal weight gain, stretch marks on her abdomen, and facial hair. Her past medical history is positive for systemic lupus erythematosus. Her medications include high-dose daily prednisone and oral contraception. A picture of this patient is shown below (Figure 13). What is the most likely cause of her symptoms?

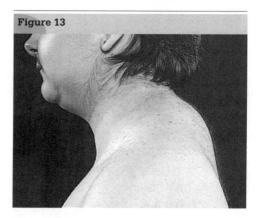

Figure 13

A. Adrenal neoplasm

B. Ovarian neoplasm

C. Pituitary adenoma

D. Polycystic ovary syndrome

E. Prednisone

126. A 4-year-old is brought to his pediatrician for evaluation. His eyes are protruding slightly. He has polydipsia and polyuria. Cardiac examination reveals tachycardia and a systolic ejection murmur. Pulmonary auscultation is within normal limits. X-ray studies reveal multiple lytic bone lesions on the calvarium and the base of the skull. What is the most likely diagnosis?

A. Eosinophilic granuloma

B. Diabetes mellitus type I

C. Hand-Schüller-Christian disease

D. Letterer-Siwe disease

E. Nephrogenic diabetes insipidus

127. A 38-year-old man, a chronic alcoholic, presents with a yellowish tint to his skin. What is the most likely pigment described?

A. Bilirubin

B. Iron

C. Keratin

D. Lipofuscin

E. Melanin

128. A 28-year-old G3P3003 woman has recently given birth. She is recovering from impaired placental separation after delivery, which resulted in massive hemorrhage. The patient reports that her previous two deliveries were by cesarean section. Which of the following diagnoses is most likely in this patient?

A. Amniotic fluid embolism

B. Chorioamnionitis

C. Placenta accreta

D. Placental abruptio

E. Placenta previa

129. Laboratory studies for a 1-month-old infant with nausea and vomiting are shown below. On the basis of these, what is the most likely metabolic explanation for this infant's condition?

Sodium, serum	133 mEq/L
Potassium, serum	3.6 mEq/L
Chloride, serum	93 mEq/L
Carbon dioxide, serum	20 mg/dL
Capillary blood pH	7.51

A. Combined metabolic and respiratory alkalosis

B. Compensated metabolic alkalosis

C. Metabolic alkalosis

D. Normal acid-base status

E. Respiratory alkalosis

130. A 33-year-old office manager with seasonal allergies experienced near-syncope after standing up from his desk. After grabbing onto the desk to steady himself, he continued on with his afternoon duties, which included running up four flights of stairs to deliver a package to an executive, visiting the building superintendent's office on the ground floor to find out why the air conditioning is not working, and distributing new computer monitors to his company's 17 employees. After placing the old monitors out on the loading dock, he ran back up to the seventh floor to participate in a buildingwide blood drive. Which of the following sets of values (compared to normal) will best correspond to those found in this man's blood?

	ADH	Osmolarity	Na+	Hematocrit
A	↑	↑	↑	↔
B	↓	↑	↑	↓
C	↑↑↑	↓	↓	↓
D	↓	↔	↓	↔
E	↑	↑	↑	↔
F	↑	↑	↑	↓
G	↑	↑	↑	↑
H	↔	↓↓↓	↔	↑

131. A 23-year-old sexually active woman presents to her family physician with fever, pelvic pain, adnexal tenderness, and vaginal discharge. The physician diagnoses pelvic inflammatory disease (PID). On additional history and clinical assessment, the physician is told of a complicated first-trimester induced abortion 3 weeks earlier. Which of the following organisms is least likely to be responsible for this patient's PID?

A. *Clostridium perfringens*

B. Coliform bacteria

C. *Neisseria gonorrhoeae*

D. Staphylococci

E. Streptococci

132. After your pediatric rotation, you decide to take some time off to work on a research project. While in clinic you had noticed many of your young patients to be diagnosed with a peanut allergy. You decide to design a research project to look at possible exposures that may have led to that diagnosis (documented peanut allergy). You hang up flyers in the pediatric clinic asking for all parents of children with a documented peanut allergy to contact you to see whether they are eligible to enroll in your project. What type of research study did you design?

A. Cohort

B. Case-control

C. Cross-sectional

D. Clinical trial

E. Experimental group

133. A 46-year-old woman who recently had a parathyroidectomy presents to the emergency department with tingling of her lips and fingers. The medical student demonstrates that when he taps on her cheek, her facial muscle begins to spasm. The sign that the medical student has shown to be positive in this patient is:

A. Chvostek's sign

B. Cullen's sign

C. Grey-Turner's sign

D. Trousseau's sign

E. Tubercular sign

134. A 55-year-old woman has developed fever, chills, and a productive cough over the past week. Physical examination reveals dullness to percussion in the left lower lung lobe. Chest x-ray confirms a lobar pneumonia. *Streptococcus pneumoniae* is the suspected organism. She is not allergic to any medications. What is the most appropriate antibiotic to treat her condition?

A. Ampicillin

B. Ceftriaxone

C. Erythromycin

D. Penicillin

E. Vancomycin

135. A 34-year-old woman presents to the ambulatory care clinic. She admits that she can now drink a twelve pack without feeling "good" when she used to feel good after only a six pack. She claims she has tried to stop drinking alcohol and will often try to limit how much she allows herself to drink. She also tells you that since she lives in a dry county, she often has to drive 20 to 30 mi just to get more beer when her stock runs out. When asked whether her drinking were getting in the way of her work and personal relationships, she says no. Which of the following is she most likely suffering from?

A. Abuse

B. Dependence

C. Intoxication

D. Withdrawal

136. A 47-year-old man presents to his primary care physician complaining of having gotten sick often over the previous 6 months. He reports no significant medical/surgical history and agrees to have some labs drawn. Studies reveal anemia, leukopenia, hypercalcemia, and Bence Jones protein in the urine. What is the next area to investigate to further confirm the presumed diagnosis?

A. Axial skeletal scan

B. Buccal swab

C. Kidney biopsy

D. Liver function tests

E. Liver ultrasound

137. A study at a local high school was conducted to determine the average intelligence of 879 students. The results were distributed according to a normal curve. The mean IQ was 113, with a standard deviation of 7. Which of the following statements is true according to the information provided and the graph in Figure 14?

A. All of the students' scores fall between 106 and 120.

B. All of the students' scores fall between 99 and 127.

C. The median score is 111.

D. 95.5% of the students' scores fall between 99 and 127.

138. A 42-year-old man presents to his primary care physician with multiple small, dark-purple skin lesions on his torso and upper extremities. He was diagnosed with HIV approximately 10 years ago and progressed to full-blown AIDS within the last year. Which of the following viruses has most likely led to these new lesions?

A. Cytomegalovirus

B. Epstein-Barr virus

C. Human herpesvirus 8

D. Human papillomavirus

E. Varicella zoster virus

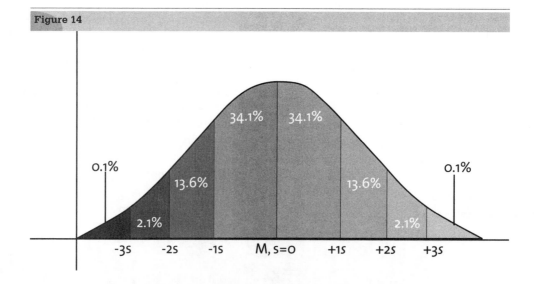

Figure 14

139. A 55-year-old woman has been experiencing feelings of guilt, lack of appetite, lack of sleep, decreased energy, and lack of pleasure for 3 weeks. She was advised by her husband to "go see someone" and presents to her primary care physician for further evaluation. Physical examination of the heart reveals no evidence of rubs, murmurs, or gallops. Pulmonary auscultation reveals no evidence of wheezes, rhonchi, or rales. Abdominal examination reveals no evidence of peritoneal signs. Bowel sounds are present. What is the most likely diagnosis?

A. Bereavement

B. Bipolar disorder type 1

C. Factitious disorder

D. Major depressive episode

E. Schizoid disorder

140. A 14-year-old boy has noticed enlargement of his scrotum and testes while his penis has remained the same size. He has also noticed some straight pubic hair at the base of his penis. What is his most likely stage of development?

A. Tanner 1

B. Tanner 2

C. Tanner 3

D. Tanner 4

E. Tanner 5

141. A 45-year-old patient with AIDS presents to his primary care physician with increasing symptoms of fatigue, weight loss, and chronic cough. After his physical exam, you order multiple blood tests, a chest x-ray, and a TB test. The next day there is reddening and an induration at the site of the intracutaneous injection of the tuberculin. What is the most likely explanation for these findings?

A. Type I hypersensitivity reaction

B. Type II hypersensitivity reaction

C. Type III hypersensitivity reaction

D. Type IV hypersensitivity reaction

E. Type V hypersensitivity reaction

142. A 19-year-old woman presents to her primary care physician with complaints of chronic sinusitis. While examining her oropharynx, you notice that her teeth are extensively decayed. Her BMI is estimated at 21. What is the most appropriate treatment for this patient?

A. Amphetamines

B. Behavioral therapy

C. Fluoride rinse

D. Imipramine

E. Thioridazine

143. A 34-year-old health professional presents to employee health services to have her yearly tuberculin test. The injection is properly placed and the patient is instructed to return in 2 days to check the results. She returns to clinic with a >10-mm indurated, red, swollen area at the site of the injection. Which of the following mechanisms is responsible for this finding?

A. Antibodies reacting with intrinsic components of cell membranes, resulting in direct damage

B. Antibodies recognizing and binding the foreign proteins and triggering cytokine release from neutrophils

C. Complement-bound aggregates of antigen-antibody complexes deposited on vessel walls and serosal surfaces, which attract neutrophils and trigger the release of lysosomal enzymes

D. IgE recognizing and binding the foreign protein and triggering mast cell degranulation and histamine release

E. Proliferation of antigen-specific CD4+ memory cells with secretion of IL-2 and other cytokines, which recruit and stimulate phagocytic macrophages

144. A 24-year-old man is hospitalized following a heroin overdose. He begins to develop severe dyspnea and labored rapid breathing. His lips and nails are blue. Blood pressure is 90/50 mm Hg. Chest auscultation reveals bilateral crackles. Blood cultures are negative. The patient eventually expires. Histological examination of lung tissue shows intraalveolar hyaline membrane composed of fibrin and cellular debris. Which of the following was the most likely cause of death?

A. Adult respiratory distress syndrome

B. Cor pulmonale

C. Pulmonary alveolar proteinosis

D. Pulmonary embolism

E. Sepsis

145. A 20-year-old college football player suffers a severe knee injury, dislocating the joint. Even after the team physician resets the knee, the pulses distal to the injury are still absent. What vessel found posterior to the knee joint is often damaged with knee dislocations?

A. Anterior tibial artery

B. Peroneal artery

C. Popliteal artery

D. Posterior tibial artery

E. Superficial femoral artery

146. A 27-year-old woman has had a pancreas transplant 12 hr earlier and is now in the surgical intensive care unit. Since age 5, she has had insulin-dependent diabetes mellitus. Her vital signs are normal, chest is clear to auscultation, and cardiac examination reveals a regular rate and rhythm. Her wound dressing is clean, dry, and intact. Which of the following is the best method of monitoring the transplanted pancreas?

A. Serum amylase level

B. Serum glucose level

C. Serum insulin level

D. Ultrasonography of the pancreatic vessels

E. Urinary amylase level

147. A 63-year-old woman is admitted to the hospital for shortness of breath, a debilitating dough-like swelling of her ankles, and—of late—the inability to catch her breath while lying supine in bed. Her daughter, who has accompanied her to the hospital, gives the admitting nurse a list of medications that her mother has been using. Later that night, the nurse notes on the chart that the physician on call has ordered even higher doses of one of these medications. What beneficial alteration in kidney function would account for the physician's decision to increase the dosage of this particular medication?

A. Decreased glomerular filtration rate (GFR) due to constriction of afferent arterioles

B. Decreased secretion of antidiuretic hormone (ADH) by mesangial cells

C. Disruption of the corticopapillary osmotic gradient

E. Impaired insertion of H_2O channels into the lumen of the proximal tubules

F. Increased concentration of urea in the renal cortex

G. Increased transport of sodium, potassium, and chloride through the thick ascending loop of Henle

148. A 16-year-old youth presents to his primary care physician for the physical examination required to participate in after-school sports. One of his shoulder blades is found to protrude more than the other. The forward-bend exam is positive. What best characterizes this disorder?

A. Best treated during growth spurt

B. Caused by carrying books or bad posture

C. Deterioration of microarchitecture from gonadal deficiency; increased incidence among Asians

D. Degeneration of synovial joints due to excessive use

E. Inflammation of sacroiliac joints with lymphocytic infiltration followed by calcification and ossification around the sites of attachment

F. Kyphoscoliosis, hearing loss, fragile bones, blue sclerae, mild short stature

G. Soft tissue swelling over sternocleidomastoid presenting with painful muscle spasms

149. A 16-year-old girl presents to her primary care physician complaining of a poorly healing painless ulcer on her labia (Figure 15). She first noticed the lesion about a week earlier. She states that she had a sexual encounter at a friend's party with an older man she didn't know very well. What is the most appropriate treatment for this patient?

A. Ceftriaxone

B. Ciprofloxacin

C. Gentamicin

D. Penicillin G

E. Tetracycline

150. A 55-year-old man who is a chronic smoker presents to his primary care physician with a long history of vascular issues and problems but has never been specifically diagnosed with any ailment. He does complain of erectile dysfunction and is treated with a phosphodiesterase type V inhibitor. Physical examination of the heart and lungs is within normal limits. Angiography reveals ring-like calcifi-

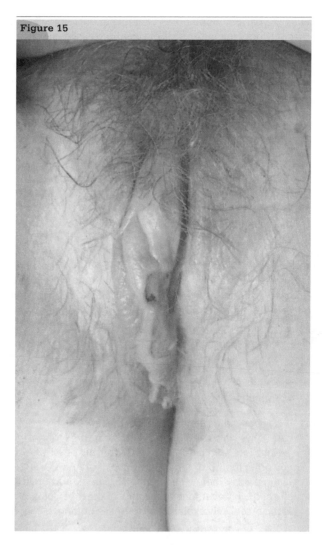

Figure 15

cations in the media of the arteries. What is the most likely diagnosis?

A. Arteriolosclerosis

B. Hyperparathyroidism

C. Mönckeberg's arteriosclerosis

D. Rheumatic endocarditis

E. Waldenström's macroglobulinemia

Block 4

151. A 16-year-old girl is on day 15 of her menstrual cycle. Which hormone is responsible for the growth and maintenance of the corpus luteum?

A. Estrogen

B. Human chorionic gonadotrophin

C. Prolactin

D. Progesterone

E. Testosterone

152. A 68-year-old woman who had a coronary artery bypass procedure 9 days earlier was started on warfarin 5 days ago. Today her international normalized ratio (INR) is 10. What treatment should she receive to prevent myocardial arrhythmia?

A. Atropine

B. Calcium

C. Fluid resuscitation with sodium chloride

D. Folate

E. Magnesium

F. Potassium

153. A 25-year-old woman presents to her primary care physician with skin thickening and darkening pigmentation of her neck, axilla and groin. Physical examination shows that she is 5 ft 4 in tall and weighs 220 lb. Cardiac, pulmonary, and abdominal examinations are within normal limits. What is the most likely diagnosis?

A. Acanthosis nigracans

B. Actinic keratosis

C. Basal cell carcinoma

D. Malignant melanoma

E. Psoriasis

F. Squamous cell carcinoma

154. A 73-year-old woman with a long-standing history of schizophrenia presents to your office with complaints of spasms in her face, neck, and tongue; a resting tremor in her hands; and a general feeling of restlessness. These symptoms have gradually been getting worse over the previous 3 months; now she seems unable to sit still and her speech is difficult to understand owing to involuntary movements of her tongue. She also has difficulty initiating movements. Her current medications are haloperidol, atorvastatin, and famotidine. She used to drink two cups of coffee a day but stopped doing so 6 weeks ago. Dysfunction in which of the following areas in the central nervous system is most likely to be causing her symptoms?

A. Caudate nucleus

B. Mesolimbic tract

C. Nigrostriatal tract

D. Prefrontal cortex

E. Tuberoinfundibular tract

155. A 46-year-old man with a 35-pack-year history of cigarette smoking developed shaking chills and shortness of breath 2 days earlier. He is on prednisone for psoriasis. His cough is productive of a yellowish sputum. Culture shows Gram-negative rods that are hard to see. What is the preferred treatment for the causative organism?

A. Azithromycin

B. Ciprofloxacin

C. Gentamicin

D. Penicillin

E. Tetracycline

156. A 15-year-old boy with a 10-year history of HIV experiences pain, limited range of motion, muscle spasms, and progressive bone damage, especially in the proximal femur. He contracted HIV during a blood transfusion. He does not know his most recent CD4 cell count. Physical examination of the heart, lungs, and abdomen is unremarkable. Which of the following is the next most appropriate course of action?

A. Continue weight-bearing exercises of the affected joint

B. Chest and lower extremity x-ray

C. Have an MRI done

D. Install stair rails

E. Reduce intake of caffeine and alcohol

F. Stop his steroids

157. A 34-year-old man presents to his primary care physician concerned about recent changes in his body. He reports that he is losing sensation in his arms and legs and is quite upset. A peripheral blood smear is shown in Figure 16. What would be the most effective treatment based on this clinical presentation?

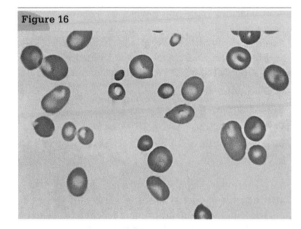

Figure 16

A. Vitamin B_{12} supplementation

B. Blood transfusion

C. Increased ingestion of red meat

D. Supplementation of intrinsic factor

E. Iron supplements

158. A 35-year-old man with a history of tonic-clonic seizures presents to his primary care physician with new growth of facial hair, double vision, and thickened gums. Which of the following medications is most likely causing his symptoms?

A. Acetaminophen

B. Carbamazepine

C. Ethosuximide

D. Phenytoin

E. Valproic acid

159. A 24-year-old sexually active woman is diagnosed by her family physician with a sexually transmitted disease that is associated with pharyngitis, proctitis, pelvic inflammatory disease, and monoarticular arthritis. With which of the following organisms is this woman most likely infected?

A. *Candida albicans*

B. *Chlamydia trachomatis*

C. *Gardnerella vaginalis*

D. *Neisseria gonorrhoeae*

E. *Trichomonas vaginalis*

160. A 63-year-old woman, a retired oil refinery worker with a BMI of 32, calls her son because she has been having headaches, dizziness and gastrointestinal disturbances. Concerned, her son takes her to their family physician. While waiting, the nurse notes that the woman's blood pressure is elevated. What elevated blood indicator is the most likely explanation for these findings?

A. Aldosterone

B. Angiotensin II

C. Antidiuretic hormone (ADH)

D. Atrial natriuretic factor

E. Cholecalciferol

F. Erythropoietin (EPO)

161. A 55-year-old man has developed polyuria, polydipsia, polyphagia, and a red, scaly rash on his face over the past 2 weeks. His fasting blood glucose is 315 mg/dL. He is thin and has never had elevated blood glucose levels in the past. What is the most likely diagnosis?

A. Glucagonoma

B. Insulinoma

C. Type I diabetes

D. Type II diabetes

E. VIPoma

162. A 44-year-old schizophrenic man is brought to the psychiatric emergency department because of delirium, fever, muscle rigidity, and autonomic instability. His current medications include haloperidol. What is the most likely diagnosis?

A. Hypertensive crisis

B. Malignant hyperthermia

C. Neuroleptic malignant syndrome

D. Serotonin syndrome

E. Tardive dyskinesia

163. A 17-year-old girl is found unconscious by her mother. An ambulance is called and she is brought to the emergency department. In the ambulance, two large-bore IV lines with normal saline are initiated. Fingerstick glucose level is 800 mg/dL. She is later diagnosed with diabetes mellitus and discharged from the hospital on an insulin regimen. Two months later she presents to her primary care physician complaining about having to take insulin at school. What drug can be added to decrease the number of insulin injections she may need?

A. Alpha glucosidase inhibitor (acarbose)

B. Glyburide

C. Lisinopril

D. Metformin

E. No oral drug should be prescribed

164. A 44-year-old man presents to his primary care physician for follow-up of hypertension. His father and brother also have hypertension. Physical examination of the heart, lungs, and abdomen is within normal limits. What is the main cause of this condition?

A. Cigarette smoking

B. Environmental exposure

C. Lack of daily exercise

D. Poor diet

E. Unknown etiology

165. A 51-year-old man presents to his primary care physician for evaluation of a skin lesion. He complains of hypopigmentation of the skin of his lower back. What cells are responsible for this condition?

A. Adipocytes

B. Keratinocytes

C. Langerhans cells

D. Melanocytes

E. Merkel cells

166. A 66-year-old retired construction worker presents to his primary care physician with ulcerated, scaling nodules on his lip, forearms, and hands. A picture of his lip is shown in Figure 17. Punch biopsy reveals nests of atypical keratinocytes forming keratin pearls. What is the most likely diagnosis?

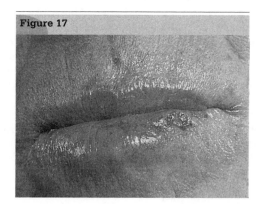

Figure 17

A. Basal cell carcinoma

B. Malignant melanoma

C. Psoriasis

D. Seborrheic keratosis

E. Squamous cell carcinoma

167. A 13-year-old boy is brought to the ambulatory care clinic complaining of anosmia after being tackled during a football game after school. He remembers feeling "knocked in the head" and is worried that he "broke something" in his skull. Based on his presentation and brief history, what would be the most likely bone that was injured/fractured?

A. Calcaneus

B. Ethmoid bone

C. Occipital bone

D. Parietal bone

E. Sphenoid

168. A common condition found in older women is the presence of varicose veins, which are abnormally dilated, tortuous veins. They typically arise due to increased intraluminal pressure from standing erect for long periods of time. Varicose veins found on the surface of the lower leg just medial to the tibial bone are drained by which vein?

A. Accessory saphenous veins
B. Anterior tibial veins
C. Great saphenous veins
D. Peroneal veins
E. Small saphenous veins

169. Bile salts are responsible for the solubilization of lipids into an absorbable form in the body. Where does this solubilization occur?

A. Hepatocytes
B. Kupffer cells
C. Micelles
D. Vacuoles

170. A 68-year-old postmenopausal woman presents to her primary care physician for a 4-month follow-up for management of her osteoporosis. Current medications include alendronate. A dual-energy x-ray absorptiometry (DEXA) scan reveals the vertebral bodies with massive demineralization, especially in L2-L5. All other bony structures are not as severely affected. She says that since beginning with the medication, she has been getting bad stomach aches and burning in her chest. She does not want to be put on estrogen replacement therapy because of the associated risks. Which of the following would be an appropriate medication to begin for the prevention of vertebral fractures in this woman?

A. Cabergoline
B. Calcitonin
C. Danazol
D. Raloxifene
E. Risedronate
F. Toremifene

171. A 54-year-old alcoholic presents to the emergency department stating that he drank what he thought was moonshine, but after finishing the bottle his friend told him that he had added rubbing alcohol for a little extra kick. What is the most appropriate treatment for this patient?

A. Administer ethanol
B. Administer normal saline
C. Call the police
D. Intravenous infusion of vitamins
E. Tell the patient to drink a cup of coffee and call a cab to go home

172. A 55-year-old woman presents her primary care physician's office with the complaint of hot flashes, along with trouble sleeping at night and mood swings. Her last menstrual period (LMP) was 8 months earlier, and periods before that, over about a year, were becoming increasingly irregular. Physical examination of the heart, lungs, and abdomen is unremarkable. Which of the following tests would most likely confirm the diagnosis?

A. hCG
B. FSH
C. LH
D. Prolactin
E. TSH

173. A 44-year-old man presents to his primary care physician complaining of a prolonged, painful erection unrelated to sexual desire. He also complains of fever, fatigue, and weight loss. Physical examination reveals nontender cervical lymphadenopathy and inguinal adenopathy. The cardiac, pulmonary, and abdominal examinations are noncontributory. Genitourinary examination reveals an erect penis that is painful to palpation along the glans and shaft. Laboratory studies reveal a white blood cell count of 45,000/mm³. A translocation between which chromosomes is probably present in this patient's leukocytes?

A. 9 and 22
B. 8 and 14
C. 15 and 17
D. 14 and 18
E. 14 and 21

174. A 38-year-old woman who used to do aqua aerobics during the week and cycle 30 mi on weekends can no longer ride or do aerobics due to severe back pain. It occurs when she gets out of bed or does water aerobics and is also exacerbated by long rides in the car. She never used to sleep on her side but must now sleep with her knees close to her chest. What is the most likely explanation for these findings?

A. Loss of horizontal trabeculae in the vertebrae and thickened vertical trabeculae
B. Surrounding soft tissue damage
C. Strong association with HLA B27; inflammation at insertion points leading to ossification
D. Tears or fissures, which may impinge on movement of nutrients and waste, proteoglycan destruction
E. Three-dimensional curvature of the spine

175. A 35-year-old man presents to the clinic with a 3-day history of a productive cough and fever. He is sexually active and has had numerous partners in the past. Culture of the sputum does not reveal any organisms. What is the most appropriate treatment for this patient?

A. Cefuroxime
B. Gentamicin
C. Penicillin
D. Tetracycline
E. Vancomycin

176. A 23-year-old African American woman presents to you, a primary care physician, as a new patient. She tells you that she was diagnosed with beta-globin hemoglobinopathy. She is understandably concerned and asks you to please clarify exactly what her diagnosis means. You proceed to tell her that she has:

A. Autoimmune hemolytic anemia

B. Beta-thalassemia major

C. Erythroblastosis fetalis

D. Hereditary spherocytosis

E. Sickle cell anemia

177. A 73-year-old Caucasian man presents to his primary care physician complaining of a 1-month history of nocturia, polyuria, and difficulty starting and stopping his urinary stream. Physical examination of the prostate shows it to be uniformly enlarged (70 g), with a rubbery texture. His prostate-specific antigen (PSA) is 6 ng/mL; urinalysis is negative. The patient is begun on finasteride. What is the mechanism of action of this medication?

A. Alpha₁ receptor agonist

B. Alpha₁ receptor antagonist

C. Androgen receptor agonist

D. Androgen receptor antagonist

E. 5-alpha reductase inhibitor

F. GnRH analog

178. A 28-year-old woman presents to her primary care physician after two consecutive missed menstrual periods. She is concerned that she may be pregnant, but home testing results have remained inconclusive. Her beta-hCG levels are measured in the office and found to be within reference range. Which of the following hormones, if found to be below normal levels, would most likely be predictive of anovulatory cycles?

A. Estrone

B. Follicle-stimulating hormone

C. Gonadotrophin hormone–releasing hormone

D. Luteinizing hormone

E. Progesterone

179. A man who has been HIV-positive for 5 years visits your office. He comes to see you regularly and has no new complaints. He is currently receiving highly active antiretroviral therapy (HAART) and his CD4 cell count has been steady around 450 for a year. The patient believes that he was infected with the virus when he was abusing heroin and was sharing needles. He currently denies any drug or alcohol use. Which of the following statements regarding HIV/AIDS transmission is true?

A. Approximately 50% of neonates born to HIV+ mothers will be seropositive at birth.

B. The average risk of being infected after a needle-stick with HIV+ blood is 1 in 50.

C. The risk from a single sexual encounter with a man who is not a member of a high-risk group is 1 in 100,000.

D. The risk of seroconversion from a blood transfusion with an HIV+ donor is 2 in 3.

E. There are no medications that can be given to decrease the rate of HIV transmission from mother to child.

180. A 4-year-old girl is brought to the emergency department by her parents, who report that their daughter has had recurrent muscle spasms in her arms. The child is of short stature and has shortened fourth and fifth phalanges on both hands. What is the cause of this child's condition?

A. 46, XO genotype

B. Dietary calcium deficiency

C. Failure of development of the third and fourth pharyngeal arches

D. Renal unresponsiveness to PTH

E. Vitamin D deficiency

181. You are treating a 74-year-old Caucasian woman for chronic myelogenous leukemia, which has progressed to the blast phase. She complains of increased confusion and urination. Physical examination is unremarkable. Laboratory studies reveal a serum sodium of 115 mEq/L and decreased serum osmolarity. Which of the following medications is most likely causing her complaints?

A. Cisplatin

B. Cyclosporine

C. Doxorubicin

D. Methotrexate

E. Paclitaxel

182. A 24-year-old man presents to you, his primary care physician, complaining of constant headaches and a feeling of pressure in his head that are not relieved by over-the-counter analgesics. A computed tomography (CT) scan reveals a cerebral tumor. Which of the following would correlate with this presentation?

A. Anosmia

B. Ataxia

C. Diplopia

D. Nystagmus

E. Papilledema

183. A 63-year-old woman presents to her primary care physician with dyspnea on exertion, which has been occurring progressively over 3 months. She has a 90-pack-year history of cigarette smoking. Physical examination of the lungs reveals decreased fremitus, hyperresonance on percussion, and diminished breath sounds. Her breaths are shallow and rapid and she has pursed lips. Her chest appears barrel-shaped. Based on this description and the image in Figure 18, which of the following would she be expected to have?

A. Decreased lung compliance

B. FEV₁/FVC ratio greater than 0.8

C. Reduced functional residual capacity (FRC)

D. Increase in elastic recoil

E. Increase in the expiratory phase of respiration

Figure 18

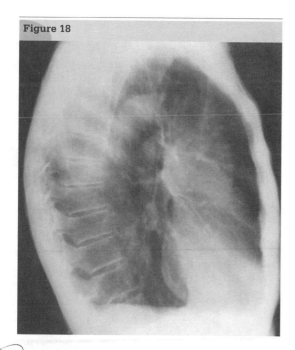

184. A 5-year-old boy is brought to the emergency department in respiratory distress and with a temperature of 103°F (39.4°C). He has difficulty swallowing and, on physical examination, an inspiratory stridor is heard. His x-ray reveals swelling of the epiglottis. The organism responsible for his symptoms can be cultured on what medium?

A. Chocolate agar with factors V and X

B. Charcoal yeast extract

C. Löwenstein-Jensen agar

D. Potato agar

E. Thayer-Martin medium

185. A 30-year-old woman with a valve replacement requires anticoagulation therapy to prevent the formation of a clot. She also informs the physician of her desire to have children in the near future. What is the most appropriate agent?

A. Abciximab

B. Aspirin

C. Heparin

D. Streptokinase

E. Tinzaparin

F. Warfarin

186. A 21-year-old woman who is a college soccer player has participated in the sport since the age of 8. She has a history of an eating disorder, menstrual abnormalities, and osteoporosis. Her menstrual cycle ranges from 14 to 39 days in duration. Her menstrual flow time ranges from 1 to 8 days. Which of the following conditions is she most at risk for?

A. Contralateral side closed head injury

B. Increased risk of fractures

C. Insomnia

D. Knee joint osteoarthritis

E. Sudden loss of vision

187. A 66-year-old man is diagnosed with internal hemorrhoids. He also has external hemorrhoids found on physical examination. These are painful to the touch. What defines the area that demarcates painful from nonpainful hemorrhoids?

A. Meissner's plexus

B. Muscularis plexus

C. Myenteric plexus

D. Pectinate line

188. A 27-year-old woman presents to her primary care physician for follow up. She was diagnosed with bipolar disorder type II 3 years earlier but is currently stabilized on medication. She does not appear well and tells you that she has been having an exacerbation of her Crohn's disease and has been quite ill over the past few days. Also, she recently got into an argument with her mother, with whom she is quite close, and has not spoken to her in a week. On which axis would one place her Crohn's disease according to the classification of the fourth edition of the *Diagnostic and Statistical Manual of Mental Disorders* (DSM-IV)?

A. Axis I

B. Axis II

C. Axis III

D. Axis IV

E. Axis V

189. A 13-year-old boy is brought to his pediatrician complaining of fever, malaise, and periorbital edema, which developed 2 days earlier. He had a sore throat 2 weeks previously that lasted for a few days but resolved. In addition he has noticed that his urine has been darker than usual over the past 2 days. Physical examination of the heart, lungs, and abdomen are within normal limits. There is no guarding or rebound tenderness. Bowel sounds are present in all four quadrants. Which of the following would you expect to find histologically with a renal biopsy of this patient?

A. Crescent formation in Bowman's space

B. Dense deposits within the glomerular basement membrane

C. Fusion of foot podocytes

D. Mesangial deposits of IgA

E. Smooth and linear pattern of IgG in the glomerular basement membrane

F. Subepithelial humps

190. A specimen is sent from gastroenterology to the pathology department for analysis. The attached note states that the specimen was taken from the stomach of a 35-year-old woman after gastroscopy revealed a suspicious lesion. On microscopy, the pathologist notes several signet-ring cells, some of which pass through the basal lamina and into the submucosa. Which of the following is the most likely consequence of this finding?

A. Choriocarcinoma

B. Clear cell adenocarcinoma of the vagina

C. Endometrial carcinoma

D. Granulosa cell tumor of the ovary

E. Krukenberg tumors

191. A 41-year-old male schizophrenic is brought to the emergency department for evaluation of hemoptysis and hematemesis. He spends his free time in the courtyard eating dirt and grass. Examination of the oropharyngeal cavity reveals an ulcerating, necrotizing gingivitis. What is the most likely causative agent?

A. *Actinomyces israelii*

B. *Bacteroides fragilis*

C. *Borrelia burgdorferi*

D. *Fusobacterium nucleatum*

E. *Prevotella melaninogenica*

192. A 45-year-old man presents to the emergency department after suffering a laceration of his left arm. Proper measures have been taken to stop the bleeding, but excessive blood loss has continued despite the physicians' efforts. The patient becomes unconscious and is unable to answer questions. Initial laboratory studies indicate a normal bleeding time and PTT but an INR of 5.8. In addition to replacing fluids lost by this patient, the physician decides to administer which of the following treatments to correct this problem?

A. Aminocaproic acid

B. Enoxaparin

C. Protamine sulfate

D. Streptokinase

E. Vitamin K

193. A 28-year-old woman presents to the physician with a flat rash over the malar eminences, sparing the nasolabial folds, which is worse with exposure to sunlight. She has ulcers on her oral mucosa, which she says are painless; she also has tenderness and some swelling of both wrists and ankles. Laboratory studies show a high antinuclear antibody (ANA) titer along with positive anti-Smith antibodies. What is her diagnosis?

A. Dermatomyositis

B. Discoid lupus erythematosus

C. Psoriasis

D. Scleroderma

E. Systemic lupus erythematosus

194. The developing fetus depends on the mother for oxygenation of its blood. This exchange occurs in the umbilical cord, and the blood is transported back into the fetal circulation. Once the infant is delivered and takes its first breath, which structure immediately closes to block the right-to-left shunt?

A. Allantois

B. Ductus arteriosus

C. Ductus venosus

D. Foramen ovale

E. Umbilical arteries

195. A 77-year-old woman presents to the clinic with a recent onset of severe abdominal pain and fever. She had recently been at a football game, where she ate a box of popcorn. Physical examination reveals diffuse abdominal tenderness, worse in the left lower quadrant. Barium enema was obtained and is shown in Figure 19. What is the most likely diagnosis?

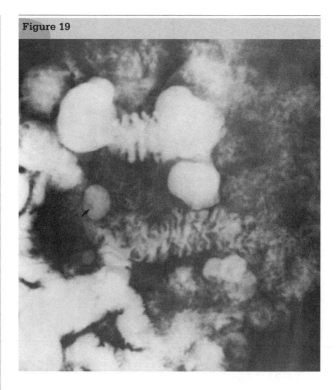

Figure 19

A. Appendicitis

B. Bowel obstruction

C. Colonic adenocarcinoma

D. Diverticulitis

E. Ulcerative colitis

196. A 34-year-old woman complains of having had burning stomach pain with eating over 3 to 4 months. She also reports a history of chronic back problems as well as a weight gain of 20 lb in the last 4 months. She denies the use of nonsteroidal anti-inflammatory agents. She denies nausea and vomiting. Physical examination of the heart, lungs, and abdomen is within normal limits. What is the most likely pathogen associated with this condition?

A. Enterohemorrhagic *Escherichia coli*

B. *E. coli*

C. *Helicobacter pylori*

D. *Shigella*

E. *Streptococcus pyogenes*

197. A 42-year-old man presents to his primary care physician for a 3-month checkup. He reports that he has had episodes of sweating, headaches, and intermittent palpitations. His blood pressure is 160/94 mm Hg. Looking back through his chart, you notice that he has had two previous episodes of elevated blood pressure that were separated by two readings. Laboratory analysis show increased levels of vanillylmandelic acid (VMA). Which of the following drugs is an irreversible alpha-adrenergic receptor blocker that is used in a condition of this kind?

A. Doxazosin

B. Phenoxybenzamine

C. Phentolamine

D. Prazosin

E. Terazosin

F. Yohimbine

198. An 84-year-old Caucasian woman is admitted to the hospital because of a left lower lobar pneumonia. Weakened by the illness, she is unable to mobilize for a week. On rising from bed, she immediately becomes short of breath. CT angiography reveals a pulmonary embolism. Anticoagulation with both heparin and warfarin is undertaken. What is the rationale for beginning both medications at the same time?

A. Heparin counteracts warfarin's initial procoagulable state of inhibiting plasmin.

B. Heparin counteracts warfarin's initial procoagulable state of inhibiting protein C.

C. Heparin counteracts warfarin's initial procoagulable state of inhibiting protein S.

D. Heparin potentiates warfarin's anticoagulant effect initially by blocking antithrombin III.

E. Heparin potentiates warfarin's anticoagulant effect initially by blocking factor VII.

199. A 20-year-old woman presents to her primary care physician with a single lesion on her left labium. It is very tender. Initially it appeared as a papule but now it is a nonindurated ulcer. Physical examination reveals bilateral inguinal adenopathy. Gram's stain reveals organisms associated in clumps that appear to follow each other across the slide. What is the most likely etiology?

A. Chlamydia trachomatis

B. Haemophilus ducreyi

C. Herpes simplex virus 1

D. Neisseria gonorrhoeae

E. Treponema pallidum

200. An irritable 6-month-old boy who has been vomiting for a day is brought to the emergency department. He has recently become extremely difficult to rouse. Lab tests show hyperammonemia, hypoglycemia, and, given the hypoglycemia, abnormally low serum ketones. Further lab tests reveal an error in fatty acid oxidation. What is the most likely diagnosis?

A. Acetyl-CoA carboxylase deficiency

B. Glucose-6-phosphate dehydrogenase deficiency

C. Glycogen synthetase deficiency

D. Medium-chain fatty acyl-CoA dehydrogenase (MCAD) deficiency

E. Phosphofructokinase deficiency

Block 5

201. A 30-year-old woman presents to the local clinic with the complaint of a foul-smelling vaginal discharge. She has a prior medical history of recurrent urinary tract infections. Physical examination of the cervix reveals punctate epithelial papillae. The organisms are seen on wet prep of the discharge. What is the most likely etiology?

A. Candida albicans

B. Gardnerella vaginalis

C. Haemophilus ducreyi

D. Trichomonas vaginalis

E. Streptococcus pyogenes

202. A 32-year-old man recently underwent a left adrenalectomy. The patient had been experiencing symptoms secondary to an increase in a specific adrenal hormone. His preoperative CT scan is shown in Figure 20. The pathology report states that the area of abnormality was in the zona glomerulosa. Which of the following hormones was involved?

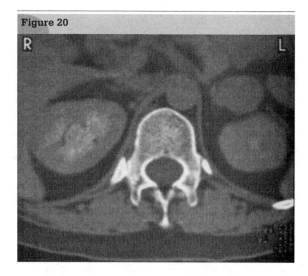

Figure 20

A. Aldosterone

B. Cortisol

C. Dehydroepiandrosterone

D. Epinephrine

E. Norepinephrine

203. A patient with dysplastic nevus syndrome presents to the clinic with a brown papular lesion on his neck. What is the most likely diagnosis?

A. Basal cell carcinoma

B. Squamous cell carcinoma

C. Malignant melanoma

D. Merkel cell carcinoma

E. Histiocytosis X

204. A 34-year-old woman presents to her primary care physician with fatigue and weakness. She explains that she cannot finish a small bowl of Grape Nuts cereal because her jaw muscles get too tired. She also complains that she cannot finish her lectures because she just gets too worn out. She is asked to lift her arms up and down repetitively. She cannot do more than four repetitions. After neostigmine is administered, she can complete twelve repetitions. What is the most likely diagnosis?

A. Becker muscular dystrophy

B. Fibrositis

C. Myasthenia gravis

D. Polymyalgia rheumatica

E. Septic arthritis

205. A 65-year-old woman is brought to the emergency department because of a 3-day history of fever, shortness of breath, and a cough productive of rust-colored sputum. Culture of sputum reveals the presence of Gram-positive cocci. The colonies are green in color and, when exposed to optochin, are inhibited. What is the most likely explanation for these findings?

A. *Peptostreptococcus*

B. *Streptococcus agalactiae*

C. *Streptococcus mutans*

D. *Streptococcus pneumoniae*

E. *Streptococcus pyogenes*

206. A 46-year-old man with no pertinent medical history presents to his primary care physician with scleral icterus, gynecomastia, and sparse pubic hair; he also reports increased bleeding upon brushing his teeth and blowing his nose. Laboratory studies reveal an AST 320, ALT 160, and increased PT; other lab values within range. On biopsy, 2-mm liver papules are appreciated. He denies any drug use or recent changes in his lifestyle. The patient should be questioned about which of the following topics to assist with formulating the diagnosis?

A. Alcohol history

B. Psychiatric/hormonal issues

C. Recent trauma

D. Sexual history

207. A 1-week-old infant remains in the intensive care unit because of cyanosis and failure to thrive. The infant has paroxysms of tachypnea, which occur concomitantly with the cyanosis. What is the most appropriate explanation for these findings?

A. Aortic stenosis

B. Atrial septal defect

C. Patent ductus arteriosus

D. Situs inversus

E. Tetralogy of Fallot

F. Ventricular septal defect

208. A 25-year-old man presents to his primary care physician complaining of difficulty with an exercise regimen. He is able to run on a treadmill for no more than 5 min (at a pace of 4 mi/hr) without developing severe calf pain. Deficiency of which enzyme will lead to this situation?

A. Alpha 1,6 glucosidase

B. Glucose-6-phosphatase

C. Glycogen phosphorylase

D. Lysosomal alpha 1,4 glucosidase

E. Pyruvate dehydrogenase

209. A 32-year-old woman in her thirty-second week of pregnancy develops an acutely painful calf while resting in bed awaiting the birth of her child. She has not been active in the last few days and has been out of bed only once in the last 3 days. She has a prior 10-pack-year history of smoking; however, she quit smoking when she became pregnant. Physical examination reveals a tender left calf and a positive Homans' sign. Which of the following can be a safe and effective agent to prescribe to this woman in the next few hours to prevent the occurrence of deep venous thromboses?

A. Aspirin

B. Garlic

C. Heparin

D. Urokinase

E. Warfarin

210. A 58-year-old African American man complains of pain in his eyes and cannot go outside without sunglasses. He also has lower back pain, which wakes him up in the middle of the night. Whenever he sits for long periods, his pain gets worse. However, on walking a bit, the pain subsides significantly. Which test for this patient might have a positive result?

A. anti-dsDNA

B. antinuclear antibodies

C. anti-Scl-70

D. HLA-B27

E. Tensilon test

211. A 45-year-old woman with a history of Crohn's disease presents to the emergency department after several days of nausea and diarrhea. Physical examination reveals an elevated blood pressure, orthostatic hypertension, tachycardia, delayed capillary refill, and poor skin turgor. Serum blood urea nitrogen and creatinine are both elevated. Which of the following urinary laboratory values would most likely correlate with the patient's acute renal failure?

A. Blood urea nitrogen/creatinine ratio < 15

B. Urinary fractional excretion of sodium < 1%

C. Urinary fractional excretion of sodium > 2%

D. Urinary osmolality < 350

E. Urinary sodium > 20

212. A 32-year-old sexually active woman presents to her family physician complaining of a painful sore on her vulva. Examination reveals a 1 cm round, shallow, nonelevated ulceration on the inner surface of the left labia majora. If biopsied, which of the following characteristics would you expect the cells of the lesion to exhibit?

A. Antoni B inclusions

B. Cowdry type A inclusions

C. Koilocytosis

D. Negri bodies

E. Owl's-eye inclusions

213. A 22-year-old woman who delivered a healthy child 2 weeks earlier is now experiencing feelings of hopelessness and helplessness. She also complains that she feels no joy in activities that used to make her happy. Her general appearance is unkept, suggesting poor hygiene. Her hair is unbrushed; her clothes are wrinkled and stained. What is the most likely explanation for these findings?

A. Brief psychotic disorder

B. Major depressive episode

C. Postpartum blues

D. Postpartum psychosis

E. Pregnancy-induced bipolar disorder

214. A 37-year-old man is brought to the emergency department after having been found unconscious at his home. After waking up in the emergency department, he reveals that he has been chronically dependent on alcohol for 17 years. He says he normally drinks a pint of whiskey every day. After 3 days in the hospital, the patient's heart rate and blood pressure increase quickly. He seems very confused and tells you the electric cord on the floor is a snake. A CT scan is performed (Figure 21). Which of the following drugs should the patient be given immediately?

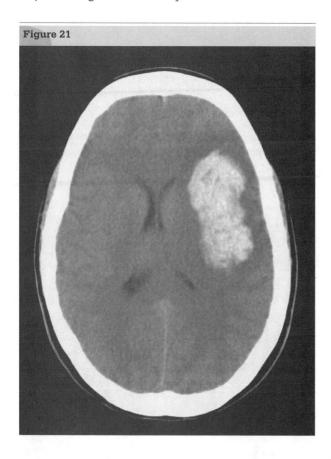

Figure 21

A. Clozapine

B. Diazepam

C. Lithium

D. Meperidine

E. Thiopental

215. A 55-year-old woman presents to her primary care physician saying her heart seems to be racing a lot, she has lost weight despite eating well, and lately tends to feel unusually nervous. Physical examination reveals a heart rate of 115 bpm. Her skin is warm. Bilateral proptosis is noted. Radioactive uptake is uniformly increased throughout the thyroid gland. In this condition, B- and T-cell mediated autoimmunity are known to be directed primarily against which protein?

A. Sodium-iodide importer

B. Thyroglobulin

C. Thyroperoxidase

D. Thyroid-stimulating hormone receptor

E. Vanillylmandelic acid importer

216. The medical intensive care unit at a local hospital has five beds, all of which are filled with critically ill patients. All patients will require nutritional support to prevent metabolic consequences of their respective diseases. Which of the following patients have the highest increase in energy expenditure above the basal rate because of their illness?

A. A 19-year-old man with a subdural hematoma following blunt head injury

B. A 44-year-old man who underwent right hemicolectomy

C. A 56-year-old man who has a fractured right femur

D. A 60-year-old woman who suffered blunt trauma to the abdomen in a motor vehicle accident

E. A 71-year-old man with pneumococcal pneumonia and bilateral subphrenic abscesses

217. A 45-year-old man who has a history of recurrent gastric ulcers presents to his primary care physician reporting that he has been vomiting up bright red blood and is unable to sweat. His doctor decides to do an upper gastrointestinal series as well as a CT scan. Results of the CT show a solid tumor in the apex of the left lung. Which of the following is the most likely consequence of this tumor?

A. Cushing's syndrome

B. Horner's syndrome

C. Paraneoplastic syndrome

D. Pleural effusion

E. Superior vena cava syndrome

218. A 55-year-old woman presents to her primary care physician with uncontrollable asterixis of the hands and progressive dementia. She also has circumferential deposits in the subcutaneous tissues around her eyes. What is the most appropriate treatment for this patient?

A. Azithromycin

B. Ciprofloxacin

C. Epinephrine

D. Penicillamine

E. Tetracycline

219. A 53-year-old man has been complaining of dysuria and frequency along with tenderness of the glans penis. He makes an appointment to see his primary care physician. On exam, testes are found to be descended bilaterally without masses. The penis is uncircumcised; on retraction of the foreskin, the physician notices an erythematous plaque on the glans. What is the most likely diagnosis?

A. Bowen's disease

B. Bowenoid papulosis

C. Condyloma acuminatum

D. Erythroplasia of Queyrat

E. Syphilitic chancre

220. A 7-year-old girl is brought to her pediatrician with a 6-month history of intermittent wheezing, especially at night. Physical examination of the heart is within normal limits. Pulmonary auscultation confirms wheezes in both lung fields. She also has decreased breath sounds at both lung bases. Abdominal examination reveals evidence of a healed right inguinal hernia. A methacholine challenge test proves positive for asthma. She is begun on a treatment regimen with inhaled corticosteroids. What is the mechanism of action for this medication?

A. Blocks acetylcholine signaling in bronchial airways

B. Helps to relax bronchial smooth muscle by activating beta$_2$ receptors

C. Inactivates NF-kB and thus the production of TNF-alpha

D. Inhibits phosphodiesterase, thus decreasing cAMP hydrolysis

E. Prevents release of mediators from mast cells

221. A 39-year-old man with metastatic renal carcinoma opts for a protocol of immunotherapy. He is to receive combination immunotherapy with external beam radiation over a 6-month period. The immunotherapeutic agents given will include interleukin-1, interleukin-2 and interleukin-6. Which of the following describes the potential of interleukin-2 as the key agent in this therapeutic trial?

A. Ability to cause proteolysis

B. Ability to serve as an endogenous pyrogen

C. Ability to serve as an immunostimulant

D. Ability to stimulate the hypothalamus

E. Ability to synthesize hepatic acute-phase proteins

222. A 33-year-old woman presents to her family physician after suffering her third consecutive miscarriage in 6 years. Her past medical history is significant for a deep venous thrombosis at the age of 26. She has no prior history of smoking or use of oral contraceptives and is not currently on any medications. Physical examination reveals no abnormalities. She does have some erythema of both cheeks. Laboratory studies are normal except for a prolonged PTT. What is the likely cause of this woman's miscarriages?

A. Abruptio placentae

B. Antiphospholipid-antibody syndrome

C. Factitious use of heparin or enoxaparin

D. Placenta accreta

E. Placenta percreta

223. A 36-year-old man with type IV Ehlers-Danlos syndrome presents to his primary care physician for a follow-up examination. He has no complaints. Physical examination of the heart, lungs, and abdomen is noncontributory. Which of the following is a likely complication of this disease?

A. Bilateral ocular lens dislocations

B. Multiple herniated disks in the lumbar spine

C. Multiple bone fractures found on x-ray

D. A holosystolic heart murmur with a midsystolic click

E. Rupture of the small intestine after eating a meal

224. An 18-year-old girl presents to her primary care physician for a sports physical. Physical examination reveals a continuous systolic murmur, but her doctor is unsure of the cause. He asks the patient to stand next to the examining table and valsalva while he listens to her heart, then he asks her to relax and squat down while he listens. The following observations are made: while the patient is standing, the intensity of the murmur decreases, but while she is squatting, the intensity of the murmur increases. What is the cause of this murmur?

A. Aortic stenosis

B. Hypertrophic cardiomyopathy

C. Innocent murmur

D. Mitral valve prolapse

E. Mitral stenosis

225. A 65-year-old shipbuilder presents to his primary care physician with difficulty breathing. A chest x-ray is obtained and is shown in Figure 22. Spirometry reveals reduced expansion of the lungs and reduced total lung capacity. Microscopic examination of sputum reveals rod-shaped objects with clubbed ends that stain positively with Prussian blue. This man has most likely developed which of the following as a result of his occupational history?

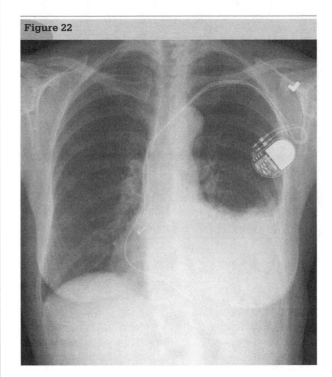

Figure 22

A. Bronchogenic carcinoma

B. Malignant mesothelioma

C. Progressive massive fibrosis

D. Squamous cell carcinoma of the larynx

E. Tuberculosis

226. An 18-month-old infant is brought to the pediatrician after her mother noticed a mass protruding from her vagina. The remainder of the physical examination (heart, lungs, and abdomen) is within normal limits. Pelvic examination of the external genitalia confirms the above finding. A biopsy of the mass is taken. The pathology reveals desmin within the tumor's stroma. What is the most likely diagnosis?

A. Adenomatoid tumor

B. Dermoid cyst

C. Dysgerminoma

D. Gestational choriocarcinoma

E. Leiomyoma

F. Rhabdomyosarcoma

227. The epithelium of the choroid plexus creates the blood-brain barrier. This is the barrier between the cerebral capillary blood and the cerebrospinal fluid. Which of the following substances is most likely to be excluded from passage through this barrier?

A. Carbon dioxide

B. Cholesterol

C. Glucose

D. Lipid-soluble drugs

E. Oxygen

228. The patient, a G1P0 at 14 weeks' gestation, begins experiencing abnormal uterine bleeding as well as the passage of a watery fluid and small, grapelike masses from her vagina. Physical examination shows that fetal heart tones are not heard with the Doppler. What finding would confirm the diagnosis of partial mole rather then complete mole?

A. Elevated serum human chorionic gonadotrophin

B. Fetal parts

C. One year later, the woman is diagnosed with chorio-carcinoma

D. Trophoblast proliferation

E. Villous edema

229. A 65-year-old man presents to his primary care physician complaining of having had a cough and shortness of breath for 2 days. He has worked with air conditioners for 30 years. A sputum culture is obtained and stained with silver stain. Gram's stain reveals Gram-negative rods. What is the most likely causative agent?

A. *Haemophilus influenzae*

B. *Legionella pneumophila*

C. *Mycoplasma pneumoniae*

D. *Staphylococcus aureus*

E. *Streptococcus pneumoniae*

230. A 43-year-old man presents to his primary care physician with the following triad: micronodular pigment cirrhosis, diabetes, and changes in skin color/pigmentation. He also complains of difficulty catching his breath when climbing stairs and has noticed increased swelling in his ankles at the end of the day. What is the most likely diagnosis?

A. Alcoholic hepatitis

B. Budd-Chiari syndrome

C. Congestive heart failure

D. Hemochromatosis

E. Tuberculosis

231. A 26-year-old Caucasian man has had a painless enlargement of his right testis for 2 months. He had a cryptorchid right testis as an infant, which was corrected surgically. A scrotal ultrasound confirms the presence of a right intra-testicular mass. What is the most likely diagnosis?

A. Choriocarcinoma

B. Embryonal carcinoma

C. Endodermal yolk-sac tumor

D. Seminoma

E. Teratoma

F. Leydig cell tumor

232. A 34-year-old man who is trapped in a burning building calmly explains to the other people trapped with him how the fire will spread through the building and the mechanics of the conflagration. What is the defense mechanism utilized by this individual?

A. Humor

B. Identification

C. Intellectualization

D. Isolation of affect

E. Projection

233. A 9-year-old girl is brought to her primary care physician because of a history of inattentiveness at school. During your examination, you witness what appears to be a staring spell, which prompts you to order an EEG. This shows a 3-Hz spike-and-wave pattern. You begin treatment with an antiepileptic drug. Some 2 weeks later, this patient presents to the emergency department with a rash of sudden onset (red lesions that include papules, vesicles, bullae, and targets) with an accompanying fever, malaise, and mucosal erosion. What is the most appropriate treatment for this patient?

A. Carbamazepine

B. Diazepam

C. Ethosuximide

D. Lamotrigine

E. Phenytoin

F. Topiramate

G. Valproate

234. An 8-year-old boy is brought to the pediatrician by his parents. They are concerned by his recent growth spurt. The pediatrician notices that he is above the ninety-ninth percentile on the growth curve for height and weight, whereas he had always been in the sixtieth to seventieth percentiles. Physical exam reveals a Tanner Stage 1 male. The best initial test to determine the etiology of his condition would be which of the following?

A. Have his parents keep a log of everything the boy eats in a 2-week time period

B. Measure serum ACTH levels

C. Measure fasting serum glucose levels

D. Measure serum levels of growth hormone (GH)

E. Measure serum levels of insulin-like growth factor (IFG-1)

235. An embryo is exposed to a particular teratogen during development. This teratogen will affect only organs that participate in hematopoiesis. If any and all hematopoietic organs are susceptible to the effects of this teratogen at any time during the embryo's development, which will be the very first organ affected?

   A. Bone marrow

   B. Liver

   C. Spleen

   D. Thymus

   E. Yolk sac

236. A 9-year-old girl presents to her primary care physician with multiple pigmented macules on the vermilion borders of her upper and lower lips. The lesions are 2 mm in diameter and appear clustered. The patient has also recently complained of abdominal pain. Sigmoidoscopy reveals multiple pedunculated polyps in the sigmoid colon. What is the most likely diagnosis?

   A. Familial adenosis polyposis

   B. Gardner's syndrome

   C. Hereditary nonpolyposis colorectal cancer

   D. Peutz-Jeghers syndrome

   E. Turcot's syndrome

237. An 18-year-old basketball player is brought to the emergency department because of a knee injury. He claims that he feels no pain but that he heard a popping sound when his body twisted in a different direction than his feet. Physical examination reveals that his right knee is filled with fluid. The physician bends the patient's right knee about 30 degrees, stabilizes the femur, places one hand behind the proximal tibia, and pulls forward. Approximately 1 cm of translation is found on the right knee, whereas there is no translation on the left. What ligament was most likely damaged?

   A. Anterior cruciate ligament

   B. Lateral collateral ligament

   C. Medial collateral ligament

   D. Posterior cruciate ligament

   E. Talar ligament

238. A 27-year-old woman is brought to the emergency department after a motor vehicle accident. She has a suspected high-impact skull fracture and is experiencing lucid intervals. A CT of the head is obtained and is shown in Figure 23. What is the associated blood supply that is suspected of sustaining the laceration?

   A. Bridging vein

   B. Circle of Willis

   C. Middle cerebral artery

   D. Middle meningeal artery

   E. Superior cerebral vein

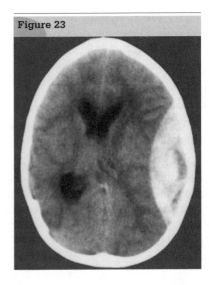

Figure 23

239. A 4-week-old infant is brought to the emergency department because of difficulty breathing, feeding, and failure to gain weight. Physical examination reveals tachypnea, a weak femoral pulse, and a 35 mm Hg difference in systolic pressure between the upper and lower limbs. What is the most likely diagnosis?

   A. Aortic regurgitation

   B. Aortic stenosis

   C. Coarctation of the aorta

   D. Hypovolemia

   E. Left-sided heart failure

240. A 31-year-old woman is 11 weeks pregnant by dates. She denies any prior medical or surgical history. Doppler ultrasound reveals evidence of fetal heart tones. Abdominal examination reveals normoactive bowel sounds with a nonpalpable fundus. Which of the following pelvic types is most favorable for a vaginal delivery of her newborn?

   A. Android

   B. Anthropoid

   C. Gynecoid

   D. Platypelloid

   E. Polypoid

241. A 35-year-old man presents to his primary care physician with bilateral breast enlargement and nipple soreness over the past few months. Physical examination confirms the presence of gynecomastia. Cardiac examination reveals no evidence of rubs, murmurs, or gallops. Pulmonary and abdominal examinations are noncontributory. A scrotal ultrasound reveals a left testicular mass. Which of the following histological characteristics would most likely be associated with this testicular mass?

   A. Auer rods

   B. Birbeck granules

   C. Call Exner bodies

   D. Charcot-Leyden crystals

   E. Mallory bodies

   F. Reinke crystals

242. A single mother is trying to teach her 6-year-old son to pick up his clothes and clean his room. His mom makes sure to thank and praise him immediately each time he shows the behavior she is trying to enforce. Which of the following methods of operant conditioning is being utilized in this situation?

A. Extinction

B. Negative reinforcement

C. Positive reinforcement

D. Punishment

E. Stalling

243. While working in a small community hospital, a physician notices a 6-year-old child who appears distinctly bow-legged. The child also complains of muscular weakness. In an adult, this child's disorder would be called which of the following?

A. Osteogenesis imperfecta

B. Osteomalacia

C. Osteomyelitis

D. Osteoporosis

E. Rickets

244. A 2-year-old girl is brought to the emergency department with a suspicious lesion on her forearm; it is diagnosed as an abscess. The mother notes that this is the tenth time they have had to come into the emergency room for the same reason. Culture of the skin abscess reveals *Staphylococcus aureus*. The doctor then orders a nitrozolium blue test, which turns out to be negative. The enzyme missing from this child's leukocytes is:

A. Glucose-6-phosphate dehydrogenase (G6PD)

B. Hexokinase

C. Myeloperoxidase

D. NADPH oxidase

E. Pyruvate kinase

245. A 28-year-old woman presents to her primary care physician with a 2-month history of increasing weakness, especially in getting up from a chair, climbing stairs, and combing her hair. She also has a rash above her eyelids, which is lilac in color. A picture of her eyelid is shown in Figure 24. She is given the tentative diagnosis of dermatomyositis. Which of the following tests would provide a definite diagnosis?

A. Antinuclear antibodies

B. CT of the abdomen

C. Muscle biopsy

D. Rheumatoid factor

E. Skin biopsy of rash lesion

246. A 55-year-old postmenopausal woman has been feeling depressed for 3 weeks. She has finally elected to see a psychiatrist about her problem and hopes to get started on a medication. Her doctor examines her and tells her about the possibilities of medication. The one she decides to prescribe has as its major side effect a decrease in sexual function. What neurotransmitter is most likely involved?

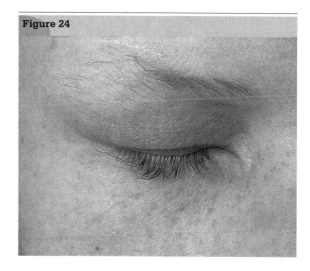
Figure 24

A. Glycine

B. Histamine

C. Serotonin

D. Tyrosine

247. A 56-year-old alcoholic with severe liver disease presents to his physician with what he refers to as strange-looking skin marks on his chest. Physical examination reveals several pulsatile erythematous lesions that blanch when light pressure is applied. Which of the following hormones is linked with this condition?

A. Cortisol

B. Estrogen

C. Growth hormone

D. Progesterone

E. Testosterone

248. A 28-year-old man who was recently diagnosed with asthma is brought to his primary care physician for evaluation. He has been experiencing increasingly worse dyspnea and cough. His medications include albuterol as well as aspirin for his history of coronary artery disease. He is placed on zafirlukast and an inhaled corticosteroid. He is also advised to stop taking aspirin. The most likely effect of this new regimen will be to:

A. Antagonize LTD_4 receptors

B. Inhibit 5-lipoxygenase

C. Inhibit phosphodiesterase

D. Inhibit phospholipase A_2

E. Stimulate beta$_2$ receptors

249. A 10-month-old infant is brought to the emergency department with severe jaundice. Testing shows deficiency in UDP-glucuronyl transferase and high levels of unconjugated bilirubin. What is the most likely explanation for these findings?

A. Crigler-Najjar syndrome

B. Dubin-Johnson syndrome

C. Gilbert's syndrome

D. Reye's syndrome

E. Rotor syndrome

250. An 84-year-old nursing home resident was bathed 3 days earlier by a newly hired licensed practical nurse. After retracting his foreskin to clean the glans penis, she neglected to replace it in its original position. Since then he has been complaining of extreme pain in his penis and urinary retention. What is the most likely explanation for these findings?

A. Balanoposthitis

B. Epispadias

C. Hypospadias

D. Paraphimosis

E. Phimosis

Block 6

251. A 33-year-old man presents to the emergency department complaining of visual changes. When the eye exam is performed, it is noted that the right eye has normal motor function, but the left one continues to look in an inferior and lateral direction. Damage to which cranial nerve is responsible for the appearance of the left eye?

A. Cranial nerve I

B. Cranial nerve II

C. Cranial nerve III

D. Cranial nerve IV

E. Cranial nerve VI

252. A new patient presents to a primary care physician looking for a second opinion based on some news he has just gotten. He is a 42-year-old recent immigrant from Greece. Looking over the lab and film reports he is carrying, you note the following: marked anemia, splenomegaly, increased hemoglobin F, and a generalized hemosiderosis. Physical examination reveals facial, skull, and long bone distortion. What is the most likely explanation for these findings?

A. Alpha thalassemia

B. Cooley's anemia

C. Hemoglobin E disorder

D. Pyruvate kinase deficiency (PKD)

E. Sickle cell anemia

253. A patient comes to his primary care physician complaining of a deficit in sensory perception. On examination, the deficit appears to be that of vibration and tapping. Which of the following types of mechanoreceptors are the most likely to be involved?

A. Meissner's corpuscle

B. Merkel's disk

C. Pacinian corpuscle

D. Ruffini's corpuscle

E. Sensory homunculus

254. A 45-year-old woman presents to her primary care physician complaining of unilateral headache, which she has had for 3 days. She states that the pain has become unbearable. She also states that she has episodes where she suddenly loses vision in both eyes and that her jaw hurts towards the end of a meal. Her erythrocyte sedimentation rate is 40 mm/hr. What is the most likely diagnosis?

A. Churg-Strauss syndrome

B. Giant cell arteritis

C. Lymphomatoid granulomatosis

D. Raynaud's disease

E. Thromboangiitis obliterans

255. A 14-year-old girl is having episodes of hemoptysis and lower abdominal pain. Physical examination reveals decreased breath sounds at both lung bases with scattered wheezes bilaterally. Abdominal examination is unremarkable. She is diagnosed with histiocytosis X. What is the most likely finding on skin biopsy?

A. Auer rods

B. Birbeck granules

C. Ferruginous bodies

D. Noncaseating granulomas

E. Giant cell inclusions

256. A 20-year-old Caucasian man presents to his primary care physician with complaints of low back pain, which began the previous day shortly after he lifted some kegs of beer at his place of work. He rates his pain as a 7 to 8 out of 10. It is a constant, sharp pain that does not radiate and keeps him awake at night. Generally, certain movements make it worse and ibuprofen gives some relief for short periods. He has never experienced such pain before and is unable to work because of it. He denied any costovertebral angle (CVA) tenderness, dysuria, or hematuria. He is concerned about the pain because it is preventing him from working. He wants to know what his treatment options are. Physical examination of the heart, lungs, and abdomen is within normal limits. His musculoskeletal exam reveals limited range of motion of the lumbar area and obvious muscle spasm with palpation of the left lower lumbar area. Straight leg raise is negative bilaterally. What would be the most effective first-line treatment for this patient?

A. He is malingering and needs to be referred to psychiatry.

B. No course of treatment is necessary at this time.

C. Opioids should be prescribed for persistent pain.

D. The patient needs an immediate surgery consult to have his herniated disc repaired.

E. The patient should be treated conservatively with a short period of rest, muscle relaxants, and analgesics and told that his symptoms should resolve in the near future.

257. A 71-year-old woman complains of a headache and pain in her jaw, especially when she tries to eat; she also has visual impairment. Physical examination reveals tenderness and nodules on the left side of face near her eye. Cardiac, pulmonary, and abdominal examination is within normal limits. There are good bowel sounds in all four quadrants. There is no evidence of guarding or rebound tenderness. The erythrocyte sedimentation rate (ESR) is 29 mm/hr. What is the most appropriate treatment for this patient?

A. Allopurinol

B. Heparin

C. High-dose corticosteroids

D. Monitor only at this time

E. Urokinase

258. Which of the following enzymes converts trypsinogen to trypsin?

A. Chymotrypsin

B. Enterokinase

C. Pepsin

D. Sucrase

259. A 16-year-old boy is brought to the pediatrician with a 1-month history of right knee pain and a 10-lb weight loss. He is very active and participates in many different sports, but has been unable to do so since his pain began. Both he and his mother deny any history of trauma or injury. On physical examination, he appears pale and is afebrile. All other exam components are within normal limits except for the musculoskeletal exam, which reveals localized pain with palpation of the distal femur. He is sent for x-rays, which are shown in Figure 25. What is the most likely diagnosis?

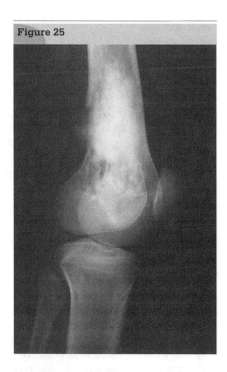

Figure 25

A. Ewing's sarcoma

B. Osteochondroma

C. Osteomyelitis

D. Osteosarcoma

E. Paget's disease

260. A 5-year-old boy presents to the family medicine clinic with an enlarged scrotal sac that, on transillumination, appears clear and translucent. What is the most likely diagnosis?

A. Hematocele

B. Hydrocele

C. Inguinal hernia

D. Spermatocele

E. Undescended testicle

261. A 21-year-old heterosexual man presents to his primary care physician because of decreased libido and erectile dysfunction. Further history reveals that he is embarrassed to take his shirt off in front of his friends because he has no chest hair and his breasts are slightly enlarged. Physical examination reveals bilateral gynecomastia, sparse body hair, and small, firm testicles. Cardiac examination reveals no evidence of rubs, murmurs, or gallops. Pulmonary auscultation reveals no wheezes or rhonchi. Abdominal examination reveals no evidence of hepatosplenomegaly. What is the most likely diagnosis?

A. Female pseudohermaphroditism

B. Fragile X syndrome

C. Klinefelter's syndrome

D. Male pseudohermaphroditism

E. Turner's syndrome

262. After being discharged from the emergency department several days earlier, a 45-year-old man returns with severe, watery diarrhea. He states that he has been taking antibiotics for the past 10 days to treat an intraabdominal infection. Flexible sigmoidoscopy reveals yellow plaques covering the colonic mucosa. What is the most likely diagnosis?

A. *Clostridium difficile*

B. *Clostridium perfringens*

C. *Corynebacterium diphtheriae*

D. *Helicobacter pylori*

E. *Shigella dysenteriae*

263. A 28-year-old woman presents to her physician for an infertility workup. She and her husband have been having unprotected intercourse for the past 2 years without being able to conceive. She reports irregular menstrual periods that are occurring less frequently over time. She has noted hot flashes and vaginal dryness as well. Physical and pelvic examinations reveal no abnormalities. Blood tests show normal luteinizing hormone (LH), normal dehydroepiandrosterone-sulfate (DHEAS), normal testosterone, normal prolactin, and markedly increased follicle-stimulating hormone (FSH). Urine β-hCG is negative. What is the most likely diagnosis?

A. Adrenal hyperplasia

B. Endometriosis

C. Ovarian failure

D. Polycystic ovary syndrome

E. Pseudocyesis

264. A 9-year-old girl's parents present to the pediatrician to discuss the IQ results they received from their child's school. They explain that their child received a score of 67 on her standardized IQ exam and are concerned about the meaning of this number. You explain that a score of 67 is equated with the following classification of mental retardation:

A. Mild   50 -70

B. Moderate   35 - 55

C. Severe   20 - 40

D. Profound   < 20

E. Unclassified

265. A 71-year-old man with progressive dyspnea and hemoptysis undergoes a bronchoscopy and lung biopsy. Specimen from the biopsy is sent for pathologic analysis. What is seen in Figure 26?

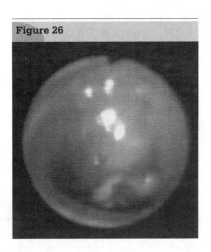

Figure 26

A. Alveoli

B. Bronchi

C. Bronchioles

D. Larynx

E. Trachea

266. A 62-year-old man with a history of myocardial infarction presents to the emergency department with a sudden onset of a severe retroorbital headache and nausea. He reports increased fatigue and decreased libido, which he attributes to normal aging. His blood pressure is 122/80 sitting and 98/50 standing, while his heart rate increases from 72 sitting to 94 bpm standing. His skin is pale and axillary pubic hair sparse. Bitemporal hemianopsia is noted on visual field testing. MRI shows a 1.9-cm suprasellar mass, compression of the optic chiasm, and bilateral invasion of the cavernous sinuses. After the administration of contrast, evidence of a large area of hemorrhage within the mass becomes evident. What is the most likely diagnosis?

A. Carotid artery embolism

B. Epidural hemorrhage

C. Pituitary apoplexy

D. Sheehan's syndrome

E. Subdural hemorrhage

267. A 73-year-old man with diabetes mellitus and hypertension presents to his primary care physician complaining of a painful right foot, which he has had for 1 week. Physical examination of the right foot reveals several toes with painful black-and-blue areas. Sensation is diminished as compared with the contralateral foot. What is the most likely explanation for these findings?

A. Digital arteries are embolized

B. Digital arteries are thrombosed

C. Femoral vein thrombosis

D. Inferior vena cava thrombosis

E. Thrombophlebitis of the lower extremity veins

268. A 47-year-old woman with herpes simplex type 1 (HSV-1) presents to her primary care physician for a follow-up examination. She also has a history of diabetes mellitus, hypertension, hypothyroidism, and endometriosis. HSV-1 can remain latent in which of the following areas?

A. Dorsal root ganglia

B. Mesenteric ganglion

C. Sacral nerve ganglia

D. Thoracic root ganglion

E. Trigeminal root ganglion

269. A 38-year-old Caucasian man comes to the ambulatory care clinic for follow-up of a lesion on his hand. A dysplastic nevus was suspected on his last visit. Since then, the lesion has changed color, changed in contour, increased in depth, increased in diameter, and is not filled with fluid. Which of these findings correlates with risk of metastasis?

A. Change in color

B. Change in contour

C. Increase in depth

D. Increase in diameter

E. Not being fluid filled

270. A 62-year-old woman presents to her primary care physician for a routine yearly physical examination. She has no particular concerns but then mentions that she recently went to her ophthalmologist and was told that she had presbyopia. Being nervous, she failed to ask what her condition indicated and does not understand. You proceed to tell her that presbyopia is corrected with:

A. Biconcave lenses

B. Convex lenses

C. Cylindrical lenses

D. Daily eye drops

E. Laser surgery

271. A 28-year-old woman presents to her primary care physician with a reddish area over her nasal bridge and cheeks. She also complains of muscle aches and joint pains. Physical examination of the heart reveals a regular rate and rhythm. Pulmonary auscultation reveals no evidence of wheeze, rales, or rhonchi. Abdominal examination reveals no evidence of guarding or rebound tenderness. Antihistone antibodies are positive. Which of the following is a major side effect of a drug that is known to elicit this reaction?

A. Cinchonism

B. Disulfiram-like reaction

C. Nephrogenic diabetes insipidus

D. Pellagra

E. Reddish discoloration of tissues

272. A 69-year-old man presents to his primary care physician because of progressive dysphagia. He was diagnosed many years ago with a heart valve abnormality. He is not aware of his diagnosis and the only information he can provide is that he has a heart murmur. He has not seen his primary care physician a checkup for more than 5 years. Physical examination reveals a delayed, rumbling, late-diastolic murmur. The patient's ECG is shown in Figure 27. What underlying heart defect is causing his dysphagia?

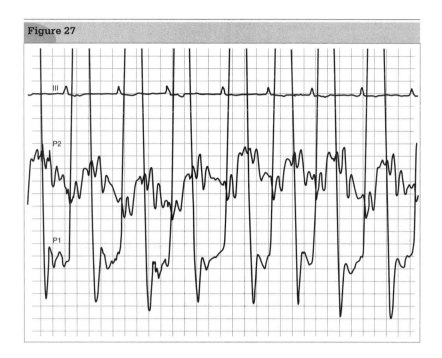

Figure 27

A. Aortic stenosis

B. Mitral regurgitation

C. Mitral stenosis

D. Tricuspid stenosis

E. Ventral septal defect

273. The roommate of a 22-year-old college senior came home and found her friend unconscious on the floor. She was unable to arouse the girl and was unsure of how long she had been unresponsive. After minor investigation, she discovered an empty, unlabeled bottle lying near her. Which of the following substances would most likely be responsible for this woman's overdose?

A. Amphetamines

B. Barbiturates

C. Benzodiazepines

D. Marijuana

E. Opioids

274. A 45-year-old man presented to the emergency department with severe right-sided lower-quadrant abdominal pain. The presumptive diagnosis was acute appendicitis and he was sent directly to the operating room. Prior to intubation, he was given atropine and an intravenous bolus of succinylcholine. He then underwent induction of general anesthesia with pancuronium. During the operation he develops a temperature to 39°C (102.2°F) and muscular rigidity is noted. What is the most appropriate treatment for this patient?

A. Atropine

B. Dantrolene

C. Dopamine

D. Epinephrine

E. Neostigmine

F. Nicotine

G. Norepinephrine

H. Pyridostigmine

I. Rocuronium

J. Scopolamine

275. A 63-year-old man collapses and dies in a shopping mall. An autopsy is performed and reveals hyaline thickening of the small arteries of the kidney and spleen. What is the most likely explanation of these findings?

A. Arteriosclerosis

B. Arteriolosclerosis

C. Potential myocardial infarction

D. Pulmonary emboli

E. Swiss-type agammaglobulinemia

276. A 65-year-old woman presents to the ambulatory care clinic complaining of morning stiffness, which she says improves after a few hours of walking around and doing work. She states that the stiffness is equal on both sides of her body and mainly affects her wrists, ankles, and feet. Physical examination reveals prominent nodules in her metacarpophalangeal and proximal interphalangeal joints. Her hands appear to have an ulnar deviation. Which of the following findings is likely to be present in this patient?

A. Abnormal D-xylose test

B. Heberden's nodes

C. Noncaseating granulomas

D. Pannus eroding cartilage

E. Rhomboid crystals in the joint spaces

277. A 68-year-old man presents to his primary care physician complaining of progressive dyspnea on exertion. His breathing is shallow and rapid and he purses his lips to control his breaths. His chest appears barrel-shaped. He has a 75-pack-year history of cigarette smoking. Physical examination of the lungs reveals decreased fremitus, hyperresonance on percussion, and decreased breath sounds. Which of the following is responsible for his pursed lips?

A. Decreased functional residual capacity (FRC)

B. Decreased intrapleural pressure

C. Decreased lung compliance

D. Increased airway resistance

E. Increased lung compliance

278. The main purpose of the HMP (hexose monophosphate shunt) is which of the following?

A. Breakdown of glycogen to glucose under hormonal control

B. Oxidation of acetyl-CoA to CO_2 and transfer of electrons to NAD^+ and FAD

C. Oxidation of NADH and $FADH_2$ to form three and two molecules of ATP respectively

D. Production of NADPH and/or ribose from glucose

E. Reduction of ADH

279. A 59-year-old man with diabetes mellitus, hypertension, and angina presents to the emergency department complaining of crushing chest pain that radiates to his left arm. His current medications include an oral hypoglycemic, a calcium channel blocker, and sublingual nitroglycerine. Cardiac auscultation reveals a loud murmur with a palpable thrill. To what grade would this murmur be assigned?

1-3) No thrill

A. Grade 2   *No thrill, heard c stetch*

B. Grade 3   *" " , moderately loud murmur.*

4-6, thrill

C. Grade 4   *Loud murmur + thrill heard c steth.*

D. Grade 5 ↑↑   *" " + " " " " " partly off chest*

E. Grade 6 ↑↑↑   *" " + " heard c out steth.*

280. A 53-year-old man with diabetic ketoacidosis presents to the emergency department with progressive dyspnea. Arterial blood gas measurement is ordered. Which of the following arterial blood gas changes would most likely be representative of a patient in uncompensated diabetic ketoacidosis?

A. Decreased pH, decreased P_{CO_2}, decreased HCO_3

B. Decreased pH, increased P_{CO_2}, increased HCO_3

C. Increased pH, decreased P_{CO_2}, decreased HCO_3

D. Increased pH, increased P_{CO_2}, increased HCO_3

E. Increased pH, increased P_{CO_2}, increased P_{O_2}

281. A 10-year-old girl whose mother was taking her to the emergency room because of vomiting, diarrhea, and cyanosis began to have tonic-clonic seizures and died on the way to the hospital. Her mother reported that 2 hr prior, she was fine. There was no evidence of trauma and no significant medical history other than a sore throat a few days earlier. An autopsy was done, which revealed enlarged, hemorrhagic adrenal glands. No cardiac or cerebral pathology was found. Which of the following most likely caused these findings?

A. Myocardial infarction

B. Cerebral vascular accident

C. Cytomegalovirus infection

D. *Neisseria meningitidis* infection

E. *Mycobacterium tuberculosis* infection

282. A 12-year-old girl presents to the pediatrician's office with her parents. They are concerned, as their daughter has been going through periods of sleeping excessively and having a ravenous appetite. The parents say that these cycles last about 7 to 21 days each and seem to subside on their own. What is the most likely diagnosis?

A. Circadian rhythm sleep disorder

B. Kleine-Levin syndrome

C. Nocturnal myoclonus

D. Restless legs syndrome

E. Sleep drunkenness

283. A 21-year-old man is brought to the emergency department after sustaining a gunshot wound to the abdomen. After initial evaluation, the patient is taken to the operating room for exploration. It is apparent that he has suffered a ruptured spleen as a result of his injury. The surgeon must ligate the blood supply to the spleen. At what structure does the splenic artery originate?

A. Abdominal aorta

B. Celiac trunk

C. Left gastroepiploic artery

D. Right gastric artery

E. Superior mesenteric artery

284. An 87-year-old man with coronary artery disease is currently on digoxin, furosemide, and captopril. He is unable to walk from his living room to his kitchen, approximately 25 ft, without getting short of breath. His ejection fraction is 35%, his heart rate is 88 bpm, and his blood pressure is 135/87 mm Hg. Physical examination reveals no evidence of ankle edema, minor crackles on pulmonary examination, and no audible bruit in the carotid arteries bilaterally. What is the next most appropriate treatment for this patient?

A. Add albuterol

B. Add beta-blocker

C. Add nitroglycerin

D. Add prazosin

E. Add spirolactone

285. A 27-year-old G1 is in her fortieth week of gestation. The fetus's weight has been estimated to be 4,400 g. Both the patient and her obstetrician would like to avoid a cesarean section, so the decision is made to induce labor. What is the most appropriate hypothalamic or pituitary hormone to be administered to this patient?

A. Adrenocorticotropic hormone

B. Gonadotropin-releasing hormone

C. Growth hormone

D. Growth hormone-inhibiting hormone

E. Human chorionic gonadotropin

F. Oxytocin

286. Autopsy of a 56-year-old obese male cadaver reveals concentric onionskin thickening of his arteriolar walls. Various deposits of fibrinoid material in his arterioles are noted, as well as areas of severe vascular necrosis and inflammation. In life, this patient was noted to have suffered from chronic malignant hypertension. What is the most likely diagnosis based on the above presentation?

  A. Hemangioendothelioma

  B. Hyaline arteriolosclerosis

  C. Hyperplastic arteriolosclerosis

  D. Hypersensitivity vasculitis

  E. Polyarteritis nodosa

287. A 2-year-old infant with a history of failure to thrive is seen in follow-up by his pediatrician. He has proteinuria of +7 g/day. Renal biopsy is performed. Based on the information given and the images in Figure 28, what is the most likely diagnosis?

  A. Alport's disease

  B. IgA nephropathy

  C. Membranous glomerulonephritis

  D. Minimal change disease

  E. Poststreptococcal glomerulonephritis

288. A 25-year-old college student notices a spotted rash on his groin and leg. He presents to the ambulatory care clinic for further evaluation. Physical examination reveals ataxia when walking, swollen joints, and decreased vibration and proprioception. Gram's stain of the rash is negative. What is the most likely causative agent?

  A. *Borrelia burgdorferi*

  B. Measles

  C. *Staphylococcus aureus*

  D. *Streptococcus pneumoniae*

  E. *Treponema pallidum*

289. A 56-year-old woman presents to her primary care physician for her annual checkup. Her only complaints are intermittent constipation, some recent fatigue, and occasional bone pain. She quit smoking 5 years earlier, tries to eat a healthy diet, and exercises three times a week. Her physical exam is normal. She is sent for routine labs, which reveal a serum calcium level of 11 mg/dL and serum phosphate of 1.3 mg/dL. Her 24-hr urine studies reveal hypercalciuria. What is the most likely diagnosis?

  A. Addison's disease

  B. Parathyroid adenoma

  C. Parathyroid carcinoma

  D. Tuberculosis

  E. Vitamin D intoxication

290. A parent brings her newborn infant to the pediatrician. She is worried about a recent outbreak of rotavirus and is very concerned about her child's health. You reassure her that her asymptomatic child will be fine. You base your information upon the knowledge that:

  A. Infants are not susceptible to rotavirus infection.

  B. Infants are immunized at birth against rotavirus.

  C. Rotavirus is virtually benign and "nothing to worry about."

  D. Secretory IgA to rotavirus is commonly present in colostrum of lactating mothers.

  E. Transmission occurs sexually.

291. An 82-year-old man presents to his primary care physician with dyspnea and swelling of the lower extremities. He has been ill for several years. Echocardiography is remarkable for left ventricular hypertrophy, pulmonary hypertension, and right ventricular hypertrophy. What is most likely the cause of his right ventricular hypertrophy?

  A. Dilated cardiomyopathy

  B. Left-sided heart failure

  C. Pulmonary hypertension

  D. Pulmonary valve stenosis

  E. Tricuspid disease

Figure 28

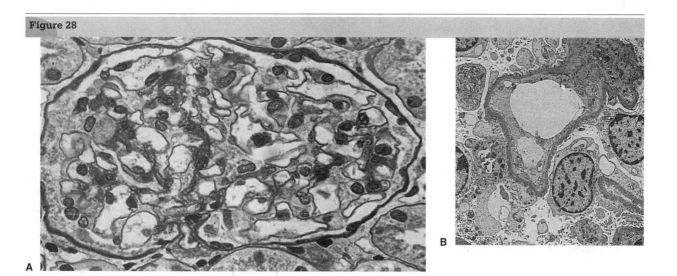

A

B

292. A 24-year-old woman who is a postpartum G1P1001 has been diagnosed by her delivering obstetrician with acute endometritis secondary to postpartum retention of placental fragments. Which of the following organisms is most commonly associated with this diagnosis?

  A. *Candida albicans*

  B. *Chlamydia trachomatis*

  C. *Gardnerella vaginalis*

  D. *Mycobacterium tuberculosis*

  E. *Staphylococcus aureus*

293. A 29-year-old man with a history of asthma presents to the emergency department complaining of severe dyspnea. Testing of his arterial blood gases (ABGs) reveals a pH of 7.32, a CO_2 level of 45, and a bicarbonate level of 29. Which of the following is most responsible for the patient's condition?

  A. Aspirin ingestion

  B. Hyperventilation

  C. Hypoventilation

  D. Renal failure

  E. Water intoxication

294. A 23-year-old woman is 20 weeks pregnant and presents to her primary care physician for treatment of knee pain. She wants something to relieve her pain but is worried about drug toxicity. Which of the following anti-inflammatory drugs could cause cardiovascular complications for the fetus?

  A. Acetaminophen

  B. Cortisone

  C. Hydrocortisone

  D. Indomethacin

  E. Prednisone

295. A newborn has a heart rate of 120 bpm, regular respirations, and some muscle tone. She grimaces in response to stimulation and her pallor is pink throughout. What is her Apgar score?

  A. 6

  B. 7

  C. 8

  D. 9

  E. 10

296. A 58-year-old man with a long history of obstructive voiding symptoms is currently taking finasteride and tamsulosin to control his symptoms. At last follow-up, his urinary flow rate had improved as well as his nocturia. His prostate gland has decreased in size by 20%, and his serum PSA is now 3.1 ng/mL. What is the mechanism of action by which finasteride can improve the patient's voiding symptoms?

  A. Blocks the production of weak adrenal androgens such as DHEA

  B. Competitively blocks androgen receptors in the prostate gland

  C. Inhibits 5-alpha reductase, preventing the conversion of testosterone to dihydrotesterone

  D. Inhibits LH and FSH when given in a continuous fashion by acting as a GN-RH agonist.

  E. Reduces the production of LH and FSH by negative feedback inhibition on the pituitary.

297. A 26-year-old sexually active woman presents to the emergency department with increasing pelvic pain, an increased hCG, and no apparent pregnancy on intravaginal ultrasound. Which fallopian tube abnormality is most commonly a direct cause of her diagnosis?

  A. Adenomatoid tumor

  B. Hematosalpinx

  C. Hydrosalpinx

  D. Pyosalpinx

  E. Tuboovarian abscess

298. A 68-year-old woman in the hospital's intensive care unit is found to have suffered a ruptured Charcot-Bouchard aneurysm. What is the most likely predisposing factor that led to her intracerebral hemorrhage?

  A. Diabetes

  B. Genetic predisposition

  C. Hypertension

  D. Tobacco use

  E. Work environment

299. A 45-year-old man is admitted to the hospital's psychiatric ward after coming to the emergency room with suicidal ideation. He gives a history of alcoholism since age 19. He states that he has been drinking a fifth of vodka and a six-pack of beer daily for 2 months. He has received three citations for driving under the influence (DUI) in the past 15 years and had his license suspended twice. He has lost several jobs and been divorced twice because of his alcohol dependence. The patient states that he has tried to quit drinking several times on his own but has been unable to stay sober. He says he wants to quit and asks about disulfiram (Antabuse). Which of following statements regarding this is true?

  A. Disulfiram decreases the psychological desire to drink by inhibiting dopamine release.

  B. Disulfiram inhibits aldehyde dehydrogenase, causing acetaldehyde to accumulate.

  C. Disulfiram inhibits aldehyde dehydrogenase, causing acetic acid to accumulate.

  D. Topical alcohols like aftershave will not produce a reaction similar to liquor.

  E. The patient does not need to attend psychotherapy or a 12-step program.

300. A 32-year-old woman presents to her primary care physician with complaints of proximal forearm pain exacerbated by use. The pain originates at the lateral aspect of the proximal forearm and radiates down the forearm and into the dorsal aspect of her wrist. She denies any recent trauma to the area but is an avid racquetball player. Physical examination reveals swelling over the lateral aspect of her elbow, and pain is elicited with extension of the wrist against resistance with elbow extension. No obvious ecchymosis or erythema is noted. What is the most likely diagnosis?

A. Biceps tendinitis

B. Carpal tunnel syndrome

C. Lateral epicondylar tendinitis

D. Medial epicondylar tendinitis

E. Olecranon bursitis

Block 7

301. A 65-year-old man presents to his primary care physician complaining of recent onset of ringing in his ears and nausea. He also states that he has been having difficulty hearing the television and has to turn the volume up higher than usual. His current medications include diazepam for insomnia, quinidine for atrial fibrillation, ibuprofen for arthritis, and a daily multivitamin. He has recently started a 10-day course of ciprofloxacin for a urinary tract infection. What is the most likely explanation for these findings?

A. Ciprofloxacin

B. Ibuprofen

C. Multivitamin

D. Quinidine

E. Phenytoin

302. A 46-year-old obese woman presents to the emergency department complaining of excruciating pains and a tearing sensation in her chest that is bringing her to tears. Immediately you realize that she is experiencing which of the following:

A. Arteriovenous fistula

B. Berry aneurysm

C. Descending abdominal aortic aneurysm

D. Dissecting aneurysm

E. Syphilitic aneurysm

303. An 8-year-old boy presents to his primary care physician complaining of hoarseness. Laryngoscopy reveals multiple lesions on his true vocal cords. Physical examination of the heart and abdomen is unremarkable. There is no evidence of guarding or rebound tenderness. Bowel sounds are present in all quadrants. What is the most likely diagnosis?

A. Glottic carcinoma

B. Laryngeal papilloma

C. Singer's nodule

D. Subglottic carcinoma

E. Supraglottic carcinoma

304. At the arteriolar end of a capillary, the capillary hydrostatic pressure is 40 mm Hg, the capillary oncotic pressure is 38 mm Hg, the interstitial hydrostatic pressure 0 mm Hg and the interstitial fluid oncotic pressure is 4 mm Hg. What is the net pressure?

A. 2 mm Hg

B. 4 mm Hg

C. 6 mm Hg

D. 10 mm Hg

E. 14 mm Hg

305. A 65-year-old man presents with severe right arm pain that started about 3 weeks earlier. He notes that he cannot get around as he used to and that he has been extremely lethargic of late. The physician orders a series of blood tests, noting that the white blood cell count is 40,000 and the hemoglobin and hematocrit are abnormally low. An x-ray of the arm is shown in Figure 29. An unchecked proliferation of what type of cell is responsible for this man's symptoms?

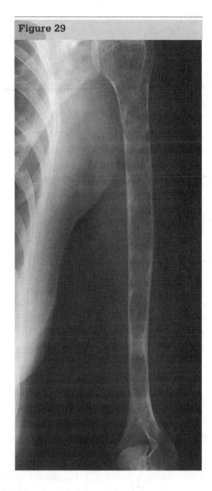

Figure 29

A. Cytotoxic T lymphocyte

B. Erythrocyte

C. Helper T lymphocyte

D. Mast cell

E. Plasma cell

306. A husband and wife, both 43 years old, present to the local emergency department complaining of vomiting, headache, and constitutional symptoms, along with watery diarrhea. They mention having been on a cruise and returning home 2 days ago. Based on the information given, what is the primary working diagnosis?

A. Herpes simplex I

B. Herpes simplex II

C. *Giardia lamblia*

D. Norwalk virus

E. Tuberculosis

307. A 35-year-old man presents to his primary care physician complaining of painless enlargement of his testicles. He reports no other symptoms. Physical examination reveals an enlarged, nodular right testicle. Ultrasound confirms the presence of a hypoechoic mass in the right testicle. What is the most probable classification of this testicular tumor?

A. Embryonal carcinoma

B. Leydig cell tumor

C. Seminoma

D. Teratoma

E. Yolk sac tumor

308. A 26-year-old man presents to his primary care physician with pneumonia and recent episodes of blood-tinged sputum. Antibodies are reported in the glomerular and pulmonary alveolar basement membranes as well as IgG linear immunofluorescence. What is the most likely explanation for these findings?

A. Alport's syndrome

B. Berger's disease

C. Goodpasture's disease

D. Lupus nephropathy

E. Tuberculosis

F. Uremia

309. A 45-year-old man presents to his primary care physician for a checkup. His past history is not significant for any illness. Physical examination reveals that the man is tall, with large hands. He has a prominent mandible and coarse facial features. His voice is deep, and he has macroglossia. His point of maximal auscultable cardiac impulse (PMI) is displaced 2 cm laterally. What is the most likely diagnosis?

A. Acromegaly

B. Amyloidosis

C. Familial prognathism

D. Gigantism

E. Hypothyroidism

310. A 3-year-old girl and her mother seek counseling regarding a recent diagnosis. A geneticist informed the mother that her daughter suffers from a congenital disorder known as chronic granulomatous disease. The mother wants to know more about the disease and what it means for the future of her daughter. She wants to know about the defect involved as well as what type of illness her daughter may suffer. What is the most appropriate response to the mother?

A. "The defect is impaired chemotaxis. Your daughter will have an increased susceptibility to viral infections."

B. "The defect is impaired chemotaxis. Your daughter will have an increased susceptibility to bacterial infections."

C. "The defect is deficient activity of NADPH oxidase. Your daughter will have an increased susceptibility to viral infections."

D. "The defect is deficient activity of NADPH oxidase. Your daughter will have an increased susceptibility to bacterial infections."

E. "The defect is impaired leukocyte adhesion. Your daughter will an increased susceptibility to viral infections."

F. "The defect is impaired leukocyte adhesion. Your daughter will an increased susceptibility to bacterial infections."

311. A 38-year-old woman presents to her primary care physician complaining of generalized weakness and feelings of lethargy. She is a happily married mother of two and denies any past medical or surgical history. Social and family histories are noncontributory. She reports that her difficulties seem to be getting slowly worse and wants to know whether there is any test that can diagnose her problem. What is the most appropriate next step in the management of this patient?

A. Complete blood count

B. CSF immunoglobulin electrophoresis

C. CT of abdomen and pelvis

D. Hemoglobin electrophoresis

E. Urinalysis

312. A 16-year-old youth presents to his pediatrician because he has developed a rash. He tells you that he noticed it a week after his camping trip in the northeastern part of the country. He cannot recall if he was bitten by any insects or animals. The patient states that he has also had a fever and runny nose for 2 days. Physical examination reveals a rash and an erythematous ring with central clearing. What is the most likely explanation for these findings?

A. *Borrelia burgdorferi*

B. *Brucella* species

C. *Francisella tularensis*

D. *Pasteurella multocida*

E. *Rickettsia rickettsii*

313. A 35-year-old woman who was working out in her garden was pricked by a rose thorn. She washed the wound with soap and water and the next day developed an ulcerated papule and became short of breath. She denies any fever or cough. What is the most likely etiology of her condition?

A. *Bacillus anthracis*

B. Blastomycosis

C. Histoplasmosis

D. *Sporothrix schenckii*

E. *Staphylococcus aureus*

314. A 54-year-old man presents to clinic with complaints of ankle pain. The pain developed shortly after he stepped into a hole in the ground while mowing his lawn. He promptly treated the injury with ice and took some ibuprofen. However, the next day his ankle was swollen, bruised, and so painful that he could not walk. Physical examination shows that the lateral aspect of the right ankle is edematous and ecchymotic. Both the anterior and lateral aspects of the ankle are tender to palpation, and inversion of the ankle is painful. What is the most likely diagnosis?

A. Achilles' tendon rupture

B. Ankle sprain

C. Plantar fasciitis

D. Stress fracture of the fifth metatarsal

E. Tarsal tunnel syndrome

315. A 59-year-old man loses consciousness in a shopping mall. He is brought to the emergency department for evaluation. He is alert and awake but oriented only to person. Review of his MedicAlert bracelet reveals that he has a medical history of unstable angina, diabetes mellitus, and atrial fibrillation. His current medications include warfarin (Coumadin) and nitroglycerin. Physical examination reveals atrial fibrillation. His pulse oximetry on room air is 91%. The main cause of ischemic heart disease in this patient is which of the following?

A. Carbon monoxide poisoning

B. Occlusion of the coronary sinus

C. Narrowing of the coronary arteries

D. Plaque accumulation in the left anterior descending artery

E. Poor oxygen-blood concentration

316. A 4-year-old boy from a Caribbean nation is brought to the local clinic by his mother, who reports that he is not developing intellectually like other boys of his age. Physical examination reveals an enlarged tongue and protruding abdomen. Which of the following treatments would be appropriate for this child?

A. Levothyroxine

B. Methimazole

C. Propylthiouracil

D. Vitamin B_6

E. Vitamin B_{12}

317. A 27-year-old woman presents to her primary care physician because of difficulty sleeping. She is having trouble staying awake at work and sometimes while driving. She reports that she has no trouble falling asleep, but once she is asleep she experiences vivid, life-like visions immediately. These visions are very frightening and wake her up immediately. She denies drinking caffeine and denies any illicit drug use. What is the name of the episodes this patient experiences while falling asleep?

A. Delusions

B. Hypnagogic hallucinations

C. Hypnopompic hallucinations

D. Illusions

E. Loose associations

318. A 31-year-old man with severe allergies is brought to a new physician for evaluation. He is believed to have a deficiency in IgA production. Which of the following is the major area of IgA production in the small intestine?

A. Adipose cell

B. Epithelium

C. Lamina propria

D. Mucous glands

E. Villi

319. An 8-year-old boy presents to his pediatrician with non-pruritic lesions on the back of his hand. Physical examination of one lesion reveals a 3-mm flesh-colored papule with central umbilication. The lesion is pictured in Figure 30.

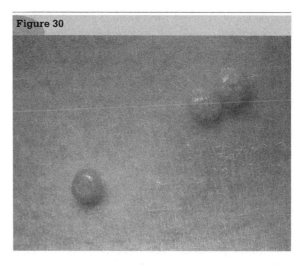

Figure 30

Which of the following virus types is most responsible for the development of these lesions?

A. Ambisense single-stranded RNA virus

B. Double-stranded DNA virus

C. Negative-sense single-stranded RNA virus

D. Positive-sense single-stranded RNA virus

E. Single-stranded DNA virus

320. A 15-year-old girl is diagnosed by her gynecologist with an ovarian tumor. She has a prior medical history of recurrent urinary tract infections and had nocturnal enuresis until age 7. Physical examination of the heart and lungs is within normal limits. Which of the following ovarian tumors is homologous to a testicular seminoma?

A. Dysgerminoma

B. Endodermal sinus (yolk sac) tumor

C. Immature teratoma

D. Mature teratoma (dermoid cyst)

E. Monodermal teratoma

321. A 35-year-old woman with peptic ulcer disease is currently treated with sucralfate. She complains of diffuse abdominal pain. Which drugs would be problematic for this patient?

A. Lactose to decrease constipation symptoms

B. Methylcellulose to increase the bulk of the stool

C. Milk of magnesia to relieve constipation

D. Omeprazole to decrease acid in the stomach

E. Scopolamine to decrease the patient's nausea

322. A fourth-year medical student is conducting a mental status examination on a 39-year-old man who complains of having felt sad and emotionless for 5 months. When the patient is asked where he was born, he replies that he was born in a house with walls. The walls hold up the house, and without walls, the house would come apart. The most likely explanation of this patient's response is:

A. Aphasia

B. Clanging

C. Circumstantial thinking

D. Tangential thinking

E. Thought blocking

323. A newborn baby is delivered, and discovered to have hydrocephalus and suspected mental retardation. Periventricular calcifications are noted on the radiograph, specifically in the cerebral cortex. The parents ask what may have caused this problem. What is the most likely response to this question?

A. Alcohol ingestion

B. Exposure to aniline dyes

C. Exposure to sick children during pregnancy

D. Pets at home (specifically cats)

E. Smoking in the house

324. A 2-year-old boy who has had no prior medical care is brought to a pediatrician by his parents. They are concerned about an abnormal structure at the back of his tongue. This boy has been slow to develop speech and moves much more slowly than other boys his age. What is the likely diagnosis of the structure at back of his tongue?

A. Brachial cleft cyst

B. Choanal atresia

C. Congenital pyloric stenosis

D. Meckel's diverticulum

E. Thyroglossal duct cyst

325. A 35-year-old runner presents to his primary care physician with complaints of severe foot pain that is worse in the mornings. He has been training for a marathon and denies any recent trauma. His foot pain is at its worst when he steps out of bed; it subsides after a few minutes of walking. Physical examination reveals that pain is elicited with palpation over the medial aspect of the heel. No swelling or ecchymosis is present. What is the most likely diagnosis?

A. Achilles' tendon rupture

B. Ankle sprain

C. Medial meniscus injury

D. Patellofemoral syndrome

E. Plantar fasciitis

F. Stress fracture

G. Tarsal tunnel syndrome

326. A 53-year-old obese man complains of chest pain and is brought to the emergency department for evaluation. Physical examination reveals a man who appears to be his stated age in acute distress. Vital signs reveal a blood pressure of 150/90 mm Hg and a pulse of 110 bpm. During what time period would you expect to see the serum AST level peak, a rise in the serum LDH, and a concomitant decrease in serum CPK?

A. 24 hr

B. 24 to 48 hr

C. 7 days

D. 28 days

E. 6 months

327. A 52-year-old man with a past medical history of alcoholic cirrhosis presents to the emergency department because he has been vomiting blood. Physical examination reveals diffuse abdominal tenderness without rebound tenderness. He has a positive abdominal fluid wave test. Upper gastrointestinal endoscopy reveals bleeding epigastric varicose veins. What is the best treatment for this patient?

A. Aspirin

B. Budesonide

C. Infliximab

D. Misoprostol

E. Octreotide

328. A patient with fragile X syndrome is typically mentally retarded with an intelligence quotient (IQ) in the range of 20 to 60, has a long face with a large mandible, large everted ears, and macroorchidism. In this syndrome the severity of symptoms appears to be related to the number of triplet repeats, and that clinical features worsen with each successive generation. What is the term for the above characteristics of fragile X syndrome?

A. Allelic heterogeneity

B. Anticipation

C. Pleiotropy

D. Reduced penetrance

E. Variable expressivity

329. Which of the following properties of *Streptococcus pneumoniae* allows the organism to penetrate into the respiratory epithelium to colonize mucosal surfaces?

A. Complement

B. Flagellae

C. IgA protease

D. M protein

E. Pili

330. A 72-year-old woman presents to the emergency department with expressive aphasia and weakness of the right side of her face and extremities. The right arm is affected more than the right leg. She has a prior medical history of insulin-dependent diabetes mellitus, hypertension, atrial fibrillation, hypercholesterolemia, and urinary incontinence. CT scan of the head is obtained and shown in Figure 31. Which of the following is the most likely explanation for this patient's symptoms?

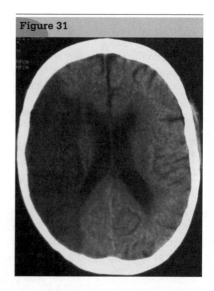

Figure 31

A. Anterior cerebral artery infarction, right

B. Middle cerebral artery infarction, left

C. Middle cerebral artery infarction, right

D. Posterior cerebral artery infarction, left

E. Posterior cerebral artery infarction, right

331. A 35-year-old woman was diagnosed with a peptic ulcer and started on omeprazole, metronidazole, amoxicillin, and bismuth subsalicylate. She has been on this regimen for 4 days. She presents to the emergency department with nausea, vomiting, hyperventilation, and vertigo. What is the most likely explanation for her symptoms?

A. Amoxicillin

B. Bismuth subsalicylate

C. Metronidazole

D. Omeprazole

E. Tetracycline

332. A 66-year-old woman presents to her primary care physician with atrophied labia bilaterally and a narrowed introitus. On histological examination of the labia, there is thinning of the epidermis and disappearance of the rete pegs with replacement of the underlying tissue with dense collagenous fibrous tissue. Which of the following diagnoses is most likely in this patient?

A. Lichen sclerosis

B. Papillary hidradenoma

C. Squamous hyperplasia

D. Vestibular adenitis

E. Vulvar intraepithelial neoplasia

333. Homicide is one of the top causes of mortality in specific age groups. Which group is the most likely to be affected by homicide?

A. 20-year-old white women

B. 20-year-old black women

C. 30-year-old black men

D. 30-year-old black women

E. 40-year-old Asian men

334. An 8-year-old boy is brought to the emergency department because of an unstoppable bloody nose over the last 4 hr. The child has a long history of easy bruising and his gums bleed when he brushes his teeth. He has never been tested or diagnosed with any blood disorders. What is the most appropriate treatment for this patient?

A. Aspirin

B. Beta-blocker

C. Cryoprecipitate

D. Desmopressin

E. Pseudoephedrine

335. A 19-year-old college student was brought to the emergency department by his friends after a party. His behavior was found to be impulsive and belligerent. He has no prior medical history. Physical examination reveals horizontal and vertical nystagmus. During the examination, he also claimed to see things on the wall that were not there. What is the most likely substance that this student abused?

A. Cocaine

B. LSD

C. Marijuana

D. Opioids

E. PCP

336. A 43-year-old woman with a history of using Pamprin (a combination of pamabrom, pyrilamine maleate, phenacetin and acetaminophen) for her severe menstrual cramps presents to her primary care physician for a checkup. Her past medical history is positive for diabetes mellitus, chronic renal infections, and mild vascular disease. In view of her comorbidities, what would be most concerning about which of the following renal disorders?

A. Cystinuria

B. Fanconi's syndrome

C. Hartnup disease

D. Necrotizing papillitis

E. Obstructive uropathy

337. An 8-year-old boy is brought to the emergency department because of a sudden onset of coughing and difficulty breathing. His mother states that she noticed he began to have difficulty breathing after holding a rabbit at the city zoo. She denies any similar events in the past. He has no current medical illnesses and takes only some over-the-counter medications for seasonal allergies. Physical examination reveals that the boy is tachypneic and tachycardic. Bilateral wheezes are heard on pulmonary auscultation. Which of the following cell levels would likely be elevated with this condition?

A. Basophils

B. Eosinophils

C. Neutrophils

D. Mast cells

E. Monocytes

338. A 71-year-old woman with new-onset open-angle glaucoma presents to her primary care physician for follow-up. She has a history of diabetes mellitus, hypertension, and temporal arteritis. Prior ophthalmoscopic examination reveals increased intraocular pressure. She is begun on therapy with brimonidine. The likely physiological change based on this medication would be which of the following?

A. Decreased aqueous humor secretion

B. Decreased aqueous humor synthesis

C. Increased aqueous humor outflow

D. Increased aqueous humor secretion

E. Increased aqueous humor synthesis

339. A 19-year-old man presents to his primary care physician with a fever and, on his left arm, a deep black lesion covering vesicular papules with a surrounding ring of inflammation. The patient is placed on ciprofloxacin. A colleague of the patient had recently developed a pneumonia that proved to be fatal. What is the most likely explanation for these findings?

    A. *Aspergillus fumigatus*

    B. *Bacillus anthracis*

    C. *Clostridium perfringens*

    D. *Pneumocystis carinii*

    E. *Pseudomonas aeruginosa*

340. A 51-year-old man and his 43-year-old wife undergo bone-density testing at a local health fair. The man has a history of diabetes mellitus and a family history of prostate cancer. The woman has a history of endometriosis. There is a discrepancy between their bone masses based on density testing. Which of the following would support an explanation for this discrepancy and be associated with an increased risk of osteoporosis?

    A. Decreased serum levels of osteocalcin in women

    B. Decrease in the number of primitive osteoblastic cells

    C. Differential ability of receptors to respond to signals

    D. Hormonal changes in pregnancy

    E. Men exercise more than women

    F. Prostate cancer treatment

    G. Women have heavier bones

341. An 18-year-old man presents to his primary care physician with a cough and a sore throat that have troubled him for a week. Physical examination reveals that he is febrile and has enlarged cervical nodes. Heterophile antibodies were detected in serum. What is the class of the most likely etiologic agent responsible for his symptoms?

    A. Adenovirus

    B. Herpesvirus

    C. Orthomyxovirus

    D. Paramyxovirus

    E. Picornavirus

342. A 42-year-old African American woman presents to her primary care physician with a rash across her nose and cheeks. She says that she also suffers from extreme fatigue but claims that she has had this problem since her early 20s. She complains of achy joints and is often feverish. A chest x-ray is obtained; it is shown in Figure 32. What is the most likely diagnosis?

    A. Angelman syndrome

    B. Hypothyroidism

    C. Reiter's syndrome

    D. Sarcoidosis

    E. Systemic lupus erythematosus

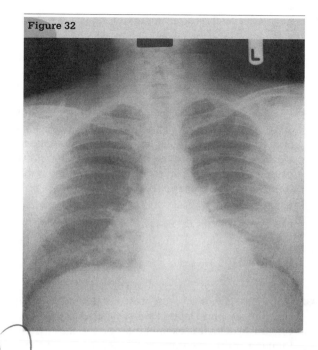

Figure 32

343. A 17-year-old woman presents for a general physical examination. During auscultation of the heart, a systolic murmur with a midsystolic click is audible. This can lead to which of the following issues?

    A. Aortic insufficiency

    B. Aortic regurgitation

    C. Mitral insufficiency

    D. Mitral stenosis

    E. Tricuspid insufficiency

344. A 62-year-old alcoholic man has cirrhosis and has developed portal hypertension. In order to relieve some of the portal hypertension, his surgeon is going to insert a portocaval shunt. Between which vascular structures will the surgeon most likely insert the shunt?

    A. Inferior mesenteric and superior mesenteric veins

    B. Left renal vein and right renal vein

    C. Right renal vein and right testicular vein

    D. Splenic vein and left renal vein

    E. Superior mesenteric and splenic vein

345. A 32-year-old G2P1001 presents to her primary care physician in her thirty-fourth week of pregnancy for a routine checkup. Her pregnancy has been unremarkable to date and she states that she feels well, but requests an ultrasound because her weight gain exceeds that expected for a normal pregnancy. The physician performs ultrasonography during the office visit, revealing dizygotic twins. Assuming that late splitting occurred (11 days after fertilization), which of the following conditions was more likely to develop than if earlier or later splitting had occurred?

    A. Conjoinment

    B. Cord strangulation

    C. Meconium ileus

    D. Potter sequence

    E. Twin-twin transfusion

346. A 35-year-old woman presents to the emergency department complaining of dysuria and lower back pain with radiation to the groin. Her past medical history is significant for squamous cell carcinoma of the lung. Physical exam reveals CVA tenderness and left lower quadrant tenderness. The rest of the exam is unremarkable. Urinalysis shows moderate blood and positive nitrite and leukocyte esterase. KUB reveals a right ureteral stone located in the midureter. What is the most likely composition of the stone?

A. Ammonium magnesium phosphate

B. Calcium

C. Cystine

D. Triamterine

E. Uric acid

347. A 24-year-old married couple has been trying to conceive for 18 months without success. Over the last 3 to 4 weeks, the wife began experiencing symptoms of morning sickness and noted a 5-lb weight gain. Repeated pregnancy tests confirm a negative result. What is the most likely explanation for these symptoms?

A. Depression

B. Ectopic pregnancy

C. Normal pregnancy

D. Postpartum syndrome

E. Pseudocyesis

348. A 65-year-old man presents to his primary care physician reporting gradual onset of shortness of breath and cough. Radiographs reveal bilateral pleural plaques and a right-sided pleural effusion. The patient's past social history is significant for employment at a shipyard for 30 years. What occupational exposure is likely to have caused this man's symptoms?

A. Asbestos

B. Beryllium

C. Carbon monoxide

D. Coal

E. Silica

F. Sulfur dioxide

349. A 24-year-old homeless man is brought to the emergency department unconscious and only minimally responsive. His clothing smells of alcohol. Which of the following symptoms would suggest the most likely diagnosis?

A. Heightened coordination

B. Hyperventilation

C. Increased anxiety

D. Inhibited behavior

E. Somnolence

350. A 60-year-old man comes to his primary care physician with the complaints of abdominal pain, weight loss, decrease in appetite, and weakness. His past medical history is significant for ulcerative colitis. He states that his father died at the age of 70 of colon cancer. He denies ever having had a colonoscopy because he was afraid of what it would show. In addition to other labs and tests, which of the following tumor markers should be measured?

A. Alpha fetoprotein

B. β-hCG

C. CA-125

D. Carcinogenic embryonic antigen

E. Prostate-specific antigen

Answer Key

BLOCK 1

1. C	**14.** E	**27.** B	**40.** B
2. A	**15.** D	**28.** D	**41.** D
3. C	**16.** B	**29.** B	**42.** B
4. E	**17.** A	**30.** C	**43.** D
5. B	**18.** B	**31.** D	**44.** E
6. A	**19.** C	**32.** B	**45.** D
7. B	**20.** A	**33.** E	**46.** B
8. C	**21.** A	**34.** C	**47.** F
9. E	**22.** A	**35.** A	**48.** E
10. A	**23.** B	**36.** E	**49.** A
11. C	**24.** B	**37.** C	**50.** A
12. C	**25.** D	**38.** D	
13. E	**26.** G	**39.** D	

BLOCK 2

51. B	**64.** D	**77.** B	**90.** A
52. A	**65.** C	**78.** E	**91.** D
53. A	**66.** E	**79.** A	**92.** E
54. A	**67.** D	**80.** B	**93.** C
55. A	**68.** E	**81.** C	**94.** E
56. A	**69.** D	**82.** E	**95.** D
57. E	**70.** E	**83.** E	**96.** C
58. A	**71.** E	**84.** B	**97.** E
59. A	**72.** E	**85.** A	**98.** E
60. B	**73.** A	**86.** A	**99.** E
61. A	**74.** E	**87.** C	**100.** D
62. E	**75.** B	**88.** C	
63. B	**76.** D	**89.** C	

BLOCK 3

101. A	**114.** D	**127.** A	**140.** B
102. A	**115.** C	**128.** C	**141.** D
103. B	**116.** E	**129.** A	**142.** B
104. A	**117.** B	**130.** E	**143.** E
105. A	**118.** C	**131.** C	**144.** A
106. C	**119.** A	**132.** B	**145.** C
107. C	**120.** D	**133.** A	**146.** E
108. D	**121.** B	**134.** D	**147.** C
109. C	**122.** D	**135.** B	**148.** A
110. B	**123.** E	**136.** A	**149.** D
111. D	**124.** A	**137.** D	**150.** C
112. G	**125.** E	**138.** C	
113. C	**126.** C	**139.** D	

BLOCK 4

151. D	**164.** E	**177.** E	**190.** E
152. F	**165.** D	**178.** D	**191.** D
153. A	**166.** E	**179.** D	**192.** E
154. C	**167.** B	**180.** D	**193.** E
155. A	**168.** C	**181.** A	**194.** D
156. B	**169.** C	**182.** E	**195.** D
157. D	**170.** D	**183.** E	**196.** C
158. D	**171.** A	**184.** A	**197.** B
159. D	**172.** A	**185.** G	**198.** B
160. F	**173.** A	**186.** B	**199.** B
161. A	**174.** A	**187.** D	**200.** D
162. C	**175.** D	**188.** C	
163. E	**176.** E	**189.** F	

Answer Key

BLOCK 5

201. D	214. B	227. B	240. C
202. A	215. D	228. B	241. F
203. C	216. E	229. B	242. C
204. C	217. B	230. D	243. B
205. D	218. D	231. D	244. D
206. A	219. D	232. C	245. C
207. E	220. C	233. C	246. C
208. C	221. C	234. E	247. B
209. C	222. B	235. E	248. A
210. D	223. E	236. D	249. A
211. B	224. A	237. A	250. D
212. B	225. A	238. D	
213. B	226. F	239. C	

BLOCK 6

251. C	264. A	277. E	290. D
252. B	265. B	278. D	291. B
253. C	266. C	279. C	292. E
254. B	267. A	280. A	293. C
255. B	268. E	281. D	294. D
256. E	269. C	282. B	295. A
257. C	270. B	283. B	296. B
258. B	271. A	284. C	297. B
259. D	272. C	285. F	298. C
260. B	273. B	286. C	299. B
261. C	274. B	287. D	300. C
262. A	275. A	288. E	
263. C	276. D	289. B	

BLOCK 7

301. D	**314.** B	**327.** E	**340.** F
302. D	**315.** C	**328.** B	**341.** B
303. B	**316.** A	**329.** C	**342.** E
304. C	**317.** B	**330.** B	**343.** C
305. E	**318.** C	**331.** C	**344.** D
306. D	**319.** B	**332.** A	**345.** E
307. C	**320.** A	**333.** C	**346.** B
308. C	**321.** D	**334.** D	**347.** E
309. A	**322.** D	**335.** C	**348.** A
310. D	**323.** D	**336.** D	**349.** E
311. B	**324.** E	**337.** B	**350.** D
312. A	**325.** E	**338.** B	
313. D	**326.** B	**339.** B	

Answers and Explanations

Block 1

1. C. Cholesterol functions as part of the lipid bilayer to maintain the structural integrity of the plasma membrane. As cholesterol increases in the membrane, the fluidity decreases. This membrane fluidity is important for exocytosis, endocytosis, membrane biogenesis, and membrane trafficking. Cholesterol does not have any involvement in cell signaling or attachment.

2. A. Cluster headaches typically present as described by the patient. Incidence is greater in males; in addition, these can be associated following consumption of alcohol, nitrates, or stressful events and have a tendency to occur in clusters. Symptoms in these patients can include unilateral facial pain, conjunctival injection, lacrimation, rhinorrhea, ptosis, congestion, and facial sweating. Giant cell arteritis, or temporal arteritis, is defined as an arterial inflammation that often involves the temporal arteries and may lead to blindness when the ophthalmic artery and/or its branches are involved. It is characterized by the formation of giant cells and may be accompanied by fever, malaise, fatigue, anorexia, weight loss, and arthralgia. Migraine is defined as a condition involving unilateral severe headache that can last several hours; it is often accompanied by nausea and vomiting and followed by sleep. There does appear to be a genetic component involved. Both types of headaches can include neurological dysfunction, including photophobia, diplopia, and weakness as well as nausea and vomiting. Patients who experience *migraine with aura* describe a subjective sensation (for example a voice, colored lights, or numbness) experienced about an hour prior to onset of the migraine.

3. C. Langerhans cells are part of the mononuclear phagocytic system and are antigen-presenting cells. They are similar in morphology and function to macrophages. Melanocytes produce melanin, a pigment. Keratinocytes produce keratin, which forms a waterproof layer. Merkel cells are epidermal cells, which function in cutaneous sensation. Adipocytes are fat-storage cells.

4. E. The alveolar P_{O_2} is decreased at high altitude due to a decrease in barometric pressure. Therefore, arterial P_{O_2} is also decreased, causing hypoxemia. Hypoxemia then stimulates peripheral chemoreceptors and increases the ventilation rate, producing primary alkalosis.

5. B. Early in the seventh week, the limbs extend ventrally and then rotate in opposite directions. Originally, the flexor aspect is ventral and the extensor is dorsal. However, the upper limb rotates so that the extensor muscles are posterior, whereas the lower limb rotates so that the extensor muscles are anterior.

6. A. Adenosine has limited uses in medicine. Its most important and effective use is in the setting of an acute arrhythmic episode due to a supraventricular tachycardia or arrhythmia. In this setting it can very transiently block the conduction through the AV node and allow for a decrease in the overstimulation from the atria. Amiodarone is a class III drug that functions mainly by blocking potassium channels, thus prolonging the action potential. It has very little effect on the atria and AV node. Flecainide falls under class Ic drugs and is commonly thought of as a last-resort drug, as it may lead to arrhythmias of its own. Lidocaine is both a local anesthetic and a class Ib antiarrhythmic. It would not be effective in this clinical scenario because most of its clinical effects are with acute ventricular arrhythmias. Quinidine is a class Ia antiarrhythmic. Typically it is used for the long-term treatment and prophylaxis of arrhythmic episodes; it has little use in the acute care setting.

7. B. Ipecac is a mixture of alkaloids that induce vomiting by stimulating the chemotactic trigger zone, which causes gastrointestinal irritation and afferent input to the vomiting center. This agent produces vomiting in the majority of patients within 20 min and is useful for removing toxins that have slow gastric transit times. Ipecac does not stimulate the gag reflex and does not suppress gastric outlet pressures or the motor cortex.

8. C. Lupus nephropathy can present with a combination of nephrotic and nephritic symptoms in conjunction with the standard presentation. There are five renal patterns with which this nephropathy can present. Type IV (diffuse proliferative) is the most severe. The finding of subendothelial immune complex deposition is pathognomonic. Diabetic nephropathy often shows signs of classic nephrotic syndrome. On light microscopy you see basement thickening and Kimmelstiel-Wilson lesions. High urine glucose/poorly controlled sugars can suggest potential diabetic comorbidities. Renal amyloidosis is due to the deposit of amyloid in the basement membrane. This will show up as apple-green birefringence on immunofluorescence.

9. E. In general, females under 18 years of age may receive confidential care for contraception, sexually transmitted diseases, or pregnancy. Despite the possible negative impacts that this could have on their sexual behavior, young women benefit from being able to adopt healthier sexual practices without having to consult their parents. This approach is thought to have drastically decreased teenage pregnancy rates and the spread of sexually transmitted diseases.

10. A. This patient likely has left ventricular concentric hypertrophy. Chest x-ray reveals cardiomegaly with enlargement of the cardiac silhouette. Chronic uncontrolled hypertension results in a pressure overload on the left ventricle and thus leads to a concentric hypertrophy of the left ventricle, with an increase in wall thickness and typically a reduced cavity diameter. Hypertrophy is defined as an increase in the size of an organ or tissue due to an increase in the size of cells. Concentric hypertrophy is typically due to a pressure overload, while eccentric hypertrophy is due to a volume overload. Hyperplasia is an increase in the number of cells in an organ or tissue. Adult cardiac myocytes cannot divide; therefore hyperplasia of the myocytes does not occur. Metaplasia is the replacement of one adult cell type for another adult cell type. This does not happen in response to pressure overload of the heart.

11. C. Renal amyloidosis is characterized by subendothelial and mesangial amyloid deposits. These deposits are reactive with stains such as Congo red, crystal violet, and thioflavin T. There is also a correlation with chronic inflammatory diseases and plasma cell disorders such as rheumatoid arthritis and multiple myeloma. Lupus nephropathy can present with a combination of nephrotic and nephritic symptoms in conjunction with the standard presentation. IgA nephropathy is associated with deposits of IgA in the glomerular basement membrane (GBM). There is no such diagnosis of RA nephropathy.

12. C. This patient likely has an insulinoma. Often these patients have become so adapted to hypoglycemia that they present with neurological symptoms of hypoglycemia (blurry vision, diplopia, seizures, confusion) rather than adrenergic symptoms (tachycardia, weakness, tremor, etc.). They have often gained weight from frequent snacking to self-treat the hypoglycemia. The glucose, insulin, and C-peptide levels clinch the diagnosis. If the patient had self-administered insulin, the C-peptide levels would have been suppressed. A cerebrovascular accident (CVA) is possible but less likely, given the rest of the information in the stem of the question. A myocardial infarction is possible, but the question stem indicates that the vital signs, ECG, and initial set of cardiac enzymes are within normal limits, making this less likely than insulinoma. Although dehydration can cause syncope, the man's blood pressure and electrolytes are normal, and based on the rest of the information, dehydration too is less likely than insulinoma.

13. E. In order to answer this question, you would have to first figure out the age of this child based on the developmental milestones he has already mastered. Based on this, you would have known that the child in question is 4 months old. The only milestone on the list that is observed in a 4-month-old is E, reaching for objects and batting at them. Cruising and taking steps alone is a milestone for 1 year of age. Drinking from a cup and pulling to stand are milestones reached at 9 months of age. Finally, cutting the first tooth usually happens at 6 months of age.

14. E. This patient most likely was given vancomycin, which is the drug of choice for methicillin-resistant *Staphylococcus aureus* (MRSA). A known complication of vancomycin treatment is flushing of the skin, commonly referred to as "red-man syndrome." This is caused by the release of histamine. Vancomycin is also known to cause dose-related hearing loss. Ampicillin and cefotaxime can cause a severe rash in predisposed individuals in addition to anaphylactic shock. Chloramphenicol is a broad-spectrum antibiotic that is useful against anaerobes. In adults with glucose-6-phosphate dehydrogenase deficiency, chloramphenicol may cause a hemolytic anemia and an aplastic anemia that can be fatal. Trimethoprim-sulfamethoxazole (TMP-SMX) is a combination of trimethoprim and sulfamethoxazole that is commonly used in the treatment of urinary tract infections (UTIs). A variety of adverse effects have been associated with TMP-SMX, including GI effects, rash, and anemia.

15. D. This patient has a paraneoplastic syndrome of the syndrome of inappropriate antidiuretic hormone (SIADH), causing increased water absorption, hyponatremia, and the resulting symptoms. The most common cancer associated with this type of paraneoplastic syndrome is small cell carcinoma of the lung. Squamous cell carcinoma of the lung causes paraneoplastic parathyroid hormone (PTH)–related peptide, leading to hypercalcemia. Clear cell carcinoma and renal cell carcinoma may be associated with paraneoplastic syndromes, but usually not SIADH. Pheochromocytomas would cause paradoxical hypertension due to excess catecholamine production.

16. B. Patients with lung disorders, especially emphysema, are at substantial risk for developing cor pulmonale. Pulmonary arterial hypertension is the most common characteristic that is indicative of the possibility of cor pulmonale. Bacterial endocarditis is related to the valvular issues and vegetation. Deep venous thrombosis and pulmonary embolism tend to be associated with hypercoagulable states, especially in bedridden patients. Mitral valve prolapse is associated with Marfan's syndrome and not necessarily with a diagnosis of emphysema.

17. A. Berry aneurysm at the circle of Willis is very common with the diagnosis of autosomal dominant polycystic kidney disease. Diabetes mellitus, renal stones, and recurrent urinary tract infections are all possible scenarios, but none is directly related to the diagnosis of adult polycystic kidney disease.

18. B. Fibroadenoma is the most common benign cause of a breast lump in a female below 30 years of age. It presents exactly as in the vignette. Fibrocystic disease presents in women 30 to 40 years of age as a cystic swelling of one breast, with pain and tenderness. Cystosarcoma phyllodes is a variant of the fibroadenoma, involving epithelial and stromal proliferation. It appears as a large, bulky, mobile mass. The overlying skin is warm and erythematous. Intraductal papilloma is a benign solitary lesion that is the most common cause of bloody nipple discharge in the absence of a concurrent mass. Mammary duct ectasia is a subacute inflammation of the ductal system causing dilated mammary ducts. It presents with nipple retraction with discharge and non-cyclic breast pain.

19. C. The correct answer is PCP. It is associated with all the symptoms described in the passage, and horizontal and vertical nystagmus is unique to PCP. LSD can produce similar symptoms but not nystagmus. Look for visual hallucinations and flashbacks with LSD. Marijuana causes paranoia and slows reaction times. Opioids are used as analgesics and are associated with respiratory depression, miosis, and constipation. Cocaine is a stimulant that causes euphoria, mydriasis, tachycardia, and hypertension.

20. A. Over 65% of ovarian tumors and over 95% of ovarian cancers arise from the coelomic epithelium on the ovary. Germ cell tumors make up only 15% of neoplasms; sex cord-stromal tumors account for 5 to 10%; Krukenberg or metastatic tumors make up only 5%.

21. A. This history is most consistent with the diagnosis of cluster headaches. They commonly occur in males and are precipitated by alcohol. The symptoms are noted in Answer 2. Migraines are more throbbing in nature and usually have an associated aura. Tension headaches are usually bilateral and feel like a tight band around the head. Sinusitis is associated with fever. There is no reason to suspect tuberculosis in this case, given the lack of exposure history and the lack of pulmonary symptoms.

22. A. With contact dermatitis, you see papules and vesicles localized to the area exposed or in contact with something. Shingles is causes by the latent varicella zoster virus, which lies dormant in ganglia. It causes a vesicular eruption along a specific dermatome and is extremely painful. Herpes simplex virus causes a vesicular eruption and is associated with pain. The most common location is along the lips. Seborrheic dermatitis presents as red, scaly lesions, usually in the nasolabial folds and scalp. This lesion is not considered to be normal.

23. B. Intussusception is the most common cause of blood in the stools and abdominal distension in a 2-year-old. On barium enema examination, you see a sausage-shaped lesion, and the stools have the characteristic currant-jelly consistency. If the child were under 1 year of age, you would diagnose volvulus as the cause. Meckel's does present with blood in stools, but it was not suggested by the findings on enema. Rotavirus is a common cause of watery diarrhea in the United States. It does not present with bloody stools. This is not a normal variant.

24. B. This boy is suffering from Duchenne muscular dystrophy (DMD), an X-linked progressive myopathy almost exclusively affecting males that is caused by mutations in the dystrophin gene. The DMD gene encodes for the protein dystrophin, which is a component of all types of muscle. In skeletal muscle, dystrophin provides stability to the sarcolemma. In males, weakness begins in the proximal muscle groups, starting with the hip girdle muscles and neck flexors, then the shoulder girdle, distal limb, and trunk muscles. By age 5, most patients will have pseudohypertrophy of the calves and be using the Gowers' maneuver to stand up. (The Gowers' maneuver involves using the arms to push the body up and walking the hands along the legs to bring the upper body erect.) Most of these patients have some associated cardiomyopathy and impaired pulmonary function. The median age at death is 18 years. The diagnosis should be made based on family history and either muscle biopsy or DNA analysis. Collagen is not defective in patients with DMD. Fibrillin is not defective and myelin levels as well as spectrin levels are normal in patients with DMD.

25. D. The patient demonstrates the typical manifestation of multiple myeloma. The mild thrombocytopenia is secondary to the increase of plasma cells, with a resulting decrease in all cell lines. The mild platelet decrease would not result in bleeding or bruising. The patient's renal insufficiency results in a qualitative platelet disorder, which is the likely diagnosis in this case. Disseminated intravascular coagulopathy, acquired factor VIII deficiency, and vitamin K deficiency can be ruled out with normal PT, PTT, and platelet count. The bone marrow aspirate reveals increased plasma cells with decreased myelopoiesis, erythropoiesis, and megakaryocytes.

26. G. Seborrheic keratosis is a benign squamoproliferative neoplasm that typically presents as in the main question stem. Microscopy reveals "horn cysts," which are filled with keratin. These may be left untreated or removed for cosmetic reasons. Acanthosis nigricans is a thickening and darkening in pigmentation of the neck, axillae, and groin most often seen as a benign condition indicating insulin resistance. Squamous cell carcinoma is most often seen among people who have heavy sun exposure and usually presents on sun-exposed areas such as the face, arms, and hands. Basal cell carcinoma is common in sun-exposed areas of the body. It is locally invasive. Psoriasis is a dermatosis characterized by koebnerization and skin scaling. Malignant melanoma is a common tumor with significant risk of metastasis. It is associated with sun exposure. Fair-skinned persons are at increased risk. Depth of tumor correlates with risk of metastases.

27. B. Babies gradually learn coordination and control of their muscles from the head down: the muscles of the neck, the shoulders and arms, and then the body. The last muscles the baby masters are those of the pelvis and legs, which make standing and walking possible.

28. D. The presentation described in this patient, known as Broca's aphasia or motor aphasia, is the inability to speak or to organize the movements of speech while the ability to comprehend is retained. Lesions to the arcuate fasciculus will produce a conduction type of aphasia or problems with repeating; these patients have good comprehension as well as fluent speech. A lesion to the amygdala is reflective of Klüver-Bucy syndrome, which involves hypersexuality and disinhibited behavior. Lesions to the basal ganglia, such as in Huntington's disease, result in tremors at rest or choreoathetotic movement. Wernicke's aphasia, or receptive aphasia, is the inability to understand spoken or written symbols and results from damage to an area of the brain (Wernicke's area) concerned with language.

29. B. This individual has evidence of diabetes mellitus of the juvenile type, a condition associated with ketoacidosis but not obesity. Ketosis is due to a decrease in insulin production and increase in glucagon levels. Ketone bodies serve as an energy source in the central nervous system. Accelerated fat breakdown does not explain the ketoacidosis of diabetes mellitus. Hepatic failure is not a consequence of ketosis. Hyperglycemia is due to a decrease in insulin production. Renal failure is a consequence of glomerulosclerosis.

30. C. The location of the right kidney is a little lower due to the presence of the liver. The right kidney is associated with the 12th rib, as the left is associated with the 11th and 12th ribs, both posteriorly. T1-T4 represents the location of the heart. S2-S4 is the pudendal nerve supply location, which is responsible for parasympathetic supply to the bladder aiding in voiding. C1-C8 indicates the range of the cervical vertebrae and has no bearing on the location of the kidneys.

31. D. Seventy-five percent of the breast, including the entire nipple and most of the lateral segment, drains lymph to the pectoral node, with minor amounts going to the remaining axillary nodes. Lymph from the pectoral node then drains into the central axillary node, along with contributions from the posterior and lateral axillary nodes. Lymph from the central axillary node then drains into the apical axillary node, which lies along the subclavian artery. The remaining 25% of the breast drains into the parasternal nodes, which lie along the internal thoracic artery.

32. B. Conduction through the AV node is represented by the PR interval. This area is commonly monitored for AV block, where signal transmission may be slowed, occasionally blocked, or completely blocked; these situations are labeled first-, second-, and third-degree blocks, respectively. The P wave represents atrial depolarization. The QRS wave represents ventricular depolarization. A wide QRS implies abnormal conduction. The QT interval represents the approximate time of ventricular systole. If it is prolonged by drug toxicity or electrolyte disturbances, arrhythmias may ensue. The T wave is the ventricular repolarization phase of the ECG. Spiked or large T waves may indicate hyperkalemia. The ECG here shows features of left ventricular hypertrophy. An area of R- and T-wave inversion is also seen.

33. E. Tetracycline acts by binding to the 30S ribosome and thus not allowing the aminoacyl-tRNA, which blocks translation, to bind. Macrolides inhibit protein synthesis (translation) by blocking the translocation step. Penicillin is responsible for inhibiting proper cell wall synthesis by blocking the transpeptidase cross-linking of the cell wall. Chloramphenicol inhibits the 50S peptidyl transferase, disrupting translation. Aminoglycosides are responsible for inhibiting the formation of the initiation complex needed to start protein synthesis.

34. C. Based on observation of this young man, he would be assigned to Tanner stage 3. His pubic hair has matured (darker and curlier), but it is in sparse distribution. The penis has grown only in length, not breadth (width), and the glans penis has yet to develop. These are all characteristics of stage 3. Tanner 1 would be a male who is preadolescent, with no pubic hair, and his penis would be of the same size and proportion as in childhood. Tanner 2 would be a male who has developed some sparse pubic hair that is straight (not curly) and only slightly pigmented. His penis would have only slight if any enlargement. A Tanner 4 male has coarse, curly hair covering a greater area but not yet including the thighs. The Tanner 4 male's penis has enlarged in both length and breadth with additional development of the glans penis. Finally the scrotal skin has darkened in a Tanner 4 male. The Tanner 5 male has pubic hair of adult quality and quantity, which spreads to the thighs. The penis and testes are of adult size and shape.

35. A. This woman is experiencing side effects of corticosteroid use, including osteoporosis, immunosuppression, and adrenal atrophy. Cretinism is caused by lack of dietary iodine, causing failure in thyroid function (usually in children), which has nothing to do with this vignette. Cushing's disease is caused by a pituitary adenoma secreting corticotrophin and would be associated with enlarged adrenal glands. Diabetes may be a common finding in the elderly but does not explain this woman's symptoms. Osteoporosis explains the compression fracture but not the other symptoms.

36. E. In the female, the ureter is accompanied in its course by the uterine artery, which runs above and anterior to it. Because of this location, it is sometimes injured by a clamp during surgical procedures and may be ligated and sectioned by mistake during a hysterectomy. The mesometrium is a major part of the broad ligament below the mesovarium. The mesosalpinx is a fold of the broad ligament that suspends the uterine tube. The rectouterine ligaments hold the cervix back and upward. The sacrocervical ligaments are firm, fibromuscular bands than extend from the cervix to the vagina.

37. C. A lacunar infarct of the internal capsule typically shows as pure motor deficits in the presenting patient. Pure sensory loss after a lacunar infarct is pathognomonic for a thalamic lesion. Infarcts of the caudate, external capsule, and putamen do not present with pure sensory or motor impingement symptoms. The MRI shown (Figure 4) confirms the findings of lacunar infarct.

38. D. This child suffers from Prader-Willi syndrome, a developmental disorder that results from loss of paternally expressed genes most often from a deletion of the 15q11-q13 chromosome. It may also result from a mutation within the imprinting control center, leading to a failure to switch maternal imprints to paternal imprints. This causes a loss of paternal imprinting. The genes within the 15q11-q13 are differentially expressed depending on whether the area is inherited from the mother or the father. Thus, a deletion in a specific region will cause inability to express that particular set of genes. The phenotype of Prader-Willi presents in early infancy with severe hypotonia, feeding difficulties, and hypogonadism with cryptorchidism. Between 1 and 6 years of age, the appetite problems resolve and transform into extreme hyperphagia and food seeking behavior. This leads to a marked obesity, which is a major cause of morbidity resulting from cardiopulmonary disease and type

2 diabetes mellitus. Most of these patients also have a delayed development and severe learning disabilities. Prader-Willi syndrome is not due to a deletion in either chromosome 5 or 22. This syndrome is not due to a loss of maternal imprinting or to a missense mutation.

39. D. Referring this patient to a general surgeon for a splenectomy offers a potential cure to her hereditary spherocytosis. The spleen becomes enlarged in this disease, as erythrocytes are trapped and destroyed in the organ. Splenectomy corrects the disease process. The administration of phenobarbital has been known to correct the hyperbilirubinemia in specific conditions such as Crigler-Najjar syndrome and Gilbert's syndrome. This could also help reduce itching, which is caused by hyperbilirubinemia. This does not provide any chance of a cure, however. Dialysis is used in patients who have kidney failure, such as patients with late-stage diabetes. A liver transplant is a treatment option for patients who have liver failure due to conditions such as primary biliary cirrhosis. Quinidine is an antiarrhythmic drug that has many side effects, including hemolytic anemia and agranulocytosis. There are no indications to give quinidine to this patient. In fact, administering this drug may cause hemolytic anemia, which is the exact disease process we are trying to overcome.

40. B. Measles is cause by the morbillivirus, a member of the paramyxovirus family. This is a highly contagious virus with the classic presentation being described above. The classic triad of symptoms is cough, coryza, and Koplik's spots, which are gray-white macules on the buccal mucosa. This disease has seen a drastic decline since the beginning of routine vaccination of children. *Staphylococcus epidermidis* can cause skin infections. Group A beta-hemolytic streptococcus causes scarlet fever. Human herpesvirus 6 causes the childhood exanthem known as roseola. Parvovirus B19 causes fifth ("slapped cheeks") disease.

41. D. This patient has Kartagener's syndrome, caused by immotile cilia due to a dynein arm defect. Patients present with bronchiectasis, recurrent sinusitis, and situs inversus. Kartagener's also results in sterility, because the sperm are immotile. An extra X chromosome in a male would result in Klinefelter's syndrome, which presents with testicular atrophy, eunuchoid body shape, gynecomastia, and a female pattern of hair distribution. An extra Y chromosome in a male would result in XYY syndrome. These men are phenotypically normal but are very tall, with severe acne, and they may exhibit antisocial behavior. C-ANCA is a strong marker for Wegener's granulomatosis. It is characterized by vasculitis, granulomas in the lung, and glomerulonephritis. Patients present with hematuria, red cell casts, sinusitis, and otitis media. P-ANCA is a serum marker commonly seen in polyarteritis nodosa. This is a necrotizing immune complex inflammation of small or medium-sized muscular arteries. It typically involves the renal and visceral vessels. Trisomy 21 is seen in patients with Down's syndrome.

42. B. Carpal tunnel syndrome occurs when tendons or ligaments in the wrist become enlarged, often from inflammation, and after being aggravated. The narrowed tunnel of bones and ligaments in the wrist pinches the nerves that reach the fingers and the muscles at the base of the thumb. The first symptoms usually appear at night. Symptoms range from a burning, tingling numbness in the fingers, especially the thumb and the index and middle fingers, to difficulty gripping or making a fist, to dropping things. Some cases of carpal tunnel syndrome are due to cumulative trauma of the wrist. The Phalen or wrist-flexion test involves having the patient hold his or her forearms upright by pointing the fingers down and pressing the backs of the hands together. The presence of carpal tunnel syndrome is suggested if one or more symptoms, such as tingling or increasing numbness, are felt in the fingers within 1 min. Lateral epicondylitis, also known as tennis elbow, is commonly seen in people who overuse their arm(s). The most common cause is overuse of the wrist extensors. All the extensor muscles of the hand attach to the lateral epicondyle; if they are strained or overused, they become inflamed. Medial epicondylitis is inflammation of the medial epicondyle.

43. D. This patient is clearly having another myocardial infarction, which has just begun. In this patient the most important therapy would be revascularization of the coronary vessels, which are currently occluded. Thrombolytic drugs such as streptokinase and tPA lead to the activation of plasmin, which digests fibrin clots, leading to reperfusion of the myocardium. Heparin is used for prophylaxis of deep venous thrombosis, pulmonary embolism, arterial embolism, and atrial fibrillation. It potentiates the activity of antithrombin III and thereby inactivated thrombin. Aspirin is a nonselective inhibitor of cyclooxygenase and inhibits platelet aggregation. It is metabolized by esterases.

44. E. The superior gluteal nerve leaves the pelvis through the greater sciatic foramen above the piriformis muscle. The sciatic nerve, internal pudendal vessels, inferior gluteal nerves and vessels, and posterior femoral cutaneous nerve leave the pelvis below the piriformis muscle.

45. D. Although type I diabetes is the most common type seen in this age group, the greater amount of obesity at younger ages is increasing the incidence of type II diabetes. The patient's weight, acanthosis nigricans, and lack of serum ketones all are clues that this is a type II pathology rather than a type I. In order to diagnose maturity diabetes of youth, the patient would have to have a significant family history of diabetes (across many generations). Hyperthyroidism and secondary diabetes are highly unlikely in this patient.

46. B. This syndrome is also known as testicular feminization. In this condition, the androgen receptors are absent. During embryogenesis, this interferes with the fusion of the labial-scrotal folds, resulting in the presence of a short vagina. The fallopian tubes, uterus, and upper portion of the vagina are absent because the testes secreted müllerian inhibitory factor early during development. The patients will have breast enlargement during puberty because the testes secrete some estradiol, and peripheral tissues convert androgens into estrogens. Anorchia and cryptorchidism are not plausible given that this patient is female.

47. F. Probenecid blocks the active reabsorption of uric acid that occurs in the proximal tubules, thereby increasing the amount of urate eliminated. It is an effective and safe agent for controlling hyperuricemia and preventing the deposition of tophi in patients who suffer from chronic gout. It is not useful in treating acute attacks or in cases of renal insufficiency when GFR have been reduced below 30 mL/min. Allopurinol reduces serum urea levels through a competitive inhibition of xanthine oxidase. This results in the reduction of the urinary concentration of uric acid and increases the excretion of the more soluble compounds xanthine and hypoxanthine. Colchicine is the first-line anti-inflammatory agent used in the treatment of acute gouty arthritis. Therapy with colchicine is usually begun at the first sign of an acute attack and is continued until symptoms subside. Indomethacin is a nonsteroidal anti-inflammatory agent. Probenecid is used in the management of chronic gout. It inhibits the resorption of uric acid and also inhibits the synthesis of penicillin. Phenylbutazone is not used in the management of this patient.

48. E. Vitiligo is a disease caused by an acquired loss of melanocytes in discrete areas of the skin, resulting in lack of pigment. It is much easier to appreciate the depigmented skin in darker-skinned individuals. Vitiligo has no relation to albinism. It can be caused by several factors, including autoimmune dysregulation, destruction of melanocytes by toxic metabolites, or by toxic intermediates of melanin production. The exact etiology of vitiligo is currently unknown. Cicatricial pemphigoid is a subset of the mucous membrane pemphigoid family. It often has ocular manifestations as well as affecting the skin and other mucous membranes. It is caused by an autoimmune reaction to adhesion molecules in the hemidesmosome-epithelial membrane complex. Erythema multiforme is associated with drug hypersensitivity. Targetoid cells are seen histologically. Bullous pemphigoid is caused by an autoimmune dysfunction whereby IgG antibodies attack the basement membranes of the epidermis, compromising the stability of the epidermis and resulting in bullae.

49. A. This patient has a carcinoid tumor, which is the most common neuroendocrine tumor, with an incidence of 1.5 per 100,000. The most common location is the appendix (40%). The tumor produces high levels of 5-hydroxytryptamine (5HT) or serotonin in the blood and high levels of 5-hydroxyindole acetic acid (5-HIAA) in the urine. It results in recurrent diarrhea, cutaneous flushing, and asthmatic wheezing. The second most common location is the ileum (30%, not given as an option), followed by the rectum (10%) and then the colon (5%). A carcinoid tumor in the esophagus is a very rare finding.

50. A. Amitriptyline is a tricyclic antidepressant that causes significant sedation, particularly in the elderly. It is not recommended as the first-line therapy of depression in the older population. Tricyclics can also cause decreased seizure threshold, cardiotoxicity, and coma. Lithium is used in the treatment of bipolar disorder. The adverse effects of lithium include tremor, ataxia, choreoathetosis, and nephrogenic diabetes insipidus. Paroxetine, a

selective serotonin reuptake inhibitor, is also used for depression and anxiety. It can cause anxiety, agitation, and sexual dysfunction. Thioridazine, a phenothiazine, is an antipsychotic medication. It may cause sedation as well as cardiotoxicity. This answer is not correct because this patient does not suffer from psychosis.

Block 2

51. B. This patient most likely has a prolactinoma that is causing amenorrhea and the breast discharge. Bilateral involvement is more suggestive of this diagnosis. It is best to obtain a prolactin level. Pregnancy is less likely due to the 4 months of amenorrhea with no palpable uterus. A TSH would be useful if she was experiencing weight changes and hot spells. LH and β-hCG would be tested if pregnancy were a concern.

52. A. REM sleep is similar on EEG to the awake period; the sleeper may experience erections, increased pulse, eye movements, and dreaming. Stage 1 is classified as light sleep, during which theta waves are seen on the EEG. Most of stage 2 is characterized by sleep spindles and K complexes. Stages 3 and 4 are classified as slow-wave sleep, during which night terrors and sleepwalking may be experienced.

53. A. Benign prostatic hyperplasia is a common disease seen in men beginning around age 50. Symptoms include increased frequency, urgency, and nocturia with difficulty initiating the urine stream. Urethral stricture can cause similar symptoms but is usually associated with anuria and pain. Urinary tract infection and pyelonephritis would include irritative symptoms such as urgency, dysuria, and hematuria. Bladder tumor is almost always associated with painless hematuria.

54. A. The patient presents with primary amenorrhea due a lack of pulsatility of gonadotropin-releasing hormone (GnRH), which is secondary to her extreme exercise. There is no reason to suspect that she is anorexic, but this should be considered. The normal cervical and bimanual exam rules out the anatomical causes. Those with gonadal agenesis do not have breast development.

55. A. This is typical of a Stills murmur, the most common of the innocent murmurs. It is a continuous murmur with a vibratory sound. It usually goes away as the child grows. A patent ductus arteriosus is a continuous murmur with a machine-like sound. A venous hum is another innocent murmur; it is systolic in nature and is heard best under the right clavicle with the patient in the supine position. It disappears when the patient lies down or the jugular vein is compressed. The murmur of a peripheral pulmonic stenosis is another innocent murmur of infancy heard best either at the sternal border or in the axilla. It will also disappear as the infant grows. There is no history to suggest uremic pericarditis in this patient.

56. A. This is a common presentation for *Chlamydia trachomatis,* which causes a urethral discharge and is not seen on Gram's stain. *Neisseria gonorrhoeae* is always susceptible to ceftriaxone. Herpes simplex virus would present with vesicular lesions. *Chlamydia psittaci* is an atypical cause of pneumonia associated with exposure to birds. *Treponema pallidum* is the etiologic agent of syphilis. This individual does not have the characteristic chancre seen in syphilis. In general, this condition is not associated with urethritis.

57. E. This is a case of heroin overdose. Heroin is classified as an opioid. The opioids lead to euphoria, analgesia, sedation, constipation, and strong miosis. With toxicity, there is severe respiratory depression, nausea, and vomiting. Naloxone is the antidote used to reverse this reaction. Atropine is used for organophosphate toxicity. Flumazenil is the antidote for benzodiazepine toxicity. Ethyl alcohol may be used as a treatment for methanol poisoning. *N*-acetylcysteine is used for the treatment of acetaminophen overdose.

58. A. This patient has Bernard-Soulier disease, which is characterized by defective platelet adhesion to the endothelial wall caused by a defect in platelet glycoprotein Ib. Bernard-Soulier disease is an autosomal recessive disorder that often skips a generation, with parents being unaffected carriers. Platelets are often unusually large. Glanzmann's thrombasthenia is a disorder characterized by poor platelet aggregation due to a defective glycoprotein IIb-IIIa. Idiopathic thrombocytopenic purpura is an acquired condition caused by antiplatelet antibodies; it leads to thrombocytopenia. Thrombotic thrombocytopenic purpura is caused by a defective enzyme; it leads to thrombocytopenia, hemolytic anemia, and the propensity to form microthrombi in blood vessels. It is also characterized by neurological problems, renal insufficiency, and fever. Thrombocytopenia is simply a decreased platelet count and is not the cause of this patient's platelet disorder, since he had a normal platelet count.

59. A. Roseola is being described in the question stem. It is characterized by a prodrome of high fever, symptoms of upper respiratory infection (URI), palpebral injection, bulging fontanelle, and leukopenia. The fever and prodromal symptoms then subside, followed by a rash that appears up to 2 days later and is described as a 2- to 5-mm erythematous maculopapular eruption that may or may not have a white halo. This rash proceeds from the neck and trunk to the face and extremities. Roseola is caused by human herpesvirus 6. Morbillivirus is a paramyxovirus and causes measles. *Staphylococcus aureus* can cause Filatow-Dukes' disease. Group A beta-hemolytic streptococcus causes scarlet fever. Parvovirus B19 causes fifth ("slapped cheeks") disease.

60. B. Osteoarthritis due to excessive wear and tear on the joint may present as dermatomal pain. There is decreased chondrocyte formation to make up for cartilage loss, which exposes underlying bone. Thus, proteoglycan and cartilage synthesis are affected. Calcium oxalate crystals are found in kidney stones and calcium apatite crystals are found when cartilage breaks down. Hyperextension of the proximal interphalangeal (PIP) joints and flexion of the distal interphalangeal joints (DIP) is seen in rheumatoid arthritis. The wrists and ankles are usually spared in osteoarthritis but are affected in rheumatoid arthritis. The x-ray (Figure 6) reveals narrowing of the DIP joint space, with subluxation and osteophyte formation.

61. A. The disease described in the question is cytomegalovirus (CMV) infection. This can result in encephalomyelitis in addition to producing lesions in other organs such as the kidneys, liver, and lungs. Histologically, CMV infection is characterized by giant cells with eosinophilic inclusions in the nucleus and cytoplasm. Generally, those who contract CMV infection are immunocompromised, such as patients with AIDS. Poliomyelitis is characterized by degeneration of spinal anterior horn cells. Kuru is a type of central nervous system (CNS) infection transmitted by ingestion of human brain (e.g., by cannibals), which has been documented in New Guinea; patients infected with Kuru present with marked tremor, ataxia, slurred speech, and progressive mental deterioration. Creutzfeldt-Jakob disease (mad cow disease), or the variant form due to the ingestion of infected beef, is characterized by ataxia, rapidly progressive dementia, and death.

62. E. This patient has chronic bronchitis. The criteria are a productive cough for > 3 consecutive months in 2 or more years. In these patients, you will find hypersecretion of mucus due to hypertrophy of the mucus-secreting glands in the bronchioles. Patients often present with wheezing, crackles, and cyanosis. Chronic bronchitis is often associated with frequent bronchial infections due to smoking. A hereditary alpha$_1$-antitrypsin deficiency is seen in panacinar emphysema. Bronchial hyperresponsiveness is characteristic of asthma. Diffuse pulmonary interstitial fibrosis with ferruginous bodies is seen in asbestosis. It is caused by the inhalation of asbestos fibers. In chronic bronchitis as in any obstructive lung disease, the FEV$_1$/FVC ratio is < 80%. A FEV$_1$/FVC ratio > 80% is seen in restrictive lung diseases.

63. B. *Cryptosporidium parvum* is a protozoan parasite causing an untreatable or very poorly treatable chronic diarrhea in AIDS patients. In healthy individuals, the diarrhea is transient. The cysts can be found in undercooked meat or water and cannot be killed by chlorination. Acid-fast oocysts can be found in the stool, and a biopsy shows cysts in the intestinal glands. *Giardia lamblia* causes giardiasis. It is transmitted by cysts in the water and is diagnosed by trophozoites in the stool. *Vibrio cholerae,* found in contaminated water, is transmitted via the fecal-to-oral route. Watery diarrhea is common. *Yersinia enterocolitica* is transmitted by pet feces.

64. D. Loop diuretics act on the thick ascending limb, blocking the cotransport system and thus facilitating the excretion of sodium, potassium, and chloride, which in turn will increase the excretion of water—hence diuresis. Loop diuretics have little to no effect on other areas of the renal system. Carbonic anhydrase (acetazolamide) inhibitors act on the proximal convoluted tubules. Thiazide diuretics (hydrochlorothiazide) decrease sodium chloride transport in the distal convoluted tubule.

65. C. Four cyclic adenosine monophosphate (cAMP) molecules complex with two regulatory subunits that are bound to two molecules of protein kinase A catalytic subunits. Binding of the cAMP molecules causes the regulatory subunits to be released from protein kinase A. This liberation of the catalytic protein kinase A subunit allows phosphorylation of cellular proteins, leading to an effect such as the release of testosterone from Leydig cells.

66. E. This scenario fits the definition of malingering, which is the conscious faking of symptoms for secondary gain. The teenager doesn't want to go to school, so he fakes a fever, night sweats, and pallor. In somatization disorder, the patient has a variety of complaints in multiple organ systems for which, on further exploration, no cause can be found. It is important to rule out any possible multiorgan diseases, such as multiple sclerosis or systemic lupus erythematosus, before labeling a person with a somatization disorder. Major depressive disorder is characterized by five symptoms for at least 2 weeks. One of the symptoms must be a depressed mood or anhedonia. Bipolar disorder is defined by the presence of at least one episode of mania cycling with major depression. Body dysmorphic disorder exists when a person believes that his or her body is malformed in some way.

67. D. The fertile period during a 28-day menstrual cycle is about 120 hr. This is the case because sperm cannot survive in the female genital tract for more than 72 hr, while the ovum, once released from the follicle, is fertilizable for 36 hr. Thus, the entire fertile period is approximately 120 hr.

68. E. Ulcerative colitis (UC) is an inflammatory disease of the colonic superficial mucosa; it is always more intense in the rectum and usually involves the colon in a contiguous manner. It occurs predominantly between the ages of 15 and 35 years and usually presents with bloody diarrhea, abdominal pain, weight loss, and sometimes fever. This pathology is virtually diagnostic for UC. Pathology will reveal a superficial "pan-fried," inflamed appearance of the mucosa from the rectum continuously to the sigmoid colon. No granulomas are noted. Crohn's disease presents very much like UC except that it can involve the small intestine, the colon, or both. Crohn's includes transmural mucosal involvement. Fistulas, skip areas, and granulomas are also commonly seen in Crohn's. Bacterial colitis usually presents in a much more acute setting. Irritable bowel syndrome does not present with blood in the stools. It is characterized by abdominal pain, alternating diarrhea and constipation, dyspepsia, anxiety, and/or depression. Diverticulitis is normally seen in an older population and does not present with this type of pathology.

69. D. Rifampin is a drug classically associated with a red-orange discoloration of body fluids such as urine, stool, sweat, and tears (thus discoloring contact lenses). The other medications listed are not associated with this side effect. Ethambutol is associated with nausea, vomiting, headache, peripheral neuropathy, thrombocytopenia, hepatotoxicity, and retrobulbar neuritis. Isoniazid has toxicities similar to those of ethambutol. Trimethoprim-sulfamethoxazole is an antibiotic useful in the management of respiratory and genitourinary infections.

70. E. This patient has symptoms of infectious mononucleosis. Patients with this disease present with fever, lethargy, and splenomegaly. A heterophil antibody test (commonly called the Monospot test) is positive in these patients. The disease is caused by the Epstein-Barr virus, which invades maturing B cells. As a result, the immune system responds by rapidly producing T cells, some of which will begin to appear atypical. Atypical B cells do not occur in infectious mononucleosis, as they are the cells that are invaded. Eosinophils, macrophages, and white blood cells are not affected in patients with infectious mononucleosis.

71. E. Ringworm, a dermatophyte infection, is caused by *Tinea corporis*. It is classically a ring-shaped erythematous lesion, which shows hyphae when viewed under the microscope with potassium hydroxide (KOH). *Sporothrix schenckii* causes sporotrichosis, a cutaneous fungal infection. *Borrelia burgdorferi* causes Lyme disease. *Plasmodium* species cause malaria. *Candida albicans* is a member of the normal flora; it can cause infections in the vagina and mouth as well as systemically.

72. E. This patient has a normal chest x-ray. The left lateral film provides an excellent check on the posteroanterior (PA) appearance of the heart. When apparent enlargement to the left in the PA view is checked on the left lateral chest film, any increase in mass of the left ventricle will extend the border of the heart posteriorly and low against the diaphragm. The pulmonary vasculature is normal in this x-ray. There is no evidence of rib notching in this patient. The cardiothoracic ratio is measured from the PA projection.

73. A. This patient presents with the classic symptoms of the acute inflammatory demyelinating polyradiculoneuropathy known as Guillain-Barré syndrome (GBS), which is a life-threatening disorder of the peripheral nervous system (PNS). GBS is characterized by a motor neuropathy that results in ascending paralysis with acute onset of weakness in distal extremities (hands, feet) and rapidly affects the proximal muscles. Diagnostic tests include lumbar puncture, which demonstrates a significant increase in protein in the CSF; electromyography (EMG), which demonstrates loss of reflexes due to nervous response; and nerve conduction velocity (NCV) study, which shows decreased velocity. GBS is very often preceded by a viral upper respiratory tract infection and can affect individuals of any age, race, or sex. Trauma injuries that can lead to a demyelinating disorder have not been documented. The history of recurrent exacerbations with asymptomatic remissions and a progressive course describes multiple sclerosis, another demyelinating disease that usually presents with weakness in all aspects of the lower extremities. Mutations in the APP gene of chromosome 21 have been linked to the familial inheritance Alzheimer's disease. A long-standing history of alcoholism can lead to Wernicke's disease, or alcoholic encephalopathy. It is due to the combined effects of alcohol and thiamine deficiency and is characterized by marked atrophy of cerebral cortex, pons, cerebellar vermis, mamillary bodies, and other areas of gray matter.

74. E. Squamous cell carcinoma is the most common type of cancer of the larynx. Cigarette smoking is the most important risk factor. Laryngeal polyps are small and benign. They are usually associated with chronic irritation from excessive use or heavy cigarette smoking. Mucoepidermoid carcinoma and adenocarcinoma of the larynx are not as common as squamous cell carcinoma and do not have dysplasia as a precursor. Laryngotracheobronchitis is acute inflammation of the larynx, trachea, and epiglottis. It is most often caused by a viral infection.

75. B. Osteogenesis imperfecta is an inherited disorder that causes a generalized decrease in bone mass, which makes bones brittle. This condition is frequently associated with blue sclerae, dental abnormalities, progressive hearing loss, and a positive family history. Patients with osteoarthritis (OI) have defects in the genes that code for collagen. There are four different classifications of OI, each with several subtypes. The disease is variable and can be very mild or result in death in utero, at birth, or shortly thereafter. Often, x-rays reveal decreased bone density. Child abuse is defined as any interaction or lack of interaction between family members that results in nonaccidental harm to the child's physical or developmental well-being. Abuse should be suspected in any child presenting with failure to thrive, apparent soft tissue injury, broken bones, and/or a story (told by the parent) that does not fit the injuries. Osteopetrosis, also known as Albers-Schönberg or marble bone disease, is a condition in which there is increased bone mass secondary to a defect in bone resorption. Although these patients are also more prone to sustain fractures, their x-rays appear hyperdense. Osteosarcoma is the most common malignancy of bone and typically presents with pain and swelling in a bone or joint (especially the knee). Radiographs reveal both bone destruction and production as well as periosteal elevation. Scurvy is a nutritional deficit of vitamin C and results in bleeding gums, impaired formation of mature connective tissue, impaired bone growth, and ultimately failure to thrive (if not corrected).

76. D. This patient consumes 50 g of carbohydrate at 4 kcal/g or 200 calories. He consumes 10 g of protein at 4 kcal/g or 40 calories and consumes 20 g of fat at 9 kcal/g or 180 calories. In summary, he consumes 200 + 40 + 180 = 420 calories per day.

77. B. This patient has an amniotic fluid embolism. The underlying cause of this is infusion of the amniotic fluid into the maternal circulation due to a tear in the placental membranes and rupture of the uterine veins. This has a mortality of rate of about 80% or greater. It is an important cause of maternal mortality because many other obstetric complications have been managed with medical intervention. Fat emboli are associated with long bone fractures. Tumor emboli can result from primary cardiac tumors, such as myxoma. Thrombus can originate in the deep veins of the lower extremities.

78. E. This woman most likely has a leiomyoma, or uterine fibroid. Leiomyomas are the most common uterine tumors as well as the most common tumors in women. The incidence of leiomyoma is increased in African American women. They are benign neoplasms with a very low malignant transformation rate, much less than 15%. Leiomyosarcomas arise de novo and are almost never caused by malignant transformation of leiomyomas. Leiomyomas usually occur in multiple foci simultaneously and are estrogen-sensitive tumors that often increase in size during pregnancy and almost always

decrease in size during menopause. The most common manifestation of leiomyoma is menorrhagia.

79. A. This patient is suffering from primary cortical insufficiency, which is most commonly caused by acute adrenal crisis secondary to destruction of the adrenal cortex. This leads to increased production of adrenocorticotropic hormone (ACTH) with decreased glucocorticoid, androgen, and mineralocorticoid production. Owing to the low level of cortisol, increased ACTH attempts to stimulate the cortisol. The ACTH contains melanin-stimulating hormone factors, which accounts for the "sunless" tanning. The aldosterone deficiency is responsible for hyperkalemia, hypotension, and metabolic acidosis. Conn's syndrome is characterized by increased aldosterone levels with hypertension (HTN) and potassium wasting. Hemochromatosis is a genetic disorder of iron metabolism leading to the accumulation of iron in different organs. One usually sees a bronze color of the skin but there will also be cardiac and liver involvement. Pineal gland tumor will produce excess melatonin, not melanin, which is responsible for regulating the sleep-wake cycle. Wermer's syndrome is a multiple endocrine neoplasia characterized by pituitary, parathyroid, and pancreatic involvement.

80. B. Osteomalacia (the adult form of rickets) is a disorder in which mineralization of the organic matrix of the skeleton is defective; it is caused by a number of different conditions associated with vitamin D deficiency or resistance. The presenting symptoms are usually bone pain and muscle weakness. Osteomalacia secondary to chronic renal failure results in a state of hyperphosphatemia, hypocalcemia with a normal 25(OH)D and low 1,25(OH)$_2$D levels. In secondary hyperparathyroidism, one is likely to see normal to elevated levels of 1,25(OH)$_2$D. In vitamin D deficiency due to dietary lack, inadequate sunlight exposure, or intestinal malabsorption calcium levels may be low or normal, while phosphorus and 25(OH)D levels are low. In a patient with nephritic syndrome, one would see low 25(OH)D levels secondary to urinary losses of vitamin D–binding protein-bound 25(OH)D. Patients with renal tubular disorders will have normal serum calcium levels and hypophosphatemia.

81. C. This patient most likely has dermatitis herpetiformis. This disease is characterized by urticarial plaques and vesicles that occur in groups. Dermatitis herpetiformis is pathologically characterized by granular deposits of IgA in the tips of the dermal papillae upon immunofluorescent staining. The disease has also been consistently associated with celiac sprue (gluten-sensitive enteropathy), of which the patient shows symptoms. A netlike pattern of intercellular IgG deposits would be seen with the multisystem disease systemic lupus erythematosus. Extensive parakeratosis would be seen with any form of dermatitis and psoriasis. HLA-B27 positivity is found with ankylosing spondylosis, which involves the sacroiliac joint. Linear deposition of immunoglobulin along the basement membrane would be seen with Goodpasture's syndrome, which presents with pulmonary and renal manifestations.

82. E. This infant has a tracheoesophageal fistula. This is an abnormal communication between the trachea and esophagus by a malformation of the tracheoesophageal septum. Along with the symptoms described above, it results in reflux of the gastric contents into the lungs. In the most common variant, the lower portion of the esophagus communicates with the trachea near the tracheal bifurcation. This is associated with maternal polyhydramnios. Neonatal respiratory distress syndrome is due to a surfactant deficiency that leads to an increased surface tension and ultimately respiratory collapse. Pulmonary hypoplasia occurs when lung development is stunted. Predisposing factors are congenital diaphragmatic hernia and bilateral renal agenesis. Pyloric stenosis is caused by hypertrophy of the muscular layer of the pylorus. It causes projectile vomiting in the first 2 weeks of life. Barrett's esophagus is columnar metaplasia of the esophageal squamous epithelium, which can be caused by reflux. Such patients have an increased risk of adenocarcinoma.

83. E. Quinidine is a drug associated with idiopathic thrombocytopenic purpura (ITP), along with heparin, quinine, phenytoin, carbamazepine, penicillin, and most sulfa drugs. The remaining drugs on the list are not associated with ITP. Lidocaine and mexiletine are analogs of lidocaine. Side effects can include drowsiness, dizziness, paresthesias, and euphoria.

84. B. Vulvar cancer is most closely related to cervical cancer, and HPV DNA is commonly found in both cancers. Because the patient did get some relief from the single dose of fluconazole, the likelihood of this being a benign condition is increased. This patient is too young to have malignant breast cancer. She is more likely to have a fibroadenoma, a benign lesion. Colon cancer is unlikely given the patient's age and lack of gastrointestinal symptoms. Endometrial cancer is rare in patients under 30 years of age. Ovarian cancer is also unlikely, given this patient's age.

85. A. Acute attacks of gout commonly present in middle-aged men and affect the first metatarsophalangeal joint. Gout is caused by hyperuricemia secondary to overproduction or underexcretion of uric acid. Risk factors for gout include alcohol consumption, medications (especially diuretics, cyclosporine, low-dose aspirin, and niacin), myeloproliferative disorders, and chronic renal disease. In the acute phase of gout, as in this patient, aspiration of the joint will show negatively birefringent, needle-like crystals found free or within neutrophils; these findings confirm the diagnosis.

Allopurinol is a xanthine oxidase inhibitor and functions to lower plasma and urinary uric acid concentrations. This drug is a useful maintenance drug in the treatment of uric acid overproduction. It is not useful in the setting of an acute attack, and empiric treatment does not confirm the diagnosis. Both intravenous and oral corticosteroids can be used to treat the inflammation of acute attacks of gout; however, steroids treat only the symptoms and have no role in diagnosis. The radiologic appearance of gout is highly variable, especially in acute attacks. With chronic tophaceous gout, one will generally see lesions in the subchondral bone. Radiologic studies are useful in determining the extent of damage to a joint, but they do not confirm the diagnosis. Determination of the serum urate concentration is useful in the management of gout if the level is obtained within the first 24-hr of the attack. However, uric acid levels do not confirm the diagnosis of gout.

86. A. The correct answer is that she does not need to worry. Since she is having a boy, there is no risk. The distinguishing feature of an X-linked dominant condition is that *all* of the daughters and *none* of the sons of an affected male with a normal mate will have the condition. It is safe to assume that the son of this couple will not have the disease. However, if the mother were affected as well as the father, the risks would change. There would be a 100% chance if they had a girl and a 50% chance if they had a boy.

87. C. This patient most likely has developed thrombotic thrombocytopenia purpura (TTP) secondary to ticlopidine administration following coronary artery stent placement. Thus, discontinuing ticlopidine and starting plasmapheresis is the best approach to treatment. Atenolol is a beta-blocker and is not associated with the development of thrombotic thrombocytopenic purpura. Nitrates are not associated with development of TTP. This condition is not infectious and is not likely to improve with antibiotic therapy. Administration of platelets is unlikely to be of immediate benefit to this patient.

88. C. The reflection coefficient is a number between 0 and 1 and indicates the ease with which a solute can pass through a membrane. If the reflection coefficient is 1, the solute will cause water flow. The solute is probably a large molecule, such as albumin, which is impermeable. The solute will not generate an osmotic effect. The solute is completely impermeable. The solute is similar in size to albumin.

89. C. Hyperosmotic volume contraction. Sweat is hyposmotic compared to the amount of water lost, so the osmolarity of the extracellular fluid (ECF) increases as the ECF volume decreases. Owing to the increased ECF osmolarity, water shifts out of the intracellular fluid (ICF) into the ECF, thus decreasing the volume of the ICF.

90. A. This patient has acute bacterial endocarditis, classified as endocarditis with large vegetations on otherwise normal valves. It has a very rapid onset and is caused by *Staphylococcus aureus*. A 6-hour acute onset makes this answer stand out. *Streptococcus viridans* is the cause of subacute bacterial endocarditis. This type of endocarditis has the same presenting symptoms but has a much more insidious onset. The echocardiogram reveals the vegetation attached to the anterior leaflet of the mitral valve. *Streptococcus pneumoniae* is not a cause of endocarditis; it usually causes meningitis and pneumonia in older children and adults. *Streptococcus pyogenes* causes rheumatic fever after a pharyngeal infection. It has a late onset and does not present with a new heart murmur and rapid onset. *Treponema pallidum* causes syphilis and the aorta can be affected in the tertiary form of the disease. This does not have a rapid onset and it does not present with a new heart murmur.

91. D. Polycystic ovary syndrome characteristically occurs in young women and is an important cause of infertility. It is clinically characterized by amenorrhea, obesity, and hirsutism. It may be caused by excess luteinizing hormone (LH) and androgens and is associated with insulin resistance and an increased risk of diabetes mellitus. It is believed that the hyperinsulinemia may lead to increased androgen production, which in turn may lead to increased LH. Chocolate cyst is a blood-containing cyst due to ovarian endometriosis. Corpus luteum cyst is due to hemorrhage into a persistent corpus luteum. Follicular cyst is distension of an unruptured graafian follicle. Theca lutein cyst is associated with choriocarcinoma or molar pregnancy.

92. E. This woman is suffering from somatization disorder. She has a variety of complaints in multiple organ systems and, with further exploration, no cause can be found. It is important to rule out any possible multiorgan diseases, such as multiple sclerosis or systemic lupus erythematosus, before labeling a person with somatization disorder. Obsessive-compulsive disorder is characterized by obsessions, which are recurrent intrusive thoughts, and compulsions, which are repeated actions done in order to reduce the anxiety from the compulsions. Schizotypal personality disorder is characterized by interpersonal awkwardness and odd thought patterns and behaviors. Schizophreniform disorder is similar to schizophrenia, but the duration of symptoms is from 1 month to 6 months, whereas schizophrenia has symptoms present for > 6 months.

93. C. Pregnenolone is the result of the enzyme desmolase acting on cholesterol. All of the other choices are precursor hormones in the adrenal steroid pathway. 17 hydroxypregnenolone is converted to dehydroepiandrosterone (DHEA), which can then be converted to androgens. 17 hydroxyprogesterone can be converted to androstenedione and then to estrone. 17 hydroxyprogesterone can also be converted to cortisol via the 11 deoxycortisol pathway.

94. E. The patient described presents with the classic triad (confusion, ataxia, ophthalmoplegia) symptomatic of alcoholic encephalopathy or Wernicke's syndrome. This condition is caused by the combined effects of alcoholism and thiamine deficiency. The degeneration of lateral corticospinal tracts describes amyotrophic lateral sclerosis (ALS). Depigmentation of the substantia nigra and locus ceruleus is characteristic of Parkinson's disease. Huntington's disease is characterized by increased numbers of CAG trinucleotide repeats in the huntingtin gene of the short arm of chromosome 4. Marked cortical atrophy significant in the temporal and frontal lobes is found in Pick's disease.

95. D. Studies have shown an increased occurrence of patent ductus arteriosis in pregnant mothers living in elevated/higher altitudes. A possible explanation is fetal oxygen deprivation. Atrial septal defect has not been shown to correlate with increased altitudes. Down's syndrome tends to be associated with advanced age of the birth mother. Mitral valve prolapse is associated with rheumatic fever, with no bearing in elevation.

96. C. Antagonists at the 5HT3 receptor include agents such as ondansetron (Zofran), which is highly effective in the treatment of nausea and vomiting associated with chemotherapy. This agent inhibits receptors for 5HT3 in the area postrema, which will prevent nausea and vomiting and might have an added effect by reducing peripheral sensation of pain. The 5HT1 receptors cause smooth muscle contraction, especially in the carotid artery, as well as platelet aggregation. The dopamine receptors play a minor role in the treatment of chemotherapy-associated nausea and vomiting.

97. E. 21 β-Hydroxylase deficiency is the most prevalent biochemical abnormality of the steroid-producing pathway. The enzyme block prevents the production of the aldosterone and cortisol precursors. There are increased levels of ACTH due to the lack of cortisol inhibition. Meig's syndrome is associated with the triad of ovarian fibroma, ascites, and hydrothorax. Polycystic ovary syndrome (Stein-Leventhal syndrome) is associated with increased levels of LH due to peripheral estrogen production, which leads to anovulation. It is manifest clinically by amenorrhea, infertility, obesity, and hirsutism. Virilization is simply the possession of mature masculine features as a result of gonadal or adrenocortical deficiency.

98. E. Disease-modifying antirheumatic drugs (DMARDs) are medications employed in the treatment of rheumatoid arthritis. The effect of these drugs does not manifest until weeks or even months after therapy is initiated. These drugs slow the course of disease and may actually put a patient with a rheumatologic condition into remission. Some drugs in this category include methotrexate, leflunomide, hydroxychloroquine, gold salts, sulfasalazine, minocycline, azathioprine, D-penicillamine, cyclosporine, and cyclophosphamide. Indomethacin is a nonsteroidal anti-inflammatory drug (NSAID) commonly used in the treatment of pain and inflammation. It inhibits cyclooxygenase 1 and 2 (COX-1 and COX-2). Lisinopril is an angiotensin-converting enzyme (ACE) inhibitor that functions to lower blood pressure by reducing peripheral vascular resistance. It accomplishes this by blocking ACE, which cleaves angiotensin I to form the potent vasoconstrictor angiotensin II. Metformin is a biguanide used in the treatment of type II DM. It acts by decreasing hepatic glucose output by inhibiting gluconeogenesis, thereby decreasing the level of glucose in the blood. It also aids in the reduction of hyperlipidemia (low-density lipoprotein [LDL] and very low density lipoprotein [VLDL] fall, high-density lipoprotein [HDL] rises). Premarin is an estrogen/progestin combination given to postmenopausal women to help control menopausal symptoms and prevent osteoporosis.

99. E. Rheumatoid arthritis is a chronic systemic inflammatory disease of unknown cause chiefly affecting synovial membranes of multiple joints. If affects 1 to 2% of the general population and is found in women three times as often as in men. Clinical manifestations are highly variable but often include malaise, weight loss, and vague periarticular pain or stiffness. There is characteristically symmetrical joint swelling with associated stiffness, warmth, tenderness, and pain. The condition can be hereditary.

Ankylosing spondylitis is a chronic inflammatory disease of the spinal sacroiliac joints. It can result in a stiff spine, uveitis, and aortic regurgitation. Reiter's syndrome is associated with urethritis, conjunctivitis, and arthritis. Osteoarthritis is associated with mechanical wear and tear of the joints, leading to destruction of articular cartilage, subchondral bone formation, and osteophytes. Rheumatoid arthritis is an autoimmune disorder that affects the synovial joints (MCP, PIP), giving rise to rheumatoid nodules, ulnar deviation, and subluxation.

100. D. The correct answer is paracentric inversion. An inversion is a chromosomal rearrangement in which there are two breaks on a single chromosome with inverted reincorporation of the segment. There are paracentric inversions and pericentric inversions. Paracentric inversions do not include the centromere and both breaks occur on one chromosomal arm. Pericentric inversions *do* include the centromere and there are breaks in each chromosomal arm. An isochromosome is a chromosomal mutation where one arm is missing and the other is duplicated in a mirror-image fashion. A ring chromosome results when a deletion occurs at both ends of a chromosome with fusion of the deleted ends. A deletion is a loss of a section on a chromosome. An insertion is the gain of a section on one chromosome from another chromosome.

Block 3

101. A. This patient has Crohn's disease, based on the skip lesions and cobblestone appearance. Erythema nodosum is an extraintestinal manifestation of Crohn's disease. Pseudopolyps and *Clostridium difficile* are more commonly associated with ulcerative colitis. Sarcoidosis is not associated with Crohn's disease. Anemia may be present due to chronic blood loss, but it would not be a megaloblastic anemia. Figure 11 shows the slide of this patient's colonoscopy of the right colon. Cobblestoning and ulceration are noted.

102. A. Alcohol is the only substance listed here that is associated with congenital anomalies (fetal alcohol syndrome and cardiac defects). Cocaine use has been associated with CNS effects and developmental delay in the exposed child. Tobacco use has been associated with small for-gestational-age fetuses and increased respiratory disease in childhood. Opiates and caffeine do not have any particular fetal effects, although fetuses exposed to opiates during pregnancy need to be weaned off after delivery.

103. B. Conversion disorder is characterized by symptoms suggesting a motor or sensory neurological or physical disorder but tests and physical exam are negative. The symptoms are usually preceded by some stressful situation. PTSD is a diagnosis that requires the person to have been exposed to some stressor causing actual or threatened harm. Symptoms usually persist for > 1 month. Somatization disorder is characterized by a variety of complaints in multiple organ systems. Adjustment disorder relates to a stressor, but symptoms start within 3 weeks and end within 6 weeks of the end of the stressor. Hypochondriasis is a condition in which one misinterprets normal physical findings, leading to a preoccupation with and fear of having a serious illness.

104. A. Adenomyositis is the extension of endometrial glands in the uterine musculature. These patients usually present with dysmenorrhea. Asherman's syndrome causes secondary amenorrhea. It is characterized by the formation of intrauterine adhesions or synechiae. It is unusual to find it causing dysmenorrhea. Pregnancy would not be associated with a period. She is not in the age range for uterine carcinoma, so this is not probable. A urinary tract infection usually presents with dysuria along with hematuria.

105. A. Salicylates are the drugs of choice in the treatment of the milder forms of inflammatory disease. This includes acute rheumatic fever, rheumatoid arthritis, osteoarthritis, and mild systemic lupus erythematosus. Common adverse effects include GI disturbances (heartburn, indigestion) and peptic ulcers. Methotrexate is currently recommended for adults with severe active rheumatoid arthritis who have demonstrated an insufficient response to nonsteroidal anti-inflammatory agents.

106. C. The correct answer is maternal inheritance of a mitochondrial mutation. The ovum, not the sperm, supplies the developing zygote with *all* of its mitochondria. Therefore, if the mother has a mutant mitochondrial DNA (mtDNA), all of her children will acquire the mtDNA. However, if the father has an mtDNA, none of his children will acquire the condition. The clinical scenario presented above is typical of maternal inheritance of mitochondrial mutations. All of Susan's children have the disease, whereas Sam's children are fine. Specifically, the disease described here is Leber's hereditary optic neuropathy. This condition is not inherited in either an autosomal dominant or recessive fashion or in an x-linked fashion.

107. C. This patient has idiopathic thrombocytopenic purpura (ITP). Although it is called idiopathic, the disease is autoimmune in etiology. The diagnosis is one of exclusion. In ITP, all blood cell lines are normal except for a decreased platelet count. In thrombotic thrombocytopenic purpura (TTP), along with a decreased platelet count, PT and PTT values are usually elevated. Disseminated intravascular coagulopathy presents with similar symptoms but also manifests increased PT, PTT, platelet count, and fibrin split products. Acute myelogenous leukemia is excluded because of a normal white blood cell count and differential. Pseudothrombocytopenia results from clotting and gathering of platelets in the tube.

108. D. The described structure is a pacinian corpuscle and is primarily responsible for serving as a deep pressure receptor for mechanical and vibratory pressure. These structures are characteristically onion-shaped and are usually found in the deeper dermis of the skin. Electromagnetic radiation receptors are the rods and cones located in the retina of the eye. Fine touch receptors are the Meissner's corpuscles. These are located in the dermal papillae and appear as tapered cylinders oriented perpendicular to the skin surface. Hot temperature receptors are essentially free nerve endings that are distributed throughout the dermal layer of the skin. Although one may think that there are sound receptors located in the ear, there are not. The hair cells of the organ of Corti actually respond to the mechanical deformation produced by sound waves.

109. C. The child described most likely has developed a neural tube defect, which is characterized by the failure of closure and can be found on physical exam as dimpling along the vertebrae. These congenital defects are associated with maternal folic acid deficiency. Risk for these disorders, such as spina bifida, can be decreased with prenatal supplements. Fetal alcohol syndrome is associated with excessive alcohol abuse by the mother and is characterized by abnormal facies, microcephaly, atrial septal defect, mental and growth retardation, as well as other anomalies. Amniocentesis is the surgical insertion of a needle through the abdominal wall and into the uterus of a pregnant female to obtain amniotic fluid in order to specifically examine the fetal chromosomes for an abnormality and for the determination of sex. Measles mumps rubella (MMR) vaccination prior to pregnancy is protective against congenital rubella, which puts the fetus at increased risk for a variety of problems, including deafness, heart problems, cataracts, mental retardation, and other developmental defects. Monitoring for hypertension is a good way to assess preeclampsia, a toxic condition developing in late pregnancy that is characterized by a sudden rise in blood pressure, excessive gain in weight, generalized edema, albuminuria, severe headache, and visual disturbances. Preeclampsia has the potential to progress to eclampsia, or a convulsive state.

110. B. DiGeorge's syndrome results in thymic hypoplasia due to the lack of development of pharyngeal pouches 3 and 4. Truncus arteriosus is most commonly associated with this syndrome, along with abnormal facial features and hypocalcemia. A cleft lip is caused when the maxillary prominence fails to fuse with the medial nasal prominence. It commonly occurs with cleft palate, which arises when the palatine shelves fail to fuse with each other or the primary palate. Ankyloglossia occurs when the tongue is not freed from the floor of the mouth. The most common variation occurs when the frenulum extends to the tip of the tongue. Craniosynostosis is caused by the premature closure of one or more sutures in the skull. Pharyngeal pouches 3 and 4 differentiate into the parathyroid glands and the thymus. Failure of this process causes DiGeorge's syndrome, which is characterized by lymphopenia, recurrent viral and fungal infections, and tetany.

111. D. This patient has osteosarcoma caused by radium exposure from well water. Excessive levels of radium can be found in drinking water from deep wells, especially in New Jersey and Wisconsin. Radium exposure increases the risk of developing osteosarcoma. This main malignancy affects long bones and presents on x-ray with elevation of the periosteum, called Codman's triangle. Ewing's sarcoma, due to expression of C-*myc*, is also associated with a periosteal reaction but presents in children as an onionskin-like bone deposition on x-ray. Fibrous dysplasia, or lack of differentiation seen on x-ray, shows defined margins and a ground-glass appearance. Chondrosarcoma, or proliferation of growth-plate cartilage, is seen in 20- to 40-year-olds. *Staphylococcus aureus* will show a lytic core surrounded by sclerosis.

112. G. Ventricular septal defect is the most common congenital cardiac defect. The size of these defects is often variable; they may decrease in size as patients grow older. This accounts for the presentation of a murmur early in childhood that later disappears. Often these defects are insignificant and lack a detectable murmur. If large enough, a left-to-right shunt will occur until pulmonary hypertension is reversed; the right-to-left shunt causes more severe cyanotic episodes. Atrial septal defect is associated with a left-to-right shunt, which results in late cyanosis. The S_1 heart sound is loud and there is wide splitting of a fixed S_2. Patent ductus arteriosus (PDA) is also associated with a left-to-right shunt and late cyanosis. The PDA can be closed with indomethacin treatment. Tetralogy of Fallot is the most common cause of early cyanosis. It is the result of a right-to-left shunt and results in early cyanosis.

113. C. Membranous glomerulonephritis commonly occurs in teenagers and young adults. There is also an association with hepatitis B, malaria, and syphilis infection. Renal biopsy can reveal a "spike and dome" appearance. IgG and C3 deposits on immunofluorescence are generally characteristic of immune complex diseases, such as this one. This condition is slowly progressive and often refractory to steroids. Minimal change disease is a nephrotic syndrome. Most often it is seen in young children and less commonly in adolescents and adults. Pathological findings include lipid-laden renal cortices, most commonly in the proximal convoluted tubular cells. The images shown (Figure 12) are typical of membranous glomerulonephritis. The silver-stain images show spikes outside the capillary loop. The electron microscopic image shows immune deposits as black lumps on the basement membrane, and the immunofluorescence stain shows trapping of IgG in the basement membrane.

114. D. Peutz-Jeghers syndrome is inherited in an autosomal dominant fashion and is characterized by intestinal polyposis and mucocutaneous hyperpigmentation. Polyps are hamartomas most commonly found in the jejunum and ileum. The malignant potential of these polyps is low.

115. C. *Haemophilus ducreyi* is a sexually transmitted disease common in tropical areas but rare in the United States. It is characterized by a soft, painful, ulcerated lesion that differs from the chancre of syphilis, which is firm and painless. *Calymmatobacterium granulomatis* is a Gram-negative rod that is probably sexually transmitted. It appears initially as a papule, which becomes superficially ulcerated. It progresses as adjacent lesions coalesce to form large genital or inguinal ulcerations. Gonococcal infections are associated with the Gram-negative diplococci. *Chlamydia trachomatis* causes nongonococcal urethritis, which is treated with tetracycline or erythromycin. Herpes simplex virus would be associated with the characteristic lesion of grouped vesicles on an erythematous base.

116. E. Granular deposits of IgG, IgM, and C3 are characteristic of poststreptococcal glomerulonephritis, in this case due to an infected insect bite. The organisms involved are almost exclusively group A beta-hemolytic strains of *Streptococcus;* such glomerulonephritis is thus also seen more classically 1 to 2 weeks after infection of the pharynx. Impetigo may also serve as a starting point for the disease. Most cases resolve, but a small minority of patients may develop rapidly progressive glomerulonephritis. Linear immunofluorescence as a result of deposition of anti–basement membrane antibody is seen in Goodpasture's syndrome. Trophozoites of *Giardia lamblia* may be found on diarrhea stool cultures, but neither the organisms nor their spawn are normally found in urine. The finding of intracellular bacteria in macrophages is suggestive of *Brucella;* bacteria in capillary endothelial cells suggest *Rickettsia*. Although both of these organisms may be acquired in mountainous areas, they are not the causative agents of disease in this young explorer.

117. B. This patient has Kallman's syndrome, an autosomal dominant condition characterized by anosmia and decreased production of GnRH by the hypothalamus. This patient's mother also had anosmia and difficulty in trying to conceive, indicating the autosomal dominant pattern of inheritance. Clomiphene, a GnRH agonist, can be given in a pulsatile fashion to increase the patient's chances of conceiving. Polycystic ovary syndrome is another cause of failure to conceive and often leads to obesity and hirsutism. It is believed to be caused by an increase in the secretion of LH and a decrease in that of FSH. Klinefelter's syndrome causes infertility in males and is caused by an XXY genotype, which leads to hypogonadism. Turner's syndrome causes infertility in females and is caused by an XO genotype, which often leads to atrophic ovaries, shortened stature, and a webbed neck. XYY syndrome is a cause of mental retardation in males, which may be associated with acne and an increased tendency toward criminal activity or antisocial behavior.

118. C. The only exceptions to confidentiality are that (1) the potential of harm to others is serious, (2) the likelihood of harm to self is great, (3) no alternative means exist to warn or protect those at risk, and (4) the physician can take steps to prevent harm. Suspected child and/or elder abuse falls under the above exceptions. You must report suspected abuse in order to protect the victim and others against potential harm. In the other three cases, the patient's confidentiality must be upheld until the patient gives you permission to reveal certain details.

119. A. Allopurinol is the drug of choice in the treatment of chronic tophaceous gout and is especially useful in those patients whose treatment is complicated by the presence of renal insufficiency. Allopurinol reduces serum urea levels through a competitive inhibition of xanthine oxidase. This results in a reduction of the urinary concentration of uric acid and increases the excretion of the more soluble compounds xanthine and hypoxanthine. Colchicine is the first-line anti-inflammatory agent used in the treatment of acute gouty arthritis. Therapy with colchicine is usually begun at the first sign of an acute attack and is continued until symptoms subside. Indomethacin is a nonsteroidal anti-inflammatory agent. Probenecid is used in the management of chronic gout. It inhibits resorption of uric acid and also inhibits the synthesis of penicillin. Phenylbutazone is not used in the management of this patient.

120. D. Gravida refers to the number of pregnancies including whether the woman is currently pregnant. Parity refers to the number of deliveries. If delivery occurs from 37 to 42 weeks, the number goes in the space immediately following the P. From 28 to 36 weeks, it goes two spaces next to the P. If any abortions/miscarriages occurred, the number goes in the third space after the P. The number of living children goes in the fourth space after the P. Twins count as only 1 pregnancy. Since this woman is in her sixth pregnancy and has had two term births, one twin birth under 36 weeks, two miscarriages, and has four living children, she is a G6P2124.

121. B. B cells and other professional antigen-presenting cells possess both major histocompatibility complex (MHC) I, which recognizes CD8+ T cells, and MHC II, which recognizes CD4+ T cells. All the other cell types in the answer choices only possess MHC I, as this is present on all nucleated cells.

122. D. The ligamentum flavum unites the laminae of adjacent vertebrae and would be pierced during lumbar puncture to obtain CSF. The anterior and posterior longitudinal ligaments are located on the anterior and posterior sides of the vertebral bodies and would not be pierced during this procedure. The conus medullaris is the terminal end of the spinal cord and would certainly not be pierced during lumbar puncture. The dentate ligaments separate the ventral and dorsal roots and also help to stabilize the spinal cord. They would not have to be pierced during this procedure.

123. E. IgM is the first immunoglobulin to appear after the primary exposure to an antigen. It has a half-life of approximately 10 days. Therefore if elevated levels of IgM are detected, recent exposure to an antigen or infection is suggested. IgG is the antibody that is formed late in the primary immune response (approximately at day 10).

However, IgG is the primary antibody produced in the secondary immune response to an antigen that has already been presented to the host. Therefore, had this been the second time the young girl were exposed to the chickenpox virus, she would have had higher levels of IgG. IgE is the main antibody released in response to allergic reactions. IgA is an important component of mucosal immunity and is found primarily in secretions from respiratory and intestinal membranes as well as in tears and saliva. The function of IgD is unknown.

124. A. This is the presentation of osteoporosis, which can be caused by chronic steroid use and is often seen among body builders. The wrist fracture was the initial sign of osteoporosis. This condition stems from a reduction in bone mass in spite of normal bone mineralization. Type I osteoporosis occurs in postmenopausal women and results in increased bone resorption due to decreased estrogen levels. Type II occurs in patients over the age of 70. Caucasians are affected more than African Americans.

125. E. This patient complains of abdominal obesity, striae, and hirsutism and has Cushing's syndrome. The use of glucocorticoids, such as prednisone, is the most common cause of Cushing's syndrome. Long-term use of glucocorticoids can produce a variety of symptoms including abdominal obesity, moon facies, muscle weakness, bone destruction, and immune suppression. Ovarian neoplasms can produce an excess of estrogen or testosterone, depending on the type of tumor involved. For instance, a granulosa cell tumor would produce an excess of estrogen. Ovarian tumors do not produce Cushing's syndrome because they do not produce an excess of cortisol. This patient's symptoms could be caused by a pituitary adenoma, in which excess ACTH is produced, leading to an increase in the adrenal production of cortisol. Whenever a pituitary adenoma is the cause of the symptoms, the condition is referred to as Cushing's disease. Whenever any other cause exists, the condition is called Cushing's syndrome. A cortisol-producing adrenal adenoma could also be the cause of this patient's condition. However, given the history of prednisone usage, neoplasms are less likely to be responsible. Polycystic ovary syndrome (PCOS) is a condition that is often found in obese females and is associated with an increase in estrogen and testosterone. Patients with PCOS often manifest obesity and hirsutism, like this patient, but often do not have the same distribution of fat deposition as do patients with Cushing's syndrome. Cushing's syndrome patients have abdominal obesity, moon facies, and a buffalo hump, whereas PCOS patients typically have fat distribution in a pattern consistent with high estrogen, which tends to be in the hips, buttocks, and thighs.

126. C. This boy has Hand-Schüller-Christian disease, a form of Langerhans cell histiocytosis (histiocytosis X). Langerhans disease comprises a group of clinical diseases associated with the proliferation of Langerhans cells. These cells contain granules called Birbeck granules, which resemble tennis rackets. The peak age for Hand-Schüller-Christian disease is 2 to 6 years. It is characterized by diabetes insipidus, exophthalmos, and lytic bone lesions in the calvarium and at the base of the skull. The lesions are caused by a proliferation of Langerhans cells. Lesions around the hypothalamus lead to decreased ADH production, which results in the symptoms of diabetes insipidus. The other two forms of Langerhans cell histiocytosis are Letterer-Siwe disease and eosinophilic granuloma. Letterer-Siwe disease affects children < 3 years old. It is characterized by cutaneous lesions that resemble seborrhea, hepatosplenomegaly, and lymphadenopathy. Eosinophilic granuloma is seen in older patients. It is characterized by granulomas containing Langerhans cells, monocytes-macrophages, lymphocytes, and eosinophils. Diabetes mellitus type I is due to a failure of insulin synthesis. Patients present with polyuria, polydipsia, polyphagia, and weight loss. They do not have lytic bone lesions. Nephrogenic diabetes insipidus is a rare congenital and familial form of diabetes insipidus, resulting from failure of the renal tubules to absorb water. There is excessive production of antidiuretic hormone, but the tubules fail to respond to it. Lytic bone lesions would not be present.

127. A. This patient is most likely suffering from jaundice, which is caused by an accumulation of bilirubin in the body. Bilirubin is a breakdown product of hemoglobin and is normally recycled and excreted. The patient is a chronic alcoholic, which most likely has led to cirrhosis of the liver. This impairs the ability of the liver to conjugate and eliminate bilirubin. Unconjugated bilirubin accumulates in the blood and gives a yellowish tint to the skin. Lipofuscin, commonly called the "wear-and-tear pigment," is an intracellular pigment composed of polymers of lipids and phospholipids complexed with protein. It is a normal accumulation in cells.

128. C. Placenta accreta is the attachment of the placenta directly to the myometrium. It manifests clinically by impaired placental separation after delivery, often with massive hemorrhage. Endometrial inflammation and old scars from prior cesarean sections are predispositions to it. Placental abruption is premature separation of the placenta, an important cause of antepartum bleeding and fetal death. It is often associated with disseminated intravascular coagulation (DIC). Placenta previa is attachment of the placenta to the lower uterine segment, partially or completely covering the cervical os. It often manifests by bleeding. Amniotic fluid embolism is caused by a tear in the placental membranes and rupture of maternal veins; is characterized by sudden peripartum respiratory difficulty, progressing to shock and often DIC and death. Chorioamnionitis often follows premature rupture of membranes and is caused by ascending infection from the vagina or cervix.

129. A. This child has gastric outlet obstruction, which is characterized by a hypochloremic, hypokalemic metabolic alkalosis. Crying causes hyperventilation and creates a respiratory alkalosis, which is suggested by the capillary pH of 7.51. Thus, this child has a combined metabolic and respiratory alkalosis.

130. E. Even basic activities of daily living can lead to significant dehydration if fluid intake is not maintained. With only moderate loss of water through sweat, however, serum ADH, osmolarity, and sodium will increase. As water osmotically leaves red blood cells, hematocrit, which might be expected to change, remains the same.

131. C. Pelvic inflammatory disease (PID) is a common disorder characterized by fever, pelvic pain, adnexal tenderness, and vaginal discharge. *Neisseria gonorrhoeae* continues to be a common cause of PID; *Chlamydia trachomatis* infection is now another well-recognized cause. Besides these two, infections after spontaneous or induced abortions and normal or abnormal deliveries are also important in the production of PID. Such forms of PID are polymicrobial and caused by staphylococci, streptococci, coliform bacteria, and *Clostridium perfringens*. In contrast to this route of infection, *Neisseria gonorrhoeae* usually begins in Bartholin's gland and other vestibular or peri-urethral glands and ascends to more superior organs, such as the cervix, fallopian tubes, and tuboovarian region.

132. B. The research study described in this question is a case-control study. Case-control studies are observational studies in which the subjects are chosen based on the presence (cases) or absence (control) of disease. Information is then collected about possible risk factors or exposures that were present in the past. You will pick your subjects based on the fact that they have a peanut allergy and then look for a possible exposure. Cohort studies look at known risk factors that your subjects have and follow them over time to watch for the development of disease. Cross-sectional studies look at a population at one point in time. These are usually inexpensive but not good for studying rare exposures or the effects of exposures over time. Clinical trials are experimental studies. They usually compare the therapeutic benefit of two or more treatments. A common example is the efficacy of a new drug.

133. A. Chvostek's sign: facial twitching, especially around the mouth, is induced by gently tapping the ipsilateral facial nerve as it courses just anterior to the ear. Trousseau sign: carpal spasm is induced by inflating a blood pressure cuff around the arm to a pressure 20 mm Hg above obliteration of the radial pulse for 3 to 5 min. Grey-Turner's sign: bluish discoloration of the flank, as seen in pancreatitis. Cullen's sign: bluish discoloration of the periumbilical area caused by the retroperitoneal leak of blood from the pancreas in hemorrhagic pancreatitis.

134. D. Penicillin remains the first-line treatment for *Streptococcus pneumoniae* infection provided that the patient is not allergic to any antibiotics. Third-generation cephalosporins are not indicated for pneumococcal infections. Ampicillin is more of a broad-spectrum antibiotic, reserved for Gram-positive and negative infections not including *Streptococcus pneumoniae*. Erythromycin is reserved for penicillin-allergic patients, while vancomycin is used when penicillin-resistant organisms are found.

135. B. The correct answer is dependence. It is defined as a maladaptive pattern of substance use with three or more of the following over a 1-year period: tolerance, withdrawal, substance taken in larger amounts than intended, persistent attempts to cut down, increased energy spent trying to obtain substance, use continued in spite of knowing the problems it can cause, and social, occupational, or recreational activities given up due to that substance. Abuse is a pattern of recurrent substance use that results in failure at work, home, school, and other areas. We know this woman doesn't have abuse because she states that things are fine at work and with her personal relationships. Intoxication, a reversible symptom caused by substance use, results in "maladaptive behavior." Withdrawal is a substance-specific syndrome of symptoms that develops with cessation of use.

136. A. This patient is showing the signs of malignant myeloma (MM), and the finding of punched out lesions, which are lytic lesions in the bone, would help solidify the diagnosis of MM. A buccal swab would help if DNA issues were of concern, but they are not applicable to the diagnosis here. Kidney biopsy, secondary to the urine protein findings, might seem logical, but this would not be the first-line test to run. Liver function tests and liver ultrasound wouldn't necessarily provide more confirmatory information in relation to the current presentation.

137. D. Subtracting two standard deviations $(113 - 7 - 7)$ would give 99 and adding two standard deviations $(113 + 7 + 7)$ would give 127. The first standard deviation includes 34.1% of the population, and the second standard deviation includes 13.6% of the population. So the range of scores within two standard deviations on either side $(34.1\% + 34.1\% + 13.6\% + 13.6\%)$ of 113 will include 95.5% of the scores. Therefore the range of scores within two standard deviations of the mean (113) will be 99 to 127. The range of scores from 106 to 120 includes the scores within one standard deviation of the mean and 68.2% of the scores.

138. C. This patient is presenting with Kaposi's sarcoma, a common consequence of HIV infection. The skin lesions usually present late in the course of infection, usually after the patient has progressed to AIDS. Kaposi's sarcoma is a tumor of unknown histogenesis and may result in plaques, patches, and nodules on the skin. Until the AIDS epidemic, it was seen mostly in older Mediterranean men. Now it is recognized as a sexually transmitted disease affecting immunocompromised individuals. Cytomegalovirus (CMV), Epstein-Barr virus (EBV), and varicella zoster virus (VZV) are all herpesviruses that may affect an immunocompromised person with HIV. However VZV is the only one likely to cause a skin infection. These lesions will have a different history of onset; they are painful and distributed in a dermatomal pattern. Human papillomavirus (HPV) infection is another sexually transmitted disease that affects all persons, not just the immunocompromised, who come into contact with the virus. HPV results in wart-like lesions referred to as condyloma acuminata.

139. D. A major depressive episode is characterized by five symptoms, one of which has to be either a depressed mood or anhedonia for at least 2 weeks. If the episodes recur, it is diagnosed as major depressive disorder. Bereavement is a natural grieving process due to the loss of a loved one. Symptoms usually don't last longer than 6 months. Factitious disorder exists when a person consciously creates symptoms in order to assume the sick role and to get medical attention (secondary gain). With bipolar type 1 disorder, one must have documented one episode of mania (impulsiveness, decreased need for sleep, and racing thoughts). Such a person can also present with depressive symptoms. Schizoid disorder is a personality disorder characterized by voluntary social withdrawal and limited emotional expression.

140. B. This individual is at Tanner 2: enlargement of the testes and scrotum, penis the same in size, some straight pubic hair at the base of the penis. Tanner 1 = young child's penis, scrotum, and testes; no pubic hair. Tanner 3 = enlargement of penis and testes, scrotum descends, dark, curly pubic hair. Tanner 4 = further enlargement of the penis with dark, curly pubic hair but not beyond the inguinal fold. Tanner 5 = penis reaches to the bottom of the scrotum, hair spreads to medial surface of the thighs.

141. D. The classic example of a type IV reaction is the tuberculin reaction in a previously sensitized individual. AIDS patients, with their suppressed immune systems, often fall victim to a new TB infection or a reactivation of a previously latent infection. In a previously sensitized individual, a tuberculin injection would result in an indurated and reddened area at the site of injection after 8 to 12 hr. This arises because of the accumulation of lymphocytes, monocytes, and some neutrophils as well as the production of fibrin. Type I hypersensitivity reactions are otherwise known as anaphylactic reactions and arise when an antigen (in this case penicillin) reacts with IgE bound to the surface of basophils or mast cells in individuals previously sensitized to the antigen.

142. B. This patient with sinusitis and tooth decay but normal body weight most likely has bulimia nervosa. Behavioral therapy or psychotherapy are accepted nonpharmacological treatments for bulimia. Antidepressants can be used, but fluoxetine or monoamine oxidase inhibitors (MAOIs) are considered most appropriate for this disease. Tricyclic antidepressants, such as imipramine, are very lethal in overdose and should be used with caution in patients who may demonstrate high levels of impulsivity, as many bulimic patients do. Amphetamines are useful in the treatment of attention deficit hyperactivity disorder (ADHD). Fluoride rinse is useful in preventing tooth decay but does not address this patient's underlying psychiatric illness. Typical antipsychotics such as chlorpromazine, thioridazine, and haloperidol are useful for psychosis but not for bulimia nervosa.

143. E. The tuberculin test is used to check for exposure to *Mycobacterium tuberculosis*. The tuberculin will trigger a delayed type IV cell-mediated hypersensitivity response if there has been any past exposure to *M. tuberculosis*. This response involves CD4+ T lymphocytes recognizing the antigen and causing a release of inflammatory cytokines. Answers A and B are a type II hypersensitivity reaction seen in hemolytic anemia and Goodpasture's syndrome. Answer C is a type III hypersensitivity reaction seen in serum sickness, polyarteritis nodosa, and systemic lupus erythematosus (SLE). Answer D is a type I hypersensitivity reaction seen in allergic asthma and anaphylactic shock.

144. A. This patient has adult respiratory distress syndrome (ARDS), which can be caused by a variety of situations, including shock, sepsis, heroin overdose, acute pancreatitis, and trauma. ARDS is produced by diffuse alveolar damage resulting in increased capillary permeability. This causes leakage of protein-rich fluid into the alveoli. This fluid inhibits the passage of oxygen from the air into the bloodstream. Patients present with severe respiratory insufficiency and hypotension. The histological specimen would be characteristic of ARDS. Pulmonary alveolar proteinosis is characterized by the accumulation of phospholipids in the alveolar spaces. It affects mostly 30- to 50-year-olds. Patients present with cough, dyspnea, fatigue, and weight loss. Cor pulmonale is heart disease secondary to disorders of the lungs. It is characterized by pulmonary arterial hypertension. Patients with pulmonary emboli present with symptoms similar to those of this patient, but you would not see hyaline on histological examination. The blood culture would be positive with sepsis.

145. C. A large portion of the circulation of the lower extremity begins with the superficial femoral artery, which forms the popliteal artery passing behind the knee joint. This vessel then branches into the anterior tibial, posterior tibial, and peroneal arteries. With knee injuries, the popliteal artery is often damaged owing to its location just posterior to the joint. Because of the extensive supply of the popliteal artery, it is important always to palpate for a pulse in this artery, not just in knee injuries but in all patients, in order to determine vascular supply to the distal leg.

146. E. The exocrine pancreas is anastomosed to the bladder, and by measuring the pancreas's exocrine product, amylase, one can monitor the functioning of the graft. Unless the patient had a pancreatectomy, the native pancreas may be making amylase. For the first several days after surgery, the serum glucose may not stabilize and insulin may be required. The native pancreas may make a variably small amount of insulin, so direct measurement of the graft is not possible. The graft may have good blood flow but may not be functioning well due to microvascular damage.

147. C. Furosemide may be used in cases of congestive heart failure because of its ability to rapidly induce diuresis and its good capacity for diuretic action. The drug works by *inhibiting* a Na+/K+/2Cl– cotransporter in the thick ascending loop of Henle. This is essential to maintenance of the corticopapillary osmotic gradient, which determines the kidney's ability to create either concentrated or diluted urine. The presence of aldosterone increases the concentration of urea in the renal medulla, which increases the gradient and leads to concentrated urine. Water in the proximal tubule is reabsorbed into the plasma isosmotically. Water channels (aquaporins) are found in the collecting duct and are inserted in the tube wall by the action of ADH. ADH is not secreted by the mesangial cells but by the posterior pituitary. GFR might decrease as a result of the constriction of afferent arterioles, but this would hardly help to remove excess fluid from the woman's interstitium.

148. A. The best time to treat scoliosis is during a growth spurt. Scoliosis is not caused by carrying books or bad posture. Osteoporosis, which is typically asymptomatic until a fracture occurs, may be caused by decreased estrogen levels resulting in accelerated bone loss. Caucasians are at risk as well as Asians. Osteoarthritis causes decreased mobility and is a result of excessive use. Fusion of bones, uveitis, and aortic regurgitation occur in ankylosing spondylitis. Blue sclerae occurs in osteogenesis imperfecta. Mainly autosomal dominant, osteogenesis affects infants or fetuses in utero because of defects in collagen synthesis. In torticollis, a patient has involuntary painful muscle spasms of the neck, causing him or her to bend or twist the neck.

149. D. Penicillin G is the treatment of choice for infection with *Treponema pallidum* (syphilis). The picture of the labia (Figure 15) shows the chancre of primary syphilis. Tetracycline is sometimes prescribed to patients who are allergic to penicillin. Ceftriaxone is a third-generation cephalosporin useful in the management of Gram-negative infections. Ciprofloxacin is an antibiotic that inhibits DNA gyrase. It is useful in the management of genitourinary and respiratory infections. Tetracycline binds to the 30S ribosomal subunit and prevents the attachment of aminoacyl-tRNA. It has limited penetration into the CNS.

150. C. Mönckeberg's arteriosclerosis, also known as medial calcific sclerosis, is the correct diagnosis for this presentation. This disease usually involves the muscular arteries, especially the radial and ulnar arteries. Arterial flow remains uncompromised because of the involvement of the media and not the intima. Hyperparathyroidism is associated with altered levels of calcium absorption from bone and not necessarily calcium deposits in the arterial media. Rheumatic endocarditis has no bearing on the above presentation. Waldenström's macroglobulinemia is an increase in the production of IgM, producing lymphoid cells.

Block 4

151. D. Progesterone is increased, as ovulation occurs around day 14 of the menstrual cycle. It is elevated during the secretory phase and helps maintain the corpus luteum during this phase. Estrogen is elevated before ovulation in the proliferative phase and causes proliferation of the endometrium. hCG is produced by the placenta and helps maintain the corpus luteum during the first trimester of pregnancy. Prolactin is produced by the anterior pituitary and is responsible for inhibiting the synthesis and release of gonadotropin-releasing hormone (GnRH), which inhibits ovulation. Testosterone is found in the ovaries and is converted into estrogen in adipose tissue.

152. F. Potassium should be given to reverse the effect of warfarin. All of the other agents would not help do this. There is no reason to give calcium to this patient without knowing whether or not the serum calcium is low. Fluid resuscitation should not be given without knowing this patient's volume status. There is no evidence to suggest folic acid deficiency. Magnesium should not be given to patients unless their serum magnesium levels are low.

153. A. Acanthosis nigricans is a thickening and darkening in pigmentation of the neck, axillae, and groin, which is most often seen as a benign condition indicating insulin resistance. This patient is obese and should be evaluated for conditions such as diabetes mellitus or polycystic ovary syndrome, which cause insulin resistance. It is important to note is that there is a malignant form of acanthosis that is associated with underlying visceral adenocarcinoma nigricans. Seborrheic keratosis is a benign squamoproliferative neoplasm that typically presents as in the main question stem. Microscopy reveals "horn cysts," which are filled with keratin. These may be left untreated or removed for cosmetic purposes. Squamous cell carcinoma is most often seen among people who have heavy sun exposure and usually presents on sun-exposed areas such as the face, arms, and hands. Basal cell carcinoma is common in sun-exposed areas of the body. It is locally invasive. Psoriasis is a dermatosis characterized by koebnerization and skin scaling.

154. C. This patient is suffering from dystonia, pseudoparkinsonism, and akathisia resulting from the use of high-potency antipsychotic medications such as haloperidol. Blockage of dopamine pathways in the nigrostriatal tract causes such extrapyramidal side effects. Lower-potency antipsychotics such as chlorpromazine are associated with a lower incidence of extrapyramidal symptoms but are more likely to cause anticholinergic side effects. Another common side effect of antipsychotics is hyperprolactinemia, which results from inhibition of dopamine pathways in the tuberoinfundibular tract. Dopamine inhibition in the prefrontal cortex reduces the negative symptoms of schizophrenia, while inhibition of the mesolimbic tract reduces the positive symptoms of schizophrenia. The caudate nucleus becomes atrophied in Huntington's disease; this may become manifest with choreiform movements of the body and extremities.

155. A. This is a pneumonia caused by *Legionella* species. It most commonly affects smokers and immunocompromised patients. The drug of choice is azithromycin and the second-line treatment is a fluoroquinolone. Tetracycline is not used for *Legionella* pneumonia because it offers no coverage for this species. Gentamicin is used for Gram-negative enteric infections. Penicillin is used for Gram-positive infections, typically *S. pneumoniae*.

156. B. Osteonecrosis and osteoporosis occur at higher rates among HIV-positive patients and correlate with the length of HIV infection. This patient has osteonecrosis, and the best way to diagnosis osteonecrosis at this late stage is by x-ray. An x-ray taken at an early stage will not show evidence of osteonecrosis. Continuing weight-bearing exercise is treatment for osteoporosis. Although this patient may well have osteoporosis, a patient with necrotic bone who continues to exercise may cause harm. MRI is most diagnostic of osteonecrosis, especially when an x-ray shows no evidence of damage; at this late stage, an x-ray is the most appropriate modality and a less expensive diagnostic approach than MRI. The use of bed rails is an appropriate preventive measure for elderly patients with osteoporosis. A reduced intake of caffeine does not affect the disease; however, cutting down on alcohol *will* reduce the risk. Steroid intake is a risk for osteonecrosis; however, HIV patients use steroids to treat *Pneumocystis carinii* pneumonia (PCP), and the benefits of taking the medication outweigh the risks.

157. D. Lack of intrinsic factor is the primary cause of pernicious anemia, secondary to a chronic gastritis. Supplementation of the missing intrinsic factor would certainly aid in the uptake of B_{12} and help to alleviate the problem. Intrinsic factor is mainly secreted in the stomach; therefore blood transfusion would not have much value. Increased ingestion of red meat as well as iron supplements would increase the available iron, but low iron is really not an issue in this situation. The peripheral smear shows oval macrocytosis, poikilocytosis, and anisocytosis.

158. D. Phenytoin is used in the treatment of grand mal and tonic-clonic seizures. Hirsutism, diplopia, and gingival hyperplasia are classic side effects of phenytoin. It can also cause nystagmus, ataxia, sedation, and enzyme induction. Ethosuximide is used only for absence seizures and causes GI distress, headache, and lethargy. Valproic acid can be used for all seizure types with side effects of hepatotoxicity and GI distress. Carbamazepine can also produce diplopia but does not have the other side effects presented in this case. It may also cause ataxia and blood dyscrasias. It is used in the treatment of tonic-clonic and partial seizures.

159. D. *Neisseria gonorrhoeae* is a frequent cause of pelvic inflammatory disease. Other causes include *Chlamydia trachomatis* and enteric bacteria. *N. gonorrhoeae* is associated with pharyngitis due to orogenital sexual contact and proctitis due to anogenital intercourse. Ophthalmia neonatorum is a neonatal conjunctival infection acquired at delivery. *N. gonorrhoeae* is associated with a purulent arthritis caused by blood-borne infection, which is almost invariably monoarticular and involves large joints, such as the knee. Candidiasis, or moniliasis, is the most common form of vaginitis and is caused by *Candida albicans*, a normal component of the vaginal flora.

160. F. Polycythemia and hypertension secondary to increased production of erythropoietin is an unusual yet important paraneoplastic syndrome associated with renal cell carcinoma. Obesity and exposure to petroleum products are considered risk factors along with the most significant risk, tobacco smoking. Hypovolemic shock will also result in increased serum levels of aldosterone as the body tries to maintain what little fluid and sodium remains in the vascular space.

161. A. This patient has a glucagonoma—a tumor produced by pancreatic alpha cells that increases glycogenolysis and gluconeogenesis and leads to increased blood glucose levels. Glucagonomas are associated with necrolytic migratory erythema, a characteristically red, scaly rash usually located on the face but also in other locations. Because this patient has never had diabetes, is not obese, and presents with a new onset of symptoms of hyperglycemia, a glucagonoma should be suspected. An insulinoma would produce symptoms of hypoglycemia, such as dizziness, diaphoresis, anxiety, and tremor, because of the increased production of insulin. Symptoms rapidly reverse with intravenous glucose. A type I diabetic is often thin, like this patient, but would have had symptoms of hyperglycemia long before the age of 55. A type II diabetic would most likely be obese and experience a gradual onset of symptoms of hyperglycemia over time. Patients with a VIPoma, which is a rare vasoactive intestinal peptide (VIP) tumor, are said to have Verner Morrison disease and have WDHA symptoms. WDHA stands for watery diarrhea, hypokalemia, and achlorhydria.

162. C. This man's schizophrenia is being controlled with haloperidol, an antipsychotic or neuroleptic medication. One of its more serious side effects is neuroleptic malignant syndrome. It is characterized by hyperpyrexia (fever), rigidity, delirium, and autonomic instability. Some patients are genetically far more vulnerable than normal patients to develop malignant hyperthermia. Treatment is cessation of the drug and administration of dantrolene. Serotonin syndrome occurs when a person is taking a selective serotonin reuptake inhibitor (SSRI) along with a monoamine oxidase inhibitor (MAOI); it consists of hyperthermia, muscle rigidity, and cardiovascular collapse. Malignant hyperthermia is also treated with dantrolene but it is caused by halothane (an anesthetic agent) plus succinylcholine. It develops because Ca^{2+} is unable to leave the sarcoplasmic reticulum of skeletal muscle. Hypertensive crisis can occur when a person who is taking an MAOI ingests food containing tyramine. Tardive dyskinesia is caused by neuroleptic drugs, but its symptoms consist of stereotypic oral-facial movements probably due to dopamine receptor sensitization secondary to prolonged use of an antipsychotic.

163. E. This girl has diabetes mellitus type 1, diagnosed by her young age and the fact that she presented with ketoacidosis. These patients cannot be treated with oral antidiabetic agents. All the other choices are used in type 2 diabetics. Metformin has a mechanism of action that may act by inhibiting gluconeogenesis and increasing glycogenolysis. This will decrease serum glucose levels. Alpha glucosidase inhibition serves to delay hydrolysis of sugars and absorption of glucose. Lisinopril is an ACE inhibitor used to manage hypertension.

164. E. Essential hypertension is caused by an unknown etiology. Cigarette smoking, lack of exercise and poor diet have all been reported and proven to be contributory factors in essential hypertension, but none of the above is actually the "direct causative" agents primarily responsible for the increased blood pressure. Environmental factors can certainly be contributory factors in elevated blood pressure, such as stress and physical exertion, but again, neither of which can be attributed as a primary causative agent.

165. D. Melanocytes produce melanin and are chiefly responsible for pigmentation of the skin. They are of neural crest origin. One of the diseases associated with melanocytes is vitiligo, which is characterized by flat, well-demarcated zones of pigment loss. Keratinocytes produce keratin, which forms a waterproof layer. Langerhans cells are antigen-presenting cells. Merkel cells are epidermal cells that play a role in cutaneous sensation. Adipocytes are fat storage cells.

166. E. Squamous cell carcinoma is most often seen among people who have heavy sun exposure and usually presents on sun-exposed areas such as the face, arms, and hands. Prognosis is good in that this condition rarely metastasizes and can be cured with complete excision. Seborrheic keratosis is a benign squamoproliferative neoplasm. Basal cell carcinoma is common in sun-exposed areas of the body. It is locally invasive. Psoriasis is a dermatosis characterized by koebnerization and skin scaling. Malignant melanoma is a common tumor with significant risk of metastasis. It is associated with sunlight exposure. Fair-skinned persons are at increased risk. Depth of tumor correlates with risk of metastasis.

167. B. Classically, a fracture of the ethmoid bone causes anosmia, or loss of smell. The calcaneus is located in the foot and is nowhere near the sense of olfaction. The occipital bone is posterior. Cranial nerve I is the only cranial nerve that projects into the forebrain. The parietal and sphenoid, both being cranial bones, also have no bearing on the sense of smell.

168. C. The great and small saphenous veins begin, respectively, as the medial and lateral extensions of the dorsal venous arch of the foot. The tributaries of the great saphenous gather on the anterior (dorsal) aspect of the foot and progress upward, anterior to the medial malleolus. The tributaries of the great saphenous vein serve to drain all of the superficial tissues of the lower limb except those on the side of the foot and the posterolateral aspect of

the leg. The small saphenous vein extends upward into the leg by passing behind the lateral malleolus and extending upward, usually uniting with the popliteal vein. The accessory saphenous veins are located on the proximal and medial aspect of the thigh. The anterior tibial and peroneal veins are deep veins that do not drain superficial tissues.

169. C. The nature of bile salts is amphipathic: they are able to function in both hydrophilic and hydrophobic conditions. The solubility reactions occur in the micelles. The other areas have no bearing on the actual biochemical reaction of the lipids.

170. D. Raloxifene, while less effective than estrogen replacement therapy or bisphosphonates, has been shown to be effective in the prevention of vertebral fractures in osteoporosis. Risedronate, while associated with fewer adverse effects than alendronate, is also associated with gastritis. Toremifene is, like raloxifene, a selective estrogen reuptake modulator (SERM); however, it is at present approved only for the treatment of metastatic breast cancer. Intranasal calcitonin is a common adjunctive treatment in osteoporosis, but it has not been shown specifically to prevent vertebral fractures in these patients.

171. A. Ethanol prevents the metabolism of methanol to its toxic metabolite. The patient may need vitamins, but this is not the most pressing issue at this time. Normal saline is an important adjunct to be added to increase volume. The patient needs stabilization in the hospital after ethanol is administered and should be monitored until this is achieved. Therefore the patient should not be advised to drink a cup of coffee and be discharged home.

172. A. An elevated level of FSH is used to confirm menopause when one is uncertain. An hCG level would serve to confirm pregnancy. Prolactin and TSH would be used to rule out sources of secondary amenorrhea of unknown etiology.

173. A. Over 75% of cases of chronic myelogenous leukemia are characterized by a translocation of chromosomes 9 and 22, producing a hybrid gene called *bcr-abl*. This gene causes an overproduction of mature polymorphonuclear leukocytes (PMNs). The 9:22 translocation is referred to as the Philadelphia chromosome. The 8:14 translocation is implicated in Burkitt's lymphoma. The 15:17 translocation is implicated in the promyelocytic variety of acute myelogenous leukemia. The 14:18 translocation is implicated in mantle cell lymphoma. The 14:21 translocation, also called the Robertsonian translocation, is implicated in hereditary Down's syndrome.

174. A. Degenerative disk disease affects men and women equally. The age at diagnosis is most often around 40 years. Anterior parts of the spine carry the majority of weight, especially in sitting. Activities that involve twisting, sitting up, or vibration in a car tend to amplify pain along the outer annular wall, where innervation is present. Although there are better forms of load-bearing exercise to prevent osteoporosis and loss of horizontal trabeculae than water activities and cycling, there is no history of steroid use, anorexia, or calcium disorders that would cause osteoporosis in a 40-year-old woman. Excessive sudden stretch or contraction of muscle may result in a tear or sprain; here, however, there is no history of sudden onset. Ankylosing spondylitis with uveitis, aortitis, and amyloidosis affects young men around 20 years of age; kyphosis, stiff posture, and tenderness at the Achilles tendon are also seen in these patients. Three-dimensional curvature of the spine is scoliosis.

175. D. This patient is susceptible to chlamydial infection. The drug of choice for this organism is tetracycline. The only other possibility would be using erythromycin. Cefuroxime is a cephalosporin that does not cover *Chlamydia*. Gentamicin is an aminoglycoside antibiotic that is associated with ototoxicity, nephrotoxicity, and neuromuscular blockade. Vancomycin is a parenteral antibiotic with good coverage for *Staphylococcus*.

176. E. This patient is suffering from sickle cell anemia, which is a mutation in the coding of the beta-globin gene. There is a GAG = > GTG switch, which changes glutamine to valine and creates the "sickling" of red blood cells (RBCs). Autoimmune hemolytic anemia occurs when IgG and the RBC surface antigens cross-react and the RBCs are destroyed. Beta thalassemia major results in decreased production of beta-globin genes. Erythroblastosis fetalis is a disease of the fetus and would not affect a nonpregnant woman. Hereditary spherocytosis is due to membrane protein abnormalities.

177. E. Finasteride is a 5-alpha reductase inhibitor used in the symptomatic treatment of benign prostatic hypertrophy (BPH); it blocks the conversion of testosterone to dihydroxytestosterone (DHT) in target tissues. Since DHT is the major intracellular androgen in the prostate, finasteride is effective in suppressing DHT as well as the growth and secretory function of the prostate.

178. D. Throughout the follicular phase, estradiol levels increase, resulting in uterine proliferation; the resultant feedback suppresses the secretion of FSH and LH by the anterior pituitary. A burst of estradiol synthesis at the end of the follicular phase results in a positive feedback on the anterior pituitary, causing the characteristic surge in LH. The suddenly increased LH levels then induce ovulation. Without this surge in LH, ovulation would not occur. Although the lack of other hormones could also result in anovulatory cycles, LH is most directly related to ovulation and hence is the best option for this question. Note that the option of estradiol was not included, since low levels of this form of estrogen are also strongly correlated with anovulatory cycles.

179. D. Approximately two of every three patients who receive blood from an HIV-positive donor will themselves become infected with the virus. The risk of transmission from a single sexual encounter with a man from a low risk group is 1 in 5 million. The risk of being infected with HIV from a needle-stick depends on the viral load of the blood that one is stuck with. The risk of seroconversion from a patient with a low viral load is 1 in 1,000; if one is infected

with blood from a patient whose viral load is high, the risk rises to 1 in 100. All newborns born to HIV-positive mothers will be seropositive and about 20% of those infants will remain positive after 1 year. Azidothymidine (AZT) reduces this rate to 10% after 1 year and AZT in combination with a cesarean delivery reduces the rate even further, to 5%. Nevirapine given to the mother during labor and to the child after birth also reduces the rate to 10%.

180. D. This patient has Albright's syndrome, or pseudohypoparathyroidism, which is caused by renal unresponsiveness to PTH. This condition is inherited in an autosomal recessive pattern, in which both parents are unaffected carriers of the gene. Albright's syndrome can present with hypocalcemia, leading to tetany, shortened height, and shortened fourth and fifth phalanges. A 46, XO genotype would cause Turner's syndrome. Patients with Turner's syndrome are female, short in stature, have webbed necks, and are infertile. A dietary calcium deficiency is rare in the United States but can produce tetany and inadequate mineralization of bones. DiGeorge's syndrome is caused by failure of development of the third and fourth pharyngeal pouches, which leads to agenesis of the thymus and parathyroid glands as well as to T-cell deficiencies and recurrent infections and tetany due to hypocalcemia. A vitamin D deficiency causes rickets, or inadequate calcification of bones, in children. These patients may have shortened stature, protrusion of the sternum, bowing of the legs, and other skeletal abnormalities.

181. A. This patient is presenting with the syndrome of inappropriate antidiuretic hormone secretion (SIADH). SIADH caused by this tubulin-binding neoplastic drug, which prevents microtubular polymerization. Some other chemotherapeutic drugs that can cause SIADH include cyclophosphamide and vincristine. Cyclosporine is an immunosuppressive agent. Doxorubicin is an antineoplastic agent that noncovalently intercalates DNA and inhibits replication and transcription. Free radicals are generated. Methotrexate is an S-phase–specific antimetabolite. It is a folic acid analog that inhibits dihydrofolate reductase.

182. E. Papilledema is the most likely corresponding clinical feature, along with a resultant choked optic disk. Anosmia is not likely to be an issue unless the tumor lies specifically on the pathway of the first cranial nerve. All of the other visual issues would require the tumor to be directly on one of the areas mentioned above.

183. E. This patient has emphysema, an obstructive pulmonary disease, most likely caused by her long smoking history. In emphysema there is a destruction of alveolar septa and thus a decrease in elastic recoil. This causes small airways to collapse. Patients will prolong expiration (pursed lips) to prevent that. Lung compliance and FRC will increase. The patient's chest has become barrel-shaped to accommodate this new volume. The FEV_1/FVC ratio is less than 0.8 with obstructive lung diseases.

184. A. Chocolate agar with factors V and X is required to culture *Haemophilus influenzae,* the causative agent of epiglottitis. *Neisseria gonorrhoeae* is cultured using Thayer-Martin medium. *Mycobacterium tuberculosis* can be cultured on Löwenstein-Jensen agar. Charcoal yeast extract is used to culture *Legionella pneumophila.*

185. G. No agent is without complications. In the setting of pregnancy, any of the anticoagulants could pose problems with the pregnancy. Thus, none should be given unless required for a particular reason. Although warfarin is the anticoagulant of choice for long-term therapy, it would not be indicated in this patient owing to its teratogenic effects. Although the administration of heparin by injection is difficult, it would be needed if the patient were to become pregnant. Heparin is used for prophylaxis of deep venous thrombosis, pulmonary embolism, arterial embolism, and atrial fibrillation. It potentiates the activity of antithrombin III and thereby inactivates thrombin.

186. B. The "female-athlete triad" consists of an eating disorder, menstrual abnormalities, and osteoporosis. Eating disorders may be from 5 to 60 times more common among female athletes than in the general population. These women are at increased risk for osteoporosis and fractures. "Waddell's triad" applies to a child who has been struck by a motor vehicle, sustaining thoracic, femoral, and contralateral closed head injuries. A patient whose pain interferes with normal activities may complain of suffering, sleeplessness, and pain. The "unhappy triad" refers to injury of the medial collateral ligament, anterior collateral ligament, and medial meniscus, which predisposes a patient to eventual osteoarthritis. "Charcot's triad" consists of intention tremor, scanning speech, and nystagmus; it is associated with multiple sclerosis (MS). Although MS does substantially increase morbidity and mortality, playing soccer is not associated with increased rates of MS.

187. D. The pectinate line demarcates the transitional area between somatic and visceral innervation of the rectum. Above the pectinate line, no pain or sensation is felt, but below that area, pain is appreciated. The myenteric plexus is part of the digestive tract anatomy and is affiliated with Auerbach's plexus; it controls outer longitudinal motility. Meissner's plexus controls secretions. The muscularis plexus controls mucosal motility.

188. C. The correct answer is axis III. Any physical disorders or conditions are classified on axis III. Axis I is for clinical psychiatric disorders such as major depressive disorder, schizophrenia, bipolar disorder, and so on. Axis IV is for psychosocial and environmental problems. Since this patient has recently been in an argument with her mother, you could diagnose "Family stressors" on axis IV. Axis V is for the global assessment of functioning (GAF). It is scored on a scale of 100 to 1. A score of 100 represents superior functioning, a score of less than 50 represents serious symptoms, and a score of less than 10 represents persistent danger of hurting self or others.

189. F. The correct answer is subepithelial humps. The history suggests a streptococcal pharyngitis with a poststreptococcal glomerulonephritis 2 weeks later. The classic presentation is a young child with fever, malaise, periorbital edema, hypertension, and smoke-colored urine 2 to 4 weeks after a throat infection. The characteristic electron microscopic findings are discrete, amorphous, electron-dense deposits on the epithelial side of the membrane, often having a "humped" appearance, presumably representing the antigen-antibody complexes at the epithelial surface. Crescent formation in Bowman's space is a light-microscopic histological feature of rapidly progressive glomerulonephritis. Dense deposits within the glomerular basement membrane is an electron-microscopic characteristic of membranoproliferative glomerulonephritis type II. Fusion of foot podocytes is an electron-microscopic characteristic of minimal change disease. Mesangial deposits of IgA is an immunofluorescence pattern characteristic of Berger's IgA nephropathy. Smooth and linear pattern of IgG in the glomerular basement membrane is an immunofluorescence pattern characteristic of Goodpasture's syndrome.

190. E. A Krukenberg tumor is defined as the bilateral involvement of the ovaries by metastatic carcinoma of the stomach. These cells often possess a copious amount of mucin, which displaces the nucleus to the periphery and thereby creates the classic appearance of the signet-ring cell. Clear cell adenocarcinoma is associated with maternal use of diethylstilbestrol during pregnancy. The rest of the options are primary tumors of the female reproductive system.

191. D. This patient has evidence of Vincent's angina, a necrotizing and sometimes ulcerating gingivitis. It can occur in patients who eat dirt and grass. *Fusobacterium nucleatum* is an anaerobe that is common in the oral flora but may act in synergy with oral spirochetes to erode the oral mucosa and cause this condition. *Bacteroides fragilis* is an anaerobic bacterium. It is difficult to culture. It also causes the foul smell of some infections.

192. E. The INR, or international normalized ratio, creates a standardized value of the prothrombin time, or PT. An INR level is ordered in patients who are taking warfarin (Coumadin), an oral anticoagulant. Warfarin works by inhibiting the gamma carboxylation of the vitamin K–dependent clotting factors II, VII, IX, and X. An INR level of 5.8 is excessive and places the patient at significant risk of bleeding. Administering vitamin K reverses the effect of warfarin. Enoxaparin is a low-molecular-weight heparin that has similar effects as heparin. Heparin is especially helpful in patients who develop deep venous thrombosis and works by inhibiting antithrombin III. Although it will not lyse clots, it will prevent new ones from forming. A patient taking heparin has an elevated PTT. An overdose of heparin is reversed by protamine sulfate. Streptokinase is a thrombolytic agent that lyses clots by activating plasminogen.

193. E. This patient has the constellation of systemic and cutaneous symptoms and signs that are common for systemic lupus erythematosus. Other manifestations of the disease are renal, neurological, hematologic, and immunologic. Scleroderma is a multisystem disease characterized by abnormalities of small blood vessels, fibrosis of the skin and internal organs, immune system activation, and autoimmunity. Discoid lupus erythematosus (DLE) is not a systemic disease. Its manifestations are limited to the skin involvement presented in this case. Psoriasis is associated with scaly lesions, with arthritis developing later in some cases. Dermatomyositis is associated with proximal muscle weakness and a heliotrope rash.

194. D. On delivery, the infant takes its first breath, which leads to a chain reaction resulting in the closure of the foramen ovale. With oxygen in the lungs, the pulmonary vasculature expands and there is decreased resistance. This leads to a change in the pressure difference between the left and right atrium. Now that the pressure of the right atrium is less than that of the left atrium, the foramen ovale closes and forms the permanent structure called the fossa ovalis. In the event that this structure does not fully close, indomethacin may be used in the same manner as with the closure of the ductus arteriosus. The ductus arteriosus eventually is closed off due to the increase in oxygen, causing a decrease in prostaglandin synthesis. The allantois is the embryologic structure responsible for urine evacuation. Its remnant is the median umbilical ligament. The umbilical arteries soon lose their blood flow and become the medial umbilical ligaments. The ductus venosus connects the umbilical vein with the vena cava and eventually becomes the ligamentum venosum.

195. D. The best answer to this question is diverticulitis. The barium enema confirms the diagnosis. This condition is common in the elderly. The condition is typically exacerbated by eating nuts and popcorn, which can become entrapped in the diverticulum, leading to infection and inflammation. Appendicitis would produce more right-sided abdominal pain. A bowel obstruction would present with constipation and decreased bowel sounds. Adenocarcinoma would most likely not present with such abrupt symptoms. Ulcerative colitis would present with bloody mucoid diarrhea.

196. C. Because the symptoms are initiated with food intake and weight gain, a preliminary differential diagnosis of *Helicobacter pylori* would be appropriate. Treatment with the "triple therapy" of bismuth salicylate, metronidazole, and an antibiotic such as amoxicillin would be in order. *Escherichia coli* tends to cause a more acute infection. *E. coli* is associated with bloody diarrhea; shigellosis also presents with abdominal cramping and diarrhea.

197. B. Phenoxybenzamine is an irreversible and nonselective alpha-adrenergic blocker used in the treatment of pheochromocytoma. It controls episodes of hypertension and sweating in affected patients. Phentolamine is also an alpha$_1$-adrenergic blocker used in the treatment of pheochromocytoma. It is not an irreversible alpha-blocker and is therefore not the correct answer. Doxa-

zosin, prazosin, and terazosin are alpha$_1$-selective blockers used in the treatment of hypertension in patients with BPH. These drugs should be given at night before the patient goes to sleep because they can cause orthostatic hypotension. Yohimbine is an alpha$_2$ selective agent that has sometimes been used in the treatment of impotence. Its use is controversial.

198. B. For the first 48 to 72 hr, heparin must be used in order to prevent the hypercoagulable state created by warfarin. Protein C is affected first by warfarin because it has the shortest half-life of all the vitamin K–dependent factors. This inhibition of protein C allows factors V and VIII to go relatively unchecked. Heparin does not inhibit plasmin.

199. B. This is a classic example of chancroid, which is caused by *Haemophilus ducreyi*. It causes the symptoms noted above. Herpes simplex virus causes genital lesions but is not seen on Gram's stain. Syphilis is associated with a nontender ulcer, not a tender one. Such an ulcer is called a chancre. *Neisseria gonorrhoeae* and *Chlamydia trachomatis* do not cause the symptoms noted above. They are associated with sexually transmitted diseases that cause urethral discharge.

200. D. MCAD deficiency is the most common genetic disorder of fatty acid metabolism. Most tissues rely on fatty acid oxidation as the primary fuel source for the production of ATP during fasting. When MCAD is deficient, medium-chain fatty acid CoA accumulates in the cytosol as well as the mitochondrial matrix. This leads to hepatic resynthesis of triacylglycerides in the cytosol, causing fatty liver. ATP production and ketogenesis are decreased, slowing the activity of the urea cycle and gluconeogenesis. This leads to hyperammonemia and hypoglycemia, respectively. The other choices are enzyme deficiencies found with glycogen storage diseases.

Block 5

201. D. This is a classic description of *Trichomonas* infection, giving the cervix a strawberry appearance. Diagnosis is confirmed by wet prep. *Gardnerella vaginalis* is associated with bacterial vaginosis and is confirmed by a positive "whiff test." Clue cells are seen with this infection. The history is not consistent with *Candida*. With a candidal yeast infection you see a thick, curdy discharge and diagnosis is confirmed by KOH prep.

202. A. The zona glomerulosa is responsible for producing aldosterone. Although the history does not give any clues to the patient's symptoms, knowing the histology of the adrenal glands is the key to answering this question. This patient likely has Conn's syndrome, which is caused by an aldosterone-secreting adenoma. Treatment is surgical removal of the tumor. Spironolactone, an aldosterone antagonist, also provides symptomatic relief. Cortisol is produced in the zona fasciculata. Dehydroepiandrosterone, which is a weak androgen, is produced in the zona reticularis. Epinephrine and norepinephrine are catecholamines produced in the adrenal medulla.

203. C. Although normal individuals will develop nevi (moles) in sun-exposed areas, patients with dysplastic nevus syndrome have an increased risk of spontaneously developing malignant melanoma. Malignant melanomas are the most likely primary skin tumors to metastasize systemically. Patients who chew tobacco for long periods are at increased risk of developing squamous cell carcinomas near or in the oral cavity. Basal cell carcinomas are the most common skin tumors. They tend to involve sun-exposed areas most often in the head and neck. Grossly, they are characterized by pearly papules with overlying telangiectatic vessels. The lower lip is actually the most common site for a squamous cell carcinoma due to tobacco use. Malignant melanomas are the most likely primary skin tumors to metastasize systemically. Histiocytosis X (Langerhans cell histiocytosis) is caused by a proliferation of Langerhans cells, which are normally found in the epidermis. These cells are CD1a-positive, and Birbeck granules are seen on electron microscopy.

204. C. Myasthenia gravis is an autoimmune disorder caused by autoantibodies to acetylcholine receptors of the neuromuscular junction. It is characterized by muscle weakness that is intensified by muscle use, with recovery on rest. Patients frequently present with ptosis or diplopia and can have difficulty chewing, speaking, or swallowing. When drugs with anticholinesterase activity, such as neostigmine, are administered, dramatic improvement results. This condition is three times more frequent in women than in men. Muscular dystrophy is caused by multiple loss-of-function mutations in muscle protein. There is no evidence to suggest the diagnosis of septic arthritis in this patient. Patients with polymyalgia rheumatica often have an elevated erythrocyte sedimentation rate suggestive of the underlying inflammatory process.

205. D. This woman has a pneumonia caused by *Streptococcus pneumoniae*. This organism undergoes alpha hemolysis and is sensitive to optochin. *Streptococcus agalactiae* is a group B beta-hemolytic species that is resistant to bacitracin. *Streptococcus pyogenes* is a group A beta-hemolytic species that is inhibited by bacitracin. *Streptococcus mutans* is an alpha-hemolytic organism that is not inhibited by optochin. *Peptostreptococcus* is an anaerobe that does not undergo hemolysis.

206. A. This presentation is classic for cirrhosis/portal hypertension secondary to alcohol abuse. The patient's symptoms are all related to liver failure. The elevated AST/ALT ratio (2:1) is a red flag for alcohol-induced liver damage. Micronodular papules (< 3 mm) that are uniform in size are commonly associated with excessive alcohol usage. Sexual/drug history could possibly point to a liver insult from the transmission of hepatitis B, but this would present with nodules > 3 mm. This patient denied any recent trauma; to requestion him would be unwarranted. Because of the gynecomastia, possible hormonal factors may be involved. However, in view of the other symptoms considered this is not the most likely area to investigate.

207. E. This is a common presentation for tetralogy of Fallot. These patients have ventricular septal defect, pulmonic stenosis, an overriding aorta, and right ventricular hypertrophy. This combination of defects results initially in a left-to-right shunt. Following right ventricular hypertrophy, the shunt changes to a right-to-left shunt. Following this right-to-left shunt, pulmonic stenosis will often develop. Surgery is the only treatment. Atrial septal defect is associated with a left-to-right shunt, which results in late cyanosis. The S_1 heart sound is loud and there is wide splitting of a fixed S_2. Ventricular septal defect is associated with late cyanosis because of the left-to-right shunt. Patent ductus arteriosus (PDA) is also associated with a left-to-right shunt and late cyanosis. The PDA can close with indomethacin treatment.

208. C. This is also known as McArdle's disease, which is caused by a defect in glycogen phosphorylase. Glycogen is the primary form of glucose storage in muscle tissue. During exercise, other metabolic fuels cannot be transported to the muscles fast enough, so a stored reserve of glucose, glycogen, is used first. In McArdle's disease, this glycogen cannot be used because it cannot be broken down into glucose. Therefore other sources of energy are used, such as the degraded ATP and creatine phosphate. However, this process cannot be maintained, leading to severe pain within several minutes of exercise. The disease is not detected until the patient reaches his or her twenties or thirties. It is less severe in children. Treatment involves exercise management, dietary management, and gene therapy. Lysosomal alpha 1,4-glucosidase deficiency is a glycogen storage disease known as Pompe's disease. It causes damage to the heart, liver, and muscles. Glucose 6-phosphatase deficiency is a glycogen storage disease known as Von Gierke's disease. Signs of this condition include fasting hypoglycemia and increased glycogen accumulation in the liver.

209. C. Heparin can be given during pregnancy to provide effective anticoagulation and does not pose any teratogenic risk to the developing fetus. It does not cross the placenta and is therefore the agent of choice for anticoagulation in a pregnant woman. Aspirin increases bleeding time by irreversibly inhibiting platelets, but it would have little therapeutic benefit in this patient, who requires a more effective anticoagulant. Garlic has been reported to increase bleeding potential, but it would also be ineffective here. Urokinase is a thrombolytic agent sometimes used to treat myocardial infarction when cardiac catheterization and angioplasty are unavailable. Warfarin (Coumadin) is extremely teratogenic and should be avoided during pregnancy, as it can cross the placenta and cause significant birth defects.

210. D. Ankylosing spondylitis is a systemic disease, meaning that it can affect the entire body. It can cause fever, loss of appetite, and fatigue, and it can damage other organs besides the joints, such as the lungs, heart, and eyes. Most often though, only the low back is involved. The eye is the most common organ affected by ankylosing spondylitis. Eye inflammation (iritis) occurs from time to time in one-fourth of people with ankylosing spondyli-tis. Iritis results in a red, painful eye that also leads to photophobia, or increased pain when looking at a bright light. The inflammation in ankylosing spondylitis usu-ally starts around the sacroiliac joints, areas where the lower spine is joined to the pelvis. The pain associated with ankylosing spondylitis is worse during periods of rest or inactivity. People with this condition often wake up in the middle of the night with back pain. Typically, symptoms lessen with movement and exercise. About 90% of people diagnosed with ankylosing spondylitis test positive for the HLA-B27 gene. Anti-dsDNA is spe-cific for systemic lupus erythematosus (SLE). Antinuclear antibodies are specific for SLE. Anti scl-70 is associated with scleroderma. The Tensilon test is used to diagnose myasthenia gravis.

211. B. Acute renal failure (ARF) presents as a rapidly rising cre-atinine or a decline in urinary output. The approach to patients with ARF is simplified by classifying it as prere-nal, intrinsic, or postobstructive. This patient is suscep-tible to prerenal azotemia, which is the clinical result of renal hypoperfusion due to a decrease in effective arte-rial blood volume. In prerenal states the kidney avidly retains sodium, usually resulting in a high urine osmo-lality > 500, a low urine sodium < 20, and a fractional excretion of sodium < 1%. Intrinsic renal failure results from a variety of injuries to the renal blood vessels, glomeruli, tubules, or interstitium. Intrin-sic urinary laboratory examination reveals urine osmo-lality < 350, urinary sodium > 20, a fractional excretion of sodium > 2%, and a BUN/Cr ratio < 15. Postobstructive ARF develops with bilateral obstruction secondary to stones, BPH, or neoplasia. Urinary laboratory examina-tion reveals urine osmolality < 350, urine sodium > 40, fractional excretion of sodium > 4%, and a BUN/Cr > 15.

212. B. The keys to answering this question are that the ulcer is painful and nonelevated herpes simplex virus (HSV) must therefore be suspected. The most common histo-logic findings of cells infected with HSV are the pres-ence of multinucleated giant cells and Cowdry type A intranuclear inclusions. Antoni B histologic patterns are most commonly seen with schwannomas and some cases of neurofibromatosis. Owl's-eye intranuclear inclusions are most commonly seen in cytomegalovirus (CMV) infection. Koilocytosis is the typical histologic feature seen in HIV infection, and Negri bodies are the definitive cytoplasmic inclusion bodies seen in rabies virus infection.

213. B. Major depressive disorder would be the most accurate diagnosis based on the given information. It may also be called postpartum depression. It occurs in only 0.1 to 0.2% of delivering mothers and can last up to 1 year post-partum. Brief psychotic disorder and postpartum psy-chosis present with the same signs and, in this scenario, indicate essentially the same condition. This involves hallucinations, delusions, and a potential for infant harm by the mother. It can last usually up to a month. The onset of postpartum blues is the first few days after

delivery and usually resolves within a week postpartum. Symptoms include a highly emotional state and crying but with maintenance of proper hygiene.

214. B. The patient is suffering from delirium tremens (DTs), a life-threatening alcohol withdrawal syndrome that usu-ally presents 2 to 5 days after the patient takes his or her last drink. Initial symptoms can present 7 to 10 days after the patient's last drink. The syndrome can also present with symptoms of alcohol withdrawal (tremor, tachy-cardia, nausea, diaphoresis, anxiety, insomnia), mental status changes (agitation, confusion, hallucinations, delusions, delirium), and seizures. Diazepam is a benzo-diazepine used to taper patients going through alcohol withdrawal. Both alcohol and benzodiazepines increase GABA. Clozapine is an atypical antipsychotic that blocks serotonin and dopamine receptors. Lithium is a mood stabilizer for bipolar affective disorder; its mechanism is not known. Meperidine is an opioid agonist. Thiopental is a barbiturate. The patient's CT scan (Figure 21) shows an intracerebral hematoma. It is a noncontrast CT scan of the head showing the presence of blood in the frontal lobe. The cause of the problem in this case may ulti-mately have been an arteriovenous malformation.

215. D. This is a description of a patient with Graves' disease. Although antibodies are produced against all four anti-gens, the main antigen against which the antibodies are directed and that is responsible for the hyperthyroidism is the thyroid-stimulating hormone receptor. Diagnos-tic testing includes ultrasound and technetium scan-ning. This testing is important to differentiate Graves' disease from adenoma. The function of the thyroid hormones is as follows. T_3 functions include brain mat-uration, bone growth, and increase in basal metabolic rate. Thyroid releasing hormone stimulates TSH release, which stimulates thyroid follicular cells. Negative feed-back is provided by T_3 to the anterior pituitary gland.

216. E. For critically ill patients, it is important to determine the increase above basal energy expenditure so that such patients can receive appropriate nutritional support. The Harris-Benedict equation or a metabolic chart can be used for these calculations. Sepsis will cause a 79% increase in energy expenditure above the basal rate and must be compensated for with appropriate nutritional supplementation. Head trauma accounts for a 61% increase in energy expenditure above the basal rate. Elective, major surgery accounts for a 24% increase in energy expenditure above the basal rate. Skeletal trauma accounts for a 32% increase in energy expendi-ture above the basal rate. Blunt trauma accounts for a 37% increase in energy expenditure above the basal rate.

217. B. Horner's syndrome, due to a Pancoast tumor, is characterized by ptosis, miosis, and anhidrosis on the same side as the lesion. This is due to involvement of the cervical sympathetic plexus. Horner's syndrome can occur with apical tumors of any type, but it occurs most often with adenocarcinomas, which are the most common peripheral tumors and therefore the most common tumors occurring in the apex. Superior vena cava syndrome results from obstruction of the superior vena cava. It results in facial swelling, cyanosis, and dilation of the veins of the head and neck. Paraneoplastic syndrome refers to the ectopic production of hormones such as ACTH and ADH by lung tumors. A pleural effusion is fluid in the pleural spaces. It results in decreased breath sounds over the effusion, dullness to percussion, and decreased fremitus. Cushing's syndrome results from an excess production of cortisol. Symptoms include weight gain, central obesity, moon facies, fatigue, and weakness.

218. D. Penicillamine is used to chelate the copper and enable its excretion into the blood as ceruloplasmin. The diagnosis of Wilson's disease would be in order, as it explains the accumulation of copper in the liver and sclerae. The ring deposits, known as Kayser-Fleischer rings, are pathognomonic for this condition as well. Azithromycin, a well-known macrolide antibiotic, would have no place in the treatment of this condition. Epinephrine would be more warranted in cases of throat closure or inability to breathe, possibly secondary to an acute allergic reaction, and not a chronic condition such as Wilson's disease. Ciprofloxacin is commonly used in the treatment of respiratory and sexually transmitted disease and has no bearing or efficacy in this situation.

219. D. Erythroplasia of Queyrat is penile carcinoma in situ occurring usually in the fifth decade. It predominately affects uncircumcised men and is prone to involve the glans penis or prepuce. Grossly, it usually presents as a single shiny erythematous plaque on the glans penis or prepuce. This is not associated with visceral malignancies and progresses to invasive squamous cell carcinoma in 10% of the cases. Based on this presentation, there is no reason to suspect syphilis. The classic chancre is not present on examination. Condyloma acuminata are genital warts. The examination of this patient fails to reveal the presence of warts.

220. C. Corticosteroids are now recommended as first-line therapy in the treatment of asthma. They act by inactivating the transcription factor NF-kB (which normally induces the production of the proinflammatory molecule TNF-α), thus inhibiting the chronic reaction of an asthma attack. Ipratropium blocks acetylcholine signaling. Theophylline inhibits phosphodiesterase. Cromolyn prevents mast cell mediator release, and albuterol activates beta-2 receptors.

221. C. Interleukin-2 is a true lymphokine because it has the ability to serve as a T-cell growth factor. Production of this immunoglobulin is impaired in patients with thermal injuries. Interleukin-1 has the ability to induce proteolysis and can serve as an endogenous pyrogen. It also stimu-

lates the hypothalamic-pituitary axis. Interleukin-6 promotes the synthesis of hematic acute-phase proteins.

222. B. Antiphospholipid antibody syndrome is also called lupus anticoagulant syndrome and is often discovered in young women who have had multiple unexplained miscarriages. This patient had lupus, as suggested by her rosy red cheeks. Antiphospholipid antibody syndrome is found not only in patients with lupus but also in those who take certain medications. The name "lupus anticoagulant syndrome" is actually a paradox because people with the condition have the propensity to form clots. The word *anticoagulant* in the name comes from the fact that they have an increased PTT. Abruptio placentae is an obstetric catastrophe and is a cause of miscarriage. It is not likely that a patient would suffer three consecutive miscarriages due to abruptio placentae. Placenta accreta and placenta percreta refer to the invasion of the placenta into the uterine wall. Placenta accreta refers to the placenta invading the uterine wall superficially, while placenta percreta refers to the placenta invading through the serosa of the uterus. Placenta percreta can be associated with uterine rupture, hemorrhage, and failure to deliver the placenta. Even though she had an elevated PTT, this patient was not factitiously taking heparin or enoxaparin because she had the propensity to clot, which would not occur with the use of either of these medications.

223. E. Statistical studies show that rupture of the small intestine may occur in as many as 50% of the patients diagnosed with type IV Ehlers-Danlos syndrome. Other complications may include dysfunction of any structure with type III collagen, such as rupture of blood vessels and the uterus. Bilateral lens dislocations occur in patients with Marfan's syndrome due to a defect in the synthesis of fibrillin. The herniation of multiple disks in the lumbar spine is not associated with any classic pathology and can have many etiologies. Multiple bone fractures may be associated with osteogenesis imperfecta, a type I collagen defect usually diagnosed in childhood. A holosystolic heart murmur with a midsystolic click is indicative of mitral valve prolapse, which can be found in patients with Marfan's syndrome.

224. A. The cause of this patient's murmur is aortic stenosis. The maneuver described can help distinguish hypertrophic cardiomyopathy from aortic stenosis. When a person stands, the venous return to the heart decreases, causing a decrease in blood pressure, stroke volume, and volume of blood in the left ventricle, while squatting has the opposite effect. During times of decreased blood flow, the murmur of aortic stenosis will decrease in intensity, while an increase in flow will cause the murmur to increase in intensity. Mitral prolapse is the most frequent valvular lesion. It produces a characteristic systolic murmur with a midsystolic click. Hypertrophic cardiomyopathy can result in left ventricular outflow obstruction. The murmur would have the opposite qualities of that heard with aortic stenosis, having increased intensity while the person is standing and decreased intensity when he or she is squatting. Innocent murmurs result from turbulent blood flow. You would not expect the quality of the murmur to change from the maneuver described. Mitral stenosis produces a diastolic murmur.

225. A. Shipbuilders are at high risk of asbestos exposure. The ferruginous bodies present in this patient's sputum suggest that he has been exposed to asbestos. Although mesothelioma is a dreaded disease often associated with asbestos exposure (and in fact almost never occurs in the absence of asbestos exposure), bronchogenic carcinoma is a far more common cancer in those exposed to asbestos. Fibrosis is associated with restrictive lung disease and can be associated with occupational exposures. Squamous cell carcinoma is correlated with cigarette smoking. Tuberculosis is associated with a positive Mantoux test. The chest x-ray reveals a large left-sided pleural effusion that effaces the left costophrenic angle.

226. F. Embryonal rhabdomyosarcoma, also known as sarcoma botryoides when found in this location, is a rare tumor that occurs in children under 5 years of age and is often visualized as a "bunch of grapes" (*L. botryoides*) protruding from the introitus. It is characterized histologically by small round blue cells of the skeletal muscle lineage. The cells also express proteins native to skeletal muscle and therefore stain positive for desmin. Dermoid cyst can be demonstrated on ultrasound as complex cystic masses. Adenomatoid tumor can occur in men and is common in the epididymis. Choriocarcinoma would be associated with elevated hCG levels. Leiomyoma would be associated with a mass on ultrasound and pathology would reveal muscle and fat cells.

227. B. Lipid-soluble substances freely cross the blood-brain barrier and equilibrate between the blood and CSF. Protein and cholesterol molecules are excluded from the CSF because of their large size. Carbon dioxide, glucose, lipid-soluble drugs, and oxygen cross the blood-brain barrier freely.

228. B. Fetal parts are found only in partial moles. In complete moles, embryonic development does not occur. This woman presented with the typical findings of hydatidiform mole: absent fetal heart tones, abnormal uterine bleeding, and the passage of grapelike masses. Other findings seen with moles are hyperthyroidism from hCG cross-reacting with TSH receptors, fundal height larger then expected, and pregnancy-induced hypertension in the first trimester. Trophoblast proliferation, while greater and more diffuse in complete mole, also occurs in partial mole. All villi are edematous in a complete mole, while only some are edematous in a partial mole. Both complete and partial moles can cause an abnormally high increase in hCG levels. Choriocarcinoma can occur after a complete or partial mole, but the risk is greater in choriocarcinoma.

229. B. This is typical of Legionnaires' disease, found in individuals who work around a contaminated water source. Silver stain is positive and Gram-negative rods are visible. There is no person-to-person transmission. *S. aureus* is associated with hospital-acquired pneumonia and is characterized by Gram-positive cocci in clusters. *S. pneumoniae* is a Gram-positive organism found in chains. It is the most common cause of community-acquired pneumonia in the general population. *H. influenzae* also causes a community-acquired pneumonia. It is cultured on chocolate agar with factors V and X. *Mycoplasma pneumoniae* causes "walking pneumonia," characterized by a dry, nagging cough and a chest x-ray showing interstitial infiltrates bilaterally.

230. D. This triad is classic for hemochromatosis. Iron is deposited in various organs and causes the resulting "triad" symptoms. Alcoholic hepatitis can have definite associated liver changes but not those listed above. Budd-Chiari syndrome is caused by occlusion of the inferior vena cava or hepatic veins. It is associated with polycythemia vera, pregnancy, and hepatocellular carcinoma. Congestive heart failure is definitely present here but is secondary to the hemochromatosis and not a primary diagnosis.

231. D. More than 90% of testicular tumors derive from germ cell tumors; the remainder are gonadal stromal tumors or metastatic from another site. The most common solid tumor in men between the ages of 15 and 40 is a seminoma. Age, race (Caucasians have a higher incidence), and cryptorchidism are the only known risk factors for germ cell tumors. Nonseminomatous germ cell tumors include embryonal carcinoma, choriocarcinoma, endodermal yolk sac tumor, and teratoma. Leydig cell tumors are gonadal stromal tumors that classically present with precocious puberty in children and gynecomastia in adults.

232. C. Intellectualization utilizes the mind's fund of associations to rationalize and explain a perilous situation in order to avoid experiencing the panic and distress arising the current events. Humor is used to parlay uncomfortable feelings in a less emotionally threatening way, using laughter and jokes to hide fear. Identification exists when a person takes the role of the aggressor and becomes much like that person to others later on in life. Isolation of affect is the relaying of one's own bad news in an emotionally detached manner. Projection is the irrational transference of one's own inadequacies or issues onto another: for example, with no ground or basis, a habitual liar might accuse his wife of lying to him.

233. C. Ethosuximide is an antiepileptic agent used to treat absence seizures; it inhibits calcium currents by blocking T-type calcium channels, which are thought to be responsible for absence seizures. The rash seen here is erythema multiforme; when combined with systemic symptoms, it is known as Stevens-Johnson syndrome. Lamotrigine, a drug used to treat partial and generalized tonic-clonic seizures, can also cause Stevens-Johnson syndrome. Carbamazepine is indicated for patients with partial generalized seizures as well as those with pain due to trigeminal neuralgia. Phenytoin is indicated for the treatment of status epilepticus and generalized tonic-clonic seizures. Valproic acid is indicated for the treatment of complex partial seizures and generalized tonic-clonic seizures.

234. E. This boy likely has gigantism, since he has had a rapid increase in growth that, based on the growth curve, is drastically different from his previous growth rate, and he is still prepubertal. Although this condition is due to increased levels of growth hormone, often from a GH-secreting pituitary adenoma, the measurement of growth hormone is not the best way to diagnose it. GH levels vary throughout the day. However, IGF-1 is also known to be elevated in this condition, and its levels remain relatively constant. Thus, it is a better test. Although impaired glucose tolerance can be seen in this condition, fasting serum glucose levels would be relatively nonspecific. ACTH levels are abnormal in a variety of conditions, but this would not be expected here. Having the parents keep a log of the boy's food intake might be helpful if it were only a matter of weight gain, but with the rapid growth, such a log would be noncontributory.

235. E. This question tests your ability to remember the order of hematopoiesis in a developing embryo. The first organ involved in hematopoiesis is the yolk sac, so this is what the teratogen would affect first. The second organ to be affected would be the liver, as this organ takes over for the yolk sac about 1 or 2 months of gestation. The spleen would be affected next, as this organ begins hematopoiesis at about 3 or 4 months of gestation. The bone marrow would be the final organ affected, as it starts hematopoiesis at about 4 months of gestation. The thymus is not involved in hematopoiesis.

236. D. The patient suffers from Peutz-Jeghers syndrome. Patients with this condition present with multiple pigmented macules around the lip and also with multiple hamartomatous colonic polyps, which may cause abdominal pain. Familial adenomatous polyposis (FAP) is an inherited disorder characterized by the development of multiple colonic polyps, usually by the age of 40. Patients with FAP are at a substantially increased risk of developing colonic carcinoma. Gardner syndrome is a variation of FAP, characterized by the development of colonic polyps as well as multiple osteomas, epidermal cysts, and fibromatosis. Hereditary nonpolyposis colorectal cancer is an inherited disorder characterized by an increased risk of multiple colorectal malignancies without preceding polyps. Turcot syndrome is characterized by the presence of multiple colonic polyps along with a variety of central nervous system tumors.

237. A. The anterior cruciate ligament (ACL) is most often stretched, torn, or both by a sudden twisting motion (for example, when the feet are planted one way and the knees are turned another way). The posterior cruciate ligament is most often injured by a direct impact, as in an automobile accident or football tackle. Injury to the cruciate ligament may not cause pain. Rather, the person may hear a popping sound, immediately followed by swelling, and the leg may buckle when he or she tries to stand on it. To diagnose an injury, the doctor may perform several tests to see whether the parts of the knee stay in proper position when pressure is applied in different directions. Patients with ACL tears usually describe a twisting or hyperextension of the knee. Typically, there is a significant effusion when the patient is first evaluated. The Lachman test is the best way to assess a knee for an acute ACL rupture. Abnormal passive abduction indicates a torn medial collateral ligament.

238. D. The middle meningeal artery would be the most likely source of blood in the above scenario, where a branch laceration of the artery has caused an epidural hematoma. The short period of consciousness is indicative of this diagnosis, pointing to cerebral compression. Berry aneurysm is most commonly associated with the circle of Willis, which may be affected by a subarachnoid hemorrhage. The middle cerebral artery and bridging veins are the same blood supply and are connected with a subdural hematoma. The CT of the head confirms the findings of an epidural hematoma.

239. C. Coarctation of the aorta is a constriction that usually occurs distal to the subclavian artery. Thus the artery branches carrying blood to the head and upper extremities are not affected. However, the lower extremities are affected. The kidneys respond to the lower pressure in the renal arteries and cause renal retention of salt and water to restore pressure to the kidneys but result in hypertension in the upper body. None of the following—hypovolemia, aortic regurgitation, left-sided heart failure or aortic stenosis—would result in a 35 mm Hg difference in systolic pressure between the lower and upper limbs.

240. C. The gynecoid pelvis is the most favorable pelvis for vaginal delivery. This pelvis type is seen in 50% of women and is characterized by an oval inlet, straight side walls, nonprominent ischial spines, a wide subpubic arch, and a concave sacrum. The android pelvis is wedge-shaped with convergent pelvic sidewalls and prominent ischial spines. The anthropoid pelvis is very common in African American women and is marked by an oval inlet with divergent pelvic side walls. The platypelloid pelvis is rare and characterized by the wide transverse diameter of the inlet.

241. F. Leydig cell tumors are sex cord stromal tumors and most frequently produce testosterone; however, a feminizing syndrome is common. This syndrome is probably secondary to aromatization of the testosterone moiety, leading to increases in estrogenic steroids, although the tumors can produce estradiol. Gynecomastia, breast tenderness, and infertility are the common presenting symptoms in adults. Histologically, 30% of Leydig cell tumors will have intracytoplasmic rod-shaped crystalloids of Reinke. Auer rods are associated with acute myelogenous leukemia. Birbeck granules are associated with histiocytosis X. Call-Exner bodies are associated with granulosa cell tumors. Mallory bodies are associated with alcoholic cirrhosis. Charcot-Leyden crystals are associated with bronchial asthma.

242. C. Positive reinforcement is the form of behavior modification used by this mother in order to encourage her son's appropriate behavior. Extinction uses the idea of ignoring inappropriate behavior to encourage its cessation.

Negative reinforcement is similar in that it uses discouragement to deter unacceptable behavior immediately after the event occurs. Punishment attempts to eliminate the behavior by imposing negative consequences after unwanted actions in order to prevent future recurrences. Stalling is a made-up term of no significance.

243. B. Osteoporosis is due to decreased bone mass, which results in thin, fragile bones. It usually occurs in postmenopausal women and the elderly, and patients typically present with bone pain and fractures. Osteogenesis imperfecta is a hereditary defect resulting from abnormal synthesis of type I collagen. It presents with brittle bones, recurrent fractures, and abnormally thin sclerae with a blue hue. Osteomyelitis is infection in the bone causing localized pain, swelling, fever, and leukocytosis. Rickets and osteomalacia are diseases of decreased mineralization of newly formed bone, usually caused by vitamin D deficiency. Rickets is the childhood form, often presenting with skull deformities as well as bowing of the legs. The adult form, osteomalacia, typically involves bone pain and fractures of the vertebrae, hips, and wrist. Treatment is with vitamin D and calcium.

244. D. This child has chronic granulomatous disease (CGD), which is characterized by a lack of NADPH oxidase. This allows organisms that possess peroxidase, such as *Staphylococcus aureus,* to continually degrade the peroxides that NADPH oxidase utilizes to generate bactericidal molecules. The nitrozolium blue test is negative in patients with CGD. G6PD deficiency leads to a hemolytic anemia upon exposure to various chemicals, such as antimalarial drugs and fava beans. Pyruvate kinase also causes a hemolytic anemia, although this disease is not as common as G6PD deficiency. A deficiency of myeloperoxidase would cause the symptoms shown above, but the nitrozolium blue test would be positive in this child. Hexokinase deficiency would not affect lymphocytes but would cause severe nutritional deficiency, as hexokinase is needed for glucose metabolism.

245. C. A muscle biopsy would likely show necrosis of types I and II fibers, phagocytosis, variation in fiber size, and perivascular inflammatory infiltrate. CT scan of the abdomen and skin biopsy have no place in the diagnosis of dermatomyositis. Antinuclear antibodies and rheumatoid factor are not used to diagnose dermatomyositis. Other useful tests in diagnosis would be a creatine kinase level and electromyography. The picture (Figure 24) shows the classic heliotropic rash characteristic of this condition.

246. C. SSRIs are first-line treatment in this age group. Because of their minimal side-effect profiles, these are very safe drugs. They do, however, cause a decrease in sexual function. Serotonin is present in high concentrations in the brainstem. This neurotransmitter is formed from tryptophan and is converted to melatonin in the pineal gland. Glycine is an inhibitory neurotransmitter found in the spinal cord and will increase the conductance of chloride. Histamine is formed from histidine and is present in high concentrations in the hypothalamus. Tyrosine is an amino acid and is converted to L-dopa by tyrosine hydroxylase in the synthetic pathway for dopamine, norepinephrine, and epinephrine.

247. B. This patient most likely has multiple spider angiomas due to alcoholic liver disease. Spider angiomas are characterized by a central pulsating, dilated arteriole from which small vessels radiate. They are thought to arise from impaired estrogen metabolism in the damaged liver, leading to hyperestrogenemia. Patients with elevated levels of cortisol suffer from Cushing's syndrome, which is characterized by moon facies, truncal obesity, hyperglycemia, and abdominal striae. Elevated levels of growth hormone cause gigantism in individuals whose epiphyseal growth plates are still open and acromegaly in individuals whose epiphyseal plates are closed. Elevated levels of progesterone are generally not associated with any pathology. Women with congenital adrenal hyperplasia may have elevated levels of testosterone, which lead to virilization and hirsutism.

248. A. LTD$_4$ and other leukotrienes are thought to be responsible for bronchoconstriction, increased bronchial activity, increased secretion of mucus, and edema. Zafirlukast interrupts the leukotriene pathway. Aspirin (acetylsalicylic acid, or ASA) is a nonsteroidal anti-inflammatory agent responsible for decreasing the production of prostaglandins, which serves to limit the inflammatory response. ASA also shifts the pathway to the leukotriene side, thus favoring bronchoconstriction. These agents do not inhibit the lipoxygenase pathway or phosphodiesterase. Sildenafil is an inhibitor of the type V phosphodiesterase.

249. A. Crigler-Najjar syndrome is diagnosed by the absence of UDP-glucuronyl transferase. Death follows within 1 to 3 years of onset. Patients can be treated with plasmapheresis and phototherapy to conjugate the bilirubin. Dubin-Johnson syndrome is caused by increased levels of conjugated bilirubin in serum due to defective liver excretion. A grossly black liver is also a common finding. Gilbert's syndrome is marked by mildly decreased UDP-glucuronyl transferase and patients are asymptomatic, with no known mortality risk. Reye's syndrome is a fatal childhood hepatoencephalopathy induced by ingestion of aspirin during viral infection.

250. D. Paraphimosis results from forcibly retracting the prepuce over the glans penis without replacing it in its original position. This condition may lead to marked swelling of the glans, which can cause extreme pain and urinary retention through urethral constriction. Phimosis is a condition in which the prepuce is too small to permit normal retraction. This may result from a congenital anomaly but is more commonly caused by repeated infections that cause scarring of the prepuce. Hypospadias is a condition in which the urethral opening is located abnormally on the ventral surface of the penis. The less common epispadias occurs when the urethral opening is abnormally located on the dorsal surface of the penis. Balanoposthitis may result from infection of the glans and prepuce by a variety of organisms, such as *Candida albicans, Gardnerella,* and anaerobic bacteria. Balanoposthitis is a common cause of phimosis.

Block 6

251. C. Cranial nerve (CN) III is the affected nerve; as a result, the corresponding eye will appear in the down and out position. CN I is the olfactory nerve and is not related to the ocular muscle movement. CN II is the optic nerve and functions in the capacity of vision, not motor movement. CN IV and CN VI are trochlear, which controls the superior oblique, and abducens, which controls lateral rectus, respectively. CN IV and CN VI are responsible for pulling the eye into its current position, as they are unopposed because of the lesion.

252. B. Based on the reports and the patient's country of origin, a likely diagnosis is Cooley's anemia, also known as Mediterranean anemia, which is beta thalassemia major. Alpha thalassemia is highly prevalent in Southeast Asia and is manifest as a "duplication of the globin" gene. Hemoglobin E disorders are becoming increasingly prevalent in the United States, with a presentation akin to that of hemoglobin C disorders. PKD presents as a congenital spherocytic hemolytic anemia, which is chronic and nonepisodic.

253. C. Pacinian corpuscles are onion-like structures in the subcutaneous skin that are specific for vibratory and tapping sensation. Meissner's corpuscles are located in "non-hair containing" skin and note velocity. Merkel's disks are transducers on epithelial cells and serve to note location. Ruffini's corpuscles are encapsulated and note pressure changes. The sensory homunculus is a somatotrophic map of the body located in the cerebral cortex.

254. B. This patient has the typical symptoms of temporal arteritis, one of the giant cell arteritides. It is characterized by granuloma formation with giant cells in the medium- to large-sized arteries. Biopsy of the temporal artery is used to confirm the diagnosis. Churg-Strauss syndrome is a necrotizing vasculitis that is prominent in the respiratory tract and is often associated with asthma. Lymphomatoid granulomatosis is characterized by infiltration of arteries by atypical lymphocytoid and plasmacytoid cells. Headache, vision changes, and jaw claudication are not common manifestations. Raynaud's disease is the recurrent vasospasm of small arteries and arterioles, which causes pallor and cyanosis. This mainly affects the digits. Thromboangiitis obliterans, also known as Buerger's disease, is a painful ischemic disease of medium-sized vessels that is associated with smoking. It is more commonly seen in young men. Headache, visual changes, and jaw claudication are not common manifestations.

255. B. This disease is due to the proliferation of histiocytic cells that are closely related to the Langerhans cells of the skin. Birbeck granules are characteristic of the disease. They resemble tennis racquets under electron microscopy. Auer rods are characteristic of acute myelogenous leukemia. Ferruginous bodies are seen in asbestosis. Non-caseating granulomas are seen with sarcoidosis. Giant cell inclusions are seen with herpetic infection.

256. E. This patient presents with an acute low back strain. The pain seems to be muscular in nature in that it does not radiate anywhere and is localized and reproducible. Current recommendations for the treatment of acute low back pain include a short period of rest, muscle relaxants, and analgesics as well as education regarding proper lifting techniques, posture, and back exercises. In addition, the patient should be advised that in the majority of cases of low back pain, the pain resolves with time. Surgical treatment of back pain is reserved for patients with neurological signs and clear pathological processes seen on imaging studies. Occasionally, in the treatment of chronic, intractable back pain, opioids are prescribed to help control the pain. However, they are not used as first-line treatments. Given that the pain is affecting the patient's daily activities, including work, some type of treatment should be offered. Malingering, at least at this point, does not seem to be the case, given that the injury occurred the day before and the patient is seeking help for his pain. He does not appear to have any ulterior motive, since he has not asked for time off of work or worker's compensation.

257. C. This patient has the characteristic signs of temporal arteritis, the most frequently occurring form of systemic vasculitis. It is most commonly seen in elderly persons and usually affects branches of the carotid artery, particularly the temporal artery. It constitutes a medical emergency, as it can occlude the ophthalmic artery, resulting in blindness. It responds well to steroids. Urokinase is a thrombolytic agent that cleaves thrombin and fibrin clots. Heparin is used in immediate anticoagulation for pulmonary embolism, stroke, angina, myocardial infarctions, and so on. Allopurinol is used to treat gout. It inhibits xanthine oxidase, thus lowering uric acid levels.

258. B. Enterokinase, which is found in the small intestine, converts trypsinogen to trypsin almost 2,000 times faster than the autocatalytic actions of trypsin. Pepsin is most specific for aromatic amino acids, with an optimal pH of 1 to 4. Sucrase cleaves sucrose into glucose and fructose. Chymotrypsin is a proteolytic enzyme that ultimately aids in the formation of alpha chymotrypsin.

259. D. Osteosarcoma is a spindle cell neoplasm that produces osteoid (unmineralized bone) or bone. About 60% of all osteosarcomas occur in children and adolescents in the second decade of life, and males are affected twice as often as females. A patient usually presents with pain and swelling of the affected area, which is most often the distal femur, proximal tibia, or proximal humerus. Classic x-ray findings include bone destruction, soft tissue with "sunburst" appearance, and a Codman's triangle (periosteal elevation that forms an angle with the cortex of the bone). Treatment usually includes chemotherapy; however, the prognosis is generally poor. Ewing's sarcoma is common in adolescence and generally affects the diaphyseal region of long bones and flat bones. Radiographs show a characteristic "onion peel" periosteal reaction with a generous soft tissue mass. Osteochondromas are hereditary multiple, bony metaphyseal projections capped with cartilage. They may or may not be symptomatic and may result in a deformity that compromises the blood supply to the bone. Osteomyelitis usually presents with a fever, localized pain, erythema, and swelling. This patient is afebrile, which most likely rules out this condition. Paget's disease is due to excessive bone resorption with replacement by soft, poorly mineralized osteoid in a disorganized fashion. It most often affects the skull, pelvis, femur, and vertebrae. It generally presents in the fifth or sixth decade of life. Malignant transformation into osteosarcoma is seen in 1% of cases.

260. B. It is most often secondary to infection or lymphatic blockage by a tumor. The lesion described is a hydrocele, which is composed of serous fluid that distends the tunica vaginalis. It is most often idiopathic but may sometimes be secondary to infection or lymphatic blockage by a tumor. A hydrocele can usually be clinically distinguished from solid testicular tumors by physical examination and transillumination. Hematoceles will not transilluminate clear fluid. Inguinal hernia and undescended testicle are unlikely, given the examination findings.

261. C. Klinefelter's syndrome is a common cause of male hypogonadism caused by meiotic nondisjunction, the karyotype most commonly being 47XXY. History usually includes complaints of fatigue, weakness, erectile dysfunction, academic difficulty, subnormal libido, poor self-esteem, and behavior problems. Clinical findings include testicular atrophy, infertility, eunuchoid body shape, high-pitched voice, female pattern of hair distribution, and gynecomastia. Female pseudohermaphroditism is manifest in a genetic female 46XX with female internal gonads but ambiguous or virilized external genitalia. Fragile X syndrome is an X-linked defect of the FMR1 gene associated with mental retardation, macroorchidism, and an enlarged face and ears. Male pseudohermaphroditism is manifest in a genetic male 46XY with normal testes but ambiguous or female genitalia. Turner's syndrome is a common cause of female hypogonadism with the karyotype 45XO, which presents clinically as short stature, ovarian dysgenesis, neck webbing, primary amenorrhea, and failure to develop secondary sex characteristics.

262. A. *Clostridium difficile* is a Gram-positive spore-forming rod that causes an antibiotic-associated diarrhea with yellow plaques on the colon referred to as pseudomembranous colitis. The antibiotics that most often lead to this condition are clindamycin, cephalosporins, amoxicillin, and ampicillin. Metronidazole and vancomycin are used for treatment. *Clostridium perfringens* is a large Gram-positive spore-forming rod that causes both gas gangrene and a self-limiting noninflammatory watery diarrhea resulting from reheated meats. *Helicobacter pylori* is associated with peptic ulcer disease. *Shigella* is associated with bloody diarrhea.

263. C. Premature ovarian failure is essentially menopause occurring in women < 40 years of age. The normal physical exam and symptoms of menopause further support this etiology. The elevated FSH accompanied by normal levels of the other hormones clinches this diagnosis.

Adrenal hyperplasia can be a cause of amenorrhea. However, it would be associated with symptoms of Cushing syndrome, such as hirsutism, increasing abdominal girth, abdominal striae, easy bruising, glucose intolerance, etc. While endometriosis can be associated with infertility, it usually causes dysmenorrhea, not amenorrhea, and would not be associated with elevated FSH levels. Polycystic ovary syndrome (PCOS) is a common cause of infertility and menstrual disturbances. These patients often manifest hirsutism and obesity. Furthermore, they would have increased LH, normal or decreased FSH, and increased DHEAS or testosterone. Pseudocyesis, or false pregnancy, is associated with amenorrhea, but it is also associated with weight gain, breast enlargement and engorgement, and abdominal enlargement.

264. A. Mild retardation would be the correct answer, as the ranges for classification of mental retardation are as follows:

Mild	(IQ 50 to 70)
Moderate	(IQ 35 to 55)
Severe	(IQ 20 to 40)
Profound	(<20)

265. B. The endoscopic image (Figure 26) shows the trachea dividing into two bronchi. There is a lung carcinoma protruding into the bronchi. The bronchioles do not have cartilage and submucosal glands. The entire respiratory tree except the vocal cords is lined by pseudostratified columnar ciliated epithelial cells.

266. C. Pituitary apoplexy is the sudden onset of meningeal pain, visual loss, and ophthalmoplegia due to infarction of a pituitary adenoma, producing compression of the chiasm and cavernous sinus and some subarachnoid hemorrhage. The patient's fatigue and lack of libido are due to pituitary hormonal deficiencies. Carotid artery embolism would not show hemorrhage on the MRI and would have different CNS manifestations. In an epidural hemorrhage, there is an accumulation of blood between the dura and the skull. A subdural hemorrhage would show blood between the dural and subarachnoid membranes. Sheehan's syndrome is postpartum necrosis of the pituitary gland.

267. A. This patient has evidence of small-artery microembolism. These emboli are composed of fibrin or cholesterol. They can be due to atherosclerosis of the aortoiliac or femoral arterial vessels. This is an embolic condition, not a thrombotic one. There is no clinical information about the femoral veins to suggest a diagnosis of femoral vein thrombosis. Vascular studies were not performed, therefore the diagnosis of inferior vena cava thrombosis is unlikely.

268. E. There are several types of herpesvirus that manifest in different forms. Herpes simplex type 1 is most commonly known as oral herpes, which is associated with gingivostomatitis and recurrent cold sores on the skin or lips. It can remain latent in the trigeminal root ganglion and cause recurrent attacks in times of stress. Herpes simplex 1 does not typically remain latent in the dorsal root, mesenteric, or sacral root ganglia.

269. C. This patient likely has melanoma, which is a malignant skin cancer posing a high risk of metastasis. It is associated with sunlight exposure and is more commonly seen in fair-skinned individuals. Depth of tumor correlates with risk of metastasis. Change in color, change in contour, increasing size, and the fact that it is not fluid filled are all signs of malignancy; however, these signs do not correlate well with metastasis.

270. B. Her condition is caused by a loss of accommodation power of the lens. This usually occurs with normal aging and is not an issue of major concern. A biconcave lens would be used to correct a condition called myopia, which is nearsightedness. A cylindrical lens is used for astigmatism to correct the curvature of the lens. Eye drops would be useful in rehydrating dry eyes but are not applicable in this situation. Laser surgery can be used as well, but because that is an invasive technique, it would not be a first-line option.

271. A. Drug-induced lupus can follow the use of several drugs, such as hydralazine, procainamide, isoniazid, chlorpromazine, methyldopa, quinidine, ethosuximide, and D-penicillamine. Cinchonism is a condition that may follow quinidine use; it includes deafness, roaring in the ears, and vertigo. A disulfiram-like reaction is due to inhibition of acetaldehyde dehydrogenase and is associated with metronidazole. Nephrogenic diabetes insipidus is the loss of large amounts of free water in the urine and is a side effect of lithium. Pellagra is a condition of dermatitis, diarrhea, and dementia due to niacin deficiency. Rifampin is a drug used against tuberculosis that is known to temporarily impart a reddish color on soft tissues of the body.

272. C. This patient has mitral stenosis, which has not been treated. It has caused enlargement of his left atrium, the most posterior chamber of the heart; when it is enlarged, it can cause dysphagia. A late diastolic murmur is the murmur heard with mitral stenosis. Aortic stenosis would cause enlargement of the left ventricle, and this would not cause dysphagia. The left ventricle is more anterior. An untreated ventricular septal defect (VSD) would also cause hypertrophy of the left ventricle; the murmur associated with it is holosystolic. Mitral regurgitation could cause some left atrial enlargement, but the murmur is holosystolic. From the question stem, therefore, this should be eliminated. Tricuspid stenosis would cause enlargement of the right atrium. The right atrium is not in the posterior part of the heart. Enlargement of the right atrium would not cause dysphagia. The ECG reveals a prominent P wave as well as evidence of right ventricular hypertrophy.

273. B. Barbiturates are the most commonly used drugs in attempted suicide. They have a low safety margin and readily cause respiratory depression, which can lead to death. Amphetamines can drastically increase heart rate and cause cardiac arrest, but they are not used nearly as often as barbiturates. Benzodiazepines have a high safety margin and are relatively safe unless they are combined with another sedative, such as alcohol. Marijuana is not commonly used in attempted suicide.

Opioids can also cause respiratory depression and death, but they are not usually used in this context.

274. B. The patient is experiencing malignant hypothermia, which can lead to lactic acidosis. Dantrolene acts by blocking Ca^{2+} release from the sarcoplasmic reticulum. Atropine acts by inhibiting actions of acetylcholine stimuli at postganglionic cholinergic receptors (glands, smooth muscle, and CNS sites). Neostigmine and pyridostigmine both inhibit the destruction of acetylcholine by cholinesterase. Nicotine, epinephrine, norepinephrine, and dopamine are all stimulators but are not indicated in this patient. Scopolamine competitively inhibits the action of acetylcholine at muscarinic receptors and is used mainly in ophthalmology. Rocuronium is another nondepolarizing blocker used in anesthesia.

275. A. Arteriosclerosis is a broad term used to identify several types of vascular disease characterized by sclerosis and increased blood vessel thickness. Arteriolosclerosis is noted by increased hyaline thickening of the small arteries and arterioles, usually in the kidney. It is certainly associated with an increased risk of myocardial infarction because of the issues mentioned, but that itself is not a diagnosis. Pulmonary embolism is a serious issue, usually secondary to a hypercoagulable state, which has not been indicated here, and there have been no indications of cyanosis or breathing difficulties. Swiss-type agammaglobulinemia is noted by decreased numbers of B and T cells and has no bearing on vascular issues.

276. D. This patient has the typical symptoms of rheumatoid arthritis. Pannus tissue eroding the cartilage is a characterization of chronic rheumatoid arthritis. This granulation tissue with inflammatory, fibroblastic, and vascular properties, destroys the articular cartilage, leaving scar tissue, which is often responsible for joint ankylosis and the symptoms seen in the metacarpophalangeal (MCP) and proximal interphalangeal (PIP) joints. An abnormal D-xylose test is seen in celiac sprue, which is characterized by gliadin sensitivity, leading to steatorrhea. Heberden's nodes are nodules seen in the distal interphalangeal (DIP) joints, which is characteristic of osteoarthritis. The DIP joints are spared in rheumatoid arthritis. Noncaseating granulomas are seen in sarcoidosis. Rhomboid crystals in the joint spaces are seen with pseudogout, which is caused by deposits of calcium pyrophosphate crystals in the joint spaces. Larger joints, such as the knee, are often the targets of these deposits.

277. E. Pursed lips are a learned mechanism used to prevent airway collapse associated with a forced expiration. With emphysema, airway resistance is increased, causing this forced expiration, which raises intrapleural pressure to a positive value. Increased compliance is associated with the barrel-shaped chest. FRC increases with an obstructive lung disease such as emphysema.

278. D. The hexose monophosphate shunt produces two NADPH and/or ribose molecules from glucose. It is also known as the pentose shunt or phosphogluconate oxidative pathway. The oxidation of acetyl-CoA to CO_2 and transfer of electrons to NAD^+ and FAD is handled by the tricarboxylic acid (TCA) cycle. The oxidation of NADH and $FADH_2$ to form three and two molecules of ATP, respectively, is carried out by the electron transport chain. The breakdown of glycogen to glucose under hormonal control is carried out by glycogenesis.

279. C. A grade 4 murmur is described as being loud, with a palpable thrill. Murmurs 1 through 3 do not have palpable thrills, whereas murmurs 4 through 6 do. Grade 2 murmurs are quiet but heard immediately after placing stethoscope on the chest. Grade 3 murmurs are moderately loud. Grade 5 murmurs are very loud, with a thrill; they may be heard when the stethoscope is partly off the chest. Grade 6 murmurs are very loud, with a thrill, and may be heard with the stethoscope entirely off the chest.

280. A. A metabolic acidosis is a process that causes a primary decrease in the serum bicarbonate from either a gain of acid or loss of bicarbonate. Diabetic ketoacidosis generates excessive amounts of ketoacids from the incomplete oxidation of fatty acids that accumulate in the serum and cause a metabolic acidosis. The respiratory compensation for metabolic acidosis is increased ventilation, which produces a secondary decrease in $Paco_2$. To determine whether respiratory compensation is adequate, the Winter formula can be applied as follows: (measured bicarbonate) $\times 1.5 + 8 +/- 2.5 = Paco_2$.

281. D. This patient had Waterhouse-Friderichsen syndrome, more than likely caused by a *Neisseria meningitidis* infection. The classic presentation is a child with vomiting, diarrhea, extensive purpura, cyanosis, and tonic-clonic seizures who may have had a recent respiratory infection. Circulatory collapse and hemorrhage into the adrenal glands are classic with this syndrome. Myocardial infarction and stroke are extremely unlikely to occur in a 10-year-old. These conditions are more common in older adults.

282. B. This patient is suffering from Kleine-Levin syndrome, which is more common in the adolescent population, as the primary age of onset ranges from 10 years of age to the early twenties. Circadian rhythm sleep disorder is marked by delayed sleep and leads a person to fall asleep and wake up later than he or she had intended. Restless legs syndrome causes uncomfortable leg pains and forces the patient to keep moving his or her legs. This makes it difficult to fall asleep and wakes patients up during the night. Sleep drunkenness is a genetically inherited disorder that causes difficulty in arising from a full night's sleep; its presentation can be confused with that of actual drunkenness and hangover.

283. B. The celiac trunk originates at the abdominal aorta at the level of the T12-L1 intervertebral disc. It then gives rise to the splenic artery, which is the major blood supply to the spleen. The splenic artery also gives rise to the gastroepiploic artery, which supplies the left greater curvature of the stomach. The abdominal aorta gives rise to the celiac artery, which then gives rise to the splenic artery, but it is not the direct origin of the splenic artery. The superior mesenteric artery comes off the abdominal

aorta and supplies the duodenum, jejunum, ileum, and the proximal two-thirds of the transverse colon. The right gastric artery supplies the right lesser curvature of the stomach and does not give rise to any other arteries.

284. C. A low-dose beta-blocker (metoprolol) would help bring this patient's heart rate down to between 50 and 60 bpm and decrease his blood pressure to between 90 and 110 systolic. None of the other choices will decrease the work of this patient's heart as well as a beta-blocker would.

285. F. Oxytocin is a hormone of the posterior pituitary and is now administered to patients in synthetic form. It is used in obstetrics to stimulate uterine contractions, thus inducing or reinforcing labor. Toward the end of pregnancy, the sensitivity of the uterus to oxytocin is increased, as the uterus is under estrogenic dominance. Oxytocin can also be used to promote the ejection of breast milk, as it causes contraction of the myoepithelial cells around the mammary alveoli. Adrenocorticotropic hormone acts on the adrenal cortex to produce cortisol. Gonadotrophin-releasing hormone acts on the male testis to produce testosterone. Additional testosterone production occurs in the adrenal gland. Growth hormone-releasing hormone acts on the pituitary gland to produce growth hormone. Human chorionic gonadotrophin is elevated in tumor states such as testis tumors, specifically choriocarcinoma.

286. C. Hyperplastic arteriolosclerosis is the most accurate choice for the above situation. It is marked by necrotizing arteriolitis and onionskin thickening of the arteriolar walls; this condition is known as malignant nephrosclerosis in relation to its effect on the kidney. Hemangioendothelioma is a malignant tumor of the vascular system and does not present like the above pathology. Hyaline arteriolosclerosis is characterized by hyaline thickening of arteriolar walls and is known as benign nephrosclerosis in the kidneys, producing hypertension. Hypersensitivity vasculitis is caused by inflammation of the small blood vessels. Polyarteritis nodosa produces aneurysmal nodules secondary to destruction of arterial media and internal elastic lamellae.

287. D. Minimal change disease is a nephrotic syndrome. It is most often seen in young children and less commonly in adolescents and adults. Pathological findings include lipid-laden renal cortices, most often in the cells of the proximal convoluted tubule. The glomeruli appear normal, while the epithelial foot processes become fused. Adrenal steroid intervention is usually the method of treatment. Alport's disease is a hereditary nephritis associated with nerve deafness. One classically sees a split lamina densa of the glomerular basement membrane (GBM). IgA nephropathy has the classic picture of deposits of IgA in the GBM. Poststreptococcal glomerulonephritis (GN) is typically seen in children after infection with *Strep. pyogenes*. The slides shown illustrate minimal change disease. While Figure 28A shows a normal glomerulus on light microscopy, the electron microscopic image shows fusion of the foot processes.

288. E. This is delayed response to infection with *Treponema pallidum,* which causes syphilis. These symptoms are indicative of tertiary syphilis. Staphylococcal and streptococcal infections cause only skin infections, not any of the neurological symptoms. Measles is characterized by a maculopapular rash on the face and trunk without the neurological symptoms. *Borrelia burgdorferi* is the causative agent of Lyme disease, characterized by a bull's-eye rash, flu-like symptoms, and cardiac problems.

289. B. The most likely cause of primary hyperparathyroidism is a parathyroid adenoma. Hypercalcemia secondary to a parathyroid adenoma is usually discovered accidentally by routine chemistry panels. Most patients are asymptomatic and the adenoma is usually so small and deep in the neck that it is almost never palpable. Symptoms of hypercalcemia are best remembered by the saying, "Bones, stones, abdominal groans, psychic moans, with fatigue overtones." Parathyroid hormone usually stimulates renal tubular reabsorption of calcium and excretion of phosphate. In a state of hyperparathyroidism, the increase of calcium in the glomerular filtrate overwhelms tubular resorptive capacity and results in hypercalciuria on top of the hypercalcemia. Serum phosphate remains low secondary to increased excretion. Hypercalcemia is common in untreated Addison's disease; however, this patient did not have any other signs of adrenal insufficiency, such as weakness, skin pigmentation, weight loss, hypotension, and anorexia. A parathyroid carcinoma could cause the same clinical picture; however, such tumors are very rare and thus would not be the most likely cause of this patient's problem. Tuberculosis and other granulomatous disorders are known to cause hypercalcemia; however, this patient did not present with any other symptoms of TB. Ingestion of large amounts of calcium (antacid) or vitamin D can cause hypercalcemia. However, this patient had no history of excessive use of antacids or vitamins.

290. D. Secretory IgA to rotavirus is commonly present in the colostrum of lactating mothers and may persist in breast milk for many months postpartum. Infants are highly susceptible, as it is a highly common cause of gastroenteritis. There is no immunization against rotavirus, so this would be false. Rotavirus can cause dehydration, electrolyte imbalance, and possibly the need for hospitalization.

291. B. The most common cause of right-sided heart failure is left-sided heart failure. This is an important association. Right-sided heart failure results in right ventricular hypertrophy. Pulmonary hypertension can cause right-sided heart failure, but this is usually caused by left-sided heart failure as well. There is no evidence that this patient has a dilated cardiomyopathy, but this can be a cause of right-sided heart failure. Tricuspid disease and pulmonary valve stenosis cause right-sided heart failure, but not as often as left-sided heart failure.

292. E. Acute endometritis is most often related to intrauterine trauma from instrumentation, intrauterine contraceptive devices (IUDs), and complications of pregnancy, such as postpartum retention of placental fragments. Acute endometritis is most often caused by *Staphylococcus aureus* and *Streptococcus* species. A granulomatous endometritis known as chronic specific endometritis is usually caused by *Mycobacterium tuberculosis. Candida albicans* is associated with pseudohyphae on KOH preparation. *Chlamydia trachomatis* is associated with nongonococcal urethritis. Treatment is tetracycline or erythromycin.

293. C. Asthma is associated with a respiratory acidosis due to hypoventilation of the lung leading to retained CO_2, which causes a decrease in the pH. In acute respiratory acidosis, the compensation occurs in two steps. The initial response is cellular buffering, which occurs over minutes to hours. Cellular buffering elevates plasma bicarbonate (HCO_3^-) only slightly, approximately 1 mEq/L for each 10-mm Hg increase in $Paco_2$. The second step is renal compensation, which occurs over 3 to 5 days. With renal compensation, renal excretion of carbonic acid and bicarbonate reabsorption are both increased. In renal compensation, plasma bicarbonate rises 3.5 mEq/L for each increase of 10 mm Hg in $Paco_2$. The ingestion of aspirin and hyperventilation both cause a respiratory alkalosis by means of a decreased CO_2. Renal failure is associated with a metabolic acidosis and an increased anion gap.

294. D. Indomethacin is a nonsteroidal anti-inflammatory drug (NSAID) that causes premature closure of the patent ductus arteriosus, which can be detrimental to the fetus. Acetaminophen (Tylenol) does not cause any ill effects to the fetus. Prednisone crosses the placenta in only small amounts. Hydrocortisone and cortisone are inactivated when they cross the placenta.

295. A. The Apgar score is calculated by assigning a score of 0 to 2 for five separate categories at both 1 and 5 min. Ten is a perfect score. Color (0 = blue/pale, 1 = trunk pink, 2 = all pink); heart rate (0 = 0 bpm, 1 ≤ 100 bpm, 2 ≥ 100 bpm); reflex irritability (0 = none, 1 = grimace, 2 = grimace and cough); muscle tone (0 = limp, 1 = some, 2 = active); respiratory effort (0 = none, 1 = irregular, 2 = regular).

296. B. Finasteride inhibits the enzyme 5-alpha reductase, which normally converts testosterone to dihydrotestosterone (DHT). DHT is the strongest androgen in the body, and blocking its production decreases the size of the prostate gland because there is then less androgenic stimulus on the prostate. Finasteride is also marketed as a drug to reduce hair loss, as DHT has been proven to have a role in male-pattern baldness. Finasteride has no effect in blocking the adrenal production of androgens. In addition, Finasteride has no role in blocking androgen receptors. The drug flutamide is a competitive androgen receptor blocker that has been shown to have a role in treating prostatic adenocarcinoma. The mechanism of action being described in choice D belongs to the drug leuprolide. When given in a continuous fashion, leuprolide inhibits LH and FSH by acting as a GN-RH agonist and can be used to treat prostatic carcinoma. Finasteride does not inhibit the production of LH and FSH.

297. B. This young woman's presentation is most consistent with ectopic pregnancy. Hematosalpinx is bleeding into the fallopian tubes and is most often caused by an ectopic pregnancy. Adenomatoid tumor is a benign tumor and can be found commonly in the epididymis. There is no evidence to suggest hydrosalpinx or pyosalpinx in this patient. These would be associated with ultrasound findings of increased tubal fluid, which would be less echogenic if associated with hydrosalpinx than with pyosalpinx.

298. C. The most likely predisposing factor that led to this hemorrhage is that of long-standing hypertension. HTN is often complicated by minute dilations at small artery bifurcations. These Charcot-Bouchard aneurysms may be sites of hemorrhagic rupture; they occur most often in the basal ganglia/thalamus. Diabetes can cause vascular compromise and injury but is not specifically linked with Charcot-Bouchard aneurysm formation. Genetic predisposition is a significant cause in many medical issues but is not the strongest related causality in this condition. Tobacco use is linked with pulmonary issues and can also cause vascular compromise, but not necessarily with this specific issue.

299. B. Disulfiram produces a sensitivity to alcohol resulting in a highly unpleasant reaction when the patient under treatment ingests even small amounts of alcohol. Disulfiram blocks the oxidation of alcohol at the acetaldehyde stage. During alcohol metabolism after disulfiram intake, the concentration of acetaldehyde occurring in the blood may be 5 to 10 times higher than that found during metabolism of the same amount of alcohol alone. Disulfiram does not appear to influence the rate of alcohol elimination from the body. Even small amounts of aftershave or other forms of alcohol (e.g., mouth wash, cough medicines, vinegars) can cause a reaction with the disulfiram. Disulfiram is not a long-term cure for alcoholism. It is to be used as an aid in the management of selected chronic alcoholic patients who want to remain in a state of enforced sobriety so that supportive and psychotherapeutic treatment may be applied to best advantage.

300. C. Lateral epicondylar tendinitis, or tennis elbow, is a painful condition involving the soft tissue over the lateral aspect of the elbow. The pain originates at or near the site of attachment of the common extensors to the lateral epicondyle and may radiate into the forearm and dorsum of the wrist, as in this patient. The condition is thought to be caused by small tears of the extensor aponeurosis resulting from repeated resisted contractions of the extensor muscles. Passive flexion of the fingers and wrist and having the patient extend the wrist against resistance can elicit the pain. Biceps tendinitis is caused by friction on the tendon of the long head of the biceps as it passes through the bicipital groove. A patient will experience anterior shoulder pain that radiates down the biceps into the forearm. Carpal tunnel syndrome results from compression of the median nerve in the carpal tunnel. It is manifest as numbness and pain in the thumb as well as the second and third fingers and the radial half of the fourth. It is sometimes accompanied by thenar atrophy. Medial epicondylar tendinitis or golfer's elbow is a similar disorder of the common flexor muscle group at its origin, the medial epicondyle of the humerus. Pain can be elicited by resisting wrist flexion and pronation with the elbow extended. Olecranon bursitis is an inflammation of the bursa over the olecranon process caused by acute or chronic trauma, rheumatoid arthritis, or infection. Patients experience pain and swelling over the affected bursa.

Block 7

301. D. The classic signs of cinchonism due to overdose of quinidine are decreased auditory acuity, headache, vertigo, and lupus-like syndrome and a widened QRS complex. Phenytoin can cause similar symptoms but not the decreased auditory acuity. The others do not commonly cause the symptoms that this patient is experiencing. Ciprofloxacin is not associated with CNS effects as described in this question. Multivitamins when taken at recommended doses are not associated with CNS effects.

302. D. A dissecting aneurysm usually presents with tearing chest pain: it results in aortic rupture and, soon after, death. It is a longitudinal intraluminal tear in the wall of the ascending aorta. Syphilitic aneurysm is associated with tertiary syphilis and is caused by syphilitic aortitis; it involves the ascending aorta. Berry aneurysm occurs in the circle of Willis and usually hemorrhages into the subarachnoid space. Arteriovenous fistula is a miscommunication between an artery and a vein.

303. B. Laryngeal papillomas are benign neoplasms usually located on the true vocal cords. In children, they present as multiple lesions and are usually caused by HPV. In adults, they occur as single lesions and sometimes undergo malignant change. A singer's nodule is a small benign laryngeal polyp associated with chronic irritation from excessive use or heavy cigarette smoking. It is usually found on the true vocal cords. Squamous cell carcinomas of the larynx include glottic, supraglottic, and subglottic carcinomas. They are usually seen in men over age 40 who have a history of smoking and alcoholism. Glottic carcinomas are the most common and have the best prognosis.

304. C. The net pressure is determined by the Starling equation, which states the following: The capillary hydrostatic pressure minus the plasma interstitial pressure, in this case $40 - 0$, is subtracted from the capillary oncotic pressure minus the interstitial fluid oncotic pressure, in this case $38 - 4$. The net result is $+6$, which means that there will be a net filtration (movement of solutes out of the capillaries).

305. E. This patient has multiple myeloma, characterized by the overproliferation of plasma cells. He presents with classic symptoms of multiple myeloma, including low back pain from bone lesions caused by the release of osteoclast activating factor by the plasma cells. His lethargy can be caused by a lack of erythrocytes as the plasma cells "take over" the bone marrow. Cytotoxic T lymphocytes and helper T lymphocytes may be overly abundant in other lymphoid neoplasms but not in multiple myeloma. Mast cells and erythrocytes may actually be lacking, not overly abundant in multiple myeloma. The x-ray of the arm (Figure 29) reveals lytic areas and endosteal scalloping.

306. D. Norwalk virus's presentation has the classic presentation outlined here, especially among passengers on a cruise ship. Also prone to outbreaks are recreational camps, schools/colleges, and nursing homes. Tuberculosis presents with night sweats, cough, fevers, and shortness of breath. An initial outbreak of herpes simplex I can present with fever, malaise, and overall dysphoria, but not necessarily the above symptoms. *Giardia* is commonly found in streams and rivers, which is possible in a vacation scenario, but the cruise points to Norwalk.

307. C. Seminoma presents as the most frequently occurring germ cell tumor in 40% of the cases. It is a malignant germ cell tumor and is radiosensitive and often highly curable, with a peak occurrence in the mid-thirties. Embryonal carcinoma is also malignant, presents with pain and metastasis, and has a much worse prognosis than seminoma. Leydig cell tumors are usually benign and often cause precocious puberty. Teratoma is a germ cell tumor derived from more than one layer and is usually malignant. Yolk sac tumor usually presents with an increase in serum alpha-fetoprotein and peaks in early childhood.

308. C. This presentation is classic for Goodpasture's disease. Males in their mid-twenties have the highest reported incidence. Pulmonary involvement is common. Goodpasture's affects the kidneys and lungs, along with the linear IgG immunofluorescence would be indicative of the diagnosis. Alport's syndrome is a hereditary nephritis with nerve deafness. Berger's disease, better known as IgA nephropathy, is commonly found in children with recurrent hematuria following an infection and characterized by deposition of IgA along the mesangium. Lupus nephropathy is mainly present with nephrotic signs and possibly combined with nephritic features.

309. A. Acromegaly is associated with hypersecretion of growth hormone after closure of the epiphysis. It is most often caused by a pituitary adenoma and is characterized by macroglossia, tall stature, large hands, a prominent mandible, wide-spaced teeth, and carpal tunnel syndrome. Gigantism is associated with hypersecretion of growth hormone but occurs before closure of the epiphyses. Amyloidosis is caused by deposition of fibrin within certain organs. Macroglossia can be seen with it. Hypothyroidism can be associated with macroglossia. Coarse features may run in families with familial prognathism.

310. D. The defect is deficient activity of NADPH oxidase. The daughter will have an increased susceptibility to bacterial infections. Chronic granulomatous disease is characterized by the inability of polymorphonuclear leukocytes to kill ingested bacteria. In this disease, leukocytes are deficient in NADPH oxidase, an enzyme normally used by the cell to generate oxygen metabolites. These oxygen metabolites are then used to kill the ingested bacteria. Therefore, patients with chronic granulomatous disease have an increased susceptibility to bacterial infections due the decreased production of oxygen metabolites. These patients are not at risk for increased viral infections.

311. B. A CSF immunoglobulin would be used to potentially detect multiple oligoclonal bands, which would be indicative of multiple sclerosis and would help with the diagnosis. A complete blood count is nonspecific and might provide some information but not enough to aid in diagnosis. CT of abdomen and pelvis would provide little to no information based on the above clinical presentation. Hemoglobin electrophoresis is useful in identifying blood disorders, such as sickle cell anemia. A urinalysis would help in a genitourinary situation; it would not be relevant in this case scenario.

312. A. The patient is showing symptoms typical of Lyme disease (named after where it was first discovered, in Lyme, Connecticut). Lyme disease is caused by *Borrelia burgdorferi*, which is transmitted by the *Ixodes* tick. There are three stages of Lyme disease: erythema chronicum migrans ("bull's-eye" lesion) and flu-like symptoms, neurological and cardiac manifestations, and an autoimmune migratory polyarthritis. *Brucella* is responsible for brucellosis and is associated with unpasteurized dairy products. *Francisella tularensis* is responsible for tularemia. *Pasteurella multocida* causes a cellulitis that is usually due to an animal bite. *Rickettsia rickettsii* causes Rocky Mountain spotted fever, which manifests itself as a migratory rash starting on the palms and soles and moves to the trunk.

313. D. This is the classic example of rose gardener's disease, caused by *Sporothrix schenckii*. There is commonly a local pustule with some lymphangitis. Histoplasmosis and blastomycosis are two examples of respiratory infections caused by fungi, most commonly acquired through airborne exposure. *Bacillus anthracis* is acquired through soil but presents with a black eschar. *Staphylococcus aureus* is not the most likely culprit here.

314. B. Ankle sprains are very common and most often involve the lateral ligament complex, particularly the anterior talofibular ligament. Up to 85% of the time, the sprain is an inversion injury and pain will be elicited with this motion. The injured ligament is often tender to palpation, ecchymotic, and swollen. Treatment usually involves the employment of rest, ice, compression, and elevation (remembered by the acronym RICE) and time. Rupture of the Achilles' tendon may occur during running or jumping and causes a palpable defect—swelling, and tenderness of the tendon. Plantar fasciitis causes pain over the medial aspect of the plantar fascia. The pain is usually worse in the morning and subsides with a few minutes of ambulation. Stress fractures occur with overuse and generally present with chronic localized pain over the fracture site that becomes manifest with use. Tarsal tunnel syndrome occurs with entrapment of the posterior tibial nerve in the tarsal tunnel. Pain and numbness are experienced in the soles of the feet, toes, and medial malleoli.

315. C. Narrowing of the coronary arteries by atherosclerosis is the main cause of ischemic heart disease. All of the other answer choices could very well contribute to ischemic cardiac issues, but the main cause—the one that is most prominent and common—would be atherosclerotic narrowing of the coronary arteries.

316. A. Levothyroxine (Synthroid) is used to replace thyroid hormone whenever endogenous production is insufficient. This child has cretinism and his description gives the classic picture. Patients with cretinism have severe mental retardation, enlarged tongues, and umbilical hernias. The condition is rare in the United States because of screening tests. Methimazole and propylthiouracil are used in the treatment of hyperthyroidism. Although they work by slightly different mechanisms, they both act to decrease the synthesis of thyroid hormones. They are used in hyperthyroid conditions such as Graves' disease. Vitamin B_6, or pyridoxine, is given to replace a deficiency of vitamin B_6 caused by an inadequate dietary intake or by a medication such as pyridoxine. Signs and symptoms of vitamin B_6 deficiency are cheilosis, glossitis, anemia, and neurological dysfunction. Vitamin B_{12} can be used to treat megaloblastic anemia caused by a vitamin B_{12} deficiency.

317. B. Hypnagogic hallucinations are unpleasant experiences that a person can have while falling asleep. In a hypnagogic state, a person can have life-like visions or even full-body paralysis. The frightening part, in many cases, is the individual's inability to react to these hallucinations, even being unable to make a sound. Hypnagogic hallucinations are not uncommon, as some 30 to 40% of people experience them at least once in their lives. However, they can be a sign of narcolepsy or temporal lobe epilepsy. A hypnopompic hallucination is similar but occurs when a person is waking from sleep. A delusion is a disorder of thought content in which a person has a fixed, false belief that is not shared with other members of the culture yet that is firmly maintained even on questioning. Illusions are misinterpretations of actual external stimuli. Loose associations are disorders in the form of thought, or the way that ideas are connected by an individual.

318. C. The lamina propria is highly cellular, with numerous IgA-producing plasma cells, macrophages, eosinophils, lymphocytes, lymphatic ducts, and lymphoid nodules. Epithelium contains goblet cells and enterocytes. The villi contain lymphatic lacteals, with smooth muscle attached to the villus's tip. Mucous glands, which are also known as "crypts of Lieberkühn", serve mainly for cell and fluid replacement.

319. B. This patient presents with classic signs of molluscum contagiosum, which is characterized by flesh-colored papules with central umbilication. Molluscum contagiosum is caused by a poxvirus, which is a complex double-stranded DNA virus. Ambisense double-stranded RNA viruses include bunyaviruses and arenaviruses. Negative-sense single stranded RNA viruses include the paramyxoviruses, rhabdoviruses, filoviruses, and orthomyxoviruses. Positive-sense single-stranded RNA viruses include the picornaviruses, flaviviruses, calciviruses, togaviruses, coronaviruses, and retroviruses. The only known single-stranded DNA virus is the parvovirus.

320. A. Dysgerminomas are tumors of germ cell origin. Such tumors make up 25% of ovarian tumors and account for most ovarian tumors occurring in women > 20 years of age. Dysgerminomas are malignant tumors that are homologous to testicular seminomas. Yolk sac tumors are associated with elevated alpha-fetoprotein levels. Teratomas constitute 90% of germ cell tumors of the ovary. They involve all three germ cell layers. Mature teratomas (dermoid cysts) are benign. Immature teratoma is an aggressive malignant tumor. Monodermal teratoma (struma ovarii) is typically composed only of thyroid tissue.

321. D. Sucralfate is used as a prophylaxis of stress-induced gastritis. This drug should not be used in conjunction with proton pump inhibitors because sucralfate adheres to the ulcer in the acidic gastric juice, forming a protective layer that serves as a barrier against acid, bile salts, and enzymes in the stomach and duodenum. If a proton-pump inhibitor is used, there will be no acid in the gut to allow this drug to work. All the other drugs would be acceptable in this patient.

322. D. This patient has evidence of tangential thinking. This disorder of thought process involves loosening of associations. Each thought is connected to the one preceding but the overall topic diverges from the initial point. Aphasia is defined as a transient disruption of one's speech. Clanging is when a person makes associations based on sounds. Circumferential thinking is when someone uses excessive amounts of detail that are irrelevant in order to answer the question. Thought blocking is when a person's train of thought is blocked for some time and he or she is unable to finish the statement that had been begun.

323. D. Exposure to animal urine or feces during pregnancy is associated with an increased incidence of *Toxoplasma gondii* infection, which can cross the placenta and cause neurological abnormalities in the fetus. Smoking can lead to decreased birth weight and various birth defects, but not specifically those listed above. Exposure to aniline dyes has been linked to bladder cancer. Alcohol exposure can lead to birth defects and anencephaly. Exposure to sick children during pregnancy has no bearing on this clinical scenario.

324. E. This patient has a thyroglossal duct cyst. Because the thyroid gland begins its development behind the tongue before it descends to its position in the neck, it can remain behind the tongue if it does not migrate along the thyroglossal duct. This child has signs of hypothyroidism, which are due to failure of his thyroid hormones to be absorbed adequately into the circulation. A brachial cleft cyst can be caused by a persistent cervical sinus and would be present more laterally in the neck, near the sternocleidomastoid muscle. Choanal atresia is a closure of the nasal passageway. Congenital pyloric stenosis is a narrowing of the pyloric sphincter in the pylorus of the stomach, which is suspected in young children who vomit their food immediately after eating. Meckel's diverticulum is caused by failure of regression of the vitelline duct, which forms an outpouching in the ileum and can present with diarrhea and blood in the stools. Some types contain different kinds of tissue from different parts of the body, such as the pancreas.

325. E. Plantar fasciitis is the most common cause of foot pain in outpatient medicine. It results from constant strain on the plantar fascia at its insertion into the medial tubercle of the calcaneus. Patients report severe pain on the bottoms of their feet in the morning, but the pain subsides after a few minutes of walking. The diagnosis is confirmed by palpation over the plantar fascia's insertion on the medial heel. Radiographs serve no purpose in this diagnosis. Rupture of the Achilles' tendon may occur during running or jumping and causes a palpable defect: swelling and tenderness of the tendon. Ankle sprains generally involve the lateral ligament complex and present with swelling, ecchymosis, tenderness, and loss of function. Medial meniscal injuries are the most common knee injuries encountered in primary care. A patient will present with joint lock or instability, recurrent swelling with activity, and pain in the affected knee. Patellofemoral syndrome is also a common cause of knee pain, more so among adolescents and young adults. The presenting complaint is anterior knee pain, thought to be due to roughening of the cartilage on the patella's posterior surface. Stress fractures occur with overuse and generally present with chronic localized pain over the fracture site that manifests itself with use. Tarsal tunnel syndrome occurs with entrapment of the posterior tibial nerve in the tarsal tunnel. Pain and numbness are experienced in the soles of the feet, toes, and medial malleoli.

326. B. The time frame of 24 to 48 hr would be the ideal time to draw blood to note the peak rise of AST, a steady increase in the LDH, and the slow decrease in the serum levels of CPK. CPK peaks at 24 hr, as AST is continuing to rise. By the time 7 days have passed, CPK is normal, AST is normal, and LDH begins a steady decline back to normal as well. After the first 7 days, all levels are back down or very close to "normal."

327. E. Octreotide is a synthetic somatostatin analog that decreases splanchnic circulation and therefore reduces portal pressures. Aspirin will only increase the bleeding. Budesonide, a synthetic corticosteroid, is used in Crohn's disease. Infliximab is a mouse-human monoclonal antibody to human TNF-α and can decrease signs and symptoms in Crohn's disease. Misoprostol an analog of prostaglandin E and is used for prevention of ulceration induced by NSAIDs.

328. B. The correct answer is anticipation. Fragile X syndrome arises due to a CGG expansion. Clinical features of fragile X increase in severity with each successive generation and the amplification of the CGG repeats. In other words, the more CGG repeats a patient has, the more likely his or her mental retardation will be more severe. Other diseases such as Huntington's disease (CAG repeat), myotonic dystrophy (CTG repeat), and Friedreich's ataxia (GAA repeat) have similar characteristics, and clinical symptoms worsen with each successive generational expansion of the triplet. Variable expressivity is said to occur when two patients have the same genotype but the severity or phenotype of the disease differs. Pleiotropy refers to the ability of a single abnormal gene to produce multiple phenotypic effects. Allelic heterogeneity refers to different mutations at the same locus. Reduced penetrance refers to patients that have the genotype for a specific disease but the expression of the phenotype is less than 100%.

329. C. IgA is an immunoglobulin found in secretions and is responsible for preventing any organisms from entering into the respiratory tract. Some organisms produce IgA protease, which cleaves the IgA, preventing it from functioning. *Streptococcus pneumoniae, Neisseria meningitidis, Neisseria gonorrhoeae,* and *Haemophilus influenzae* all have this capability. Pili are used for communication between two organisms for reproductive purposes. Flagellae are part of a microtubular system, allowing the movement of organisms. M protein is found on *Streptococcus pyogenes;* when antibodies bind to it, it plays a role in host defense. Complement plays a role in the immunological response to invading organisms.

330. B. This patient likely has suffered a left-sided infarction of the middle cerebral artery. These infarctions typically affect the arms and face more than the leg. Anterior cerebral infarctions typically affect the leg more than the arm. The lesion is on the left side of the brain. This patient's posterior circulation is likely to be intact. The CT scan obtained (Figure 31) confirms the finding of a middle cerebral arterial infarct.

331. C. The correct answer to this question is metronidazole. This is an example of the Antabuse reaction that occurs when patients taking metronidazole consume alcohol. The first step of the reaction involves conversion of ethanol to acetaldehyde by alcohol dehydrogenase. The second step of the reaction involves conversion of acetaldehyde to acetate by acetaldehyde dehydrogenase. It is this enzyme that is inhibited by disulfiram (Antabuse) that leads to acetaldehyde accumulation and symptoms of hangover.

332. A. Lichen sclerosis may occur in any age group but is most common after menopause. It can lead to atrophy, fibrosis, and scarring and is also called chronic atrophic vulvitis. In lichen sclerosis, the skin becomes pale gray, the labia atrophy, and the introitus is narrowed. On histologic examination, there is usually thinning of the epidermis, with disappearance of the rete pegs and replacement of the underlying dermis by dense collagenous fibrous tissue. There is often marked hyperkeratosis and a mononuclear cell infiltrate around blood vessels. Vulvar intraepithelial neoplasia is diagnosed by vulvar biopsy. Vestibular adenitis is an inflammatory condition. A papillary hidradenoma is identical in appearance to intraductal papillomas of the breast.

333. C. Males in all racial groups face a greater risk of becoming victims of homicide. Blacks have greater risks than whites, and the highest risk occurs between the ages of 15 and 39 years. Thus, the 30-year-old black male has the highest risk of becoming a homicide victim because of his age, race, and gender.

334. D. Desmopressin would be a primary choice, as its administration will stimulate the release of von Willebrand factor from storage sites and curtail the bleeding. A beta-blocker would be of no use in this situation, as the issue is hematologic and not cardiac. Cryoprecipitate would be useful if there were no storage of von Willebrand factor in the body, and it may be used as a second-line treatment. Aspirin is completely contraindicated, as it will anticoagulate the blood and, in effect, exacerbate the bleeding. Pseudoephedrine will have no pronounced effect on the problem at hand.

335. C. The correct answer is PCP. It is associated with all the symptoms described in the passage; moreover, horizontal and vertical nystagmus is unique to PCP. LSD can produce similar symptoms, but not nystagmus. Look for visual hallucinations and flashbacks with LSD. Marijuana causes the user to become paranoid and experience slowed reaction times. Opioids are used as analgesics and are associated with respiratory depression, miosis, and constipation. Cocaine is a stimulant that causes euphoria, mydriasis, tachycardia, and hypertension.

336. D. Necrotizing papillitis, an ischemic necrosis of the renal papillae, is commonly induced by long-term chronic use of phenacetin, which is found in analgesics such as Pamprin. Diabetes mellitus is also a known predisposing factor, along with renal infections and vascular compromise. Cystinuria is a tubular inability to reabsorb cystine, resulting in the formation and excretion of cystine stones. Fanconi's syndrome, in which the proximal renal tubule fails to absorb glucose, amino acids, phosphate, and bicarbonate, presents clinically as increased glucose, phosphate, and amino acids in the urine and decreased phosphate in the blood.

337. B. This boy is suffering from an asthma attack, a bronchial disorder characterized by inflammation, reversible smooth muscle contraction, and mucus production. It leads to airway obstruction and difficulty breathing. Asthma is the most common chronic condition of childhood. Key asthma triggers include airway irritants, allergies (pets, pollens, and so on), and exercise. A complete blood count would most likely show an increase in eosinophils (eosinophilia). Basophilia is rare but is indicative of a myeloproliferative disorder. Elevated neutro-

phils signify an acute bacterial infection. A monocytosis, or increase in monocytes, is indicative of a chronic infection. Mast cell levels are not measured in standard laboratory evaluations.

338. B. Brimonidine is an alpha agonist that acts to decrease the synthesis of aqueous humor, thus providing relief for glaucoma. This agent can also cause some adverse effects, such as hyperemia, itchiness, and eyelid discomfort. Epinephrine and diuretics act to decrease humor secretion, and cholinomimetics act to increase humor outflow. Agents such as pilocarpine and carbachol increase aqueous humor outflow.

339. B. This patient suffers from the cutaneous form of anthrax, which is acquired by contact with a painless malignant pustule. Anthrax is caused by the Gram-positive rod *Bacillus anthracis*. The patient's colleague likely inhaled spores of *Bacillus anthracis* and developed woolsorter's disease, a pulmonary anthrax. *Aspergillus fumigatus* is an opportunistic fungus that causes a fungal pneumonia; however, it has no cutaneous form other than causing an ear fungus on occasion. *Clostridium perfringens* is a Gram-positive rod that causes enteritis necroticans in the GI tract and gas gangrene in tissues of the extremities. *Pneumocystis carinii* is a protozoan that causes pneumonia more commonly in patients with AIDS; however, it would not cause the dermal lesion described here. *Pseudomonas aeruginosa* is responsible for causing many diseases such as pneumonia, sepsis, otitis externa, and urinary tract infections, among others. However, *P. aeruginosa* does not cause the dermal lesion described in the question.

340. F. Men and women have different estrogen receptors, which may explain the higher prevalence of osteoporosis among women. Serum levels of osteocalcin are used to diagnose osteoporosis; higher levels correlate to more severe disease, but this alone does not explain gender differences. Osteoblasts decrease with age in both genders. Hormonal changes in menopause, not during pregnancy, are another explanation for this difference. Lack of exercise would result in increased fractures in both genders and does not explain a biochemical gender difference. Prostate cancer treatment with hormones will increase the risk of osteoporosis. Women going through treatment that suppresses hormones would also be at high risk for osteoporosis. Women have thinner and lighter bones than men.

341. B. One must determine the causative agent first. In this situation, the man has been infected with mononucleosis caused by Epstein-Barr virus, a herpesvirus. This infection usually occurs in 15- to 20-year-olds and presents with a sore throat, fatigue, and posterior cervical lymphadenopathy. Heterophile antibodies are also present. Influenza virus belongs to the Orthomyxovirus family and causes cold-like symptoms. Paramyxovirus is associated with four types of infection, but these do not resemble mononucleosis. Adenovirus does cause a sore throat but not lymphadenopathy or a positive heterophile Ab test. Rhinovirus, a picornavirus, is responsible for the common cold.

342. E. This woman most likely has systemic lupus erythematosus (SLE), which is a chronic autoimmune disorder that can affect virtually any organ of the body. In lupus, the body's immune system, which normally functions to protect against foreign invaders, becomes hyperactive, forming antibodies that attack normal tissues and organs, including the skin, joints, kidneys, brain, heart, lungs, and blood. SLE is characterized by periods of illness, called flares, and periods of wellness, or remission. Some 90% of lupus patients are women, and the onset of the disease usually occurs in the prime of life, between the ages of 15 and 44. African American women are three times more likely to get lupus than Caucasian women. Most people with lupus test positive to the antinuclear antibody (ANA) test. The chest x-ray shown (Figure 32) reveals volume loss and small reticulonodular densities in both lung bases consistent with SLE. Angelman's syndrome is an imprinting error because of a difference between phenotype and maternal origin mutation. Hypothyroidism is associated with the symptoms displayed by this patient (slow, sluggish, tired) and decreased T_3 and T_4 blood levels. Sarcoidosis is an important cause of hypercalcemia associated with the formation of inflammatory granulomas.

343. C. Mitral insufficiency is closely associated with mitral valve prolapse, which is indicated by this patient's clinical findings. This patient would also be at an increased risk for developing infective endocarditis, and arrhythmias. The systolic murmur with a "midsystolic click" is pathognomonic for mitral valve prolapse. Each of the other valvular lesions has specific sounds associated with it as well. The main cause of mitral stenosis is rheumatic fever. Tricuspid valve disease is rare in isolation and is usually associated with a history of rheumatic fever, in which case left-sided valve disease is usually present.

344. D. The correct answer is splenic vein–left renal vein. The splenic vein drains into the portal system and the left renal vein drains directly into the inferior vena cava. Both the left and right renal veins drain into the caval system. The right testicular vein drains into the caval system. The superior mesenteric vein drains into the portal system.

345. E. If splitting occurs at days 9 to 12 after fertilization, there is a greater likelihood that monochorionic/monoamniotic placentation will occur as compared to earlier splitting. These twins share a common placenta with vascular communications between the two placentas, which can sometimes result in twin-twin transfusion. If splitting occurs later than 12 days, the risk of conjoined twins increases. Cord strangulation, meconium ileus, and Potter sequence have no direct correlation with the timing of dizygotic twin splitting.

346. B. Calcium stones, which are composed of calcium oxalate or calcium phosphate, make up 80 of 85% stones that are formed. They are radiopaque and strongly associated with hypercalciuria. Uric acid stones are associated with hyperuricemia, secondary to gout in almost 50% of the patients. Ammonium magnesium phosphate stones are formed second only to calcium. They are associated with *Proteus* and staphylococcal infections and have a tendency to form staghorn calculi. Cystine stones are predominantly associated with cystinuria or aminoaciduria due to a genetic predisposition.

347. E. Pseudocyesis is the presence of many symptoms of pregnancy even though conception has not actually taken place. This usually occurs in women who have a strong desire to become pregnant and also in those who have a strong fear of becoming pregnant. Depression can cause weight gain, but it is not necessarily associated with morning sickness–like symptoms. Normal and ectopic pregnancy can cause the above symptoms, but in the presence of a negative pregnancy test, it is best to look at other potential answers.

348. A. This patient's symptoms and radiographic findings support the diagnosis of mesothelioma. Malignant mesothelioma arises in the thorax from either the visceral or parietal pleura and typically results in pleural effusions and bilateral pleural plaques. Mesothelioma is linked to asbestos exposure and typically arises 25 to 45 years after the exposure. Few victims of this disease survive longer then 2 years. Coal dust exposure is linked to coal workers' pneumoconiosis and causes fibrosis of the lungs. Silica exposure can lead to silicosis, which is also a slowly progressive fibrosing pneumoconiosis. Beryllium causes berylliosis and can either cause acute pneumonitis or pulmonary and systemic granulomatous lesions that resemble sarcoidosis. Sulfur dioxide inhalation can cause localized airway inflammation. Finally, carbon monoxide inhalation can lead to headaches, dizziness, and finally coma.

349. E. The effects of alcohol, which is a sedative and nervous system depressant, would cause somnolence. Increased anxiety, inhibited behavior, and hyperventilation would be more in line with ingestion of a stimulant, not a depressant. Heightened coordination would be an effect directly opposite to that of alcohol consumption, as the depressant would decrease coordination and reflexes and would not increase reaction time and accuracy.

350. D. CEA, or carcinoembryonic antigen, while nonspecific, is produced by nearly 70% of colorectal and pancreatic cancers. It would be beneficial to see if this patient had an elevated level so that one could follow his progress once treatment had been started. AFP, or alpha-fetoprotein, is normally made by the fetus. It may be elevated in hepatocellular carcinomas or nonseminomatous germ cell tumors of the testis. β-hCG is beta human chorionic gonadotropin, a marker seen with hydatidiform moles, choriocarcinomas, and gestational trophoblastic tumors. CA 125, or cancer antigen 125, may be elevated in ovarian and malignant epithelial tumors. PSA, or prostate-specific antigen, is a marker of prostate cancer. Tumor markers should not be used as a primary tool for diagnosing a certain type of cancer. They can be used to *confirm* a cancer and to monitor for recurrence or response to therapy.

Content Index

STEP 1

Chapter 1   General Principles

Questions

1. A 26-year-old G1P0 female at 34 weeks' gestation presents to the clinic for routine prenatal care. Her pregnancy has been complicated only by pregnancy-induced hypertension. She has no complaints of leakage of fluid, vaginal bleeding, decreased fetal movement, or vaginal discharge. Physical examination finds her blood pressure to be 155/105 mm Hg and significant edema is noted. Analysis of a 24-hr urine sample finds > 300 grams/day of protein. What is the most likely diagnosis?

   A. Chronic hypertension
   B. Eclampsia
   C. Hydatidiform mole
   D. Preeclampsia
   E. Pregnancy-induced hypertension

2. An 11-year-old girl visits the school nurse complaining of severe abdominal pain. She is also very sleepy and has been having behavioral problems. Physical examination shows that her skin and mucous membranes are pale. Cardiac, pulmonary, and abdominal examinations are within normal limits. A blood smear reveals basophilic stippling. She is diagnosed with poisoning. What is the most likely poison?

   A. Arsenic
   B. Cyanide
   C. Lead
   D. Mercury
   E. Silicon

3. A 65-year-old man with a 30-year history of smoking presents to his primary care physician complaining of chronic cough. Sampling of the epithelial cells in this patient's trachea and bronchi would reveal what pathological change?

   A. Dysplasia, specifically stratified squamous epithelial cells replacing normal columnar ciliated epithelial cells
   B. Dysplasia, specifically columnar ciliated epithelial cells replacing normal stratified squamous epithelial cells
   C. Hyperplasia, specifically stratified squamous epithelial cells replacing normal columnar ciliated epithelial cells
   D. Hyperplasia, specifically columnar ciliated epithelial cells replacing normal stratified squamous epithelial cells
   E. Metaplasia, specifically stratified squamous epithelial cells replacing normal columnar ciliated epithelial cells
   F. Metaplasia, specifically columnar ciliated epithelial cells replacing normal stratified squamous epithelial cells

4. Over the weekend, a 23-year-old college student attends a party and drinks a large amount of alcohol. The liver metabolizes the alcohol to acetaldehyde. In which component of the cell does this oxidation reaction occur?

   A. Golgi apparatus
   B. Mitochondria
   C. Peroxisome
   D. Ribosomes
   E. Smooth endoplasmic reticulum

5. In the evaluation of a 30-year-old male athlete who is preparing to run a marathon, the skeletal and smooth muscles are compared. The following statements are true of smooth muscle as opposed to skeletal muscle:

   A. It cannot be regenerated.
   B. Contraction in smooth muscle lasts longer and is slower.
   C. It has multiple nuclei.
   D. It is activated by calcium binding to troponin C.
   E. It is striated.

6. A 39-year-old woman complains of visual field defects, which are determined to be bitemporal hemianopsia. Plain-film x-rays reveal calcifications. What is the most likely diagnosis?

   A. Acanthosis nigricans
   B. Corticotropic adenoma
   C. Craniopharyngioma
   D. Pheochromocytoma
   E. Tuberous sclerosis

7. A 39-year-old man with a history of headaches and seizures undergoes a magnetic resonance imaging (MRI), which reveals an intracerebral mass lesion (Figure 1-1). He undergoes stereotactic resection of the lesion. Pathology reveals a poorly differentiated tumor composed of astrocytes. The intermediate filament that provides structural support to astrocytes is which of the following?

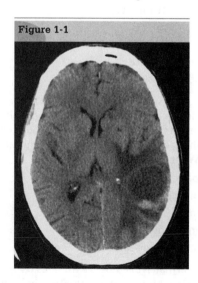

Figure 1-1

   A. Desmin
   B. Glial fibrillar acidic protein
   C. Keratin
   D. Neurofilaments
   E. Vimentin

8. Parents of a newborn child are concerned because of his appearance. He presents with a round, full face, upslanting palpebral fissures, a flattened nasal bridge, low-set ears, a broad tongue, and a single palmar crease. Physical examination of the heart reveals a systolic ejection murmur. Pulmonary auscultation is within normal limits. This child has a congenital anomaly that most likely arose from what meiotic error?

   A. Deletion

   B. Insertion

   C. Inversion

   D. Nondisjunction

   E. Translocation

9. A 16-year-old boy is brought to his primary care physician for evaluation of ataxia, muscle wasting, and myoclonic seizures. He has mildly elevated levels of lactate in his blood and cerebrospinal fluid. He has an uncle who died from a myopathic disorder in which ragged-red fibers were found in some muscle groups. This patient's disease is most likely the result of:

   A. Autosomal dominant inheritance

   B. Autosomal recessive inheritance

   C. Chromosomal deletion

   D. Mitochondrial inheritance

   E. X-linked recessive inheritance

10. Two patients arrive for their appointments at the outpatient clinic. One presents with dozens of benign fleshy skin tumors and a malignant sarcoma of the upper extremity. The other appears healthy, with a few hyperpigmented spots on the torso and freckles in the armpits that have become more noticeable. Both have the same genetic disorder. Their presentations can be explained by which of the following genetic principles:

    A. Mitochondrial inheritance

    B. Nondisjunction

    C. Reduced penetrance

    D. X-linked dominance

    E. Variable expression

11. A mother brings in her week-old newborn for a checkup because he has developed some bruising, which concerns her. She reports that he wakes up in the morning with new bruises. She had a home delivery without any medical intervention. What is the most likely diagnosis?

    A. Hemophilia A

    B. Vitamin A deficiency

    C. Vitamin C deficiency

    D. Vitamin K deficiency

    E. Von Willebrand disease

12. A 35-year-old man is diagnosed with sinusitis by his primary care physician. After careful evaluation, he is given a prescription for amoxicillin and told to follow up in three weeks. Penicillins affect bacterial growth by:

    A. Blockage of 50S ribosome

    B. Engulfment of bacteria

    C. Formation of pores in the cell membrane

    D. Interruption of cell wall synthesis

    E. Interference with the action of DNA gyrase

13. While working abroad in a pediatric hospital, you see several children with significant growth retardation, dermatitis, and hypogonadism. They also tell you that they have trouble tasting foods. Which of the following should be added to their diets as a supplement?

    A. Copper

    B. Manganese

    C. Iron

    D. Selenium

    E. Zinc

14. After living on a flat land for most of her life, a 41-year-old woman decides to move to the mountains of Colorado. What change would you expect to see in her after she has lived there for a couple of weeks?

    A. Decreased cardiac output

    B. Decreased red blood cell mass

    C. Hypoventilation

    D. Respiratory acidosis with partial compensation

    E. Respiratory alkalosis with partial compensation

15. A 6-year-old African American girl undergoes an appendectomy. A computed tomography (CT) scan (Figure 1-2) is obtained and pathology reveals suppurative appendicitis. At 6-month follow up, there is a large, raised, tumor-like scar on her abdomen where the surgical incision was made. What complication in normal wound healing occurred?

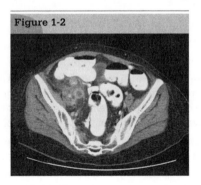

Figure 1-2

    A. Contracture

    B. Dehiscence

    C. Excessive collagen formation

    D. Infection

    E. Ulceration

16. The patient, a 60-year-old man, has spent most of his life working in a rubber factory at which several workers recently became ill and had to quit their jobs. He asks if there is anything he should be concerned about. Which of the following considerations should be discussed with this patient?

    A. Basal cell carcinoma

    B. Bladder cancer

    C. Liver angiosarcoma

    D. Lung cancer

    E. Squamous cell carcinoma

17. What structure is found in Gram-negative but not in Gram-positive bacteria?

   A. Capsule

   B. Cell wall

   C. Cytoplasmic membrane

   D. Outer membrane

   E. Flagellum

18. A family of four presents to the emergency department with a recent onset of severe watery diarrhea and abdominal cramping. They ate dinner the night before at a new seafood restaurant in town. The father, 41 years old, has a history of erectile dysfunction. The mother, 44 years old, has a history of endometriosis and hypertension. The children, both male and aged 16 and 19, are healthy. What is the most likely cause of this family's symptoms?

   A. *Bacillus cereus*

   B. *Campylobacter jejuni*

   C. *Helicobacter pylori*

   D. *Proteus vulgaris*

   E. *Vibrio parahaemolyticus*

19. A 39-year-old woman has a carbuncle on her left arm and also complains of a sore throat. Her past medical history is unremarkable. What test can be used to distinguish the causes of these conditions?

   A. Coagulase test

   B. Gram stain

   C. Hydrogen peroxide

   D. Immunofluorescent stain

   E. L-pyrrolidonyl-beta-naphthylamide (PYR) test

20. A 50-year-old man presents to his primary care physician with severe pain on one side of his face. He has a rash covering only that area of the face and nowhere else. He is extremely uncomfortable and flinches when you try to touch his face. What is the most likely diagnosis?

   A. Coxsackievirus

   B. Epstein-Barr virus

   C. Measles

   D. Rubella

   E. Varicella zoster

21. A 25-year-old soldier presents to the emergency department complaining of a three-week history of a dry, hacking cough and episodic headache. A chest x-ray is obtained (Figure 1-3). What organism is most likely responsible for this patient's condition?

   A. *Chlamydia pneumoniae*

   B. *Haemophilus influenzae*

   C. *Legionella*

   D. *Mycobacterium*

   E. *Mycoplasma pneumoniae*

   F. Rhinovirus

   G. *Staphylococcus aureus*

   H. *Streptococcus pneumoniae*

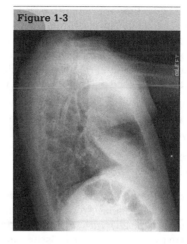

Figure 1-3

22. A 41-year-old HIV-positive man with right-upper-quadrant pain is evaluated for hepatitis. Serologic testing is ordered, the results of which are as follows: HBs antibody, negative; HBs antigen, positive; and HBc antibody, positive. What conclusion may be drawn?

   A. The patient is a chronic carrier of hepatitis B virus.

   B. He is immune to hepatitis B.

   C. More test results are needed for an accurate diagnosis.

   D. The patient has never been exposed to hepatitis B.

   E. He has recently been vaccinated for hepatitis B.

23. Which of the following types of human papillomavirus are closely associated with an increased risk of cervical cancer?

   A. HPV 1

   B. HPV 4

   C. HPV 1 and 4

   D. HPV 6 and 11

   E. HPV 16 and 18

24. A 50-year-old man presents to his primary care physician for evaluation of a 10-year history of gastroesophageal reflux disease, the symptoms of which have recently worsened. Owing to his history, you are concerned about the possibility of which of the following?

   A. Hyperplasia of intestinal cells

   B. Intestinal metaplasia

   C. Ulceration of the pharyngeal mucosa

   D. Uncontrollable growth of mucosal cells

   E. Tearing of the esophageal wall

25. A 50-year-old man with a history of coronary atherosclerotic disease presents to the emergency department with symptoms of a heart attack. Studies reveal that his left anterior descending artery is completely blocked by a thrombus. What pathological change in the myocytes would support an irreversible cell injury?

   A. Decreased oxidative phosphorylation

   B. Detachment of ribosomes from the endoplasmic reticulum

   C. Failure of the cell membrane Na^+, K^+-ATPase pump

   D. Loss of the cellular ultrastructure, as shown by the formation of blebs

   E. Mitochondrial dysfunction, specifically increased uptake of Ca^{2+} by the mitochondria

26. A 4-year-old boy is brought to the emergency department because of a swollen, painful left toe. On questioning, the mother and father reveal that their son stepped on a tack, but they do not know how long ago this occurred. Sampling of the tissue surrounding the injury reveals a high percentage of neutrophils. When did this injury most likely occur?

A. 10 min ago

B. 6–24 hr ago

C. 25–48 hr ago

D. 1 week ago

E. 1 month ago

27. A 35-year-old woman suffers from recurrent gallstones and elects to have a cholecystectomy. The surgery is performed laparoscopically with no complications and the port sites are closed with sutures. Tissue sampling of her incision site on postoperative day three would most likely reveal:

A. Accumulation of collagen and proliferation of fibroblasts

B. Maximal neovascularization

C. Neutrophils at the margin of the incision

D. Neutrophils largely replaced by macrophages and the progression of granulation tissue into the wound

E. Tissue devoid of inflammatory infiltrate with intact epidermis

28. A 5-year-old girl is brought to her primary care physician because of a recurrent runny nose, itchy eyes, urticaria, and frequent sneezing. These symptoms are new and appear to coincide with the addition of a cat to the household. What is the main amine responsible for these physiological effects and from which cell or cells can it be released?

A. Histamine: mast cells, basophils, and platelets

B. Histamine: mast cells and basophils

C. Histamine: mast cells only

D. Serotonin: mast cells, basophils, and platelets

E. Serotonin: mast cells and basophils

F. Serotonin: mast cells only

29. A 38-year-old man with AIDS present to his primary care physician for follow-up. He does not know his most recent CD4 cell count and complains of fever and dyspnea. Physical examination of the lungs reveals bilateral rhonchi and wheezing. A chest x-ray is obtained (Figure 1-4). Which of the following cell types have a surface marker that recognizes CD4+ T cells?

A. Hepatocytes

B. B cells

C. Primary spermatogonia

D. Enteric neurons

E. Mast cells

30. A 54-year-old woman presents to her primary care physician complaining of recent changes in her bowel function. She has had adenomatous colon polyps, which have been resected annually for the last four years. Physical examination reveals no evidence of guarding or rebound tenderness. However, on digital rectal examination, a nontender mass is palpable within six cm of the anal verge. The patient's

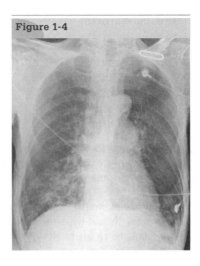

Figure 1-4

hematocrit is 28%. Of the following characteristics, which would be most indicative of a malignant colorectal tumor?

A. Absent metastasis

B. Anaplasia with pleomorphism

C. A slow-growing tumor with rare mitotic figures

D. A well-demarcated mass with little invasion into the surrounding normal tissue

E. Well-formed glands and crypts with some differentiation into mature goblet cells

31. Neurofibromatosis is a disorder of the nervous system that can present with neurofibromas in the skin, café-au-lait spots, hamartomas on the iris, as well as more severe forms mental retardation, tumors of the central nervous system (CNS), diffuse skin neurofibromas, and even the development of cancer of the nervous system and muscle. Two brothers have recently been diagnosed with this disease. The older brother's only symptoms have been café-au-lait spots and a few neurofibromas. However, the younger brother shows diffuse skin neurofibromas covering his trunk as well as multiple hamartomas on the iris and severe mental retardation. What genetic concept does this scenario illustrate?

A. Allelic heterogeneity

B. Consanguinity

C. New mutation

D. Pleiotropy

E. Variable expressivity

32. A 10-month-old infant is seen in the pediatrics clinic with his mother, who is distraught. She has just been told by a geneticist that her son suffers from a rare disease due to a deficiency in hexosaminidase A. You examine the boy and notice that there is a red spot on his macula; he also exhibits motor incoordination and muscular flaccidity. The mother is highly concerned and wants to know the risk of having more children with this same condition. She has three other healthy children and neither she nor her husband have symptoms of the disease. What is the pattern of transmission for this disease and what is the risk that this woman will have another affected child?

A. Autosomal dominant, and there is a 50% chance

B. Autosomal dominant, and there is a 25% chance

C. Autosomal dominant, and there is a 75% chance

D. Autosomal recessive, and there is a 50% chance

E. Autosomal recessive, and there is a 25% chance

F. Autosomal recessive, and there is a 75% chance

33. A 12-year-old boy with Down's syndrome is evaluated by his primary care physician. He has a history of nocturnal enuresis and recurrent otitis media. Physical examination shows that the heart and lungs are within normal limits. Recent urinalysis, complete blood count, and serum electrolytes are within normal limits. What is the most common karyotype seen in patients with Down's syndrome?

A. 47XY or -XX trisomy 18 due to mitotic nondisjunction of the chromosome 18 pair

B. 47XY or -XX trisomy 21 due to meiotic nondisjunction of the chromosome 21 pair

C. 47XY or -XX trisomy 13 due to meiotic nondisjunction of the chromosome 13 pair

D. 46XY or -XX with a Robertsonian translocation between chromosome 21q and the long arm of one of the other acrocentric chromosomes

E. 46XY or -XX with a 21q21q translocation

34. A 38-year-old man undergoes endoscopy for a six-month history of progressive dyspepsia. Biopsy specimens of the esophagus and stomach are taken. These grow urease-positive curved bacteria. What is the most likely diagnosis?

A. *Campylobacter jejuni*

B. *Clostridium perfringens*

C. *Entamoeba histolytica*

D. *Helicobacter pylori*

E. *Salmonella typhi*

35. A 28-year-old African American woman presents to her primary care physician with complaints of joint pain and dry cough. Physical examination reveals erythema nodosum of the skin. Spirometry suggests restrictive lung disease. A chest x-ray is obtained (Figure 1-5). Which of the following additional findings would be expected in this patient?

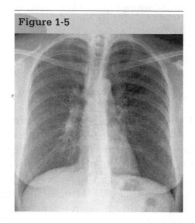

Figure 1-5

A. Hypercalciuria

B. Hypernatremia

C. Hypocalcemia

D. Hypogammaglobulinemia

E. Impaired activity of serum angiotensin-converting enzyme

36. For a given type of inheritance the phenotype typically appears in every generation, any child of an affected parent has a 50% chance of inheriting the trait, and males and females are equally likely to transmit the phenotype to children of either sex. What is the most likely inheritance described?

A. Autosomal dominant

B. Autosomal recessive

C. Mutation (cellular level)

D. X-linked dominant

E. X-linked recessive

37. Bruton's X-linked infantile agammaglobulinemia is a recessive disorder in which those affected typically suffer from repeated bacterial infections. The disorder is due to a defective gene that encodes tyrosine kinase, resulting in undetectable levels of B cells and thus antibodies. Typically infants do not present symptoms until they are about six months old, when the antibodies they had obtained during gestation begin to decline. What antibody is the primary source of protection to the infant from birth until six months?

A. Maternal IgA

B. Maternal IgD

C. Maternal IgE

D. Maternal IgG

E. Maternal IgM

38. A 71-year-old man presents to his primary care physician complaining of chronic cough and wheezing. He has a 100-pack-year history of smoking. A tissue sample taken from his lung reveals large cells with ingested carbon particles loosely attached to the epithelial cells of the alveoli or lying free within the alveolar space. What type of cell is this and from what cell line does it derive?

A. Alveolar macrophage derived from blood monocytes

B. Alveolar macrophage derived from T cells

C. Alveolar macrophage derived from NK cells

D. Kupffer cell derived from blood monocytes

E. Kupffer cell derived from T cells

F. Kupffer cell derived from NK cells

G. Microglial cells derived from blood monocytes

39. DiGeorge syndrome is a disease that results in a predisposition to serious viral, fungal, and/or protozoal infections as well as hypocalcemia and tetany. What defect is responsible for this condition?

A. Bone marrow hypoplasia

B. Complement deficiency

C. Parathyroid hypoplasia

D. Splenic hypoplasia

E. Thymic hypoplasia

F. Thymic and parathyroid hypoplasia

40. A 37-year-old man presents to the emergency department because of episodic edema of the skin and extremities. This problem first appeared 4 days after he was fired from his job. He is also having difficulty speaking. Otolaryngology consultation is obtained and nasolaryngoscopy is performed, revealing edema of the larynx. A later endoscopy of the lower gastrointestinal tract reveals edema of the ileal mucosa. The patient's father complained of similar problems and died unexpectedly at age 52 of respiratory distress. What is the primary defect in this disease?

A. Alternative complement pathway activation

B. Classic complement pathway activation

C. Combined alternative and classic complement pathway activation

D. Complement regulation, specifically C1 esterase inhibitor deficiency

E. Complement regulation, specifically decay accelerating factor deficiency

41. A 46-year-old woman with polycystic kidney disease is receiving a kidney transplant. Within minutes of anastomosis of the graft vasculature, the kidney rapidly regains a pink coloration as well as normal tissue turgor and begins excreting urine. However, 1 month after the transplant she has a serum creatinine of 3.9 mg/dL. Urine output is 20 mL/hr. Biopsy of the transplant shows extensive mononuclear cell infiltrates, edema, and mild interstitial hemorrhage. What is the most likely explanation for these findings?

A. Acute rejection

B. Chronic rejection

C. Graft versus host disease

D. Hyperacute rejection

E. A normal posttransplant process

42. A 12-year-old boy with leukemia has received a bone marrow transplant. Within 1 week of the transplant the boy begins experiencing a rash, fever, jaundice, and hepatosplenomegaly. There is little infiltration of the affected tissues with lymphocytes. What is the most likely explanation for these findings?

A. Acute graft rejection

B. Chronic graft rejection

C. Graft versus host disease

D. Hyperacute graft rejection

E. A normal, expected posttransplant process

43. A 12-year-old girl presents to her primary care physician with symptoms of severe pharyngitis, including a temperature of 40.3°C (104.5°F) and tachycardia. You decide to give her an injection of penicillin in your office. Within minutes of the injection the patient develops itching, hives, skin erythema, and respiratory distress. What is the most likely explanation of these findings?

A. Type I hypersensitivity reaction

B. Type II hypersensitivity reaction

C. Type III hypersensitivity reaction

D. Type IV hypersensitivity reaction

E. Type V hypersensitivity reaction

44. A 28-year-old African American woman presents to her primary care physician complaining of joint pain and a dry cough. Physical examination reveals erythema nodosum. Spirometry suggests restrictive lung disease. A chest x-ray is obtained (Figure 1-6). What is the most likely etiology of this condition?

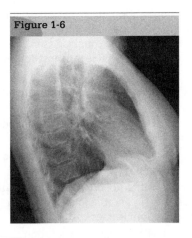

Figure 1-6

A. Exposure to free silica dust

B. History of smoking

C. Infectious agent

D. Neoplasm

E. Unknown

45. With intravenous infusion, a drug reaches 90% steady state in 12 hr. The elimination half-life of the drug is approximately:

A. 1 hr

B. 2 hr

C. 4 hr

D. 6 hr

E. 8 hr

46. A 41-year-old man with diabetes has chronic sinusitis. It has not responded to a six-week course of antibiotic therapy. Which of the following organisms should be considered?

A. *Actinomyces*

B. *Aspergillus*

C. *Cryptococcus*

D. *Mucor*

E. *Pneumocystis*

47. A 9-month-old boy is brought to his pediatrician with a 24-hr history of generalized weakness and poor feeding. The mother states that she fed the baby some honey several times to calm him. Physical examination indicates that the child appears to be its stated age. Cardiac and pulmonary examinations are unremarkable. There is no evidence of guarding or rebound tenderness. Genitourinary examination reveals bilateral descended testicles. The foreskin is phimotic and does not retract easily. The toxin responsible for causing these symptoms works by which of the following mechanisms:

A. It stimulates guanylate cyclase.

B. It blocks the release of acetylcholine from the nerve terminal.

C. It uses a subunit that inactivates an elongation factor (EF) by ADP ribosylation.

D. It blocks the release of gamma-aminobutyric acid (GABA) and glycine.

E. It stimulates the release of GABA.

48. A 61-year-old man with a history of chronic obstructive pulmonary disease presents to the emergency department complaining of headache. He has a 60-pack-year history of smoking. His blood pressure is 160/95 mm Hg. Which of the following antihypertensives is contraindicated in this patient?

A. Acebutolol

B. Betaxolol

C. Esmolol

D. Metoprolol

E. Nadolol

49. Several hospitals are coordinating a study to test the safety of a newly developed drug designed to lower blood pressure. The 25 normal volunteers receiving the drug are being followed for the pharmacokinetics of the medication and any adverse effects. Which of the following steps in the drug development and approval phase is most likely described here?

A. New drug application (NDA)

B. Investigational new drug (IND) application

C. Phase I

D. Phase II

E. Phase III

F. Phase IV

50. A 55-year-old alcoholic man presents to the ambulatory care clinic because of a wound on his thigh that will not heal. Physical examination reveals numerous ecchymoses on his legs and upper arms. He also has splinter hemorrhages in the nail beds and loosening of his teeth. Laboratory studies reveal a hemoglobin of 10 g/dL. What is the most appropriate treatment for this patient?

A. Factor VIII

B. Iron

C. Vitamin C

D. Vitamin D

E. Vitamin K

51. Shortly after the birth of her first child, a mother learns that her daughter has an inherited disorder whereby her health could be harmed by the ingestion of products that are "sugar-free" and contain aspartame. Which of the following genetic disorders does she most likely have?

A. Hyperornithinemia

B. Hyperuricemia

C. Hypervalinemia

D. Phenylketonuria

E. Wilson's disease

52. A 10-year-old boy was camping with his dad over the weekend. Upon returning home, he developed a very itchy red rash with several blisters on his legs. He said that he had walked through several bushes to get to the camp-

site. Which type of hypersensitivity is associated with this condition?

A. I

B. II

C. III

D. IV

53. A 61-year-old alcoholic man presents to the emergency department with ataxia, global confusion, and psychosis. He also has polyneuropathy and ophthalmoplegia. Which of the following would be the most suitable therapy for this patient?

A. Biotin

B. Niacin

C. Pyridoxine

D. Riboflavin

E. Thiamine

54. A mother brings her 3-year-old daughter to her primary care physician because of severe pruritus in the perianal region. Further history reveals that the child attends day care 5 days a week. A Scotch tape test reveals small operculated eggs. The primary white blood cell involved in fighting this condition uses a molecule specifically geared to this purpose. What is this molecule?

A. Heparin

B. Histamine

C. Major basic protein

D. Myeloperoxidase

E. Perforin

55. A man presents to the emergency room with a stab wound to his left side. Examination reveals a very deep wound at the left midaxillary line in the region of the ninth through eleventh ribs. The organ most likely at risk of damage from this wound has what histological feature associated with it?

A. Enterochromaffin cells — adrenal gland

B. Hassall's corpuscles — Thymus

C. Islets of Langerhans — liver

D. A periarteriolar lymphatic sheath — spleen

E. Space of Disse — Liver

56. A 65-year-old man presents with severe lower back pain that started about 3 weeks earlier. He notes that he cannot get around as he used to because he has been feeling extremely lethargic. Blood tests are ordered, which show that the patient's white blood cell count is 40,000; the hemoglobin and hematocrit are 10 mg/dL and 30%, respectively. A spinal x-ray reveals lytic lesions of the L2, L3, and L5 vertebrae. The proliferation of what type of cell is responsible for this patient's symptoms?

A. Cytotoxic T lymphocyte

B. Erythrocyte

C. Helper T lymphocyte

D. Mast cell

E. Plasma cell

57. A 2-year-old girl is brought to the emergency department; a suspicious lesion on her forearm is diagnosed as an abscess. The mother notes that this is the tenth time they have had to come into the emergency department for the same reason. Culture reveals *Staphylococcus aureus*. The doctor then orders a nitrozolium blue test, which turns out to be negative. The enzyme missing from this child's leukocytes is:

A. Glucose-6-phosphate dehydrogenase (G6PD)

B. Hexokinase

C. Myeloperoxidase

D. NADPH oxidase

E. Pyruvate kinase

58. A 45-year-old patient recently diagnosed with acute myelogenous leukemia suddenly presents to the emergency department with an uncontrollable nosebleed. Laboratory studies obtained are presented below:

Prothrombin time = elevated

Activated partial thromboplastin time = elevated

Platelets = decreased

Fibrin split products = present

Based on these data, this patient most likely has acute myelogenous leukemia of the following type:

A. M1

B. M2

C. M3

D. M4

E. M5

59. A 5-year-old child is brought to the emergency department with severe difficulty in breathing. There is no history of trauma. The family was traveling to a wedding when the child suddenly began to have this problem. The child is clothed rather formally in a dress shirt, which has spots of saliva in places and appears to be missing a button. The child's temperature is 38°C (100.4°F) orally and his throat is nonedematous. Which of the following findings would be most likely due to this child's condition?

A. Collapsed right lung with decreased blood flow in the right pulmonary artery

B. Consolidation of the left lung base with the trachea deviating to the right

C. Diffuse infiltrate in the right middle lobe with prominent air bronchograms

D. Hyperinflated right middle lobe with increased blood flow to the left pulmonary artery

E. "Thumbprint" epiglottis on radiograph

60. A 33-year-old man presents to his primary care physician with a 2-week history of low-grade fever, night sweats, and hemoptysis. His chest x-ray reveals an area of hyperdensity in the left upper lobe. Which of the following growth media would be most likely to grow cultures of the organism causing this condition?

A. Bordet-Gengou agar

B. Chocolate agar

C. Lowenstein-Jensen medium

D. Tellurite plate

E. Thayer-Martin agar

61. A 4-year-old girl is brought to the emergency department because of difficulty breathing. Her parents are refugees from Africa and speak little English; therefore a history is difficult to elicit. You notice that the child has a prominently enlarged neck and that her breathing is stridorous. She is treated empirically with erythromycin and antitoxin. A few days later the pathology lab reports that the throat swab grew black colonies. Which medium was likely used?

A. Chocolate agar

B. Löffler's coagulated serum medium

C. Lowenstein-Jensen medium

D. Tellurite plate

E. Thayer-Martin agar

62. A 32-year-old woman presents to her primary care physician complaining of increased difficulty breathing. Her face is rather pink, and she tends to exhale slowly, through pursed lips. Spirometry reveals increased total vital capacity and decreased FEV₁. Her mother suffered from a similar mysterious disease. She has never smoked or resided with anyone who smoked. Which extrarespiratory findings are likely in this patient?

A. Congenital heart defect

B. Hepatic cirrhosis

C. Infertility

D. Ovarian cysts

E. Situs inversus

63. A 33-year-old man presents to his primary care physician with a 2-week history of low-grade fever, night sweats, and hemoptysis. His chest x-ray reveals some hyperdensity in the left upper lobe. Occupational exposure to which of the following would most likely influence the development of this man's disease?

A. Asbestos

B. Coal workers' disease

C. Grain dust

D. No occupational risk is associated with this disease

E. Silica

64. Juxtaglomerular cells sense changes in sodium concentration and pressure via feedback from cells of the macula densa in the distal tubule. What is the cells' response to a decrease in sodium concentration?

A. Angiotensinogen release

B. Angiotensin-1 release

C. Direct vasoconstriction

D. Renin release

E. Somatostatin release

65. A 54-year-old obese postmenopausal woman presents to her primary care physician for an annual checkup. Her medical history is notable for hypertension and diabetes mellitus. Medications include an angiotensin-converting enzyme (ACE) inhibitor and glyburide. She complains of intermittent vaginal bleeding and states that she feels a small lump in her right breast. Physical examination confirms a 2-cm indurated breast lesion. Speculum examination of the vagina reveals blood in the vaginal vault. Overweight women are at a greater risk for endometrial and breast cancers because:

A. Adipose cells produce 5α-reductase.
B. Adipose cells produce aromatase.
C. Fat is carcinogenic.
D. They are more likely to be sedentary.
E. They are more likely to have tuberculosis.

66. A 37-year-old disheveled paranoid schizophrenic man is brought to the emergency department after being found sleeping in a doorway. He is awake, alert, and oriented to time, place, and person. His current medications include a dopamine-blocking antipsychotic agent. A potential side effect of this drug is increased production of which anterior pituitary hormone?

A. ACTH
B. FSH
C. LH
D. Prolactin
E. TSH

67. A five-year-old African American boy is brought to the emergency department after becoming unconscious in day care. Prior to collapsing he complained of unremitting pain in his back and lower extremities. Physical examination reveals an erect penis. A CT scan of the head is ordered (Figure 1-7).

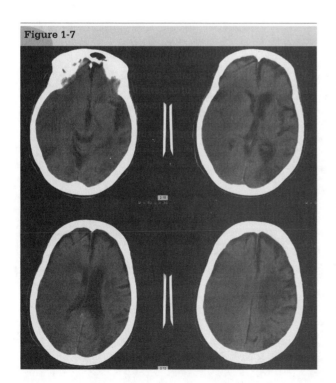

Figure 1-7

When glutamate at the sixth position of the two β chains of hemoglobin is substituted with valine, what happens?

A. Decreased polymerization of deoxyhemoglobin
B. Increased flexibility of red blood cells
C. Increased gel electrophoresis migration at pH 7
D. Increased solubility of deoxyhemoglobin
E. Primary structure is unchanged

68. Lactate dehydrogenase (LDH) is an isozyme measured to evaluate possible myocardial infarction (MI). It is composed of two different polypeptides arranged in the form of a tetramer. If all possible combinations of polypeptide chains occur, how many isozyme forms must be measured?

A. Three
B. Four
C. Five
D. Six
E. Nine

69. A 3-week-old infant is evaluated for ambiguous external genitalia, which look more like an enlarged clitoris than a penis. However, an apparent labial fusion has formed a scrotum-like structure. The karyotype is 46,XX and ultrasound reveals normal ovaries. What is the most likely explanation for these findings?

A. 17-a-hydroxylase deficiency
B. 21-a-hydroxylase deficiency
C. 11-a-hydroxylase deficiency
D. Galactose 1-P uridyltransferase deficiency
E. Turner syndrome

70. A 51-year-old woman with hypothyroidism, diabetes mellitus, hypertension, and stress urinary incontinence presents to her primary care physician for a follow-up examination. She is taking multiple medications including levothyroxine. Thyroxine (T_4) is derived from which of the following?

A. Alanine
B. Glutamic acid
C. Histidine
D. Threonine
E. Tyrosine

71. A 50-year-old white woman with chronic uncontrolled type 2 diabetes is referred to a rheumatologist because recent bone scans revealed marked osteopenia throughout her body. What is the most likely cause of this finding?

A. Chronic osteomyelitis
B. Osteogenesis imperfecta
C. Osteomalacia
D. Osteopetrosis
E. Sickle cell anemia

72. A 4-year-old girl is being evaluated for congenital deafness. Otoscopy reveals the absence of the stapes and incus bilaterally. Physical examination reveals malformation of the anterior neck: the hyoid bone cannot be palpated. A defect in which of the following aortic arches is possible?

    A. I

    B. II

    C. III

    D. IV

    E. V

73. A 45-year-old nurse with a history of chronic diarrhea presents for evaluation. She has no prior medical or surgical history. Her physical examination is unremarkable. A mucosal biopsy reveals a series of permanent folds consisting of mucosa and submucosa. Each villus contains a central lacteal, which will result in the absorption of:

    A. Bilirubin

    B. Biliverdin

    C. Cholesterol

    D. Chylomicrons

    E. Fatty acids

74. A medical student is doing a summer research project to further evaluate hypothalamic function in rodents. The project will involve chemical ablation of the hypothalamus with a pharmacologic agent—a procedure that will likely result in which of the following effects?

    A. Atrophy of the cerebellum

    B. Abnormal ejaculatory function

    C. Increased sexual behavior

    D. Defects in temperature regulation

    E. Visual hallucinations

75. A 24-year-old woman comes to her primary care physician with a complaint of fullness in her breasts, noted a few days earlier. Although the feeling is now gone, she is still concerned. Further questioning reveals that the patient began menstruating today. Sampling of this patient's breast tissue would most likely reveal which of the following?

    A. Apoptosis

    B. Caseous necrosis

    C. Coagulative necrosis

    D. Fat necrosis

Answer Key

1. D	**20.** E	**39.** F	**58.** C
2. C	**21.** E	**40.** D	**59.** D
3. E	**22.** A	**41.** A	**60.** C
4. C	**23.** E	**42.** C	**61.** D
5. B	**24.** B	**43.** A	**62.** B
6. C	**25.** E	**44.** E	**63.** E
7. B	**26.** B	**45.** C	**64.** D
8. D	**27.** D	**46.** D	**65.** B
9. D	**28.** A	**47.** B	**66.** D
10. E	**29.** B	**48.** E	**67.** C
11. D	**30.** B	**49.** C	**68.** C
12. D	**31.** E	**50.** C	**69.** B
13. E	**32.** E	**51.** D	**70.** E
14. E	**33.** B	**52.** D	**71.** C
15. C	**34.** D	**53.** E	**72.** B
16. B	**35.** A	**54.** C	**73.** D
17. D	**36.** A	**55.** D	**74.** D
18. E	**37.** D	**56.** E	**75.** A
19. C	**38.** A	**57.** D	

Answers and Explanations

1. D. The findings of edema, blood pressure > 140/90 mm Hg, and > 300 g of protein in a 24-hr urine sample define preeclampsia. Otherwise known as toxemia of pregnancy, this condition occurs in roughly 6% of pregnant women, typically in the last trimester and more commonly in primiparas than in multiparas. The diagnosis of pregnancy-induced hypertension does not include proteinuria > 300 g in a 24-hr sample. This finding automatically establishes the diagnosis of preeclampsia. The diagnosis of eclampsia is made after finding edema, blood pressure > 140/90 mm Hg, proteinuria > 300 g in a 24-hr urine sample, *and* the development of seizures or convulsions. Chronic hypertension is an incorrect diagnosis in this patient as she did not have elevated blood pressure prior to pregnancy, as indicated by her previous diagnosis of pregnancy-induced hypertension. Hydatidiform mole can lead to pregnancy-induced hypertension, but this is normally diagnosed in the first trimester and there would be no fetus or fetal movement.

2. C. Lead poisoning is the most common type of chronic metal poisoning in the United States and largely affects children in poor urban areas. Lead paint, plumbing, and leaded gasoline are possible sources. The toxicities from lead cause lethargy, behavioral problems, cognitive impairment, mental retardation, and encephalopathy. Patients present with severe abdominal pain (lead colic), renal tubular acidosis, and microcytic anemia with basophilic stippling. One may also see a "lead line" along the gingivodental line from lead deposition. Mercury poisoning causes intention tremors, dementia, and delirium. Patients with cyanide poisoning will have "bitter almond"–scented breath. Acute arsenic poisoning will cause hemorrhagic gastroenteritis, seizures, and a "garlic-scented" breath. Chronically, you will see malaise and abdominal pain with skin changes of hyperpigmentation and dermatitis. Lead poisoning may also cause transverse bands on the fingernails, called Mees lines. Silicosis is seen in sandblasters, metal grinders, and miners. It causes nodular fibrosis of the upper lung lobes, leading to dyspnea.

3. E. Metaplasia, specifically normal columnar ciliated epithelial cells replaced by stratified squamous epithelial cells. Metaplasia is the replacement of one adult cell type for another adult cell type. A common epithelial metaplasia arises in the setting of chronic irritation to the respiratory tract, as occurs in cigarette smoking. In the chronic cigarette smoker, the normal columnar ciliated epithelial cells of the trachea and bronchi are often replaced by stratified squamous epithelium. Dysplasia, in contrast, is a sometimes premalignant tissue change characterized by pleomorphism, changes in the spatial orientation of cells, and increased mitotic activity. Hyperplasia is an increase in the number of cells in an organ or tissue.

4. C. Peroxisomes, also known as microbodies, are membrane-bound cellular organelles containing enzymes that function in the detoxification of ethanol. These enzymes also oxidize long-chain fatty acids and synthesize cholesterol. Mitochondria synthesize adenosine triphosphate (ATP) via the Krebs cycle. Ribosomes are the sites where mRNA is translated into protein. The Golgi apparatus processes proteins made in the rough endoplasmic reticulum and recycles and restructures membranes. The smooth endoplasmic reticulum functions in the synthesis of steroid hormones, drug detoxification, and muscle contraction and relaxation.

5. B. Smooth muscle is composed of short, spindle-shaped cells without striations. Smooth muscle cells contain one central nucleus and can undergo extensive regeneration. It is activated by a Ca^{2+}-calmodulin complex that activates the enzyme myosin light-chain kinase. The contraction of smooth muscle is slower and lasts longer than that of skeletal muscle because its rate of ATP hydrolysis is slower. In contrast, skeletal muscle cells are long and cylindrical, with many peripheral nuclei and striations. Skeletal muscle has restricted regeneration and is activated by calcium binding to troponin C, uncovering the binding sites of myosin (active state).

6. C. The craniopharyngioma is not a true pituitary tumor. It is a benign tumor located at the base of the skull in the region of the pituitary gland. The symptoms of craniopharyngioma relate to its location and size. They include those related to increased intracranial pressure caused by blockage of cerebrospinal fluid pathways, causing hydrocephalus. Additionally, decreased vision, particularly peripheral vision, may be noted. Also, pressure on the hypothalamus and pituitary gland may cause obesity and delayed development. The most effective treatment for craniopharyngioma is surgery. Pheochromocytoma is the most common tumor of the adrenal medulla. It is derived from chromaffin cells. Tuberous sclerosis is associated with facial angiofibroma, seizures, and mental retardation. This condition is also associated with renal angiomyolipoma. Acanthosis nigricans is associated with hyperpigmentation and visceral malignancy, such as cancer of the stomach, breast, lung, and uterus.

7. B. Glial fibrillar acidic protein (GFAP) is the intermediate filament present in astrocytes, oligodendrocytes, and Schwann cells. GFAP provides structural support and serves as an immunological marker for tumors that arise from the glia. Desmin is found in muscle cells and keratin provides support in epithelial cells. Vimentin is primarily involved with fibroblasts and endothelial cells and can also be found along with desmin and GFAP. Neurofilaments are supportive for axons and dendrites in neurons.

8. D. The features described here comprise the classic phenotype for Down's syndrome, which results from trisomy 21 and is the single most common genetic cause of moderate mental retardation. In 95% of patients, the trisomy is a result of meiotic nondisjunction of the chromosome 21 pair. The error most often occurs during maternal meiosis I. Nondisjunction is the failure of a pair of chromosomes to disjoin properly during one of the two meiotic divisions, most often meiosis I.

9. D. This patient suffers from myoclonic epilepsy with ragged-red fibers (MERRF). This rare disorder is caused by mutations in mitochondrial DNA and thus is inherited maternally. The manifestations of MERRF include myoclonic epilepsy and mitochondrial myopathy with ragged-red fibers. Other possible findings are sensorineural hearing loss, ataxia, diabetes, cardiomyopathy, dementia, and renal dysfunction. Treatment is symptomatic and palliative. MERRF is not inherited in either an autosomal dominant or autosomal recessive fashion. It is not due to a chromosomal deletion and is not inherited in an X-linked recessive fashion.

10. E. Both of these patients suffer from neurofibromatosis type 1 (NF1), an autosomal dominant disease of the nervous system. This disease displays variable penetrance, meaning that its severity may vary in people who have the same genotype. Reduced penetrance refers to people who have the genotype for a particular disease and completely fail to express it. Penetrance is an all-or-none concept. The other answer choices do not involve variability in disease expression; they are related to methods of inheritance.

11. D. In newborns, vitamin K deficiency is possible for several reasons. First, the placenta does not transmit lipids well. Second, the neonatal liver is not able to synthesize prothrombin. Also, breast milk is low in vitamin K, and the neonatal gut is sterile during the first few days of life. A deficiency in vitamin K can lead to hemorrhagic disease of the newborn in the first week of life, causing cutaneous, gastrointestinal, intrathoracic, or even intracranial bleeding. At present, it is common for hospitals to administer vitamin K at birth in order to reduce the risk of bleeding, particularly intracranial bleeding from the trauma of birth. Vitamin A deficiency is associated with visual disturbances. Vitamin C deficiency can be associated with impaired wound healing and poor collagen synthesis.

12. D. Penicillin is an inhibitor of bacterial cell-wall synthesis. It works by interacting with cytoplasmic membrane-binding proteins to inhibit transpeptidation reactions necessary for cross-linking of the cell wall. The macrolides and clindamycin alter binding sites of the 50S ribosome, thus interfering with bacterial protein synthesis. The fluoroquinolones inhibit DNA gyrase, which blocks the relaxation of the coiled DNA, necessary for replication.

13. E. These children are suffering from zinc deficiency. The first signs of zinc deficiency in slightly malnourished children are suboptimal growth, impaired taste, and anorexia. Other signs and symptoms include delayed sexual maturation, hypogonadism and hypospermia, alopecia, immune disorders, dermatitis, night blindness, and impaired wound healing. The treatment is the supplementation of zinc in the diet. Iron deficiency can be associated with anemia. Wilson's disease is due to the failure of copper to enter the circulation in the form of ceruloplasmin. This leads to the accumulation of copper, especially in the liver, brain, and cornea. Hemochromatosis is the deposition of iron. It can be associated with macronodular cirrhosis.

14. E. After a few days, this patient should acclimatize to the increased altitude. This includes an initial increase in cardiac output, increased red blood cell mass, and sustained hyperventilation with persistent partially compensated alkalosis. All of these changes are important in maintaining adequate oxygenation and perfusion of body tissues.

15. C. Collagen formation is a normal part of the wound healing process. However, certain individuals seem to have an increased predisposition to excess production of collagen, the result of which is a raised tumor-like scar known as a keloid. African Americans are more frequently affected. Infection results in delayed wound healing, causing an erythematous, swollen area around the wound. Dehiscence is rupture of the wound due to increased abdominal pressure; it arises more acutely after surgery. Ulceration is discontinuity of the skin, leading to complete loss of the epidermis and often portions of the dermis or even subcutaneous fat. It is due to inadequate vascularization. Contracture stems from excessive contraction in the wound. It arises more commonly on the palms of the hands or soles of the feet or after burn injuries. The CT scan in the present case reveals evidence of acute appendicitis. The appendix is dilated and there is inflammation of the periappendiceal fat.

16. B. There are a number of industrial toxins that, with chronic exposure, may lead to carcinomas and other toxicities. Dye makers and rubber workers are at risk of bladder cancer because of exposure to B-naphthylamine. Liver angiosarcoma is a risk from contact with vinyl chloride in the plastics industry. Uranium and radon gas put miners at risk for lung cancer. Squamous and basal cell carcinomas are associated with excessive sun exposure.

17. D. Cell walls, capsules, and cytoplasmic membranes are found in both Gram-positive and Gram-negative bacteria. The presence of a flagellum depends on the specific type of bacterium. An outer membrane is found only in Gram-negative bacteria.

18. E. *Vibrio parahaemolyticus,* a flagellated Gram-negative curved rod, can cause food poisoning when present in undercooked or raw seafood. Its incubation period ranges from 5 to 94 hr (mean 24 hr). The result of infection is a self-limiting watery diarrhea with cramping abdominal pain. *Proteus vulgaris* is a highly motile Gram-negative rod associated with urinary tract infection and septicemia. *Bacillus cereus* is a Gram-positive spore-forming rod that causes vomiting and diarrhea from eating food held warm but not hot, particularly fried rice. *Campylobacter jejuni* is a motile, curved Gram-negative rod leading to an inflammatory diarrhea with blood and pus in stools; it is primarily transmitted from poultry. *Helicobacter pylori* is a Gram-negative spiral gastric bacillus that invades the stomach lining and causes chronic gastric and duodenal ulcers.

19. C. In contrast to *Streptococcus, Staphylococcus* is catalase-positive; thus, when exposed to hydrogen peroxide, *Staphylococcus* will produce a bubbling effect. *Streptococcus* will not have this effect, since it is catalase-negative. Both *Staph* and *Strep* are Gram-positive. PYR and coagulase positivity vary within both of these genera.

20. E. Varicella zoster is a herpesvirus that arises originally as chickenpox. It can remain latent in the dorsal root ganglia, erupting later in life as shingles. Shingles causes an asynchronous rash that appears in a dermatomal pattern, with severe root pain. Epstein-Barr virus causes infectious mononucleosis and Burkitt's lymphoma. It is transmitted through respiratory secretions and saliva. Measles virus is a paramyxovirus. Koplik's spots are diagnostic.

21. E. *Mycoplasma pneumoniae* is responsible for an atypical "walking pneumonia" that presents with a dry, hacking cough and an x-ray that looks much worse than the patient does. Rhinovirus is responsible for the common cold. *Legionella* is another cause of atypical pneumonia but is due to water from an infected source. *Chlamydia* also causes an atypical pneumonia but is relatively uncommon and does not fit this clinical scenario. *Mycobacterium* is associated with tuberculosis. *Staphylococcus aureus* is the most common cause of nosocomial pneumonia, and *Streptococcus pneumoniae* and *Haemophilus influenzae* are more commonly found in elderly persons with pneumonia.

22. A. The positive test for hepatitis surface antigen and the absence of the surface antibody indicate either an acute infection of very short duration or a chronic carrier state that has existed for many months. The core antibodies would not be positive if the patient had simply been vaccinated. Also, the hepatitis surface antigen would not be measurable from vaccination only. This patient is not immune to hepatitis B; he has been exposed to hepatitis B on the basis of the testing described in the question. This patient has not recently been immunized for hepatitis B.

23. E. Human papillomavirus (HPV) types 1 and 4 are associated with plantar warts. HPV types 6 and 11 are the most common benign types, causing anogenital and laryngeal papillomas. Types 16 and 18 are the most common types of HPV, leading to cervical intraepithelial neoplasia. A condition of this kind can lead to cervical cancer; therefore, infected patients should be monitored regularly for epithelial changes.

24. B. Because of the esophagus is chronically exposed to gastric secretions from gastroesophageal reflux disease (GERD), intestinal metaplasia of the squamous esophageal mucosa to a protective columnar type may result. This is referred to as Barrett's esophagus. An important concern with this condition is the associated increased risk of dysplasia and esophageal adenocarcinoma. GERD is not associated with intestinal cell hyperplasia. It can be associated with ulceration of the esophagus near the lower esophageal sphincter. There is no uncontrollable growth of mucosal cells in this condition. Mallory-Weiss tears are tears of the esophageal wall, which occur in chronic alcoholics.

25. E. The correct answer is "Mitochondrial dysfunction, specifically increased uptake of Ca^{2+} by the mitochondria." Two morphological features typically characterize irreversible cell injury: mitochondrial dysfunction and disturbances in the cell membrane. ATP depletion leads to an increase in cytosolic calcium levels, which leads to an increase in mitochondrial calcium uptake. The accumulation of increased calcium within the mitochondria activates mitochondrial phospholipases, which ultimately leads to changes in the permeability of the inner mitochondrial membrane. Ribosome detachment, formation of blebs, failure of the cell membrane pump, and decreased oxidative phosphorylation are all mechanisms of *reversible* cellular injury.

26. B. This injury occurred 6 to 24 hr ago. Neutrophils are the first inflammatory cells to show up in response to acute inflammation. They predominate typically within the first 6 to 24 hr of an inflammatory lesion. The neutrophils are short-lived at the injury site and typically undergo apoptosis and disappear after 24 to 48 hr. Although there may be some neutrophils in the affected area in the first 10 min, it takes longer for many neutrophils to accumulate, as they must undergo the steps of extravasation: adhesion, diapedesis, and migration. After 24 hr, neutrophils are replaced mainly by monocytes and macrophages. If the boy's symptoms had persisted for a week or a month, they would most likely be due to chronic inflammation. Lymphocytes are the most prominent cell in chronic inflammation.

27. D. The correct answer is "Neutrophils largely replaced by macrophages and the progression of granulation tissue into the wound." A clean, uninfected surgical incision closed with sutures is an example of healing by first intention. This type of wound healing progresses in a fairly orderly fashion. Within 24 hr, neutrophils will appear at the margins of the incision. By day 3, neutrophils are largely replaced by macrophages, and granulation tissue begins to enter the incision area. By day 5, the wound area is filled with granulation tissue and neovascularization of the wound is maximal. At approximately the second week, there is proliferation of fibroblasts and accumulation of collagen at the site. Finally, about 30 days from the initial incision, the tissue is almost clear of inflammatory infiltrate and the epidermis is intact.

28. A. The correct answer is "Histamine: mast cells, basophils, and platelets." This patient is experiencing the typical symptoms of a hypersensitivity reaction, most likely from the introduction of the cat. Histamine is the major amine released in response to an allergen. Histamine is stored and released from mast cells, basophils, and platelets. It causes increased vascular permeability. While serotonin is an amide, it is not a major player in hypersensitivity reactions. It is released from platelets.

29. B. B cells and other professional antigen-presenting cells possess both major histocompatibility complex (MHC) I, which recognizes CD8+ T cells, and MHC II, which recognizes CD4+ T cells. All the other cell types in the answer choices possess only MHC I, as this is present on all nucleated cells. The chest x-ray reveals findings of bronchopneumonia. There is patchy alveolar infiltration particularly involving the right middle lobe.

30. B. The correct answer is "Anaplasia with pleomorphism." Typically the more undifferentiated a tumor, the greater its malignant potential. Anaplasia, or complete lack of differentiation, is found in some tumors and is considered a sign of malignant transformation. Pleomorphism is another mark of malignancy and refers to the variation in size and shape that the malignant cells show as compared with neighboring healthy cells. Other signs of malignancy include increased number of mitotic figures, dark staining or hyperchromatic DNA, aggressive and invasive growth, and metastases. Benign tumors, on the other hand, are typically well differentiated and show no signs of anaplasia. Their growth is typically slower and mitotic figures are rare. The mass is well demarcated and there is little invasion into the surrounding tissue.

31. E. This scenario is an example of variable expressivity. Expressivity can be defined as the severity of expression of a specific phenotype. When two patients have the same genotype but the severity of disease differs, the phenotype is said to have variable expressivity. Neurofibromatosis type 1 is a disorder that has variable expressivity. Although penetrance for this disease is approximately 100%, the presentation of symptoms varies from only a few café-au-lait spots or hamartomas on the iris to multiple neurofibromas and even malignant sarcomas of an extremity. This variable expressivity can occur even within a family. Pleiotropy refers to the ability of a single abnormal gene to produce multiple phenotypic effects. Allelic heterogeneity refers to different mutations at the same locus. Consanguinity refers to couples who have one or more ancestors in common or are the result of inbreeding. Consanguineous breeding results in an increase risk of genetically inherited diseases, specifically autosomal recessive conditions.

32. E. The correct answer is "Autosomal recessive, and there is a 25% chance." The disease described in the 10-month-old boy is Tay-Sachs disease, which is due to a deficiency in hexosaminidase and an inability to degrade GM_2 gangliosides. Accumulation of gangliosides leads to the symptoms seen in the patient above. Tay-Sachs is an autosomal recessive disease. Autosomal recessive diseases have a recurrence risk of one in four or 25%. Any child of an affected parent with an autosomal dominant disorder, however, has a 50% risk of inheriting the trait.

33. B. 47XY or -XX trisomy 21 due to a meiotic nondisjunction of the chromosome 21 pair is the most common. Approximately 95% of all Down's syndrome cases are due to trisomy 21 resulting from meiotic nondisjunction of the chromosome 21 pair. This type of Down's syndrome carries an approximate recurrence rate of only 1%. The second most common cause of Down's syndrome is a Robertsonian translocation between 21q and the long arm of an acrocentric chromosome (typically 14 or 22). Unlike trisomy 21, this type of Down's syndrome carries a high risk of recurrence in families, especially if the mother is the carrier. The only other viable trisomies are trisomy 13 and 18. Trisomy 13 is also referred to as Patau syndrome and results in polydactyly, microphthalmia, microcephaly and mental retardation, cleft lip and palate, rocker-bottom feet, and cardiac and renal defects. Trisomy 18, also known as Edward's syndrome, results in a prominent occiput, mental retardation, low-set ears, overlapping fingers, heart defects, horseshoe kidney, and rocker-bottom feet. Trisomy 21 is the most common, occurring in approximately 1 in 700 births.

34. D. *Helicobacter pylori* is a flagellated Gram-negative spiral gastric bacillus that invades the stomach lining and causes chronic gastric and duodenal ulcers. It is urease-positive and has fecal-oral or oral-oral transmission. *H. pylori* infection can be diagnosed with a serological test, biopsy with culture, and urease breath test. *Campylobacter jejuni* is a motile, curved Gram-negative rod causing an inflammatory diarrhea including blood and pus in the stools; it is transmitted primarily from poultry. *Clostridium perfringens* is a large Gram-positive spore-forming rod that may be found in reheated meat dishes; it causes both gas gangrene and a self-limiting noninflammatory watery diarrhea. *Salmonella typhi* is a Gram-negative rod that causes typhoid fever, gastroenteritis, and septicemia. *Entamoeba histolytica* is a parasite that can produce dysentery and liver abscesses.

35. A. This patient has sarcoidosis, a disease that typically afflicts young black women and demonstrates laboratory findings of hypercalcemia, hypercalciuria, hypergammaglobulinemia, and elevated angiotensin-converting enzyme. Patients can present with abnormal chest x-rays, dyspnea, erythema nodosum, hypercalcemia, arthropathy, and skin lesions. The chest x-ray shown reveals bilateral hilar adenopathy. Full blood counts are usually normal, the erythrocyte sedimentation rate is usually elevated. A Mantoux test is negative in most patients.

36. A. In autosomal dominant inheritance, every affected person in a pedigree has an affected parent; i.e., the disease is in every generation. Each child of an affected parent has a 50% chance of acquiring the disease, and males and females are equally affected. In autosomal recessive conditions, 25% of the offspring from two carriers are affected. This is usually due to enzymatic deficiencies. X-linked recessive conditions are such that the sons of heterozygous mothers have a 50% chance of being affected. There is no male-to-male transmission.

37. D. IgG is the only antibody that can cross the placenta. Infants do not start producing their own antibodies until they are about 6 months of age. Therefore the maternal IgG that crossed the placenta is the only antibody that the infant has protecting it from infection during its first 6 months of life. In the case of Bruton's infantile agammaglobulinemia, symptoms of immune deficiency do not present themselves until after the mother's antibodies have begun to decrease and before the baby has begun to make its own antibodies. All other antibodies (IgA, IgE, IgD, and IgM) cannot cross the placenta and thus do not confer immunity to the infant.

38. A. Monocytes enter the bloodstream and differentiate into macrophages after they enter the tissues. The type of tissue they are found in determines their name. Macrophages in the lung are called alveolar macrophages. This monocyte-macrophage system is responsible for trapping and engulfing foreign substances such as carbon particles in the bloodstream and tissues. In the liver, macrophages are called Kupffer cells. In the CNS they are called microglial cells.

39. F. DiGeorge syndrome is due to failure of the third and fourth pharyngeal pouches to develop. The third pharyngeal pouch gives rise to the inferior parathyroid glands and thymus. The fourth pharyngeal pouch gives rise to the superior parathyroid glands. The absence of the thymus gland leads to T-cell deficiency and thus repeated viral, fungal, and/or protozoal infections. The absence of the parathyroid glands results in hypocalcemia and tetany. DiGeorge syndrome is not due to bone marrow hypoplasia, splenic hypoplasia, or a complement deficiency.

40. D. Hereditary angioedema is a rare autosomal dominant disorder that leads to episodes of acute inflammation and edema due to a deficiency of C1 esterase inhibitor (C1INH). C1INH prevents the activation of C1 and thus prevents the initiation of the classic complement pathway. C1INH is important for helping to prevent an overaccumulation of complement components. Decay-accelerating factor is another inactivator of the complement system; it inhibits C3 convertase. There is also a C3b inhibitor and a C6 inhibitor. Hereditary angioedema is not due to a defect in the activation of the alternative or classic complement pathways but rather to a problem in their regulation.

41. A. Acute rejection typically occurs days to months after transplantation and is characterized by the infiltration of lymphocytes and macrophages. Acute rejection is primarily T cell-mediated. These patients typically present with symptoms of acute renal failure. Hyperacute rejection occurs within minutes or hours of transplantation and is primarily antibody-mediated. In a hyperacute kidney rejection, the graft would rapidly become cyanotic, mottled, and flaccid and would not produce urine. This type of rejection is typically due to the presence of preexisting antibodies to donor antigens. A chronic rejection is primarily due to antibody-mediated vascular damage and occurs months to years after transplantation. Patients typically present clinically with a progressive rise in serum creatinine over a 4- to 6-month period. Histologically, this type of rejection is marked by vascular changes consisting of dense fibrosis in the arteries that supply the kidney. Graft-versus-host disease (GVHD) is more commonly seen after bone marrow transplantation. Symptoms of acute GVHD include fever, rash, jaundice, and hepatosplenomegaly. It arises within days to weeks of the transplant when the donor T cells recognize the recipient's human leukocyte antigens (HLA) as foreign and react against them. The symptoms and histological findings would never be considered normal following a renal transplant.

42. C. Rash, fever, jaundice, and hepatosplenomegaly are typical clinical features of GVHD, which occurs most commonly following a bone marrow transplant. Symptoms arise within days to weeks of the transplant, when donor T cells react against the recipient's cells. Principal target organs are the liver, skin, and gastrointestinal mucosa, leading to the common symptoms of jaundice, rash, mucosal ulceration, bloody diarrhea, hepatosplenomegaly, and fever. Hyperacute rejection occurs within minutes to hours of transplantation and is primarily antibody-mediated. It is typically due to the presence of preexisting antibodies to donor antigens. Acute rejection typically occurs days to months after transplantation and is characterized by the infiltration of lymphocytes and macrophages. Acute rejection is primarily T cell-mediated. Chronic rejection occurs over months to years after transplantation and is primarily due to antibody-mediated vascular damage. The symptoms presented above would never be considered normal following a bone marrow transplant.

43. A. This is an example of a type I hypersensitivity reaction, in this case an anaphylactic reaction to penicillin. Type I hypersensitivity reactions are otherwise known as anaphylactic reactions and arise when an antigen (in this case penicillin) reacts with IgE bound to the surface of basophils or mast cells in individuals previously sensitized to the antigen. The result of the antigen-antibody–mast cell complex is massive degranulation and the release of histamine and vasoactive, chemotactic, or other substances that induce smooth muscle spasm. The reaction is rapid and develops within minutes of the antigen exposure. Type IV hypersensitivity reactions, or cell-mediated reactions, occur when sensitized T lymphocytes react against antigens presented by macrophages. The result is a release of lymphokines and cell-mediated cytotoxicity.

44. E. Sarcoidosis is a disease of unclear etiology. It is common in African-American individuals. Presenting features include cough and joint pain. Physical examination can reveal erythema nodosum. Chest x-ray typically reveals bilateral (perihilar) lymphadenopathy and diffuse reticular densities. The incidence is approximately 1 in 20,000 and peaks in early adult life. The condition is more common in women than men. The prognosis is good in a young patient with an acute onset, hilar adenopathy, and erythema nodosum.

45. C. The half-life can be determined by manipulating the equation used to determine the time to reach 90% of final steady-state plasma levels. That equation is 3.3 × half-life. Thus, this problem can be solved by as follows:

$$12 \text{ hr}/3.3 = \text{half-life, or } 4.75$$
It takes four to five half-lives to reach
"clinical" steady state.

46. D. Diabetes has a strong association with chronic sinusitis due to saprophytic Zygomycetes, including *Mucor* and *Rhizopus*. It is very important to recognize this as a possibility for infection in any patient with chronic sinusitis who appears unusually ill and does not respond to antibiotics. The fungi can spread rapidly into the skull bones and brain, with potential tissue destruction and death. *Pneumocystis* is a cause of pneumonia in immunocompromised patients, e.g., those with AIDS. Members of the genus *Actinomyces* are part of the normal flora of the mouth. They may cause infection in the facial region from trauma or dental procedures and also in the lungs or abdomen after surgery or trauma. However, these organisms are not associated with diabetes. Cryptococcal infection is generally established through the respiratory tract from exposure to pigeon droppings. It would not be a specific concern for this patient with sinusitis. *Aspergillus* can be a cause of sinus problems in diabetics; however, it would not be of greatest concern.

47. B. This patient has been infected with *Clostridium botulinum*, a common contaminant in honey. The toxin blocks the release of acetylcholine, causing floppiness in an infant. Acetylcholine works at the neuromuscular junction, thus inhibition of its release will cause muscle weakness, failure to thrive, and, more critically, respiratory distress. Ribosylation of EF by adenosine diphosphate (ADP) is an action of diphtheria toxin. GABA and glycine are inhibited by *Clostridium tetani*. Stimulation of guanylate cyclase occurs through heat-stable toxin from *Escherichia coli*.

48. E. This question is concerned with the effect of nonselective beta-blockers. These medications are contraindicated in patients with lung disease because they cause bronchoconstriction by blocking the beta$_2$ receptors, which promote bronchial smooth muscle relaxation. Nadolol is a nonselective beta-blocker and therefore should not be used in patients with lung disease. Esmolol, acebutolol, betaxolol, and metoprolol are cardioselective beta$_1$ blockers that may be used in patients with lung disease.

49. C. Phase I trials are the initial phase of clinical testing. Such a trial involves approximately 20 to 30 normal volunteers who establish the safety and pharmacokinetic properties of a new drug. Phase II trials test a newly developed drug on a group of selected patients (100 to 300) in relation to therapeutic efficacy, kinetics, metabolism, and dose range. Phase III trials typically consist of 500 to 5,000 patients who participate in a double-blind controlled study. Such a trial determines whether the drug is more effective than placebo and older therapies. During this phase, drug toxicity is also monitored. The NDA contains the results of the clinical studies and must be submitted to obtain approval from the U.S. Food and Drug Administration (FDA) for marketing the drug. An IND application has to be submitted by the manufacturer to the FDA. It describes the drug's chemical makeup and behavior, data from animal testing, and designs for clinical trials.

50. C. This patient has scurvy, which results from a vitamin C deficiency. This leads to impaired hydroxylation of proline residues in the nascent procollagen chains, which weakens the walls of the blood vessels, producing such symptoms as splinter hemorrhages, perifollicular hemorrhages, ecchymoses, purpura, and hemorrhages into muscle. Patients may also experience gum changes. If supplementation of vitamin C is not given, death may occur. Iron would be of benefit in iron-deficiency anemia, which presents as a hypochromic microcytic anemia. This is not indicated in this patient. Vitamin D would be administered if there were bone disease in some form. There may be malabsorption of vitamin D or direct deficiency. Vitamin K is given in the event of a prolonged prothrombin time due to a deficiency of the vitamin. This symptom is followed by a prolonged partial thromboplastin time (PTT) and depletion of the vitamin K–dependent factors (II, VII, IX, X, protein C, and protein S). Factor VIII would be indicated in factor VIII deficiency, which also leads to a prolonged PTT, which was not noted in this patient.

51. D. The administration of aspartame, which contains phenylalanine, can be detrimental in this patient. Phenylketonuria results from impaired conversion of phenylalanine to tyrosine, which is caused by a deficiency of phenylalanine hydrolase. An increase in phenylalanine and its by-products can lead to mental retardation. Wilson's disease is an autosomal recessive condition due to an abnormality in copper excretion; it causes accumulation of copper in the brain, liver, and other organs. Hypervalinemia is an inherited disorder resulting from a defect of valine aminotransferase. It presents with mental retardation, protein intolerance, and neuropsychiatric problems. Hyperuricemia is an increased concentration of uric acid levels in the blood. It may lead to gout if persistent. Hyperornithinemia results from a defect of ornithine decarboxylase. It is also associated with mental retardation, protein intolerance, and neuropsychiatric dysfunction.

52. D. This is a contact dermatitis from exposure to poison ivy. It is a type IV or delayed-type hypersensitivity reaction resulting from a T-cell reaction with the antigen. Another example includes the tuberculin skin test. Type I hypersensitivity is an immediate, atopic, or anaphylactic reaction. It is IgE-mediated with cross-linking of IgE receptors on basophils and mast cells. There is subsequent release of a variety of mediators, including histamine. Examples include asthma, atopic dermatitis, eczema, and allergic rhinitis. Type I is characterized by hives. A type II reaction is an antibody-mediated hypersensitivity resulting from IgG or IgM antibody reacting with membrane-associated antigen on the surface of cells, leading to the complement cascade and thus cell destruction. Examples include Goodpasture's syndrome, some drug allergies, blood transfusion reactions, and hemolytic disease of the newborn. A type III reaction is an immune complex-mediated hypersensitivity caused by the formation of antigen-antibody complexes, leading to the generation of C3b and the anaphylatoxins C3a and C5a. These cause inflammation and tissue destruction. Type III reactions generally present with signs of urticaria, angioedema, fever, chills, and malaise approximately 7 to 14 days after exposure. Syndromes include serum sickness and the Arthus reaction.

53. E. This patient has symptoms of thiamine deficiency, which can lead to Wernicke encephalopathy. This condition presents as a triad of global confusion, ataxia, and ophthalmoplegia. Administration of thiamine (vitamin B$_1$) is crucial, because this deficiency is a medical emergency. Niacin deficiency presents with "the three D's": diarrhea, dermatitis, and dementia, otherwise known as pellagra. A deficiency of pyridoxine, or vitamin B$_6$, leads to peripheral neuropathy and dermatitis. A deficiency of riboflavin, or vitamin B$_2$, presents with lesions of the lips, mouth, skin, and genitalia. This results from lack of maintenance of appropriate levels of flavin mononucleotide (FMN) and flavin adenine dinucleotide (FAD). Biotin deficiency involves alopecia, muscle pain, and skin and bowel inflammation.

54. C. This child most likely has an infection with *Enterobius vermicularis*, commonly called pinworm. The perianal itching, attendance at day care (a big reservoir for pinworm), and positive Scotch tape test point to this diagnosis. The main cell involved in fighting this infection is the eosinophil, which uses major basic protein specifically. Histamine and heparin are products of mast cells and not used to fight parasites. Myeloperoxidase is a nonspecific agent used by a variety of white blood cells to fight infectious agents; however, it is not specifically geared to parasitic infections. Perforin is used by cytotoxic T cells to induce apoptosis in virally infected cells.

55. D. The organ most likely to have been damaged by a stab wound to the left midaxillary line in the region of the ninth and eleventh ribs is the spleen. Histologically, the spleen is characterized by red pulp, which consists of red blood cells removed from circulation, and also white pulp, which consists of lymphoid cells. The periarteriolar lymphatic sheath (PALS) is a collection of T lymphocytes surrounding splenic arterioles. Enterochromaffin cells are located in the adrenal gland and produce epinephrine and norepinephrine. Hassall's corpuscles are located in the thymus; their function is not entirely clear. Islets of Langerhans are collections of endocrine cells in the pancreas.

56. E. This patient has multiple myeloma, characterized by the overproliferation of plasma cells. He presents with the classical symptoms of multiple myeloma, including low back pain from bone lesions caused by the release of osteoclast activating factor by the plasma cells. His lethargy can be caused by a lack of erythrocytes as the plasma cells "take over" the bone marrow. Cytotoxic T lymphocytes and helper T lymphocytes may be overly abundant in other lymphoid neoplasms but not in multiple myeloma. Mast cells and erythrocytes may actually be lacking rather than overly abundant in multiple myeloma.

57. D. This child has chronic granulomatous disease, which is characterized by a lack of nicotinamide adenine dinucleotide phosphate (NADPH) oxidase. This allows organisms that possess peroxidase, such as *Staphylococcus aureus,* to continually degrade the peroxides that NADPH oxidase utilizes to generate bactericidal molecules. The nitrozolium blue test is negative in patients with CGD. G6PD deficiency leads to a hemolytic anemia upon exposure to various chemicals, such as antimalarial drugs and fava beans. Pyruvate kinase also causes a hemolytic anemia, although this disease is not as common as G6PD deficiency. A deficiency of myeloperoxidase would cause the symptoms shown above, but the nitrozolium blue test would be positive in this child. Hexokinase deficiency would not affect lymphocytes but would cause severe nutritional deficiency, as hexokinase is needed for glucose metabolism.

58. C. In general, acute leukemia is classified into two main categories, depending upon the lineage to which the blast cells belong: acute myelogenous leukemia (AML) or acute lymphoblastic leukemia (ALL). This patient is presenting with signs and symptoms of disseminated intravascular coagulation, a known complication of the M3 (promyelocytic) form of AML. The other forms of AML have different complications, but none has DIC as a likely complication.

59. D. This child most likely has aspirated a button from his shirt. Foreign objects are more likely to obstruct the right middle bronchus due to its more vertical orientation with the trachea. Air will be allowed into the obstructed lobe but will not be exhaled as easily, leading to hyperinflation. Ventilation of the hyperinflated lobe will be inadequate, with the resulting hypoxia leading to vasoconstriction of the pulmonary vasculature serving the affected area. Increased

resistance in the right pulmonary artery system will lead to increased flow in the left pulmonary artery system. A collapsed lung would decrease flow in the right pulmonary artery, but the history does not suggest an etiology for a collapsed lung, such as trauma. Consolidation is associated with bacterial pneumonia and usually causes tracheal deviation toward the lesion. Diffuse infiltrates are often seen with viral respiratory infections, which are not likely to present in such a sudden fashion. The "thumbprint sign" on chest x-ray would suggest acute epiglottitis, but the lack of fever and the child's age make this less likely.

60. C. *Mycobacterium tuberculosis* is classically cultured on Lowenstein-Jensen medium. However, growth of colonies is very slow and empirical treatment should begin immediately for patients with such symptoms of tuberculosis. Bordet-Gengou agar is also called potato agar and can culture *Bordetella.* Chocolate agar is used to culture *Haemophilus* species. Tellurite agar is used to culture *Corynebacterium diphtheriae.* Thayer-Martin agar is used to culture *Neisseria gonorrhoeae.*

61. D. This child is suffering from diphtheria, caused by *Corynebacterium diphtheriae.* Refugees from underdeveloped nations are often medically underserved and may be lacking in certain vaccinations. This organism characteristically grows black colonies on tellurite-containing medium. Loeffler's coagulated serum medium can also be used to grow *C. diphtheriae,* but the organisms will be notable for metachromatic granules.

62. B. Emphysema in a young nonsmoker should raise suspicion of alpha$_1$-antitrypsin deficiency, a hereditary disorder that results in reduced hepatic secretion of alpha$_1$ antitrypsin. Since this protein is secreted by the liver, reduced secretion results in hepatic accumulation, which can result in cirrhosis. Situs inversus and infertility (in males) is part of Kartagener's syndrome, a disorder of ciliary motility. Congenital heart diseases are unlikely to present in adulthood. Affected infants often present with cyanosis after birth. Problematic ovarian cysts are unlikely in patients who have no pelvic complaints.

63. E. This patient has classic signs of tuberculosis. Silicosis is associated with an increased susceptibility to tuberculosis. When this disease develops on preexisting silicosis, it is termed silicotuberculosis. Asbestosis demonstrates diffuse interstitial fibrosis of the lower lobes and dense hyalinized fibrocalcific plaques of the parietal pleura. Coal worker's pneumoconiosis is related to exposure to coal dust. Coal dust is inhaled into the alveoli and is engulfed by macrophages, which congregate around bronchioles in the upper lobes.

64. D. Renin is the enzyme secreted by juxtaglomerular (JG) cells in the afferent arteriole when macula densa cells in the distal tubule (which are in direct apposition to the JG cells forming the JG apparatus) sense a decrease in sodium concentration or pressure. Renin then cleaves angiotensinogen to make angiotensin-1. Angiotensin-1 is converted to angiotensin-2 via angiotensin-converting enzyme (ACE) primarily in the pulmonary capillary beds. Angiotensin-2 acts on adrenal cortex cells in the zona glomerulosa to stimulate the secretion of aldosterone, which then causes increased reabsorption of Na+ in the distal tubule.

65. B. Adipose cells produce the enzyme aromatase. Aromatase converts androstenedione and testosterone into estrone and estradiol, respectively. An excess of adipose cells leads to excess aromatase, which leads to the conversion of adrenal androgens into excess estrogen. Increased estrogen levels have been linked to breast and endometrial cancers.

66. D. Dopamine inhibits prolactin secretion. When CNS dopaminergic activity is blocked by drugs, the inhibition of prolactin is lifted. This leads to increased levels of serum prolactin and can manifest as side effects such as galactorrhea, amenorrhea, and sexual dysfunction. Dopamine-blocking agents will not affect levels of adrenocorticotropic hormone (ACTH). These agents will not affect levels of follicle-stimulating hormone (FSH) or luteinizing hormone (LH). There will be no change in TSH, T_3, or T_4 levels with the use of dopamine-blocking antipsychotic agents.

67. C. When uncharged valine is substituted for negatively charged glutamate, sickle cell hemoglobin is produced. The mutated hemoglobin is less negatively charged and has greater electrophoretic mobility. Sickle deoxyhemoglobin polymerizes and causes the primary structure to be altered. The insoluble, polymerized hemoglobin decreases the flexibility of red blood cells, making them brittle and likely to block capillaries.

68. C. LDH is a tetramer composed of any two combinations of polypeptides H and M. The possible combinations are M_4, H_4, M_1H_3, M_3H_1, M_2H_2. All five combinations are found in all tissues. However, M_4 predominates in the liver and skeletal muscle. H_4 is the predominant isozyme in heart muscle and is known as LDH1. After an infarction of the myocardium, H_4 (LDH1) rises and peaks within 36 hr from the initial insult.

69. B. Congenital adrenal hyperplasia is most commonly due to a deficiency of 21-α-hydroxylase. When 21-α-hydroxylase is absent, the production of aldosterone and cortisol decreases and their precursors are shunted into the pathway of sex hormone biosynthesis. This leads to masculinization of the external genitalia. This child is a female pseudohermaphrodite, as she is genetically and gonadally female with male secondary sex characteristics. Hyperkalemia and hypotension may also be seen due to a decreased synthesis of aldosterone. The karyotype for Turner's syndrome is XO. These are genotypic females with streak ovaries. Deficiencies in 17-α and 11-α hydroxylase are rare syndromes of ambiguous genitalia.

70. E. T_4 is derived from tyrosine by the iodination and joining of peptide-linked tyrosine residues of thyroglobulin. Proteolytic cleavage of thyroglobulin yields thyroxine. Thyroxine is named T_4 because of the four iodine atoms it contains. Thyroxine is not derived from alanine, glutamic acid, histidine, or threonine.

71. C. Osteomalacia as a result of renal failure from the chronic uncontrolled diabetes is the most likely cause of the marked osteopenia. The kidneys produce 1,25-dihydroxycholecalciferol, the active form of vitamin D. Because vitamin D is necessary for bone mineralization and bone is constantly being remodeled, marked osteopenia is the result of decreased vitamin D. There is no evidence to suggest chronic osteomyelitis in this patient (indium scan or elevated white blood cell count). Hemoglobin electrophoresis is used to test for sickle cell disease, but it was not performed in this patient because sickle cell disease is more common in blacks, and this patient is Caucasian.

72. B. The second aortic arch gives rise to the stapedial and hyoid arteries, which supply derivatives of the second pharyngeal arch. This arch is developmentally lacking in this patient, as evidenced by the findings of deafness and anterior neck defects. The first aortic arch gives rise to the maxillary artery. The third aortic arch gives rise to the common carotid artery and the first part of the internal carotid artery as well as the external carotid artery. The left side of the fourth aortic arch gives rise to the arch of the aorta, while the right side forms the right subclavian artery. The sixth arch gives rise to the right and left pulmonary arteries.

73. D. The lamina propria of the small intestine penetrates the core of the villi and is composed of blood vessels, lymphatics, defensive cells, fibroblasts, and smooth muscle cells. A central lacteal in the villus absorbs chylomicrons into the lymphatic circulation through its junctional gaps. Bilirubin, biliverdin, chylomicrons, and fatty acids are not absorbed through the lacteal.

74. D. Consequences of hypothalamic ablation include problems with eating, sexual activity, and regulation of body temperature as well as alteration of the sleep–wake cycle. Cerebellar atrophy is associated with ablation of the cerebellum. Increased sexual behavior is associated with ablation of the amygdala. Visual hallucinations and illusions as well as disturbances of spatial orientation are associated with ablation of the occipital lobe.

75. A. This patient was most likely feeling breast fullness due to the response of the breast tissue to the estrogen and rising progesterone levels occurring after ovulation. After ovulation, cell proliferation typically occurs in the breast, as do the number of acini per lobule. When menstruation finally occurs, the feeling of fullness typically wanes due to the fall of estrogen and progesterone and the resultant apoptosis of the epithelial cells. Although fat necrosis can occur in the breast. it typically follows a localized inflammatory reaction or injury and is more commonly unilateral. Caseous necrosis is often associated with tuberculosis and occurs as part of a granulomatous inflammation. Coagulative necrosis typically results from a sudden disruption of blood supply to an organ. Caseous and coagulative necroses do not occur in the breast.

Chapter 2   Behavioral Sciences

Questions

1. A newborn is delivered on the obstetrics ward. It is 1 min after delivery and the baby has a pink trunk with some peripheral cyanosis; it is making an irregular respiratory effort, has some muscle tone, and a heart rate of 95, as well as a cough/sneeze reflex. What is this infant's Apgar score?

   A. 4

   B. 5

   C. 6

   D. 7

   E. 8

   F. 9

   [handwritten: APGAR 1 1 2 1 1]

2. A young woman has come to the clinic for her yearly visit. Physical examination reveals that the nipples and areolas have projected to form a secondary mound (double mound) above the level of the breast. Examination of the genitalia shows her pubic hair to be coarse and curly, as in an adult, but the hair does not cover her thighs. She denies shaving any of her pubic hair. What is the most appropriate Tanner stage for this patient?

   A. Tanner 1 *[handwritten: no pubic hair]*

   B. Tanner 2 *[handwritten: pubic hair strts on labia]*

   C. Tanner 3 *[handwritten: " " on pubis]*

   D. Tanner 4 *[handwritten: " " not covering thigh]*

   E. Tanner 5 *[handwritten: " " covering medial thigh]*

3. A 51-year-old man presents to his primary care physician with feelings of anxiety. He goes on to say that since the New Year began (eight months earlier) he has worried all the time about "stupid things I have no control over." His boss has met with him several times because other workers have complained that he has become very irritable; moreover, his assignments are becoming sloppy and are often days late. He complains that he cannot sleep at night and says the reason his work has been late is that he cannot concentrate and often "hits a wall when trying to work." He denies any drug or alcohol abuse and has no current medical conditions that he knows of. What neurotransmitters are involved in this disease process and, as compared with a normal individual, what would his levels be—increased or decreased?

   A. Increased norepinephrine, decreased gamma-aminobutyric acid (GABA), decreased serotonin

   B. Decreased norepinephrine, decreased serotonin

   C. Decreased acetylcholine

   D. Decreased GABA, decreased acetylcholine

   E. Increased dopamine

   F. Decreased dopamine

4. A 59-year-old man with schizophrenia and mental retardation is admitted to the psychiatric unit. He has a history of hypertension and takes an angiotensin-converting enzyme (ACE) inhibitor. He is unemployed and lives in a group home. Under which axes would mild mental retardation be coded?

   A. Axis I *[handwritten: clinical mental disorder]*

   B. Axis II *[handwritten: personality disorder, mild mental retardation]*

   C. Axis III *[handwritten: medical]*

   D. Axis IV *[handwritten: environment]*

   E. Axis V *[handwritten: global]*

5. A 38-year-old woman complains of a preoccupation with minor symptoms and disease possibilities. She may misinterpret normal physical findings, leading to the preoccupation with and fear of having a serious illness despite medical reassurance otherwise. What is the most likely diagnosis?

   A. Conversion disorder

   B. Factitious disorder

   C. Hypochondriasis

   D. Malingering

   E. Somatization disorder

6. A pediatric patient is brought to see you. He is able to tell you his full name and speaks in complete sentences. He is able to ride a tricycle but, according to his mother and father, is still working on toilet training. He is also learning to cooperate in playing with others. He is not yet able to hop on one foot or use compound sentences. In Freudian terms, at what stage of psychosexual development is this child?

   A. Anal stage

   B. Genital stage

   C. Latent stage

   D. Oral stage

   E. Phallic stage

7. A 21-year-old college student is brought to the emergency department by a friend because he has been experiencing nausea and vomiting. Physical examination reveals pinpoint pupils. His friend says that the patient fell off a chair and hit his head on the floor. A computed tomography (CT) scan of the head is performed (Figure 2-1). With which of the following substances has this person most likely been intoxicated?

   A. Alcohol

   B. Amphetamines

   C. Caffeine

   D. Cocaine

   E. Lysergic acid diethylamide (LSD)

   F. Nicotine

   G. Opioids

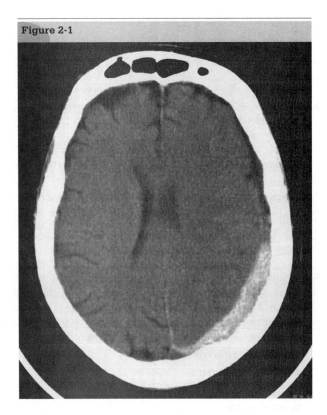

Figure 2-1

8. After being arrested for trying to rob a convenience store to get more beer, a 28-year-old man is forced to spend a couple days in jail to "dry out." On his third day in jail, one of the police officers walks by his cell and notices that the man is sitting in a corner trembling. The jail's doctor is called in. Physical examination reveals the man to be tachycardic, hypertensive, and agitated; he is also having hallucinations and delusions. What is the most likely diagnosis?

A. Amphetamine withdrawal

B. Cocaine withdrawal

C. Delirium tremens

D. Opioid withdrawal

E. Phencyclidine (PCP) withdrawal

9. A first-year medical student is given an assignment to critique a research paper. He begins to feel overwhelmed by all the statistical jargon, so he pulls out his epidemiology book to look up some definitions. He examines a 2 × 2 table to look at the probability of having a positive test result in disease-positive individuals. What is the most likely parameter he is identifying?

A. Negative predictive value

B. Positive predictive value

C. Relative risk

D. Sensitivity

E. Specificity

10. A 21-year-old college student presents to her primary care physician regarding information about contraception. She has a prior medical history of seasonal allergies and her current medications include an antihistamine. Physical examination of the heart, lungs, and abdomen is within normal limits. Pelvic examination reveals normal mucosa; there is no evidence of prolapse. Which of the following contraceptive method has the highest failure rate per 100 woman-years?

A. Estrogen-only oral contraceptive

B. Intrauterine device, copper

C. Intrauterine device, loop D

D. Vasectomy

E. Spermicide

11. A 22-year-old HIV-positive man with a CD4 cell count of 100 and his 28-year-old HIV-positive male partner with a CD4 cell count of 200 present to the outpatient clinic for evaluation. Both currently take multiple medications and have been infection-free for three weeks. Both are in the 30th percentile for height and weight. Although they are now clinically well, they are AIDS activists and encourage disease prevention and promotion. They also have an interest in world travel but have some fears of disease progression. Today they ask for information regarding the global picture of the HIV/AIDS epidemic. Which of the following countries has the largest number of adults and children who are infected with the HIV/AIDS virus?

A. Africa

B. The Caribbean

C. North Africa

D. North America

E. Southeast Asia

12. A 19-year-old college student is brought to the University Clinic by her roommate, who states that her friend has been acting oddly during the last few weeks. The roommate states that she entered the dormitory bedroom and found her friend with an open bottle of pills and several half-empty bottles of liquor. The roommate states that her friend began to act differently after the breakup of her parents a month ago, and that her grades in the current semester have been poor. Physical examination reveals a well-developed female with stable vital signs. She is alert, awake, and oriented but has alcohol on her breath. Further questioning reveals that the patient has a history of a major depressive episode, which occurred when she was 13, after the death of a close friend. Which of the following conditions is associated with the highest risk of successful suicide attempts?

A. Bipolar disorder

B. Borderline personality disorder

C. Major depression

D. Panic disorder

E. Schizophrenia

13. A 40-month-old child and his mother present to their primary care physician for a well-child examination. The child's immunizations are up to date. He is in the 40th percentile for height, weight, and head circumference. Lead testing from a prior visit was within normal limits. At today's examination, the child has a regular heart rate and rhythm. There are no rales, wheezes, or rhonchi. Both testes are descended bilaterally and the phallus is uncircumcised. The mother expresses an interest in toilet training her child. What is the most likely age at which toilet training would occur?

A. 24 months
B. 36 months
C. 48 months
D. 60 months
E. 72 months

14. A 7-year-old boy is brought to the pediatrician for evaluation. He has stereotyped body movements (finger twisting, rocking back and forth in his seat, etc.) and seems to be lacking in emotional development. However, he has normal language and cognitive development. What is the most likely diagnosis?

A. Autistic disorder
B. Asperger's syndrome
C. Childhood disintegrative disorder
D. Rett's syndrome
E. Tourette's syndrome

15. A 62-year-old woman with metastatic pancreatic cancer is admitted to a local hospice for end-of-life care. She begins to cry and plead with you, saying, "You can have all the money in my accounts, I'll give you my home and car. I'll see you every month and take any pill you give me, just make sure I live through this!" What stage of death and dying is this patient at?

A. Acceptance
B. Anger
C. Bargaining
D. Denial
E. Depression

16. A research study is trying to determine the distribution of mean arterial blood pressures in women 25 to 29 years of age. Data were collected from eight research sites and included 10,379 participants. Owing to faulty reporting, the data from 278 patients had to be removed from the study. According to the following graph (Figure 2-2), what is true of the data collected?

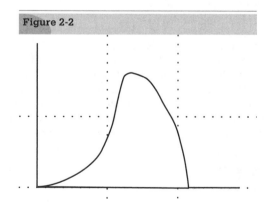

Figure 2-2

A. Mean = mode = median
B. Mean > mode > median
C. Median = mean = mode
D. Mode > mean > median
E. Mode > median > mean

17. During a well-patient evaluation of a 15-year-old boy, you discuss the dangers of cigarette smoking, including the long-term consequences. You explain that it is okay to say no to one's peers and even give some examples of how to avoid peer pressure. Which of the following methods of prevention is described?

A. Primary prevention
B. Secondary prevention
C. Tertiary prevention
D. Quaternary prevention

18. A female doctor is approached by one of her male patients after a routine office visit. She has been involved with this man's care for about 5 years and has always been careful not to send any signals to him indicating that their relationship is anything more than strictly doctor-patient. He proceeds to tell her that he has recently broken up with his long-time significant other and was wondering if she would like to go out for dinner one night. He explains that he is feeling lonely and just wants some companionship. What is the most appropriate plan of action for this woman?

A. Accept the date; if they are both single, what is the harm?
B. Scream at him, yelling that she would never date a loser like him.
C. Tell him to call her in a month and they can go out then. Right now is too close to his last exam.
D. Begin seeing him but break up with him at least 3 months before his next appointment.
E. Politely explain that it is unethical for a doctor to date a patient. If he feels he needs to talk to someone, she can put him in touch with a counselor.

19.

Disease Test		
	Positive	Negative
Positive	160	90
Negative	40	210

Which of the following values represents the sensitivity of the test?

A. 70%
B. 30%
C. 20%
D. 80%
E. 64%
F. 84%

$$\frac{160}{160+40} = \frac{160}{200} = 0.8\ldots$$

20. Which of the following definitions accurately describes lead-time bias?

    A. When a third factor is associated with both the risk factor and the disease, the study can be attributed to the third factor.

    B. The people who are selected for an intervention are different than those who are not.

    C. Because screening may diagnose a disease earlier, "survival time" appears longer, but it is not.

    D. Screening detects slowly progressive cases; those with aggressive disease are missed because they have either died or been cured.

    E. The type of people who are compliant with a regimen may be different from those who are not compliant.

    F. The data collected may depend on a patient's recollection (notoriously unreliable), and the patients may be asked more details about exposure than control.

    G. Subjects may change their behavior once they know they are being observed.

21. In a small city (population of about 50,000) there are about 2,000 cases of disease X. In the past year, there have been 500 new cases of disease X. What is the incidence of disease X in this small city?

    A. 6%

    B. 5%

    C. 4%

    D. 1%

    E. 0%

[handwritten: $\frac{500}{50,000}$ New cases / Total population]

22. A 9-year-old boy is brought in for an annual pediatric checkup. The pediatrician performs his usual exam and everything turns out normal. Upon further observation, the doctor notes that the boy was squeezing his water-filled balloon to make different shapes. The boy turned to his mother and said, "Look Mom, the water stays in the balloon but moves to the opposite side whenever I squeeze it." What is the most likely stage of this child's intellectual development?

    A. Concrete operational stage

    B. Formal operational stage

    C. Preoperational stage

    D. Sensorimotor stage

    E. Sensorineural stage

23. Which of the following would be considered a positive symptom of schizophrenia?

    A. Cognitive defects

    B. Emotional blunting

    C. Hallucinations

    D. Social withdrawal

    E. Uremia

24. A 41-year-old obese man presents to the ambulatory care clinic complaining of hypersomnia. He is admitted overnight for a sleep study. His electroencephalogram reveals beta waves. He has lost motor tone but his pulse and blood pressure are increased and variable. A full penile erection is visible. What is the principal neurotransmitter involved with the stage of sleep described in this patient?

    A. Acetylcholine

    B. Dopamine

    C. Gamma-aminobutyric acid

    D. Norepinephrine

    E. Serotonin

25. During your second year of medical school, you and a couple of your classmates decide to enroll in a research study to make some fast cash. While searching for available studies, you find one for which you qualify. This study is looking for students between the ages of 18 and 26 who consume at least ten cups of regular (caffeinated) coffee a day. The goal of the study is to follow these students for the next ten years to see what effect this large amount of caffeine has on their bodies and/or lives. Knowing that you and your fellow students drink at least that amount of coffee daily, you all decide to enroll. What is the most likely test that you have enrolled in?

    A. Cohort study

    B. Case-control study

    C. Cross-sectional study

    D. Clinical trial

    E. Primary survey

26. A 65-year-old woman visits her primary care physician for a regular checkup. For the past three weeks she has had a total loss of interest in gardening and playing bocce, which used to be her favorite hobbies. She has also lost weight even though she has not been trying to diet or exercise more. She sleeps nearly 12 hr a day but still feels that she has no energy. She often feels guilty for minor events in her past. She denies being depressed or having thoughts of hurting herself. What is the most likely diagnosis?

    A. Atypical dysthymia

    B. Bipolar affective disorder type I

    C. Bipolar affective disorder type II

    D. Major depressive disorder

    E. Schizo-affective disorder

27. A 63-year-old man who is a known alcoholic stumbles into the emergency department complaining of dysuria and urethral discharge. He has a history of type II diabetes, hypertension, prostate cancer, and schizophrenia. Laboratory testing reveals a positive Venereal Disease Research Laboratory (VDRL) test. Which of the diseases mentioned above must be reported to the county health department?

    A. Diabetes

    B. Hypertension

    C. Prostate cancer

    D. Schizophrenia

    E. Syphilis

28. A 16-year-old girl is brought to her primary care physician because her parents believe that she might have an eating disorder. She has a body mass index (BMI) of 21 and has had no recent weight gain or loss. When questioned alone, she reveals that when she starts eating, she cannot stop, even though she is no longer hungry and wants to stop eating. After these episodes, she takes laxatives to try to prevent weight gain. She does this at least 3 times a week and started these behaviors about 4 months earlier. What type of eating disorder does this patient have?

A. Anorexia nervosa, binge eating/purging type

B. Anorexia nervosa, restrictive type

C. Bulimia nervosa, purging type

D. Bulimia nervosa, nonpurging type

E. Uncontrollable eating syndrome

29. A 56-year-old schizophrenic man is brought to the emergency department from his assisted-living group home because of diffuse myalgias and decreased responsiveness, which have been present for 14 hr. He has a history of non-insulin-dependent diabetes mellitus. His surgical history is notable for resection of a poorly differentiated pancreatic carcinoma. His current medications include an antipsychotic agent, metformin, and acetaminophen. Physical examination reveals an agitated man who does not respond to verbal or tactile stimuli. His temperature is 39°C (104°F). His pulse is 140 bpm and blood pressure 160/110 mm Hg. He is diaphoretic; neurologic examination reveals increased muscular tone in all extremities. A CT scan of the head is shown in Figure 2-3. What is the most likely explanation for this patient's symptoms?

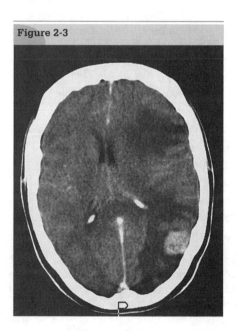

Figure 2-3

A. Acetaminophen toxicity

B. Haloperidol usage

C. Metformin toxicity

D. Underlying delirium

E. Underlying dementia

30. A 27-year-old man who works at a local car dealership has been married for 3 years. Over the past few months he has found himself flirting with an attractive coworker. He has never cheated on his wife but he does feel guilty and ashamed for his feelings toward his coworker. As a result of this guilt and shame he begins to accuse his wife of having an affair. What kind of defense mechanism is this patient using?

A. Acting out

B. Controlling

C. Displacement

D. Projection

E. Splitting

31. An 18-year-old man with a history of drug abuse and legal problems is admitting to the psychiatric ward after he carved "KILL ME" into his left forearm. The cuts were superficial and did not require stitches; they were not located near any major arteries or veins. On questioning, the patient claims that he had no intention of killing himself but wanted a "vacation" from his girlfriend. However, he is currently on probation and unable to leave his county of residence. He jokes about knowing how to "work the system" and says that he just wanted to get away for a few days. What is the most likely diagnosis?

A. Body dysmorphic disorder

B. Factitious disorder

C. Malingering

D. Pain disorder

E. Somatization disorder

32. A 31-year-old woman always keeps at least an inch of foil on her head to "prevent the aliens on Mars" from reading her thoughts. She is extremely uncomfortable in social situations and tells you that she has no close friends. When asked questions, the patient's replies are always very vague. She tells you that she does not trust her neighbors or the government. In describing either sad or happy events, she shows no change in her facial expression or tone of voice. What is the most likely diagnosis?

A. Antisocial personality disorder

B. Conduct disorder

C. Paranoid schizophrenia

D. Schizoid personality disorder

E. Schizotypal personality disorder

33. A 5-year-old boy is brought to his primary care physician. He has been waking up in the middle of the night screaming and crying inconsolably. These episodes last approximately 10 min before he is able to fall asleep again. In the morning, when asked about it, he cannot remember any such incident. During what stage of sleep and during which part of the night are these episodes most likely to occur?

A. Rapid-eye-movement (REM) sleep; first third of the night

B. REM sleep; last third of the night

C. Stages 1 and 2; first third of the night

D. Stages 1 and 2; last third of the night

E. Stages 3 and 4; first third of the night

F. Stages 3 and 4; last third of the night

34. According to research done in 1998, a home test for monitoring glucose in persons with diabetes has a sensitivity of 85%, a specificity of 92%, a positive predictive value of 90%, and a negative predictive value of 90%, and a negative predictive value of 93%. Which of the following is most likely true if the prevalence of diabetes has increased since 1998?

A. There has been an increase in the negative predictive value.

B. There has been an increase in the positive predictive value.

C. There has been an increase in the sensitivity.

D. There has been an increase in the specificity.

E. There has been a decrease in the sensitivity.

F. There has been a decrease in the specificity.

35. A 24-year-old man is committed to the psychiatric ward after being brought to the emergency department by his mother, with whom he lives. He has no pertinent past medical or psychiatric history. He states that he can hear two separate voices speaking to him almost constantly. These voices tell him about the coming apocalypse and how to protect himself. His speech is very rapid and he moves from one topic to another that is in no way related to the first. Also, his affect does not change the entire time he speaks to you, even when he is describing things that he says makes him either happy or sad. His mother says that he has been behaving this way for four months and that he hardly ever comes out of the basement. Physical examination and cranial MRI reveal no abnormalities. What is the most likely diagnosis?

A. Brief psychotic disorder

B. Delusional disorder

C. Schizoaffective disorder

D. Schizophrenia

E. Schizophreniform disorder

36. A 10-year-old girl takes a standard intelligence test and receives a score of 32, which is the median score for a 9-year-old. The median score for a 10-year-old is 35. What is this girl's most likely IQ?

A. 90

B. 95

C. 100

D. 105

E. 110

37. A 37-year-old man presents to the ambulatory care clinic with a chief complaint of depressed mood, which has lasted for a month. On questioning, he states that he eats only because his girlfriend reminds him that he has forgotten to eat. He normally lies in bed for about 5 or 6 hr before being able to fall asleep and complains of never having any energy. He claims that he has trouble focusing on the task at hand at work and that he is no longer interested in his job. Which of the following CNS neurotransmitter abnormalities is most likely to be present in this patient?

A. Decreased acetylcholine

B. Decreased GABA and acetylcholine

C. Decreased norepinephrine and serotonin

D. Increased dopamine

E. Increased norepinephrine and serotonin

38. A 27-year-old woman from Baltimore is severely depressed after the recent death of her twin brother. They were involved in a motor vehicle accident, and although she walked away from it, her brother was killed instantly. She states that her parents died about eight years earlier and he was the only family she had left. She is living alone now and is currently single. In the 3 weeks since his death she has lost 10 pounds without dieting and has been unable to sleep. She had been preparing for a marathon but has since lost interest in it as well as the energy to train. You are afraid that she might be contemplating suicide but are reluctant to suggest this as it might increase the risk. In regard to the suicide risk for this patient, which of the following is true?

A. Women have a higher rate of suicide completion than men.

B. Healthy patients are more likely to attempt suicide than those with medical problems.

C. This patient suffers from anhedonia, which is a symptom of suicide ideation.

D. Persons in the 25- to 30-year age group have the highest suicide rate.

E. The patient lives alone and will be more likely to attempt suicide than she would if she had a roommate.

39. A case-control study is attempting to determine the increased likelihood of esophageal cancer in individuals who have at least a 15-pack-year smoking history as compared with nonsmokers. The following data were collected:

	Esophageal Cancer	No Esophageal Cancer	Total
Smokers	327	992	1,319
Nonsmokers	478	344	822
Total	805	1,336	2,141

According to the table above, which of the following is true?

A. Incidence rate = (327+478)/10,000

B. Odds ratio = (327*344)/(992*478)

C. Odds ratio = (327/1,319)/(478/822)

D. Prevalence rate = (327+478)/10,000

E. Relative risk = (327*344)/(992*478)

F. Relative risk = (327/1,319)/(478/822)

40. A young boy is brought to the pediatrician. He is able to give his full name and speak in complete sentences. He is able to ride a tricycle but, according to his mother and father, is still working on toilet training. He is also learning to cooperate when playing with others. He is not yet able to hop on one foot or use compound sentences. If this child has progressed through the developmental milestones at the proper ages, how old is he?

A. 2 years old

B. 3 years old

C. 4 years old

D. 5 years old

E. 6 years old

41. A physician specializing in occupational health is preparing to start a research study to consider the incidence of cancer in a population of smokers versus a population of non-smokers. The two populations will be similar in regard to age, ethnicity, and socioeconomic status. The researcher decides to set the type I error (α error) at 0.05 and the type II error (β error) at 0.37. After the study is completed, its calculated P value is 0.02. Which of the following statements is true about this study and hypothesis testing in general?

A. Since $P \geq 0.05$ we accept the null hypothesis.

B. The power of the study can be increased by increasing the sample size.

C. The power of the study equals 0.37.

D. Type I error occurs when we fail to reject the null hypothesis when it is really false.

E. Type II error occurs when we reject the null hypothesis when it is really true.

42. According to Freud's structural theory of the mind, which of the following terms represents our sense of right and wrong and the ideals of behavior we aspire to?

A. Conscious

B. Ego

C. Id

D. Superego

E. Unconscious

43. An 87-year-old woman has a routine checkup in your office scheduled for 9:00 AM. By the time you see her it is 11:45 AM and she is very angry when you enter the room, demanding to know why she has had to wait almost 3 hr. Which of the following responses is most appropriate in this situation?

A. "I apologize, but the other patients here are much sicker than you are."

B. "I apologize. I'll speak with the nurses and receptionist."

C. "I apologize. How can we do better next time?"

D. "If you're not pleased with the quality of care here, you should find another physician."

E. "So what brings you in to the office today?"

F. "Well, you did miss your last appointment, ma'am."

44. A 30-year-old woman presents to the emergency department complaining of abdominal pain, which she has had for 3 weeks. During this time she has been drinking ipecac every other day. She was unable to give any specific reason for this but did mention that she felt at ease when she was in the hospital. What is the most likely diagnosis?

A. Factitious disorder

B. Malingering

C. Paranoid personality disorder

D. Schizoid personality disorder

E. Somatization disorder

45. A young mother brings her 2-month-old child in to the pediatric clinic for a routine examination. During the physical you lay the child supine on the table. You then lift the child by the arms until his shoulders are off the table but his head and buttocks are still touching it. You then drop the baby's arms, letting his shoulders hit the table. The baby starts crying and he adducts his upper extremities and flexes his lower extremities at the hip. What is the name of this normal infant reflex?

A. Babinski reflex

B. Grasp reflex

C. Moro reflex

D. Rooting reflex

E. Step reflex

46. A second-year medical class is attending a lecture in biostatistics. The professor puts a 2 × 2 table of disease versus test up on the blackboard. He wants to know the probability of having an MI given a positive set of cardiac enzymes. What is the most likely parameter to look at?

A. Negative predictive value

B. Positive predictive value

C. Relative risk

D. Sensitivity

E. Specificity

47. During an interview with a 51-year-old patient, she begins to scream at you, saying, "Why are you asking me these questions? You work for the government, don't you? You aren't a real doctor, you are just framing me and plan to turn me in. I know you are taping this conversation, your tie has a hidden wire!" You try to calm her down and show her your diploma to prove you are a doctor. You also give her your tie and ask her to look for the wire that she clams is hidden there. Despite all this, she refuses to believe you and tries to run from the examination room. Which of the following is she most likely suffering from?

A. Delusions

B. Hallucinations

C. Illusions

D. Loose associations

E. Sepsis

48. An 8-month-old child suddenly begins crying and withdrawing from strangers. The mother has been raising her at home, so that she has very little contact with unfamiliar people or places. The mother is concerned that her daughter may be exhibiting maladaptive behavior. What is the most appropriate explanation for these findings and the appropriate plan of action?

A. Abnormal behavior, refer to psychiatry

B. Abnormal behavior, suspect abuse, contact child protective services

C. Normal behavior, nothing to be concerned about

D. Normal behavior, but needs to be watched closely

E. Possible autistic behavior, child needs to be examined further

49. A 17-year-old girl presents to her primary care physician for a yearly physical examination. Her mother is concerned about her daughter's developmental delay. Physical examination reveals scant, straight pubic hair and only a slight elevation of breast tissue. Based on the Tanner stages of sexual development, at what stage would this girl be classified?

A. Stage 1

B. Stage 2

C. Stage 3

D. Stage 4

E. Stage 5

50. A 3-year-old boy needs to be hospitalized for observation overnight following an endoscopic procedure. The child is hysterical upon being brought into the hospital. Based on the child's age, what is the most likely cause of his fear and anxiety?

A. Fear of bodily harm

B. Fear of being lost

C. Fear of death

D. Irrational fear

E. Separation from mom and dad

51. During some time off, you design a research project dealing with heart disease and the effects of a new drug on this condition. At a meeting with the research epidemiologist, he tells you to increase your sample size. What is the purpose of increasing the sample size?

A. Increasing sensitivity

B. Decreasing sensitivity

C. Increasing power

D. Decreasing power

E. Increasing specificity

F. Decreasing specificity

52. A 56-year-old man presents to his primary care physician complaining of a general decline in muscle strength, endurance, and sexual performance. He reports noticing these changes over the past 10 years and believes that they are progressive. He has no other medical problems. Physical examination of the heart, lungs, and abdomen are within normal limits. What is the most likely explanation for these findings?

A. Climacteric

B. Depression

C. Human immunodeficiency syndrome

D. Menopause

E. Old age

53. In this disorder, patients experience loss of neurologic function with no identifiable organic pathology. Common symptoms include seizures, deafness, blindness, or paralysis. These usually occur abruptly following an acute stress. The patients suffering from this often appear indifferent to their loss of function. Tests and physical examinations performed on these patients are normal. What is the most likely diagnosis?

A. Conversion disorder

B. Hypochondriasis

C. Hypomania

D. Panic disorder

E. Pseudocyesis

54. A 43-year-old woman was recently diagnosed with inoperable brain cancer. On being told of this diagnosis, she immediately begins yelling at you, claiming "It's all your fault; you could have done more to help me," and storms out of the room. This patient is classically exhibiting which of the following stages of dying?

A. Acceptance

B. Anger

C. Bargaining

D. Denial

E. Depression

55. A 64-year-old woman is diagnosed with metastatic lung cancer; she has been a smoker for 40 years. Although she was constantly reminded of the dangers of smoking, she persisted in doing so. Suddenly, after this diagnosis, she quits smoking, joins a gym, and begins working out on a daily basis. What is the best explanation of her behavioral changes?

A. Denial

B. Depression

C. Mirroring

D. Suppression

E. Undoing

56. A couple who are first-time parents present to your office with concerns about their 3-month-old boy. They report that on being picked up from his crib, he extends his arms and legs, and they feel that this is not a natural response. You then tell them that this normal reaction is known as the:

A. Babinski reflex

B. Moro reflex

C. Palmar grasp

D. Rooting reflex

E. Tracking reflex

57. Which of the following have the highest mortality rate in the first year of bereavement?

A. Children of the deceased

B. Parents of the deceased

C. Siblings of the deceased

D. Widowed men

E. Widowed women

58. A 13-year-old boy with no past history of violence has been suspended from school for fighting with several boys in his class. He has no past record of conduct issues and his friends report that, lately, he is easily agitated and has become very aggressive. You speak with his parents, who reluctantly mention the finalization of their divorce during the previous month. What defense mechanism is this boy using?

A. Acting out

B. Altruism

C. Denial

D. Displacement

E. Dissociation

59. A 23-year-old man who was shot in the hand has, as a result, lost the use of his index finger. In speaking about this, he explains that it is for the better, because "that is the finger I used to pick my nose with, and I needed to stop anyway." What is the best classification of this behavior?

A. Rationalization

B. Reaction formation

C. Regression

D. Splitting

E. Sublimation

60. A second-year medical student is doing research on Pavlov's classical experiments with dogs. He is very unsure of the concepts of conditioned and unconditioned responses and asks a classmate for an explanation. Which of the following responses is most likely to be considered an unconditioned response?

A. Clapping hands at the end of a presentation

B. Covering one's nose when sneezing

C. Flinching at the sound of a loud car horn

D. Jumping rope

E. Saying "thank you" after having a door held open

61. A 17-year-old boy presents to his primary care physician and begins to describe a personality test that he took in school that week. He is unsure of the name of the exam but begins to describe the format. He explains that all 500 questions were of the true/false type. What is the test that this patient probably took?

A. Baltimore personality assessment

B. Minnesota Multiphasic Personality Inventory

C. Rorschach test

D. Thematic apperception test

E. Sentence completion test

62. You are performing a Mini Mental Status Exam (MMSE) and ask the patient to repeat the names of three previously stated objects. The patient is unable to recall the three objects and therefore does not receive any points for this category. In which of the following did the patient fail?

A. Attenuation and calculation

B. Construction

C. Language

D. Orientation

E. Registration

63. A 46-year-old woman presents to her primary care physician complaining of "not feeling right." She says that she is unable to enjoy anything and just doesn't find pleasure with any of her former pursuits. She reports that this has been going on for the 2 months. What is the most likely diagnosis?

A. Anhedonia

B. Dysphoria

C. Euphoria

D. Expansive mood

E. Labile mood

64. A 35-year-old man who works the night shift at a supermarket comes to the clinic for his annual examination. On observation, he appears anxious and diaphoretic. His pulse is 110 bpm and his blood pressure 136/92 mm Hg. The remainder of the examination is unremarkable. Which of the following substances is most likely being abused by this man?

A. Alcohol

B. Caffeine

C. Cocaine

D. Heroin

E. Nicotine

65. The parents of a 13-year-old girl come into your office expressing concern over their daughter's behavior. They are questioning their daughter's new friends and suspect that their daughter is using drugs. They suspect marijuana and alcohol use and want to know the time frame for laboratory drug testing. You reply that for marijuana the time window is:

A. 1 to 2 hours - alcohol,

B. 1 to 2 days - stimulants

C. 2 to 3 days

D. 1 to 2 weeks - hallucinogens

E. 1 month - marijuana

66. A patient is being monitored via electroencephalogram (EEG) in a laboratory. The frontal lobes are being monitored for periods of active mental concentration. The patient is given mathematical problems to solve. The rationale for this testing is to determine which of the following?

A. Alpha waves

B. Beta waves

C. Delta waves

D. Epsilon waves

E. Gamma waves

67. In young adults, the greatest percentage of actual sleep time is spent in which of the following stages?

A. Stage 1

B. Stage 2

C. Stage 3

D. Stage 4

E. Stage 5

68. An 85-year-old widow has been living on her own for 2 years. She finds no pleasure in activities that used to make her happy. She sleeps all day and has no interest in making new friends. A CT scan of the head is obtained (Figure 2-4). Which of the following is the most common psychiatric disorder in the elderly population?

A. Alzheimer's disease

B. Anorexia

C. Bipolar disorder

D. Bulimia

E. Depression

69. A 9-year-old boy has repetitive episodes of fright while sleeping; he then begins screaming and cannot be awakened. The following morning, he has no recollection of these events. This child's sleep disturbances may be indicative of which of the following issues?

A. Abdominal aortic aneurysm

B. Alcohol abuse

C. Autism

D. Sexual abuse

E. Temporal lobe epilepsy

Figure 2-4

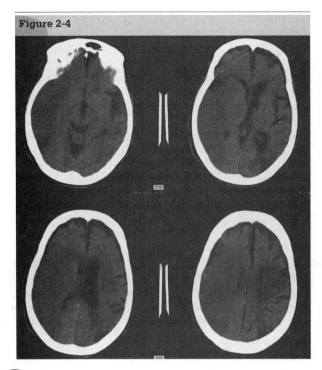

70. You are called in to see a patient who has recently arrived in the emergency department. She is a 28-year-old woman who was brought in from a local restaurant. There, she was apparently seated for dinner, and at 9 PM suddenly got up, addressed her fellow patrons, and began singing and performing. When you speak with her, she explains that she is a famous singer and was scheduled to perform that evening. Although the restaurant does not provide entertainment, she insists that she was doing this as a special favor for the owners. The restaurant's owners do not know her, and it is obvious that she is not a famous performer. From which of the following symptoms of psychosis is this young woman suffering?

A. Form of thought

B. Perception

C. Thought content

D. Thought process

E. Thought schism

71. Your anatomy professor plots your class's performance on the last anatomy examination on a perfect bell-shaped curve. The mean score was an 82 with a standard deviation of 4. What percentage of the class scored between 78 and 86?

A. 65%

B. 68%

C. 95%

D. 99%

E. 100%

72. A 13-year-old boy is brought to his pediatrician because his parents are concerned about his recent behavioral changes. The boy seemed to begin experiencing inappropriate reactions to stimuli and to laugh on hearing sad news. Lately, he has been seen removing his clothing at school and cursing

inappropriately in public. A week earlier, in broad daylight, he was found urinating on the local supermarket wall. His personal hygiene has declined and must be coaxed to take a shower and brush his hair. This boy's behavior is characteristically schizophrenic and can be further subclassified into which of the following?

A. Disorganized

B. Catatonic

C. Paranoid

D. Residual

E. Undifferentiated

73. A mother brings her 7-year-old son to the pediatrician complaining that he recently began wetting his bed at night. She explains that he was potty trained by age 4 and up to a month ago has had no problems. He had previously met all age-appropriate milestones. Review of systems reveals no pertinent information and a physical examination is normal. You begin to order a urinalysis and culture when the mother pulls you aside and says, "I really need you to fix this, I have 2-month-old twins at home and don't have time to potty train my older son all over again." What is the most likely explanation for these findings?

A. Anatomical abnormality

B. No medical problem; this child never mastered potty training

C. Regression

D. Urinary tract calculi obstructing the distal outflow tract

E. Urinary tract infection

74. An 18-year-old man is brought to the emergency department by friends who have suspected him to have a drug dependency problem. His friends are reluctant to name his drug of choice and nervously leave the hospital before you can speak with them again. After a few days in the hospital, the patient becomes febrile and has chills, a runny nose, stomach cramps, and pupil dilation; he also yawns persistently. What is the most likely explanation for these findings?

A. Alcohol withdrawal

B. Barbiturate withdrawal

C. Benzodiazepine intoxication

D. Heroin withdrawal

E. Marijuana intoxication

75. An 18-year-old college freshman presents to her primary care physician with lethargy, fevers, and anorexia. There is palpable purpura located diffusely on her trunk. The mother had been compliant with prenatal care recommendations and experienced no complications of childbirth. Lumbar puncture is performed and demonstrates a protein level of 200 g and a glucose level of 20 mg/dL in the cerebrospinal fluid. Neutrophil counts are around 70% and lymphocyte counts near 5%. What is the most likely organism responsible for this patient's condition?

A. Cytomegalovirus

B. *Escherichia coli*

C. Herpes simplex virus

D. *Neisseria meningitidis*

E. *Streptococcus pneumoniae*

Answer Key

1. C	**20.** C	**39.** A	**58.** A
2. D	**21.** D	**40.** B	**59.** A
3. A	**22.** A	**41.** B	**60.** C
4. B	**23.** C	**42.** D	**61.** B
5. C	**24.** A	**43.** C	**62.** E
6. A	**25.** A	**44.** A	**63.** A
7. G	**26.** D	**45.** C	**64.** B
8. C	**27.** E	**46.** B	**65.** E
9. D	**28.** C	**47.** A	**66.** B
10. E	**29.** B	**48.** C	**67.** B
11. A	**30.** D	**49.** B	**68.** E
12. C	**31.** C	**50.** A	**69.** E
13. C	**32.** E	**51.** C	**70.** C
14. B	**33.** E	**52.** A	**71.** B
15. C	**34.** B	**53.** A	**72.** A
16. E	**35.** E	**54.** B	**73.** C
17. A	**36.** A	**55.** E	**74.** D
18. E	**37.** C	**56.** B	**75.** D
19. D	**38.** E	**57.** D	

Answers and Explanations

1. C. Apgar (named for Virginia Apgar, a physician) stands for appearance (color), pulse, grimace, activity, and respiration. An infant is examined at 1 and 5 min after delivery in each of five categories and given a score of 0 to 2 for each of these. Scoring is as follows:

- Appearance → blue/pale = 0, pink trunk = 1, all pink = 2
- Pulse → 0 = 0, <100 = 1, >100 = 2
- Grimace/reflex irritability → no response = 0, grimace = 1, grimace/cough/sneeze = 2
- Activity/muscle tone → none = 0, some = 1, active = 2
- Respiration → absent = 0, irregular/weak crying = 1, regular/strong crying = 2

This infant received 1 point for color, 1 point for a heart rate of 95, 2 points for cough/sneeze reflex, 1 point for irregular respiratory reflex, and 1 point for some muscle tone/activity. The total Apgar score for 1 min for this infant was a 6. The infant should be reexamined at 5 min and if the score is < 7 at that time, the infant should be reassessed every 5 min for the next 20 min to assess resuscitation efforts.

2. D. This patient is at Tanner stage 4. Her breasts have a mound-on-mound appearance, which is characteristic of stage 4, and her pubic hair has the quality but not quantity of that seen in adults. An adult female's pubic hair extends onto the medial surfaces of the thigh. Females at Tanner stage 1 have no pubic hair and only an elevation of the nipple on the preadolescent breasts. Females at Tanner stage 2 have a sparse growth of long, slightly pigmented, straight pubic hair located mainly on the labia. The female at Tanner stage 2 has breast buds with a slight elevation of the nipple and breast as a small mound. The female at stage 3 has darker, coarser, curlier hair that spreads sparsely over the pubic symphysis. Her breasts show a further elevation of breast and areola, with no separation of contours. Finally, the female at stage 5 has pubic hair of adult quality and quantity that spreads to the medial surfaces of the thighs. Her breasts are mature, with projection of the nipple only; the areola has receded to the general contour of the breast.

3. A. This patient is suffering from generalized anxiety disorder. In addition to his anxiety and uncontrollable worry, he also has the following symptoms: difficulty concentrating or mind going blank, irritability, and sleep disturbances. In order to be diagnosed with generalized anxiety disorder, the previous symptoms must be occurring more days than not for at least 6 months. In anxiety disorders, norepinephrine is increased while GABA and serotonin are decreased. This explains why most anxiety disorders are treated with drugs such as benzodiazepines, which facilitate the actions of GABA by increasing the frequency of channel opening, or selective serotonin reuptake inhibitors (SSRIs), which inhibit the reuptake of serotonin, thereby increasing its availability. Decreased levels of norepinephrine and serotonin are seen in depression. Decreased acetylcholine is seen in Alzheimer's dementia. Decreased levels of GABA and acetylcholine are seen with Huntington's disease. An increase in dopamine is associated with schizophrenia, while a decrease in dopamine is seen in Parkinson's disease.

4. B. The information that this man has mild mental retardation is coded on Axis II. If he were to also have a personality disorder, this information would also go on Axis II. Axis I contains the clinical mental diagnosis, in his case the schizophrenia. Axis III includes any general medical condition, such as this man's hypertension. Any psychosocial or environmental problems, unemployment, and so on are coded on Axis IV. Finally, the global assessment of function (GAF) is coded on Axis V.

5. C. The scenario fits with hypochondriasis, in which the patient is preoccupied with the idea of having an illness despite having normal physical findings. Such patients become preoccupied with the idea of having some serious illness that they may begin to show physical symptoms of anxiety and/or depression. Malingering is the conscious faking of symptoms for secondary gain. The teenager does not want to go to school, so he fakes a fever, night sweats, and pallor. In factitious disorder, the patient fakes being sick for some unconscious gain. Such patients often require psychiatric evaluation, because they are unable to control their behavior.

6. A. According to Freud, the anal stage lasts from 18 months to around 3 to 4 years of age; and fecal retention and fecal release is a source of pleasure during this stage. The oral stage lasts from birth to age 18 months. During this stage, biting and sucking are the main sources of pleasure. The phallic stage lasts from 3 to 4 years of age to 5 to 7 years of age. The genitalia are the focus of pleasure during this time. The latent stage follows the phallic stage and ends at puberty. During this stage, Freud believed that the sexual drive was suppressed. The genital stage begins at puberty and represents the sexual drive during adolescence.

7. G. These are the classic signs and symptoms of an opioid intoxication. The signs of alcohol intoxication include disinhibition, emotional lability, slurred speech, ataxia, and blackouts. Amphetamine intoxication consists of agitation, pupil dilation, prolonged wakefulness, euphoria, and cardiac arrhythmias. Caffeine and nicotine intoxication include restlessness, insomnia, and arrhythmias. Symptoms of cocaine intoxication are euphoria, pupil dilation, hallucinations, and sudden cardiac death. LSD intoxication consists of delusions, visual hallucinations, flashbacks, and pupil dilation. In addition, this patient has suffered from a subdural hematoma. The CT scan shows a crescent-shaped hematoma in the frontoparietal region.

8. C. This man is most likely suffering from delirium tremens (DTs). This is a life-threatening alcohol withdrawal syndrome that usually peaks 2 to 5 days after the last drink. From the clinical scenario, this man is 3 days out from his last drink. Signs and symptoms of DTs include tremor, tachycardia, hypertension, agitation, and hallucinations. The signs of cocaine withdrawal include "crashing," depression, hypersomnolence, fatigue, suicidality, and malaise. Depression, lethargy, hunger, headache, and stomach cramps are seen with amphetamine withdrawal. In opioid withdrawal, the patient becomes anxious and sweaty, the pupils dilate and he or she suffers from "flu-like" symptoms—nausea, fever, and diarrhea. The signs of PCP withdrawal are recurrence of intoxication (due to re-absorption in the GI tract) and a sudden onset of severe random homicidal violence.

9. D. The correct answer to this question is D. Sensitivity is defined as the probability of a positive test when disease is present. Sensitivity involves patients with the disease. It is defined as the number of true positives divided by the number of true positives plus false negatives. It is also known as the true-positive rate. Specificity, on the other hand, is the probability of a negative test when the disease is absent. Specificity involves patients without the disease. Positive predictive value is the probability of disease being present when the test result is positive, while negative predictive value is the probability of disease being absent when the test result is negative. Relative risk is the risk of disease occurrence when a risk factor is present versus the risk of disease when the risk factor is absent. It is used in looking at cohort studies.

10. E. Spermicide use alone (without condom) has a failure rate of 11.9% per 100 woman-years. Regarding the distractor choices, all have a lower failure rate per 100 woman-years. Vasectomy has a failure rate of 0.02% per 100 woman-years, while oral contraceptives and intrauterine devices have failure rates of 1.5% or less.

11. A. According to data obtained from the Joint United Nations Program on HIV/AIDS, about 90% of people with AIDS reside in developing countries. Nearly 14 million adults and children are infected with the AIDS/HIV virus in the sub-Saharan portions of Africa. Southeast Asia has the second largest number of HIV/AIDS-affected people (nearly 5.5 million).

12. C. In evaluating the suicidal patient, it is important to perform a careful medical history with some emphasis on the psychiatric history. Several psychiatric conditions are associated with an increased risk of suicide and suicide completion. Of the conditions listed in this question, patients with major depression have an increased risk of suicide, and nearly 20% of these will succeed in killing themselves. Patients with concurrent psychoses and personality disorders also have an increased risk of suicide, and nearly 10% of these will also succeed in killing themselves.

13. C. Assuming the proper environment at home (stress- and anxiety-free), most children will be toilet-trained by 36 months of age and nearly all by 48 months. It is unrealistic to expect a 2-year-old child to be completely toilet-trained. Most children become toilet-trained when they are physically, mentally, and emotionally ready. All children mature at different times and ages. If a child is not on par for a specific milestone, this does not necessarily mean that the child is developmentally delayed.

14. B. This scenario fits the definition of Asperger's syndrome, a developmental disorder. Asperger's is just like autism in terms of stereotyped movements and delays in emotional response. But unlike autism, which also involves delays in language and cognition, patients with Asperger's are developmentally normal in these respects. In childhood disintegrative disorder, children develop normally for the first 2 years of life but then begin to lose language, motor, and others skills, all before the age of 10. Finally, Rett's syndrome is characterized by normal pregnancy, birth, and development until about 5 to 30 months of age, when growth and development begin to be lost. Stereotyped movements may accompany this disorder.

15. C. There are five stages through which people go in coping with death, dying, and loss. This woman is most likely in the bargaining stage. She is promising to be a "good patient" and will exchange anything—cars, money, etc.—just to be healed. In the acceptance stage, the patient has come to terms with the prognosis and can make and accept long-term decisions. In the stage of anger, patients may feel frustrated and angry and feel that they have bad luck. If patients are in denial, they may be in a state of shock and therefore completely deny the prognosis, stating that they are just fine and that nothing is wrong. While in the depression stage, patients may have clinical signs and symptoms similar to those seen in clinical depression, such as insomnia, hopelessness, and possibly suicidal thoughts. Even though this is a stage of death and dying, it requires psychiatric evaluation and is not normal.

16. E. The mean, median, and mode are the three most common measures of central tendency. Central tendency is a typical or representative value for a dataset. The mean is calculated by dividing the sum of the scores in a distribution by the number of scores in the distribution. This value best reflects the typical score of a dataset when there are few outliers and/or the dataset is generally symmetrical. The median is the value in a dataset that divides the scores into two equal halves and is largely unaffected by outliers. The mode is the value that occurs most frequently in the dataset. The graph above (Figure 2-2) depicts a negative distribution. In cases of negative distribution, the mode is greater than the median and the mean, in that order. In cases of positive distribution, the mean is greater than the median and mode, in that order.

17. A. This is an example of primary prevention. By explaining the risks of smoking and the associated long-term consequences, one may help to prevent disease. Education is one of the best examples of primary prevention. Secondary prevention involves the early detection of disease. Pap smears, tests for occult blood, and sigmoidoscopies are examples of this type of prevention. One is trying to find the disease and treat it at an earlier stage. With tertiary prevention, you are trying to keep a disease from getting worse. Examples of this are treatment and rehabilitation following an event such as an MI.

18. E. It is inappropriate for a physician to have any kind of romantic relationship with a patient. The physician must politely explain this. None of the other choices offers an acceptable alternative.

19. D. The sensitivity is the percentage of diseased individuals who test positive with a diagnostic test. It is found by dividing the number of true positives (block A) by the number of all people who have the disease (block A + block C). $A/(A + C) \rightarrow 160/200 = 0.8 = 80\%$. A high sensitivity is desired for a screening test so that everyone with the disease can be caught. It is a measure of how many people with a disease actually test positive for that disease.

Disease Test

A	B
C	D

20. C. Bias is the possible effect that systematic error may have on the results of a study. Lead-time bias occurs when a disease *appears* to have a longer "survival time" but in fact you have only diagnosed it earlier. Choice A describes confounding bias. B is a definition of selection bias. Length bias is described in D. E is volunteer bias. Choice F describes recall bias. Finally, G is a description of attention bias.

21. D. The incidence of a disease is the number of new cases of the disease that occur over a period of time. The formula is as follows:

Incidence = number of new cases/total population. In the above example, $I = 500/50,000 \rightarrow I = 0.01 = 1\%$. There are 500 new cases of disease X (in 1 year) in a city with a population of 50,000. Incidence does not tell you anything about the number of cases that already exist.

22. A. This describes the concrete operational phase of Piaget's stages of development, which occurs from ages 7 through 11. In this stage, the child can think logically but has not yet grasped hypothetical and deductive reasoning. He can also manage the concept of conservation of volume. In the Piaget's preoperational stage (ages 2 to 7), the child begins to think symbolically and has acquired language yet remains egocentric. During the sensorimotor stage (from birth through age 2), the child develops such skills as recognizing objects by feeling them. The last stage is called the formal operational stage (age 11 to adulthood), in which the child begins to master abstract thought.

23. C. Hallucinations are false perceptions that arise without any external stimulus. They are considered to be among the positive symptoms of schizophrenia, along with delusions and disorganized speech. The other three choices—cognitive deficits, emotional blunting, and social withdrawal—exemplify negative symptoms of schizophrenia. Schizophrenia is a psychotic disorder characterized by disturbed language, thought, and perceptions. The onset of disease may be sudden or gradual; usually these

patients are diagnosed in their twenties or thirties. An easy way to help you remember the difference between positive and negative symptoms is that negative symptoms are things that the patient lacks, such as normal emotion or the ability to sustain social interactions. The positive symptoms are extra things these people experience, such as hallucinations or delusions.

24. A. This man is experiencing rapid-eye-movement (REM) sleep. Clues that suggest this phase of sleep include the beta waves found on the EEG, penile tumescence, and variable blood pressure and pulse. Beta waves are waves of the highest frequency and lowest amplitude and are found only when patients are awake and alert or in REM sleep. This stage of sleep makes up 25% of total sleep and usually occurs every 90 min. REM sleep decreases with age. The primary neurotransmitter involved in REM sleep is acetylcholine. Norepinephrine reduces REM sleep. None of the other transmitters listed has a primary role in REM sleep.

25. A. The study that you and your classmates are about to enter is a cohort study. Cohort studies are observational studies in which the subjects are chosen based on the presence or absence of risk factors (in this case drinking large amounts of coffee). The subjects in this type of study are then followed over a certain amount of time and watched for the development of disease. These studies are often expensive and time-consuming. A case-control study is also an observational study. In this type of study, however, subjects are chosen on the basis of the presence or absence of disease. Information is then collected about risk factors or exposures that these subjects might have had. Cross-sectional studies look at a population at one point in time. These are usually inexpensive but not good for studying rare exposures or the effects of exposures over time. Clinical trials are experimental studies. They usually compare the therapeutic benefit of two or more treatments. A common example is a trial testing the efficacy of a new drug.

26. D. The *Diagnostic and Statistical Manual of Mental Disorders*, 4th edition, text revision (DSM-IV-TR), presents the criteria for major depressive disorder (MDD); this patient fits those criteria, which require five of the following: depressed mood most of the day, loss of interest/pleasure in daily activities, significant weight loss/gain or change in appetite, sleep disturbances, psychomotor retardation or agitation, feelings of worthlessness or inappropriate guilt, inability to think or concentrate, or recurrent thoughts of death during the same 2-week period. The patient *must* have either depressed mood or loss of interest/pleasure during this time period. Dysthymia is depressed mood for most of the day, for more days than not, for at least 2 years, accompanied by two of the following symptoms: change in appetite, change in sleep habits, low energy or fatigue, low self-esteem, poor concentration, or feelings of hopelessness. Bipolar affective disorder (BAD) type I presents with a manic episode, and BAD type II presents with a hypomanic episode. Schizoaffective disorder can present with a major depressive episode or manic episode with symptoms that meet criterion A of the DSM-IV-TR, such as delusions or hallucinations.

27. E. Some infectious diseases are reportable in all states. The list includes chickenpox, gonorrhea, tuberculosis, rubella, AIDS, mumps, measles, syphilis, *Shigella, Salmonella,* hepatitis A, and hepatitis B. The only disease on this list that the man in the clinical vignette has is syphilis. You know that he has syphilis because his VDRL test came back positive.

28. C. Bulimia nervosa affects 1 to 3% of young females and adolescents. It is significantly more common in females, and these patients usually maintain a normal weight or are overweight. It involves recurrent episodes of binge eating with inappropriate attempts to compensate for overeating. The binge eating and compensatory behaviors must occur at least twice a week for 3 months for this diagnosis. The purging type involves the use of laxatives, vomiting, or diuretics as a compensatory behavior; the nonpurging type involves excessive exercising or fasting. Unlike those with bulimia nervosa, patients with anorexia nervosa have a body weight that is at least 15% below normal. The binge eating/purging type of anorexia nervosa is characterized by overeating followed by excessive exercise, laxative abuse, purging, or diuretic use. Patients with the restrictive type of anorexia nervosa eat very little and exercise excessively. Uncontrollable eating is not an eating disorder.

29. B. This patient has neuroleptic malignant syndrome (NMS), which is an adverse effect of antipsychotic agents such as haloperidol. The pathogenesis involves blockade of the dopamine receptor, leading to hyperthermia and muscle rigidity. Treatment for NMS includes dantrolene, an antispasmodic, and removal of the offending agent. Acetaminophen can be toxic to the liver and cause an elevation in liver function tests (LFTs). Metformin inhibits gluconeogenesis and increases glycolysis in order to decrease blood glucose. It can be associated with lactic acidosis. The underlying delirium and dementia usually do not cause increased muscle tone. They are more associated with cognitive function. The CT scan (Figure 2-3) shows the presence of brain metastasis with bleeding. There is also surrounding cytotoxic edema.

30. D. Projection is an immature defense mechanism whereby patients deal with their own objectionable desires and thoughts by attributing them to others. In this case the husband assumes that his wife has feelings for another man just as he has for his coworker. Acting out is an immature defense mechanism whereby a patient gives in to an impulse, even if socially inappropriate, in order to avoid the anxiety of suppressing that impulse. Controlling is a neurotic defense mechanism whereby patients attempt to regulate situations and events in the external environment in order to relieve their anxiety. Displacement is a neurotic defense mechanism whereby patients shift their emotions from a difficult situation to one that is more tolerable. (For example, a child who is angry with her mother one evening may be argumentative and mean to a friend at school the next day.) Splitting is a defense mechanism whereby a patient labels another person as entirely good or entirely bad/evil. (A patient may, for example, say "You're the best doctor I've ever had, but that nurse is horrible.") Splitting is common in schizophrenia.

31. C. Malingering is the faking of physical or psychological symptoms in order to achieve personal gain. These patients are seeking secondary gain. In this case the patient had no intention of hurting himself and was not motivated to do so. Patients with body dysmorphic disorder are preoccupied with body features that they feel are not perfect. They feel that minor imperfections are hideous and are extremely self-conscious. A factitious disorder is one whereby a patient intentionally produces physical or psychological symptoms in order to achieve some gain. However, unlike malingering, these patients seek a primary gain, which is the "sick role." A patient with pain disorder has severe pain that has no medical explanation over a long period of time. A history of multiple visits to the physician is also characteristic. Somatization disorder is a diagnosis that includes multiple somatic symptoms that cannot be explained. The patient will have at least two gastrointestinal symptoms, at least one reproductive or sexual symptom, at least one neurological symptom, and at least four general pain symptoms at the same time before the age of 30.

32. E. Persons with schizotypal personality disorder display at least five of the follow characteristics: excessive social anxiety, strange thinking/speech, few close friends, odd/eccentric appearance or behavior, inappropriate or restricted affect, suspiciousness of others, unusual perceptual experiences, odd beliefs or magical thinking that is not acceptable within the person's culture, or ideas of reference. Patients with antisocial personality disorder and conduct disorder show a lack of remorse for unacceptable actions such as committing unlawful acts, lying/manipulation, impulsive behavior, aggression toward others, recklessness, and irresponsibility. Conduct disorder is the diagnosis for patients fulfilling at least three of these characteristics before the age of 18; antisocial personality disorder is the diagnosis for similar patients 18 years of age or older. Patients with paranoid schizophrenia can be distinguished from those with schizotypal personality disorder by the presence of psychotic symptoms (delusions, hallucinations, disorganized speech, grossly disorganized or catatonic behavior, or negative symptoms). Patients with schizoid personality disorder do not display the odd/eccentric behaviors that are seen in schizotypal personality disorder.

33. E. The child has a parasomnia known as sleep terror disorder. Affected children wake up in a terrified state (screaming, evincing severe anxiety, and being inconsolable). These episodes usually last 10 to 20 min before the patient is able to fall back to sleep. The patient is confused and the parent is not able to fully arouse him. This condition is most common in male children and tends to run in families. The child does not recall the incident in the morning and most children outgrow the disorder, so medication is not usually recommended. If necessary, small doses of a benzodiazepine can be given before bedtime.

34. B. An increase in prevalence will increase the positive predictive value (PPV) of the test and decrease the negative predictive value (NPV). Changes in prevalence *do not* change sensitivity and specificity. The percentages in the case are distracters and not necessary to answer the question. So remember, if prevalence increases, then ↑ PPV, ↓ NPV. And if prevalence decreases, then ↓ PPV, ↑ NPV.

35. E. This patient has schizophreniform disorder, which may occur as a brief psychotic condition lasting for 1 day to 1 month or as a lengthier psychosis lasting 1 to 6 months. Schizophreniform disorder and schizophrenia (lasting more than 6 months, including prodromal and residual periods) have the same diagnostic criteria in terms of symptoms present but are differentiated by the length of time the symptoms have been present. The criteria for these diagnoses include the presence of at least two of the following for a month resulting in significant impairment of functioning: delusions, hallucinations, disorganized speech, grossly disorganized or catatonic behavior, or negative symptoms (anhedonia, flat affect, poor attention, avolition, and alogia). Delusional disorder is considered when the delusions are not bizarre and do not result in significant impairment of function. Schizoaffective disorder requires the presence of a depressive episode, manic episode, or mixed episode and, in their absence, either hallucinations or delusions over a 2-week period.

36. A. Using the mental age method to calculate her score (mental age/chronological age × 100 = IQ), this girl's mental age correlates with that of a 9-year-old (9/10 × 100 = 90).

37. C. The patient presents with DSM-IV-TR criteria for major depressive disorder (MDD). The criteria for MDD require five of the following: depressed mood most of the day, loss of interest/pleasure in daily activities, significant weight loss/gain or change in appetite, sleep disturbances, psychomotor retardation or agitation, feelings of worthlessness or inappropriate guilt, inability to think or concentrate, or recurrent thoughts of death during the same 2-week period. The patient *must* have either depressed mood or loss of interest/pleasure during this period. Patients with MDD typically have decreased levels of norepinephrine and serotonin. Treatment approaches for MDD attempt to increase levels of these two neurotransmitters. Decreased acetylcholine is seen in patients with Alzheimer's dementia. Decreased GABA and acetylcholine are seen in patients with Huntington's disease. Patients with schizophrenia have increased levels of dopamine.

38. E. Although females are three times as likely to attempt suicide, males are four times more likely to succeed. People over 45 years of age are more likely to commit suicide than those below that age. Physical illness is a risk factor for suicide, and since this patient is training for a marathon, it is likely she is fairly healthy. Anhedonia is a symptom of major depressive disorder. Patients who live alone or are unmarried have higher suicide rates than those who live with other or are married. As a physician, you should never be afraid to bring up the subject of suicide with a patient you feel might be at risk. Patients who attempt suicide have often seen their primary care physician shortly before their attempt.

39. A. The equation odds ratio is (A*D)/(B*C). The odds ratio is used in this case because this was a case-control study. If it were a cohort study, a relative risk would have been used. The

equation for relative risk is [A/(A+B)]/[C/(C+D)]. The incidence rate is the number of new events that occur in a population. The prevalence rate refers to all persons with an event in a population. The incidence rate and prevalence rate cannot be determined with the given information.

40. B. Normal milestones for a 3-year-old include those mentioned above as well as the following: alternates feet going up stairs, copies line or circle drawings, has a fixed gender identity, has a 900-word vocabulary, cuts paper with scissors, and recognizes common objects in pictures. The ability to use compound sentences and to hop on one foot are milestones associated with 4-year-olds.

41. B. The chance of type I error (0.05 in this case) is the same number as the P-value criterion. In this case the calculated P value was less than set P value; the data are statistically significant. Therefore we would fail to reject the null hypothesis rather than accept it. We never accept the null hypothesis; rather, we either reject it or fail to reject it. A type I error (α error) occurs when we reject the null hypothesis when it is really true. A type II (β error) error occurs when we fail to reject the null hypothesis when it is really false. Type I error is generally considered worse than type II error. Power = 1 − β. In this study the power = 0.63. The power of the study can be increased by increasing the number of individuals in the study.

42. D. According to Freud, our superego represents our sense of right and wrong and the ideals of behavior we aspire to. It is made up of the conscience (sense of right and wrong) and the ego ideal (thoughts and behaviors we aspire to). The ego and id are the other two components of Freud's structural theory of the mind. The ego is the part of the mind that develops to deal with the demands of reality as well as to mediate the demands of the id and the superego. This part of the mind (the ego and superego) is mainly conscious. The id represents our primal urges and instincts. The id is mainly unconscious. The conscious, preconscious, and unconscious are part of Freud's topographic theory of the mind. The conscious represents what you are aware of in your environment. The preconscious is what you are able to make conscious with effort (like your birth date). The unconscious is the part of the mind of which you are unaware.

43. C. This answer gives some control back to the patient. Although it will be inevitable that patients have to wait, you should show empathy toward them when they do. "A" is incorrect because you are telling the patient that her care is not a priority for you at the moment. You should treat patients as if they were your primary concern. "B" is incorrect because you are shifting the blame unfairly to your staff. This depicts a level of unprofessionalism in your office and suggests you may not feel your staff to be capable of providing adequate care. Such an implication could have negative repercussions. "E" is incorrect because it ignores the patient's concerns and is likely to infuriate her even more. "D" is incorrect because the patient may feel that you are being confrontational. Your patients should be able to voice concerns over all aspects of their care freely without being spoken down to. "F" is incorrect because it shifts the blame onto the patient.

44. A. This patient has factitious disorder, whereby illness is faked for some unconscious gain. Such patients often require psychiatric evaluation because they are unable to control their behavior. In somatization disorder, patients have a variety of complaints involving multiple organ systems, and with further exploration no cause can be found. It is important to rule out any possible multiorgan diseases such as multiple sclerosis or systemic lupus erythematosus, before labeling a person with a somatization disorder. Schizoid personality disorder is characterized by social withdrawal with limited emotional expression. Paranoid personality disorder exists when someone has feelings of distrust and is very suspicious of others. The main defense mechanism at work here is projection.

45. C. The Moro reflex is elicited in the manner described in the question. This is a normal reflex in infants for the first few months of life. The presence of this reflex beyond that time is abnormal. Bilateral absence of the Moro reflex suggests damage to the CNS. A unilateral Moro reflex suggests injury to the ipsilateral brachial plexus or paralysis and must be investigated further. A Babinski reflex occurs when the outside of the sole of the foot is stroked briskly, the great toe flexes dorsally, and the remaining toes fan out. This is a normal reflex in infants up to 2 years of age; its presence after this time suggests upper motor neuron disease. The grasp reflex is elicited by placing a finger in the newborn's open palm. The hand will close around the examiner's finger; an attempt to remove the finger will cause the grip to tighten. The rooting reflex is elicited by stroking the infant's cheek. The infant will turn its head to the side of the finger and start sucking. The step reflex can be elicited by supporting the baby's weight and holding it on its feet. The child should begin stepping when its soles are touching the ground.

46. B. Positive predictive value is the probability of disease present when the test result is positive; negative predictive value is the probability of disease absent when the test result is negative. Sensitivity is defined as the probability of a positive test when disease is present. Sensitivity involves patients with the disease. It is defined as the number of true positives divided by the number of true positives plus false negatives. It is also known as the true positive rate. Specificity, on the other hand, is the probability of a negative test when the disease is absent. Specificity involves patients without the disease. Relative risk is the risk of disease occurrence when a risk factor is present versus the risk of disease when the risk factor is absent.

47. A. This woman is suffering from delusions. Delusions are false fixed beliefs, not shared by others, that are firmly maintained in spite of proof to the contrary. Even though the doctor tried to explain to the woman that he was a doctor and that his tie did not contain a wire, she refused to believe him. Hallucinations are perceptions in the absence of external stimuli; in other words, seeing things that are not there. Illusions are misinterpretations of actual external stimuli; in other words, you might see a stick in the middle of the road and mistake it for a poisonous snake. A loose association is a disorder in the form

of thought, such as the way ideas are tied together. This woman was suffering from a disorder in the content of thought, the actual idea.

48. C. This behavior, known as stranger anxiety, often begins at 7 months of age. The identification of people as strangers and unknown is completely normal and no cause for concern. This behavior also confirms that the child has formed a specific bond with her mother and is able to distinguish her from a stranger. As stated previously, there is nothing abnormal in the child's reaction and no further investigation is warranted.

49. B. Stage 2 would be the appropriate staging on the basis of the above scenario. Stage 1 genitalia are the same as in childhood, with no changes. Stage 3 is marked by the growth of curly pubic hair and enlargement of the breasts. Stage 4 in females is marked by areola rising above the breast and in males by penile growth with darkening of the scrotal skin. Stage 5 presents with adult genitalia and, in women, with areolas that are no longer elevated above the breast.

50. A. Fear of bodily harm is the greatest fear in children 2½ to 6 years of age. Fear of being separated from its parents is greatest in children from 18 months to 2½ years of age. The other fears, aside from irrational although plausible fear, are not necessarily correlated with any specific age groups. Irrational fear tends to be something on its own, and can be dealt with in an appropriate manner.

51. C. By increasing the sample size, you increase the power. The power of a test is the probability of rejecting the null hypothesis when it is in fact false. In other words, the power is the ability of a study to actually detect the difference you were looking for, and it depends on the size of the populations studied.

52. A. Climacteric is marked by the physiological changes that occur as the body enters into midlife. Hormone levels in men remain relatively stable but decreases in muscle strength, endurance, and sexual performance are quite normal and common. The signs listed above are not related to depression, and the diagnosis of depression is not indicated here. HIV infection can cause flu-like symptoms and can contribute to the above presentation, but it is not nearly the first diagnosis that would come to mind. Menopause is limited to women and therefore not applicable. Old age is a generalization and not an applicable diagnostic term.

53. A. This scenario describes conversion disorder, in which, following severe stress, patients experience a loss of some neurological function. As stated above, these patients are often indifferent to such a loss. This is known as *la belle indifference*. Malingering is the conscious faking of symptoms for secondary gain. The teenager does not want to go to school, so he fakes a fever, night sweats, and pallor. In factitious disorder, the patient fakes being sick for some unconscious gain. Such individuals often require psychiatric evaluation because they are unable to control their behavior. Panic disorder is characterized by discrete periods of intense fear and discomfort peaking within 10 min with four of the following symptoms: palpitations, abdominal distress, nausea, increased perspiration, and chest pain. Pseudocyesis is the false belief that one is pregnant associated with objective signs of pregnancy. Hypomania is like mania except that the mood disorder is not severe enough to cause marked impairment.

54. B. The classical stage of dying exhibited here is that of anger. In acceptance, the patient is calm and accepts his fate. In bargaining, the patient tries to make a deal with a higher power in exchange for resolution. In denial, the patient refuses to acknowledge or accept that she is in mortal danger. Depression is indicated by a seemingly hopeless preoccupation with death and dying.

55. E. This woman's behavior is known as undoing. In an attempt to rectify the problem at hand, she proceeds to try to alter (undo) some or all of the behaviors that she thinks may have contributed to her current situation. Suppression is blocking and failing to acknowledge the stressful or unpleasant feelings that one is currently having.

56. B. The Moro (startle) reflex is what is being described in this scenario. This reflex is commonly present until about 4 months of age. The Babinski reflex describes the dorsiflexion of the great toe when the plantar surface of the foot is stroked. This is due to partially formed neurological pathways that are usually complete by 12 months of age. Palmar grasp is a grasping reaction to objects placed in the child's palm. The rooting reflex occurs when, as the side of its face is stroked or stimulated, an infant turns its head to that side to seek a food source. The tracking reflex occurs when an infant follows with its eyes a human face or other moving object placed in its field of vision.

57. D. Widowed men tend to have the highest mortality rate of all those listed. Grief affects all the listed groups, but statistically, widowed men are the most readily affected.

58. A. Acting out is the best response for the above scenario. This behavior is utilized to deflect unwanted feelings and emotions; it channels the anger and frustration in a usually negative, attention-seeking manner. Altruism is engaging in kind acts and helping others in the hope of avoiding one's own negative feelings. Denial is the mental blocking of unwanted news or information. Displacement is a transference of anger from the appropriate party to a more acceptable and usually lower-ranking person. Dissociation is the severing of unpleasant thoughts or memories, almost disconnecting them from conscious thought.

59. A. Rationalization is the use of reasoning to justify a negative event regardless of the nonsensical nature of the rationale. Reaction formation is acting in a manner that is opposite that of one's true feelings. Regression is reversion to more child-like behavior in the face of unpleasant situations or circumstances. Splitting classifies people into one of two distinct and opposite categories (such as good and evil). Sublimation is the manifestation of an objectionable desire in a more socially acceptable manner.

60. C. Flinching at the loud sound of a car horn is a natural reflex response to being startled. It is not a learned behavior and happens instinctively. All of the other listed behaviors seem to be social graces and norms. Although pleasant and expected, they are not reflexive behaviors.

61. B. The MMPI is a true/false personality test that can be used by primary care physicians to identify and diagnose clinical issues such as depression, paranoia, and other personality-related characteristics. The Rorschach test utilizes personality projection to assess various potential thought disorders and defense mechanisms through the interpretation of symmetrical inkblot designs. The thematic apperception test asks the testee to create a story based on an ambiguous picture; the response is then analyzed. The sentence completion test presents partial sentences that the examinee is asked to complete.

62. E. Registration is the act of recalling three words that were presented previously and that the testee was asked to remember. Attenuation and calculation is doing systematic math, as in counting backwards by a certain number. Construction is manual copying of a picture or design. Orientation is knowledge of where one is and the day of the week.

63. A. Her mood would best be labeled as anhedonic, as she is experiencing the "inability to feel pleasure." Dysphoria is a generalized feeling of displeasure. Euphoria describes strong feelings of elation and joy. Expansiveness is marked by feelings of self-importance and generosity. Lability describes quick shifts in mood from euphoria to dysphoria.

64. B. Caffeine is the most widely used of all psychoactive substances. Due to his schedule at work, the man would depend on his caffeine to keep him up throughout the night. Alcohol is second only to caffeine in widespread use and has a male/female abusers ratio of 2:1. Cocaine use has steadily declined since the mid-1980s, while the use of crack has been on the increase, especially by lower socioeconomic groups, due to its lower cost. Heroin has a male/female abuse ratio of 3:1, and rates of abuse are higher in larger cities. Females have surpassed males in the number of smokers, with a prevalence of white adolescent smokers over African-American teens.

65. E. Marijuana stays in the body for up to 28 days. Opiates remain for 2 hr to 2 days postingestion. Stimulants usually last 1 to 2 days, while alcohol lasts only hours. Hallucinogens last more than 7 days, and can be detected over a longer period of time.

66. B. Beta waves are most commonly found over the frontal lobes during times of active concentration. Alpha waves tend to be found over the parietal and occipital lobes during periods of relaxation with closed eyes. Gamma, delta, and epsilon waves are not associated with frontal lobe activity.

67. B. Stage 2, which has the sleep spindle and K complex, comprises 45% of sleep time for young adults. Stage 1 is about 5%, while stages 3 and 4 would be 25% and steadily decrease with aging. Stage 5 is nonexistent. REM sleep is the final stage that is missing from this list and comprises the other 25%.

68. E. The elderly most commonly suffer from depression, usually due to loss of a spouse, friends, or family members, decreased social status, and decline in general health. Alzheimer's disease is often incorrectly diagnosed in patients with depression, as pseudodepression. Bipolar disease, anorexia, and bulimia are rarely newly diagnosed in this population. The scan shown (Figure 2-4) is a noncontrast CT of the head demonstrating a large area of hypoattenuation in the distribution of the right middle cerebral artery.

69. E. Onset of sleep terror disorder in an adolescent is indicative of possible temporal lobe epilepsy. Abdominal aortic aneurysm is rare in an adolescent and usually indicated by a tearing chest pain, which was not part of the above presentation. Autism would most likely be diagnosed at a much earlier age, and there are no indications of any autistic behaviors. Alcohol abuse is common in adolescents and teens, but the above presentation is not indicative of alcohol consumption. Sexual abuse can present with nightmares and fear but not necessarily sleep terrors.

70. C. This patient is suffering from thought content psychosis. She is experiencing false beliefs that exist only within herself and are not shared by others. She is convinced that she is a famous performer and is offering her entertainment services to a willing audience. Form of thought is more of a tangential thought process, where thoughts are loosely associated, or the drifting and distancing of the conversation from the original topic. Perception issues manifest as misperception of actual real external stimuli. Thought process disorder causes the sufferer to "invent and create" new words and leads the patient to answer questions in a very vague and ineffective manner.

71. B. One standard deviation from the mean is equal to 68% of the sample population. In the above example, one standard deviation from the mean, 82, is equal to a range of 78 to 86. This is found by taking the mean and adding one standard deviation ($82 + 4 = 86$) and then subtracting one standard deviation ($82 - 4 = 78$). This means that 68% of the class scored within that range. Two standard deviations from the mean is equal to 95%, meaning that 95% of the class would have scored in the range of 90 to 74. Three standard deviations from the mean is equal to 99%, meaning that 99% of the class would have scored in the range of 94 to 70.

72. A. This young boy is experiencing disorganized schizophrenia, as indicated by his inappropriate emotional behavior, lack of concern about his personal appearance, and lack of personal inhibition. A catatonic patient would show lethargic and slowed behavior with no related acting-out episodes. Paranoid behavior would include delusive feelings of persecution and the belief that one is being followed or watched. Residual schizophrenia would not involve any psychotic symptom, and tend to have only a minor effect. Undifferentiated schizophrenia would involve components of various subtypes of the above diagnoses.

73. C. There are two types of enuresis: primary, in which the child has never been dry, and secondary, in which the child was dry for at least 3 to 6 months before the onset of enuresis. The clinical vignette here describes a case of secondary enuresis in which the young boy was potty-trained and is now, 3 years later, suffering from urinary incontinence. Among the more common causes of secondary enuresis are psychological problems and environmental stress. Children may regress to younger behavior under certain stressors such as physical illness, punishment, birth of a new sibling, or fatigue. The child in the scenario acquired two new siblings only a month earlier, and this is most likely the cause of his enuresis. If the child were suffering from obstructing calculi or a urinary tract infection, other signs and/or symptoms would be present, such as dysuria, fever, or possibly flank pain. If an anatomical abnormality were present, the child would probably have presented at an earlier age and with primary enuresis.

74. D. Based on the above presentation, this patient is most likely suffering from heroin withdrawal. His symptoms, along with rhinorrhea and piloerection, are all associated with heroin withdrawal. Alcohol's major and most severe symptom is delirium tremens, which can be fatal if not treated. Barbiturate/benzodiazepine withdrawal causes tremor, seizures, tachycardia, and hypertension. Benzodiazepine intoxication is similar to alcohol intoxication, causing amnesia, ataxia, and minor respiratory depression. Marijuana intoxication is associated with a feeling of euphoria, anxiety, and impaired judgment; it also causes dry mouth and increased appetite.

75. D. The first question to be answered is whether the source of infection is bacterial or viral. Lumbar puncture (LP) from bacterial infections demonstrates increased neutrophils/protein and decreased glucose in the cerebrospinal fluid (CSF). LP from viral infections demonstrates increased lymphocytes and normal glucose in CSF. Therefore this infection is bacterial. The next step is to recognize the most common organisms causing meningitis based on the patient's age group. In neonates, these would be the unknown organisms causing Guillain-Barré syndrome, *Escherichia coli*, and *Listeria*. In patients 6 months to 6 years of age, the most likely organisms would be *Streptococcus pneumoniae*, *Neisseria meningitidis*, and *Haemophilus influenzae* type B. In patients 6 years to 60 years of age, the most likely organisms would be *N. meningitidis*, enteroviruses, *and S. pneumoniae*. In those above 60 years of age, the most likely organism would be *S. pneumoniae*. *N. meningitidis* affects those in close contact with the patient, specifically those staying in dorms or army barracks. One also sees purpura associated with this infection. *S. pneumoniae* causes a bacterial meningitis but is not associated with purpura.

Chapter 3   Cardiovascular System

Questions

1. A 39-year-old man presents to his primary care physician for an annual examination. His two brothers, ages 34 and 39, have both had MIs. Physical examination of the heart, lungs, and abdomen are normal. Serum lipid and lipoprotein analysis is ordered. The level of low-density-lipoprotein (LDL) cholesterol is elevated. What is the most likely familial hyperlipidemia present in this patient?

   A. Type 1
   B. Type 2a
   C. Type 2b
   D. Type 3
   E. Type 4

2. A 28-year-old man is brought to the emergency department because of fatigue and fever. He has a history of intravenous drug abuse. Blood cultures are obtained. Echocardiography suggests endocarditis of the tricuspid valve. What is the most likely etiology of these findings?

   A. Coagulase-negative staphylococci
   B. *Staphylococcus aureus*
   C. *Streptococcus pyogenes*
   D. *Treponema pallidum*
   E. *Viridans streptococcus*

3. A 36-year-old homeless man appearing to be in acute distress comes to the emergency department. Chest x-ray is obtained (Figure 3-1). Two hours after arriving, he expires owing to what appears to be an MI. The next day the county coroner performs an autopsy, which shows a ruptured ascending aortic aneurysm. The cause of death is recorded as ruptured ascending aortic aneurysm secondary to tertiary syphilis. What level of the aorta was compromised by the disease?

   A. Basal lamina
   B. Endothelium
   C. Nevus vascularis
   D. Tunica intima
   E. Tunica media

4. A 55-year-old man presents to his primary care physician because of difficulty sleeping. He uses three pillows to help with his breathing at night. What is the most likely etiology of this patient's disease?

   A. Atrial myxoma
   B. Cor pulmonale
   C. Fibrinous pericarditis
   D. Libman-Sacks endocarditis
   E. Rheumatic heart disease

5. A 25-year-old woman presents to her primary care physician complaining of progressive dyspnea on exertion. She is now unable to walk more than 100 ft without becoming winded. She has no history of congenital heart defects or other cardiac pathology. She also denies any family history of cardiac problems. Her symptoms have progressed rapidly over the last month. Her electrocardiogram (ECG) reveals paroxysms of ventricular tachycardia, and an endomyocardial biopsy shows myocyte necrosis and a lymphocytic infiltrate. Which organism is the most likely cause for these symptoms?

   A. *Borrelia burgdorferi*
   B. Coxsackievirus B
   C. *Streptococcus pyogenes*
   D. *Streptococcus viridans*
   E. *Staphylococcus aureus*
   F. *Trypanosoma cruzi*
   G. *Toxoplasma gondii*

6. An 80-year-old woman presents to the emergency department complaining of a right-sided headache and right jaw pain. Physical examination reveals induration of the left temporal artery. Laboratory studies reveal an elevated erythrocyte sedimentation rate (ESR), and biopsy of the temporal artery shows granulomatous inflammation. What class of pharmaceuticals is needed to prevent blindness in this patient?

   A. Alpha-blockers
   B. Anticoagulants
   C. HMG-CoA reductase inhibitors
   D. Steroids
   E. Thrombolytics

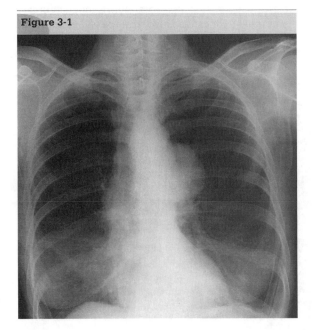

Figure 3-1

7. A 55-year-old man presents with new skin discolorations on his cheeks. His medical history is significant only for alcohol abuse and subsequent alcoholic cirrhosis. The lesions appear as small vessels radiating out from a central point that blanches when pressure is applied. What type of vascular disorder leads to these skin lesions?

  A. Hemangioma

  B. Hereditary hemorrhagic telangiectasia

  C. Kaposi's sarcoma

  D. Lymphangioma

  E. Spider telangiectasia

8. During the repair of an abdominal aortic aneurysm the anesthesiologist inserts a balloon-tipped catheter and feeds it through to the patient's pulmonary artery. Once in position, the balloon is inflated and the pressure reads a steady 5 mm Hg. What pressure is the anesthesiologist attempting to determine?

  A. Left atrial pressure

  B. Left ventricular end-systolic pressure

  C. Pulmonary artery pressure

  D. Right atrial pressure

  E. Right ventricular end-systolic pressure

9. A 72-year-old man is brought to the emergency department by ambulance after having passed out at home. His ECG reveals an arrhythmia based on the atrioventricular (AV) node. What drug would be most effective at interrupting the AV transmission and breaking the arrhythmic cycle at the AV node?

  A. Adenosine

  B. Flecainide

  C. Lidocaine

  D. Phenytoin

  E. Quinidine

10. A 55-year-old man presents to his primary care physician to follow-up on his medication for hyperlipidemia. Laboratory work suggests that his total cholesterol, LDL cholesterol, triglycerides, and high-density-lipoprotein (HDL) cholesterol are all within normal limits owing to the lovastatin he began taking 2 months ago. He has not visited the office since being given this medication. Which of the following laboratory tests should be obtained at the present office visit?

  A. ECG

  B. Hemoglobin A1C levels

  C. Liver function tests

  D. Pulmonary function tests

  E. Potassium levels

11. A 45-year-old woman presents to her primary care physician after several episodes of syncope. Physical examination reveals a plopping sound during midsystole. An ECG is obtained (Figure 3-2). What is the most likely explanation of these findings?

  A. Aortic regurgitation

  B. Aortic stenosis

  C. Atrial myxoma

  D. Heart failure

  E. Heart rhabdomyoma

12. A 56-year-old woman presents to the office with varicose veins, which have developed gradually over the past 20 years. These dilated veins are common and usually are of no significance aside from their unattractive appearance. Veins in general differ from arteries in that they have very few smooth muscle cells, which allows for easy expansion. In what histological layer would one look to compare the amount of smooth muscle present in veins and arteries?

  A. Tunica adventitia

  B. Tunica albuginea

  C. Tunica intima

  D. Tunica media

  E. Tunica serosa

13. Following an ECG, a 62-year-old man is told he has no arrhythmias and that his myocardium is conducting electricity normally. For cardiac myocytes to conduct at their high rate of velocity, special conduction apparatuses are needed. These are called intercalated disks and are composed of fascia adherens and what other junctional complex?

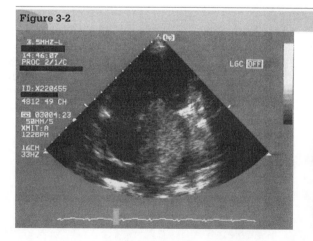
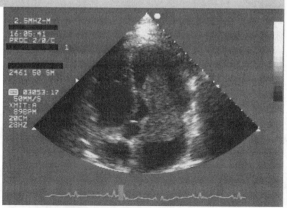

Figure 3-2

A   B

A. Adherent junction

B. Desmosome

C. Tight junction

D. Zonula adherens

E. Zonula occludens

14. A 65-year-old woman requires pacemaker implantation due to a defective sinoatrial (SA) node. The cells present at the SA and AV nodes are often referred to as pacemaker cells. They have some distinct characteristics that set them apart from the rest of the myocardium. The action potential is divided into phases 0 to 4, each of which is associated with a change in conductance or voltage. Pacemaker cells differ from the other myocytes in the pattern of these phases. Which of the following descriptions represents phase 0 in the pacemaker cells?

A. Initial repolarization from voltage-gated potassium channels

B. Plateau phase from a balance of calcium influx and potassium efflux

C. Rapid repolarization with unopposed potassium efflux

D. Rapid upstroke, referring to the opening of sodium channels

E. Slow upstroke, referring to the opening of calcium channels

15. A 48-year-old woman presents to her primary care physician with frequent episodes of syncope as well as erythema and anhidrosis on the left side of the face, neck, and chest and in the left upper limb. Measurement of her systemic blood pressure on the upper limbs reveals hypotension on the left but not on the right. Which of the following is the most likely cause of the hypotension in the left arm?

A. A stretched aortic aneurysm, which irritates and stimulates left vagus nerve

B. Atherosclerosis of the subclavian artery

C. Coarctation of the aorta

D. Multiple MIs

E. Impingement of tumor on the left sympathetic chain

16. While examining a 48-year-old diabetic woman, the physician evaluates her feet. He checks the feet for lesions and discusses the importance of proper foot care. He evaluates the dorsalis pedis pulse and finds it to be diminished bilaterally. He then checks behind the medial malleolus for the other main artery supplying the foot. Which of the following arteries is found posterior to the medial malleolus?

A. Anterior tibial artery

B. Arcuate artery

C. Medial plantar artery

D. Posterior tibial artery

E. Tibial artery

17. A 40-year-old woman presents to her primary care physician with a 1-year history of orthopnea. She has consumed five to six beers almost every night for the last 20 years. An ECG reveals an ejection fraction of 35%. What pathological process accounts for this patient's orthopnea?

A. Aortic stenosis

B. Cor pulmonale

C. Dilated cardiomyopathy

D. Hypertrophic cardiomyopathy

E. Restrictive cardiomyopathy

18. A 61-year-old man presents to his primary care physician for routine blood work to measure the levels of a drug he is taking to control his congestive heart failure. This drug functions to slow AV conduction and increase contractility. What is the most likely drug?

A. Adenosine

B. Carvedilol

C. Digoxin

D. Lisinopril

E. Warfarin

19. A 32-year-old pregnant woman presents to her obstetrician for a well-baby evaluation. Her blood pressure readings have been 165/100 mm Hg over the past two visits. The physician feels that she should be given an antihypertensive medication. A chest x-ray is obtained (Figure 3-3). What pharmacological agent is most effective and safe in pregnant women?

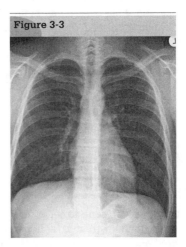
Figure 3-3

A. Furosemide

B. Hydrochlorothiazide

C. Lisinopril

D. Losartan

E. Methyldopa

20. A 57-year-old man who had an MI 5 years earlier is concerned about another such event. Currently only one drug has proven effective in decreasing the risk of MI. What is this medication?

A. Abciximab

B. Aspirin

C. Heparin

D. Streptokinase

E. Ticlopidine

21. An 80-year-old woman with a history of transient ischemic attacks begins aspirin for prophylaxis against a cerebrovascular accident but cannot tolerate the medication because it exacerbates her peptic ulcer disease. What is the most appropriate treatment?

A. Aspirin

B. Heparin

C. Streptokinase

D. Ticlopidine

E. Warfarin

22. A 41-year-old African American man is planning a visit to his parents in Brazil. Knowing the prevalence of malaria there, you begin the patient on quinine a week before he leaves. After 2 days of the medication, he returns to the office with dark urine and, on physical examination, appears jaundiced. Which of the following accounts for these findings?

A. Beta thalassemia

B. Factor V Leiden

C. Glucose-6-phosphate dehydrogenase deficiency

D. Polycythemia vera

E. Sickle cell anemia

23. A 29-year-old pregnant woman comes to the office for a well-baby checkup. It has been 34 weeks since her last menstrual period and she has had a normal pregnancy course to date. Physical examination of the heart, lungs, and abdomen is within normal limits. There is no evidence of cyanosis, clubbing, or peripheral edema. In what organ is the fetus producing most of its red blood cells (RBCs)—a process called erythropoiesis?

A. Bone marrow

B. Liver

C. Myocardium

D. Spleen

E. Yolk sac

24. A 29-year-old woman presents to her primary care physician because she has not menstruated for 6 weeks. A pregnancy test is ordered and the woman is told that it is positive. Assuming that the fetus is at least 4 weeks old, it now has a beating heart. From what embryologic layer is the heart derived?

A. Ectoderm

B. Endoderm

C. Epiblast

D. Mesoderm

E. Neural crest

25. Following an episode of pulmonary edema, a 60-year-old man is suspected of having congestive heart failure. An ECG is ordered to determine the patient's ejection fraction. During this procedure his heart rate remains at 100 bpm with an ejection fraction of 50%. Assuming that his cardiac output is 3 L/min, what is this patient's end-diastolic volume?

A. 100 mL

B. 60 mL

C. 30 mL

D. 10 mL

E. 5 mL

26. A 36-year-old woman presents to her primary care physician with jaundice and peripheral swelling. An ECG is ordered and she is determined to have right-sided heart failure with hepatic congestion and peripheral edema. No murmur is detected. What is the most appropriate explanation for these findings?

A. Aortic stenosis

B. Atrial septal defect

C. Patent ductus arteriosus

D. Situs inversus

E. Tetralogy of Fallot

F. Transposition of the great vessels

G. Ventricular septal defect

27. Upon delivery, a newborn of 38 weeks' gestation becomes cyanotic. An ECG is ordered. On the basis of its results, the infant is given prostaglandins and prepared for surgery. What is the most likely diagnosis?

A. Aortic stenosis

B. Atrial septal defect

C. Situs inversus

D. Tetralogy of Fallot

E. Transposition of the great vessels

28. A 63-year-old man with a history of hypertension presents to the emergency department complaining of chest pain. The following information is recorded in his chart:

Heart rate: 60 beats/min

Oxygen consumption: 400 mL/min

Arterial oxygen consumption: 0.25 mL O_2/min

Venous oxygen consumption: 0.15 mL O_2/min

Arterial oxygen saturation: 95%

What is this patient's cardiac output?

A. 3.5 L/min

B. 4.0 L/min

C. 4.5 L/min

D. 6.0 L/min

E. 5.0 L/min

29. A 25-year-old woman is having recurring episodes of heart palpitations and sweating. During one of these episodes her blood pressure is found to be 165/110 mm Hg. Normally her blood pressure is approximately 110/70 mm Hg. A CT scan is obtained (Figure 3-4). Urine studies reveal increased levels of metanephrine. Which of the following drugs would be best suited to control this patient's blood pressure?

A. Clonidine

B. Enalapril

C. Phenoxybenzamine

D. Reserpine

E. Verapamil

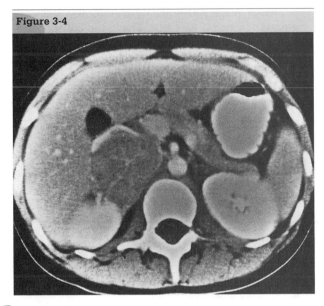

Figure 3-4

A. Left atrium

B. Left ventricle

C. Right atrium

D. Right ventricle

E. Superior vena cava

30. A 39-year-old woman has just given birth to a boy who, on physical examination, is found to have craniofacial abnormalities, including upward-slanting eyes, epicanthal folds, flat facies, small ears, and a single flexion crease in the palms of his hands. What is the mostly likely cardiac malformation associated with this condition?

A. Coarctation of the aorta

B. Patent ductus arteriosus

C. Septum primum

D. Tetralogy of Fallot

E. Ventricular septal defect

31. A 13-year-old girl has had repeated sore throats, her last one having occurred 2 weeks earlier. She now is complaining of pain in her knees and ankles. Physical examination reveals a temperature of 39°C (101.4°F), subcutaneous nodules on her shins, and a heart murmur. On the basis of this clinical presentation, what is the most likely valve causing the murmur?

A. Aortic valve

B. Mitral valve

C. Pulmonary valve

D. Tricuspid valve

E. Valve of the coronary sinus

32. On the following chest x-ray (Figure 3-5), what part of the heart is labeled?

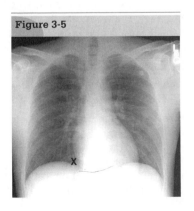

Figure 3-5

33. A 58-year-old man with a history of hypertension, diabetes mellitus, congestive heart failure, and erectile dysfunction is brought to the emergency department because of crushing chest pain. MI is suspected. When will this patient be most susceptible to rupture of the left ventricle?

A. In 12 hr

B. In 2 days

C. In 7 days

D. In 1 month

E. In 6 months

34. A 45-year-old woman has swelling and pain in her left calf—a condition that developed 16 hr ago. Physical examination reveals tenderness, warmth, and discoloration of her left leg. She has pain with palpation in the left posterior calf. A medication is given that specifically converts fibrin-bound plasminogen to plasmin. What medication was this patient probably given?

A. Aspirin

B. Calcium

C. Heparin

D. Tissue plasminogen activator

E. Warfarin

35. A 50-year-old man with a history of asthma suffers an MI. As the medical student assigned to care for this patient, you remember that the use of a class II beta-adrenergic antagonist reduces the incidence of sudden arrhythmic death after a heart attack. Which is the most appropriate choice of drug for this patient?

A. Amphetamine

B. Dobutamine

C. Metoprolol

D. Procainamide

E. Propranolol

36. A 21-year-old man presents to his primary care physician for a routine examination. His medical history is positive for hypercholesterolemia, as is his family history. Detailed serum lipid and lipoprotein analyses reveal elevated LDL cholesterol. This type of hyperlipidemia is best classified as which of the following?

A. Type 1

B. Type 2a

C. Type 2b

D. Type 3

E. Type 5

37. An 18-year-old primigravida presents for a follow-up examination. She is approximately 10 weeks pregnant by dates and has no complaints. Physical examination of her heart, lungs, and abdomen is unremarkable. At what gestational age can one expect to hear the first fetal heartbeat?

  A. 1 week
  B. 2 weeks
  C. 3 weeks
  D. 4 weeks
  E. 10 weeks

38. A 4-year-old Chinese boy is brought to his pediatrician because he has had a fever for 6 days. Physical examination reveals bilateral conjunctival injection, cervical lymphadenopathy, induration of the hands and feet with erythematous palms and soles, polymorphous exanthema, and erythematous oral pharynx. What is the most likely diagnosis?

  A. Buerger's disease
  B. Giant cell arteritis
  C. Kawasaki disease
  D. Takayasu's arteritis
  E. Temporal arteritis

39. A 23-year-old homeless man presents to the emergency department with a temperature of 102°F. Physical examination reveals tricuspid regurgitation. Blood cultures reveal *Staphylococcus aureus*. What is the most likely diagnosis?

  A. Congenital heart disease
  B. Illicit drug use
  C. Rheumatic fever
  D. Syphilitic heart disease
  E. Systemic lupus erythematosus

40. A 27-year-old black woman gives birth to a full-term male by spontaneous vaginal delivery. On examination of the newborn's umbilical cord, one umbilical artery and vein are noted. What is the significance of this observation?

  A. It is associated with congenital and chromosomal anomalies.
  B. The mother has abused drugs.
  C. It is associated with mental retardation.
  D. It is a normal variant.
  E. Renal agenesis is likely.

41. A young man presents to the emergency department after having been involved in fight. On physical examination, a 1-in stab wound is noticed at the fourth intercostal space just left of the sternum. Which chamber of the heart is most likely to have been penetrated by the knife?

  A. Left atrium
  B. Left ventricle
  C. Pulmonary trunk
  D. Right atrium
  E. Right ventricle

42. During routine screening of a 71-year-old man with refractory peripheral edema, an increase in liver function enzymes is noted. Physical examination reveals splenomegaly without hepatomegaly. Liver biopsy is performed and a chest x-ray is obtained (Figure 3-6). What is this patient's underlying condition?

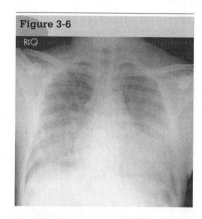

Figure 3-6

  A. Aortic stenosis
  B. Left ventricular heart failure
  C. Restrictive cardiomyopathy
  D. Rheumatic fever
  E. Right ventricular heart failure

43. A 91-year-old woman is brought to the emergency department complaining of shortness of breath. She is oriented to time and place but not to person. She has alcohol on her breath. Physical examination of the head and neck is within normal limits. Which of the following physical findings is most suggestive that she may be experiencing heart failure?

  A. Ascites
  B. Orthopnea
  C. Pulmonary wheezing
  D. S_3, a third heart sound
  E. S_4, a fourth heart sound

44. As the primary care physician of a patient who has suffered an MI, you recommend that she take an aspirin daily for prophylaxis. Aspirin is beneficial because it inhibits the formation of which of the following?

  A. Bradykinin
  B. Lipoxygenase
  C. Phospholipase A2
  D. Thromboxane A2 (TxA2)
  E. Vasopressin

45. You are the family physician of a couple who have been trying to have a baby. The woman visits your clinic for a pregnancy test and the results are positive. What can you predict about her blood pressure over the course of her pregnancy?

  A. It will decrease.
  B. It will decrease and then slowly come back to baseline.
  C. It will increase.
  D. It will increase and then slowly go back to baseline.
  E. It will not change.

46. A 2-year-old boy is brought to the emergency department because his parents found that he had turned blue. Pulse oximetry on room air is 79%. Cardiac auscultation and the

ECG reveal right ventricular hypertrophy. Which of the following etiologies can lead to this syndrome?

A. Aortic stenosis

B. Mitral insufficiency

C. Mitral prolapse

D. Patent ductus arteriosus

E. Systemic hypertension

47. A 13-year-old patient presents to the emergency department after a fall from his bicycle. There is a large hematoma in the middle of the posterior upper arm. The patient is also unable to extend his wrist. Which of the following arteries was most likely lacerated?

A. Brachial artery

B. Deep artery of the arm

C. Posterior circumflex humeral artery

D. Radial artery

E. Ulnar artery

48. A 6-year-old girl presents to a new family physician for an immunization update. On routine physical examination, the physician notes a $^2/_6$ murmur heard best along the upper right sternal border. An ECG is obtained (Figure 3-7). What is the most likely diagnosis?

A. Aortic stenosis

B. Atrial septal defect

C. Patent ductus arteriosus

D. Situs inversus

E. Tetralogy of Fallot

F. Transposition of the great vessels

G. Ventricular septal defect

49. A 58-year-old man presents to his primary care physician because of progressive dyspnea. He had rheumatic heart disease as a child. He also complains of erectile dysfunction and an intermittent decrease in his urinary stream. He has a pansystolic murmur that radiates to the axilla. What is the most likely diagnosis?

A. Aortic stenosis

B. Atrial septal defect

C. Mitral regurgitation

D. Mitral valve prolapse

E. Tricuspid regurgitation

F. Ventral septal defect

50. A researcher was doing a study on the fetal cardiovascular system and found that blood in one particular vessel had a P_{O_2} level remarkably higher than that in the rest of the fetal vessels. This finding is physiologically significant. What vessel in the fetal circulation is the researcher describing?

A. Ascending aorta

B. Ductus arteriosus

C. Ductus venosus

D. Umbilical artery

E. Umbilical vein

51. A 40-year-old construction worker presents to his primary care physician for an acute visit. He has been healthy but is now concerned because when he is out on a cold day, his fingers become extremely sensitive. Apart from this, he has no known medical problems. He is hoping that you will help him so that he will be able to work on cold days. What question should he be asked in the interview to diagnose his underlying condition?

A. Do you have a history of alcohol consumption?

B. Do you smoke, and if you do, how much do you smoke?

C. Do you have a family history of poor circulation?

D. Have you ever been diagnosed with hypothyroidism?

E. Is there any family history of diabetes mellitus?

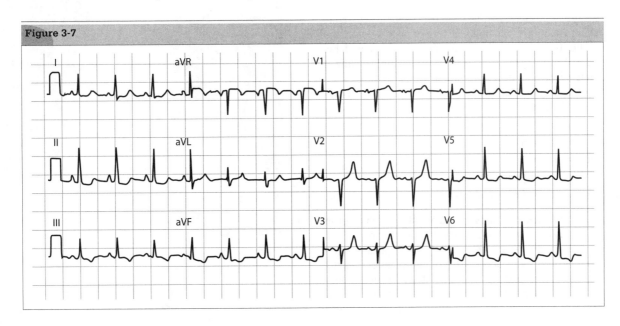

Figure 3-7

52. A female infant is noted to have swelling at the nape of her neck at birth. She is otherwise normal and has a 5-min Apgar score of 9. She is discharged after 48 hr with no complications. When she is given a routine physical examination by her pediatrician at the age of 11 years, a cardiovascular abnormality is detected. What cardiovascular abnormality would be detected during this examination?

A. Continuous machinery-like murmur

B. Carotid bruit

C. Crescendo-decrescendo murmur

D. Late systolic murmur

E. Weak pulses in the lower extremities

53. A 39-year-old man who recently went scuba diving in Hawaii presents to his primary care physician with severe substernal chest pain. What is the most likely cause of this patient's pain?

A. Air emboli

B. Amniotic fluid emboli

C. Bacteria emboli

D. Fat emboli

E. Thrombus

F. Tumor emboli

54. A 78-year-old man presents to his primary care physician for evaluation of progressive dyspnea. He has a history of MI. He has no edema in his extremities and appears to be clinically stable. Cardiac auscultation reveals an S_3 heart sound. What underlying condition should you suspect given these findings?

A. Bacterial endocarditis

B. Dilated congestive heart failure

C. Hypertrophic cardiomyopathy

D. Mitral regurgitation

E. Right heart failure

55. An infant is brought to the pediatrician for a well-child checkup. The infant has had a history of poor feeding and irritability. Birth history is unremarkable. The infant is tachycardic and tachypneic, and the liver is palpable. The infant also has bilateral rales. What other physical finding would you expect to find upon further evaluation that would confirm your diagnosis?

A. Cardiomegaly

B. Peripheral edema

C. Still's murmur

D. Total anomalous venous return

E. Transposition of the great vessels

56. A 49-year-old man who has suffered an MI is hospitalized in the coronary care unit. Cardiovascular examination reveals tachycardia and a regular rhythm. Pulmonary auscultation reveals bilateral breath sounds without wheezes or rhonchi. Abdominal examination fails to reveal the presence of peritoneal signs. Blood gas analysis reveals a Po_2 of 25 mm Hg. This implies a hemoglobin saturation that approaches which of the following?

A. 10%

B. 20%

C. 30%

D. 40%

E. 50%

57. A 21-year-old man who has suffered a gunshot wound to the back is brought to the emergency department for evaluation. A CT scan of the chest, abdomen, and pelvis reveals transection of the C7 vertebra. Which of the following sequelae of this injury is most likely to occur?

A. Bradycardia

B. Death

C. Decorticate posturing

D. Hypertension

E. Respiratory muscle depression

58. Following a complication-free delivery of a 32-week infant, care is passed on to the pediatrician. At the 2-month well-child visit, the examination reveals a holosystolic murmur with a machine-like quality. A chest x-ray is obtained (Figure 3-8). Which of the following medications is most likely to help with this infant's cardiac condition?

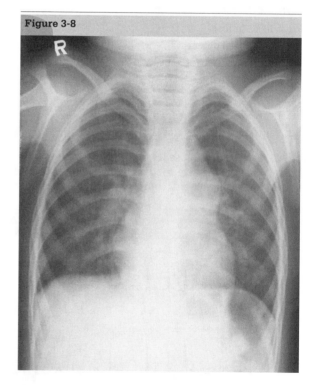

Figure 3-8

A. Hydrocortisone

B. Indomethacin

C. Mifepristone

D. Misoprostol

E. Prostaglandin E_2 (PGE_2)

59. A 41-year-old man has a resting oxygen consumption of 250 mL/min; his peripheral arterial oxygen content is 0.20 mL O_2/mL of blood. His mixed venous oxygen content is 0.15 mL O_2/mL of blood. Which of the following is his cardiac output?

A. 1.0 L/min

B. 2.0 L/min

C. 3.0 L/min

D. 4.0 L/min

E. 5.0 L/min

60. A 43-year-old man presents to his primary care physician complaining of chest tightness and chest pains. He has a medical history of hypertension, for which he takes an angiotensin-converting enzyme (ACE) inhibitor. He has a 20-pack-year history of smoking. What would be the quickest and most diagnostic test to rule out MI in this patient?

A. Auscultation of the heart

B. Examination of the deep tendon reflexes

C. Manual reproduction of the chest pain

D. Neurological examination

E. Having the patient run in place

61. A 38-year-old woman presents to her primary care physician complaining of intermittent chest pain while at rest. She reports being occasionally awakened from sleep by this pain. She says it just comes and goes. Nothing she can recall makes it better or worse. What type of angina does she most likely have?

A. Abnormal

B. Prinzmetal

C. Permissive

D. Unstable

E. Variant

62. A 44-year-old woman presents to her primary care physician visibly upset. She states that she was recently diagnosed as having had a heart attack. Review of her prior records indicates that she has had an MI that crosses the entire ventricular wall, from the endocardium through to the epicardium. What is the most likely pathophysiology of these findings?

A. Cardiac tamponade

B. Ruptured cardiac muscle

C. Subendocardial infarction

D. Transmural infarction

E. Ventricular aneurysm

63. A 7-year-old boy with fever, generalized malaise, and joint pain is brought to the emergency department. His mother mentions that he has been making weird faces and has been very moody lately. She reports that all his immunizations are up to date and denies any significant medical history aside from a case of sore throat and swollen tonsils about 3 weeks earlier. What pathognomonic lesion would be associated with this child's likely illness?

A. Aschoff bodies

B. Caput medusae

C. Parotitis

D. Pinpoint pupils

E. Sialadenitis

64. A 65-year-old man presents to his primary care physician after having had an MI. He was just discharged from the hospital 2 days earlier. How long will it take before well-developed scar tissue forms?

A. 1 to 2 days

B. 1 to 2 weeks

C. 3 to 6 weeks

D. 3 to 6 months

E. 6 months to 1 year

65. A 44-year-old man with a history of childhood rheumatic fever presents to his physician for evaluation of intermittent dyspnea and chest pressure. He has a prior medical history of erectile dysfunction. Physical examination of the heart reveals a systolic ejection murmur. What is the most commonly involved valve in rheumatic heart disease?

A. Aortic

B. Mitral

C. Myocardial

D. Pulmonary

E. Tricuspid

66. A 16-year-old immigrant presents to her primary care physician for a checkup. When questioned about her past medical history, she says that she was told of having had a heart problem at birth but is unable to offer any further detail. She is under the impression that the problem is resolved and does not think she need worry any further about it. You proceed to explain that based on her story, she may be at increased risk for which of the following conditions?

A. Acute endocarditis

B. Chronic endocarditis

C. Pericarditis

D. Rheumatic fever

E. Subacute endocarditis

67. A 69-year-old man with metastatic colon and pancreatic cancer presents to his physician for an interval examination. He complains of intermittent dyspnea and chest pain. His ECG reveals clinically small, sterile fibrin deposits on the closure line of the valve leaflets. The results show peripheral embolization with sterile emboli. What is the most likely diagnosis?

A. Acute endocarditis

B. Chronic endocarditis

C. Libman-Sacks endocarditis

D. Nonbacterial thrombotic endocarditis

E. Subacute endocarditis

68. A 24-year-old woman who admits to having worked as a prostitute presents to the emergency department; she has no insurance but complains of the treatment she received at the local free clinic. She was having chest pains and was told at the clinic that she had heart disease. She presents you with a piece of paper giving her diagnosis as syphilitic aortitis. Which of the following statements is correct about this condition?

  A. Aortic valve ring is dilated

  B. Aortic valve ring is unable to open

  C. Aortic valve is calcified

  D. Heart is functioning at 50% of capacity

  E. Heart is perfectly fine, with no issues of concern

69. A 59-year-old obese man with a history of unstable angina presents to the emergency department with an episode of chest pain. To monitor any changes in cardiac function and electric signal transmission throughout the myocardium, an ECG is ordered. A section of this ECG is shown in Figure 3-9. Which of the following corresponds to the passage of the electric signal from the atria to the ventricle via the AV node?

  A. P wave

  B. PR interval

  C. QRS wave

  D. QT interval

  E. T wave

70. A 3-year-old boy is referred to the emergency department by his pediatrician because of upper extremity hypertension and normal blood pressure in the lower extremities. Physical examination of the head and neck is within normal limits. Chest x-ray reveals notching of the ribs. What is the most likely diagnosis?

  A. Atrial septal defect

  B. Coarctation of the aorta

  C. Patent ductus arteriosus

  D. Tetralogy of Fallot

  E. Ventricular septal defect

71. Working in the coroner's office, you are presented with a male corpse which, upon examination, is found to have dilation of the left and right ventricles; therefore this individual is presumed to have suffered from bilateral heart failure. Based on this presentation, which of the following was the predisposing factor to the heart failure?

  A. Alcoholic binge drinking

  B. Congenital cardiac anomaly

  C. Intravenous heroin overdose

  D. Thiamine deficiency

  E. Ventricular septal defect

72. A patient in the intensive care unit (ICU) is in critical condition and is known to have fluid trapped in his pericardium. Some of the fluid is drawn off and sent to the laboratory for evaluation. The lab calls the ICU and reports that a clear, straw-colored fluid with protein-rich exudate was collected. Small numbers of inflammatory cells are noted to be present in the sample. On the basis of this information, what is the most likely pathological description of the fluid?

  A. Fibrinous

  B. Hemorrhagic

  C. Infectious

  D. Purulent

  E. Serous

Figure 3-9

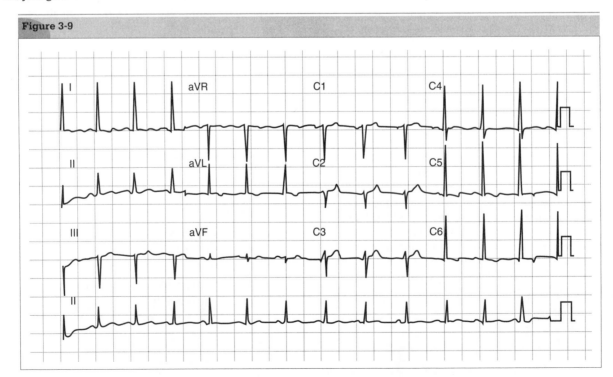

73. A 63-year-old woman is brought to the emergency department with complaints of decreased urination and peripheral swelling of the extremities due to fluid retention. Physical examination reveals distended neck veins and a liver span of 16 cm in the midclavicular line. What is the most likely diagnosis?

A. Bilateral heart failure

B. Cerebral anoxia

C. Hydrothorax

D. Left-sided heart failure

E. Right-sided heart failure

74. A 58-year-old man with a history of diabetes mellitus, hypertension, asthma, obesity, and erectile dysfunction presents to his primary care physician for follow-up. He has a 50-pack-year history of smoking. Physical examination reveals a blood pressure of 160/110 mm Hg. Cardiac auscultation reveals no murmurs or rubs. Chest x-ray reveals cardiomegaly. Which of the following is the most common direct cause of left ventricular hypertrophy?

A. Asthma

B. Chronic obstructive pulmonary disease

C. Hypertension

D. Lack of exercise

E. Smoking

75. Referring to the ventricular volume curve shown below (Figure 3-10), at what point would you first hear the first heart sound on auscultation?

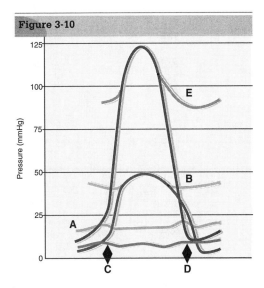

Figure 3-10

A. A

B. B

C. C

D. D

E. E

Answer Key

1. B	20. B	39. B	58. B
2. B	21. D	40. A	59. E
3. E	22. C	41. E	60. C
4. E	23. A	42. E	61. B
5. B	24. D	43. D	62. D
6. D	25. B	44. D	63. A
7. E	26. B	45. B	64. D
8. A	27. E	46. D	65. B
9. A	28. B	47. B	66. E
10. C	29. C	48. A	67. D
11. C	30. C	49. C	68. A
12. D	31. B	50. E	69. B
13. B	32. C	51. B	70. B
14. E	33. C	52. E	71. D
15. E	34. D	53. A	72. E
16. D	35. C	54. B	73. E
17. C	36. B	55. A	74. C
18. C	37. D	56. E	75. C
19. E	38. C	57. A	

Answers and Explanations

1. **B.** The various familial hyperlipidemias are classified on the basis of the presence or absence of certain lipoproteins and the patient's lipid levels. Type 2a presents with an increase in LDL only, due to a defect in either the LDL receptor or in the apolipoprotein B gene. This defect often results in the formation of atherosclerotic plaques, leading to MIs as early as age 30 in heterozygotes and even earlier in homozygotes. Type 1 represents an increase in chylomicrons and is due to a mutation in the lipoprotein lipase gene. Type 2b results from similar genetic defects as type 2a but includes increases in both LDL and very low density lipoprotein (VLDL). Type 3 includes increases in chylomicron remnants and intermediate-density lipoprotein (IDL) due to a mutation in the apolipoprotein E gene. Type 4 results in increases in VLDL only due to a mutation in the lipoprotein lipase gene; by comparison to types 1 through 3, however, it has a relatively low incidence of forming atherosclerotic plaques.

2. **B.** Patient susceptibility often plays a large part in the determination of organisms responsible for bacterial endocarditis. In this case the patient is an intravenous drug user, and these patients most often have infections of the tricuspid valve. *Staphylococcus aureus* is an extremely virulent organism and can infect both healthy and deformed valves. It is commonly found on the skin and accounts for > 60% of all endocarditis infections in intravenous drug users. Viridans streptococci, found as normal flora in the oropharynx, often infect previously damaged or abnormal valves. Coagulase-negative staphylococci are often found in patients with a prosthetic valve present. *Streptococcus pyogenes* is not a common cause of bacterial endocarditis but rather of rheumatic fever, owing to an inappropriate immune response to the M protein of *Strep. pyogenes*. *Treponema pallidum* is the spirochete responsible for syphilis, and while tertiary syphilis can lead to aortitis, it is not known to cause endocarditis.

3. **E.** This patient had a rupture of the ascending aorta due to destruction of the vasa vasorum. When the vasa vasorum (located in the tunica adventitia) become compromised by syphilis, the tunica media can no longer obtain its blood supply. It loses its elastic support and becomes dilated, producing an aneurysm. The tunica intima, endothelium, and subendothelium are the inner layers of the artery; they are not directly affected by syphilis and do not provide elasticity to the arteries. The nevi vascularis are the nerves in the tunica adventitia; they control the contraction of smooth muscle in the vessel walls and are not affected by syphilis. The chest x-ray shown reveals the presence of a thoracic aortic aneurysm.

4. **E.** This patient is describing a condition called orthopnea, which often presents with the use of multiple pillows to sit upright while sleeping. Patients need to sit more upright to decrease the pressure from fluid accumulation in the lungs. Left-sided heart failure is the cause of paroxysmal nocturnal dyspnea; of the choices listed above, rheumatic heart disease is the most likely explanation for this condition. Rheumatic heart disease can involve both mitral and aortic valves, leading to insufficiency and, over time, left-sided heart failure. Although atrial myxoma is the most common cancer of the heart, it is still rare, and the symptoms it produces would be intermittent. Cor pulmonale is the result of interstitial fibrosis of the lung, and the symptoms of restricted lung expansion would not present with paroxysmal nocturnal dyspnea relieved by sitting upright. Fibrinous pericarditis usually is not severe enough to produce symptoms of heart failure. Instead, this rare condition is likely to present with symptoms of chest pain. Libman-Sacks endocarditis is a manifestation of systemic lupus erythematosus, with the formation of small and sterile vegetations on the mitral and tricuspid valves.

5. **B.** The rapid onset of heart failure in this patient with lymphocytic infiltrate indicates a viral myocarditis. Often these infections are asymptomatic; they can, however, cause a rapid onset of symptoms. Coxsackievirus B is the most common cause of myocarditis in the United States; this usually is a self-limiting process. *Borrelia burgdorferi* is the spirochete responsible for Lyme disease. Although this disease may lead to cardiac pathology (pericarditis, myocarditis, heart block), it occurs during the secondary stage, and this patient does not have a history suggesting exposure to the spirochete. Although *Streptococcus pyogenes* may lead to rheumatic fever and symptoms of myocarditis, this patient's history does not indicate a history of infection with *Strep. pyogenes*. Viridans streptococcus and *Staphylococcus aureus* are common organisms responsible for bacterial endocarditis, not myocarditis. *Trypanosoma cruzi* leads to Chagas' disease by transmission from the reduviid bug. This infection commonly results in achalasia and dilation of the heart chambers. *Toxoplasma gondii*, the cause of toxoplasmosis, may produce a myocarditis infection, but usually only immunocompromised individuals are affected, and this patient has no such history.

6. D. This patient is presenting with temporal arteritis or giant cell arteritis, which typically affects branches of the carotid artery. If left untreated, this patient may develop occlusion of the ophthalmic artery, resulting in permanent blindness. The only medications shown to slow or stop the granulomatous occlusion of these arteries are steroids. Alpha-blockers such as phenoxybenzamine and prazosin would decrease systemic blood pressure and decrease the constriction of blood vessels, but they would not stop the progression of the granulomatous process. Anticoagulants such as heparin and warfarin would not be effective because this condition is not the result of platelet coagulation. The 3-hydroxy-3-methyl-glutaryl-CoA reductase (HMG-CoA) inhibitors, such as lovastatin, decrease the long-term occlusion of vessels by reducing the deposition of cholesterol found in atherosclerotic plaques and would not decrease the formation of granulomas. Thrombolytics such as tissue plasminogen activator (tPA) and streptokinase would not be effective because occlusion of the ophthalmic artery is not a result of clot formation.

7. E. Spider telangiectasias are nonneoplastic skin lesions commonly found in pregnant patients or those with cirrhosis. These subcutaneous arteries or arterioles tend to appear on the face, neck, or upper chest. Hemangiomas are very common neoplastic skin lesions that almost never transform into malignant tumors. These solitary lesions usually present in infancy and childhood. Hereditary hemorrhagic telangiectasia is part of the rare autosomal dominant Osler-Weber-Rendu disease and presents with telangiectases present from birth. Kaposi's sarcoma is a tumor caused by human herpesvirus 8, once found only in older men of Mediterranean extraction but now found mostly in patients who are HIV-positive. Lymphangioma is the lymphatic system equivalent of a hemangioma and would not present with a vascular lesion.

8. A. Often the pressure obtained with the balloon tip inflated is referred to as the pulmonary wedge pressure. The balloon serves to block all blood flow from the pulmonary artery in that section of the lung, leaving only the pressure from the pulmonary veins. This pressure approximates the pressure in the left atrium owing to the similar pressures in the pulmonary veins. Left ventricular pressure would be much higher and, because of the occlusion of the mitral valve at the end of systole, could not be measured from the pulmonary artery. Pulmonary artery pressure could be measured from this position if the balloon were deflated. This would allow blood flow to resume and the pressure to be measured. Right atrial pressure may be measured with a similar device. Similarly the right ventricular end-systolic pressure could be measured with a catheter for an accurate measurement. However, it could not be used while in the pulmonary artery.

9. A. The arrhythmia described involves dysfunction of the AV node, which has led to syncope in this patient. Treatment must be fast and block the AV node in order to reset the heart's normal innate automaticity. Adenosine is the best choice because of its ability to block the function of the AV node rapidly and transiently (for only 15 to 20 sec). Flecainide is a very dangerous antiarrhythmic agent and has also been shown actually to induce arrhythmias in some instances. It is still occasionally used to treat recalcitrant ventricular arrhythmias. Lidocaine is both a local anesthetic and a class IB agent for the treatment of ventricular arrhythmias. Lidocaine is generally used post-MI because it prevents the formation of arrhythmias in the infarcted tissue while also increasing the blood supply. Phenytoin is both an antiepileptic drug and a treatment for a special drug-induced arrhythmia. Phenytoin's usage as a treatment for arrhythmia is generally limited to digitalis toxicity. Quinidine is a class IA antiarrhythmic used as a long-term treatment for atrial and ventricular arrhythmias. It would not have a fast enough onset for this patient.

10. C. There are two main concerns in starting any patient on a statin: myopathy and hepatotoxicity. However, because the statins are so effective at lowering LDL and triglyceride levels, physicians still prescribe them and closely follow liver function tests and creatine kinase levels to ensure proper liver and muscle function. Although an ECG may be warranted, it is clearly not as important as looking for the toxic manifestations of lovastatin. Hemoglobin A1C would be an important monitoring test to follow a diabetic's recent sugar control. However, we have no indication of diabetes in this patient, and a hemoglobin A1C would not be used to diagnose diabetes. Pulmonary function tests are often monitored in patients who are taking drugs that can lead to pulmonary fibrosis. These include bleomycin, amiodarone, and busulfan. However, statins are not thought to be associated with pulmonary complications. Potassium levels are often checked in patients taking various diuretics: urine potassium levels increase with all diuretic classes except potassium-sparing diuretics. Statins are not associated with any changes in potassium levels.

11. C. The most frequently occurring cardiac tumor found in adults is myxoma of the left atrium. It typically occurs as a single lesion in the left atrium and can intermittently obstruct the mitral valve. The ECG shows the atrial myxoma prolapsing through the mitral valve. Aortic stenosis causes the classical crescendo-decrescendo murmur of systole. Aortic regurgitation is an early diastolic decrescendo murmur. A rhabdomyoma of the heart is most common in infants and young children. It is often associated with tuberous sclerosis. Heart failure would not cause a murmur as described.

12. D. The tunica media houses the smooth muscle cells of the arteries and veins. It is this level of musculature that facilitates the differences between arteries and veins. The multiple layers of muscle in arteries allow for strength to withstand high pressures and the ability to contract when needed. Veins, however, have a very small amount of smooth muscle, which allows for increased compliance and expansion when needed. The tunica adventitia and tunica intima are the other layers of vasculature in blood vessels and are on either side of the tunica media. The tunica adventitia consists mostly of elastic and collagen fibers and sits on the outer edge. The tunica intima is composed of metabolically active endothelial cells and lines the vessels. The tunica albuginea and tunica serosa are not associated with the layers of vessels. The term *albuginea* refers to the whitish membrane found in the corpora cavernosa of the penis. *Tunica serosa* is another name for the serous membrane and is not associated with the lining of the vessels.

13. B. The fascia adherens and desmosomes (or macula adherens) form the cell-to-cell junctions of cardiac myocytes, called intercalated disks. Another type of intracellular junction not listed, called a gap junction, also aids in the rapid conduction of electrical signals via channels called connexons. Desmosomes are small dot-like attachments composed of intermediate filaments. A tight junction, also known as a zonula occludens, is a circumferential attachment of neighboring cells. This type of attachment is often involved in the maintenance of polarity across epithelial and endothelial linings. An adherent junction, or zonula adherens, is also a circumferential attachment of neighboring epithelial cells. These attachments are associated with actin filaments, which are used in the apical contraction of epithelia.

14. E. The general pattern of action potential for a pacemaker cell is as follows: Phase 0 is represented by a slow upstroke from the opening of calcium channels that trigger the AP. This is followed by phase 3, a gradual repolarization from the closure of calcium channels and opening of potassium channels. Phase 4 is then characterized by a slow leak of sodium into the cell until there is enough of a depolarization, and phase 0 begins again. The general pattern of action potential for a regular cardiac myocyte is as follows: Phase 0 is the rapid upstroke as voltage-gated sodium channels opens (this is quite different from the slow upstroke of the calcium channels in pacemaker cells). Phase 1 is a slight repolarization from the efflux of potassium (not present in pacemaker cells). Phase 2 is the plateau phase, where voltage-gated calcium channels lead to an influx of calcium, which balances the efflux of potassium (not present in pacemaker cells). Phase 3 is very similar in that the pacemaker cells have efflux of potassium. Phase 4 is the resting state, where the cell waits at its resting membrane potential until another action potential is triggered.

15. E. The most likely cause of the hypotension in only one arm is either the increased parasympathetic output to the region or a decrease in the sympathetic output. For this question it is important to also look at the other symptoms suggesting a decrease in sympathetic output, as in Horner's syndrome. Choice A might lead to hypotension in one arm, but it could not account for the other symptoms. Atherosclerosis is a systemic process of plaque deposition and would not lead to a selective occlusion of one artery. In addition, this would still not lead to hypotension of the left arm. Coarctation of the aorta most commonly results in increased blood pressure of the upper extremities and hypotension of the lower extremities, as blood supply is cut off after the left subclavian artery. MIs, no matter how many, would not result in the symptoms present, especially not in the distribution described.

16. D. The tibial artery forms just distal to the popliteal artery as it passes posterior to the knee. This artery quickly divides into anterior and posterior segments. The anterior tibial artery passes through the interosseous membrane to run down the anterior aspect of the lower leg. After it gives off the peroneal artery in the proximal portion of the lower leg, the posterior tibial travels between the tibialis posterior and flexor digitorum longus muscles. The posterior tibial then passes behind the medial malleolus under the flexor retinaculum to supply the plantar aspect of the foot. Once on the plantar surface, the posterior tibial branches into medial and lateral plantar arteries. Arcuate arteries are anastomotic connections found in the distal portion of the foot.

17. C. This patient most likely has a dilated cardiomyopathy secondary to years of alcohol abuse. Dilated cardiomyopathy has multiple etiologies, including genetic factors, pregnancy, hemochromatosis, doxorubicin administration, cocaine abuse, and alcohol abuse. Patients can present at a wide range of ages and the initial symptomatology is usually congestive heart failure (e.g., orthopnea). These patients often develop severe systolic dysfunction, leading to drastically reduced ejection fractions. Aortic stenosis is the only other option that might produce the symptoms presented. However, the history makes aortic stenosis much less likely, owing to the onset of orthopnea at age 40. Aortic stenosis, on the other hand, would present earlier in life if it were due to a bicuspid valve or later in life if it were a result of calcific aortic stenosis. *Cor pulmonale* refers to pulmonary hypertensive disease. This eventually leads to right ventricular hypertrophy and right ventricular heart failure. Hypertrophic cardiomyopathy results in impaired compliance, leading to diastolic rather than systolic dysfunction. These patients develop hypertensive disease and would not show a decrease in ejection fraction. Restrictive cardiomyopathy is another disease similar to hypertrophic cardiomyopathy in that it also deals with impaired compliance and diastolic dysfunction.

18. C. Digoxin is a positive inotropic agent, meaning that it increases the contractility of the heart. Its mechanism of action is to block the sodium-potassium pump to block efflux of sodium out of the cell. This higher concentration of sodium in the cell increases the activity of the sodium-calcium exchanger, thus increasing the amount of calcium pumped into the cell. Ultimately the concentration of calcium in the cell is proportional to the contractility. Digoxin has a very narrow therapeutic range and its levels must be constantly measured to prevent premature beats, tachycardia, and fibrillation. Adenosine is a very short-acting blocker of conduction at the AV node and would not be useful in a CHF patient with congestive heart failure. In addition, its short half-life would prevent oral administration or home use. Carvedilol is a beta-blocker that also shares some alpha-blocking effects, and lisinopril is an ACE inhibitor. While both are commonly used for CHF patients, neither has the mechanism of action described, nor do they need close monitoring with blood work. Warfarin is the only other drug listed that requires constant monitoring with blood work. Levels of warfarin must be titrated up to a therapeutic international normalized ratio (INR). Its mechanism of action is to inhibit vitamin K–dependent clotting factors and thus prevent portions of the coagulation cascade.

19. E. Methyldopa, a centrally acting alpha$_2$ agonist similar to clonidine, is the first choice for hypertensive pregnant women and results in a decreased sympathetic output, thus reducing blood pressure. Methyldopa has shown no threatening side effects and no teratogenic effects on the fetus. Diuretics such as hydrochlorothiazide and furosemide are generally avoided owing to the electrolyte imbalances they may cause and the possibility of dehydration, resulting in compromised blood flow to the fetus. ACE inhibitors (lisinopril) and angiotensin II receptor antagonists (losartan) are both contraindicated in pregnant women. Both cross the placenta, leaving the fetus susceptible to the effects of the drug, which can lead to renal failure, anuria, and hypotension. The chest x-ray shown (Figure 3-3) is a normal posteroanterior view of the chest. There is no evidence of infiltrate or effusion.

20. B. Aspirin is currently the only medication proven to have long-term benefits for the prevention of heart attacks. Aspirin is the only medication listed for the prevention of platelet aggregation, which is thought to be the etiology of coronary artery obstruction and subsequent MIs. Tissue plasminogen activator (tPA) and heparin is the first-line treatment if the patient is having a MI. These agents serve for immediate thrombolysis if given within 6 hr of the infarct. Streptokinase is also considered to be first-line therapy to reestablish vessel patency. Heparin should be given for 48 hr after infarct if tissue plasminogen activator or streptokinase was used to lyse the clot initially.

21. D. Alternative medications used to prevent platelet aggregation are the ADP inhibitors ticlopidine and clopidogrel. Blockage of ADP blocks the cross-linking of platelets and prevents aggregation. These drugs offer an effective alternative to aspirin, especially in stroke prophylaxis. Warfarin interferes with the hepatic synthesis of vitamin K–dependent clotting factors. It is metabolized in the liver by hepatic microsomal enzymes. Streptokinase is used to lyse clots in patients with acute MI. Aspirin is a cyclooxygenase inhibitor.

22. C. Administration of quinine has elucidated a genetic defect in this patient. A deficiency of glucose-6-phosphate dehydrogenase is often discovered following a course of a pharmaceutical that causes oxidative stress. Once such stress is present, hemolysis may occur, resulting in hematuria and jaundice. Often Heinz bodies are seen on a blood smear. These pathognomonic cells are RBCs that are oxidized and have precipitated hemoglobin. Beta thalassemia is a variable genetic defect of hemoglobin formation. Heterozygous patients are often asymptomatic until challenged with strenuous exercise or oxygen deficit. Homozygotes, however, have severe pathology, with decreased oxygen perfusion and hemolysis. Homozygotes have a life expectancy of only 20 years. Polycythemia vera is a neoplastic process found in older patients who have accumulated too many RBCs. The symptoms do not match this patient. Treatment for this disorder is regular phlebotomy. Sickle cell anemia is another genetic defect involving hemoglobin. Symptoms often result from vasoocclusion. If severe enough, such an attack is called a sickle cell crisis.

23. A. Fetal erythropoiesis is a complicated process that occurs in a variety of settings in the developing fetus. All of the choices listed above except myocardium participate in RBC formation at some point during development. The first onset of erythropoiesis occurs around week 3 within the yolk sac. This coincides with gastrulation, the formation of the three germ layers, because the blood cells are derived from the mesoderm. Some time around weeks 6 to 8, the liver becomes one of the erythropoietic organs; it remains so until week 30. The spleen also produces RBCs over a similar period from weeks 9 to 28. At this point the bone and bone marrow are sufficiently developed for the bone marrow to take over as the primary erythropoietic site. The bone marrow will begin production around week 28 and continue producing RBCs from this point on.

24. D. All of the cardiovascular structures and even the blood cells are derived from mesoderm. The ectoderm, mesoderm, and endoderm form around week 3 in a process called gastrulation. Once the mesoderm layer is formed, organogenesis quickly follows, so that the heart is actually beating soon after week 4. Both the ectoderm and the mesoderm form from the epiblast, and the endoderm is a derivative of the hypoblast of the other early cell layer. The ectoderm leads to a number of structures that fall under the headings surface ectoderm, neuroectoderm, and neural crest. The endoderm is responsible for the formation of most of the gut tube and many of the abdominal and thoracic organs.

25. B. This is a complicated derivation that requires the knowledge and use of two important physiologic equations involving ejection fraction (EF), stroke volume (SV), end-diastolic volume (EDV), cardiac output (CO), and heart rate (HR). First, the equation for ejection fraction: $EF = SV/EDV$. This equation can be converted to $EDV = SV/EF$. Since we know the EF, all we need is to determine stroke volume. SV is determined by $SV = CO/HR$. We know these two parameters, and all that is left is to plug in the numbers.

$$SV = CO/HR \rightarrow SV = (3,000 \text{ mL/min})/(100 \text{ bpm}) \rightarrow SV$$
$$= 30 \text{ mL/beat}$$

$$EDV = SV/EF \rightarrow EDV = (30 \text{ mL/beat})/(50\%) \rightarrow EDV$$
$$= 60 \text{ mL/beat}$$

26. B. Atrial septal defects (ASDs) are often mild until later in life. Due to the low pressures of both atria, only a small left-to-right shunt will occur. Over time this increase in the return of blood to the right heart leads to pulmonary hypertension and right ventricular hypertrophy. Finally, right-sided heart failure will result with peripheral congestive symptoms. The only option for treatment is surgical repair. ASD is associated with a left-to-right shunt, which results in late cyanosis. The S$_1$ heart sound is loud, and there is wide splitting of a fixed S$_2$ heart sound. Ventricular septal defect (VSD) is associated with late cyanosis because of the left-to-right shunt. Patent ductus arteriosus (PDA) is also associated with a left-to-right shunt and late cyanosis.

The PDA can close with indomethacin treatment. Tetralogy of Fallot is the most common cause of early cyanosis. It is the result of a right-to-left shunt and results in early cyanosis.

27. E. This is actually a combination of two answers: transposition of the great vessels and a PDA. With transposition of the great vessels, the aorta is attached to the right ventricle and the pulmonary artery is attached to the left ventricle. This leads to two separate circuits and the inability to supply oxygenated blood to the rest of the body. This congenital defect is incompatible with life unless another defect is present to allow for exchange between the two separate circuits. The PDA serves this purpose in this patient by allowing oxygenated blood to pass from the pulmonary artery to the aortic artery. Treatment for this infant will require prostaglandins to maintain patency of the PDA until surgery can be performed to correct the transposition. Aortic stenosis is another common congenital heart defect with a bicuspid aortic valve. ASD is associated with a left-to-right shunt, which results in late cyanosis. The S_1 heart sound is loud and there is wide splitting of a fixed S_2 heart sound. Tetralogy of Fallot is the most common cause of early cyanosis. It is the result of a right-to-left shunt and causes early cyanosis.

28. B. Cardiac output in this situation can be determined by using the Fick principle. The equation is as follows:

$$\text{Cardiac output} = O_2 \text{ consumption}/(\text{arterial } O_2 \text{ content} - \text{venous } O_2 \text{ content})$$

Therefore substitution into the equation yields:

$$\text{cardiac output} = 400/(0.25 - 0.15) = 4{,}000 \text{ mL/min,}$$

$$\text{or } 4.0 \text{ L/min}$$

Heart rate and arterial oxygen saturation are not needed in this calculation.

29. C. This patient may have a pheochromocytoma. Phenoxybenzamine is an irreversible alpha$_1$ and alpha$_2$ antagonist used in the management of pheochromocytoma. The large amounts of epinephrine and norepinephrine interact with alpha$_1$ and alpha$_2$ receptors. The CT scan reveals a right adrenal mass. Often the release of these catecholamines is pulsatile and phenoxybenzamine can block the receptors, stopping the surge of the pheochromocytoma. Clonidine is a centrally acting alpha$_2$ antagonist that functions to decrease normal sympathetic output. Enalapril is an ACE inhibitor blocking the formation of angiotensin II. Angiotensin II plays no role in the pathology of a pheochromocytoma and therefore this would be of no help. Reserpine works by blocking ATP-dependent transport of norepinephrine into storage vesicles in both the peripheral nervous system (PNS) and the CNS. Although this drug would provide some protection and block some of the norepinephrine production, pheochromocytomas produce and release mostly epinephrine. Thus epinephrine would still be released. Verapamil is a calcium channel blocker, thus decreasing the contraction of both cardiac and smooth muscle. However, most of its effects on the heart serve to decrease contractility; it would therefore provide only minimal relief from the contracting blood vessels throughout the cardiovascular system.

30. C. The most common cardiac malformation associated with Down's syndrome is septum primum, a type of atrial septal defect due to abnormalities in the endocardial cushion. Because of its key location, a defect in the formation of the endocardial cushion can lead to many cardiac malformations, including atrial and ventricular septal defects as well as anomalies involving the great vessels (i.e., transposition of the great vessels and tetralogy of Fallot). However, the most common malformation in Down's patients is septum primum. Coarctation of the aorta is narrowing of the aorta; it can present with hypertension limited to the upper extremities and is often associated with Turner's syndrome. Patent ductus arteriosus is failure of the fetal ductus arteriosus to close and is not related to Down's syndrome.

31. B. Rheumatic heart disease is a potential late sequela of pharyngeal infection with group A beta-hemolytic streptococci. It is diagnosed on the basis of the Jones criteria and elevated antistreptolysin O (ASO) titers. The mitral valve is the valve affected most often, followed by aortic valve. The tricuspid valve is sometimes affected along with the mitral and aortic valves. The pulmonary valve is rarely involved. The valve of the coronary sinus is not involved.

32. C. The right lower border of the heart on an AP radiograph comprises the right atrium. The upper portion of this border comprises the superior vena cava. The left border consists of the left ventricle, left atrium, pulmonary trunk, and aortic arch. The inferior border consists of the right ventricle. The superior border is formed by the superior vena cava, aorta, and pulmonary trunk.

33. C. Left ventricular rupture is most likely between 3 and 7 days following an acute MI. This potentially catastrophic complication can result from mechanical weakening of the vessel wall due to necrosis. In addition, by the seventh day, a yellow infarct area surrounded by a red border is seen grossly; microscopically, the neutrophils are replaced by macrophages. At 12 hr, gross changes may include slight swelling and color changes. Microscopic changes include the appearance of neutrophils. By 2 days postinfarction, there is increased color and swelling with well-developed coagulative necrosis. One month after the infarction, starting between the second and fourth weeks, fibrosis will occur. Between 3 and 6 months following a myocardial infarction, a well-developed scar will have developed.

34. D. Alteplase (tissue plasminogen activator) is a thrombolytic that is claimed to convert fibrin-bound plasminogen to plasmin. Plasmin is the most important fibrinolytic protease that splits fibrin into split products. Other thrombolytic agents include streptokinase and urokinase. Heparin acts as an immediate anticoagulant by its activation of antithrombin III. Its effectiveness is monitored by the activated partial thromboplastin time (aPTT). Warfarin (Coumadin) is used for chronic anticoagulation that interferes with the vitamin K–dependent clotting factors II, V, VII, IX, and X as well as proteins C and S. Its effectiveness is monitored by prothrombin time (PT) values. Aspirin interferes in platelet interaction and can be monitored by bleeding time.

35. C. Since this man has a history of asthma, a selective beta₁ blocker is needed to reduce the risk of bronchospasm. Metoprolol is the only selective beta₁ blocker listed here and would be the best choice for this patient. Procainamide is an antiarrhythmic class I sodium-channel blocker. It is associated with a reversible systemic lupus-like syndrome. Propranolol is a nonselective beta-blocker and has the potential to cause bronchospasm. Dobutamine is predominately a beta₁ agonist used to stimulate the heart. Amphetamines, used for treatment of narcolepsy and attention deficit disorder, are indirect nonspecific agonists that cause the release of stored catecholamines.

36. B. This patient has type 2a hypercholesterolemia, classified as having elevated cholesterol in the form of LDL. It can be inherited with the problem related to a deficiency of LDL receptors. Heterozygotes for the hereditary form may develop cardiovascular disease early, at 30 to 50 years of age. Homozygotes for the disorder can develop cardiovascular disease in childhood. Type 1 is characterized by having only elevated chylomicrons. Type 2b is characterized by elevations in both cholesterol and triglycerides in the form of LDL and VLDL. Type 3 is characterized by elevations in chylomicron remnants and IDL. Type 5 is characterized by elevations of VLDL and chylomicrons.

37. D. In the fourth week the heart begins to form and starts to beat. Early development of the heart, often before some women know they are pregnant, makes the heart extremely susceptible to teratogens. Implantation in the uterus as a blastocyst occurs at 1 week. Within 2 weeks, a bilaminar disk is formed. Within week 3, gastrulation occurs while the primitive streak, notochord, and neural plate begin to form. By the tenth week, the genitalia have female or male characteristics.

38. C. Kawasaki's disease is a generalized vasculitis of unknown origin that is a leading cause of heart disease in children living in the United States. This disease rarely occurs after the age of 8, and children of Asian ancestry experience the highest incidence. Kawasaki's disease is usually self-limited, but coronary artery abnormalities can develop in 20% of untreated patients. Aspirin can be given to reduce the inflammation, and intravenous gamma globulin given within the first 10 days can reduce coronary complications. Giant cell arteritis (also known as temporal arteri-

tis) typically affects elderly females, who may present with headaches, jaw claudication, and impaired vision. Takayasu's arteritis is known as "pulseless disease"; it typically affects young Asian females. It involves thickening of the aortic arch and/or proximal great vessels and can result in weak pulses in the upper extremities. Buerger's disease is known as "smoker's disease"; it results in vasculitis of the intermediate and small peripheral arteries and veins. Treatment is to quit smoking.

39. B. Acute bacterial endocarditis involves only the tricuspid valve; its most likely etiology is the intravenous use of illicit drugs. Virulent organisms such as *Staphylococcus aureus* can infect previously normal valves, causing marked damage and potentially giving rise to septic emboli. *Staph. aureus* is commonly found on the skin and accounts for > 60% of all endocarditis infections in intravenous drug users. Rheumatic fever most commonly damages the mitral and aortic valves. Systemic lupus erythematosus causes Libman-Sacks endocarditis; valvular vegetations are usually found on both sides of the mitral valve and do not embolize. The tricuspid valve is not typically associated with congenital heart disease. A consequence of syphilis is dilation of the aorta and valve ring. This often affects the aortic root and ascending aorta.

40. A. A typical umbilical cord contains two umbilical arteries and one umbilical vein. The umbilical arteries carry deoxygenated blood from the fetus to the placenta while the umbilical vein supplies oxygenated blood from the placenta to the fetus. A single umbilical artery is associated with congenital and chromosomal anomalies. Maternal drug abuse and mental retardation are not in themselves related to a single umbilical artery. Renal agenesis is not associated with a single umbilical artery.

41. E. The right ventricle occupies most of the anterior cardiac surface. This chamber and the pulmonary artery form a wedge structure behind and to the left of the sternum. It is the mostly likely chamber to be penetrated at the described site of the stab wound. The right atrium forms the right border of the heart and is not likely to be damaged. The pulmonary trunk is located more superiorly than the described stab wound. The left atrium is mostly posterior. The left ventricle is behind the right ventricle and to the left. It forms the left lateral margin of the heart.

42. E. The presence of peripheral edema, splenomegaly, and nutmeg liver all point to right-sided heart failure. Right-sided heart failure may be a consequence of either pulmonary hypertension or left-sided heart failure. The inability of the right ventricle to clear the venous return leads to congestion of all the major blood storage sites, such as the spleen, liver, and peripheral veins. Although left-sided heart failure may eventually lead to right-sided failure, it would first present with symptoms of congestive heart failure, such as pulmonary edema. Restrictive cardiomyopathy, associated with sarcoidosis or amyloidosis, mainly decreases the compliance of the ventricles, impairing their ability to fill. Owing to the nature of restrictive cardiomyopathy, such a patient would likely present with left-sided heart failure in addition to manifesting the systemic effects associated with sarcoidosis or amyloidosis. Rheumatic fever follows infection with *Streptococcus pyogenes.* Aschoff bodies in the myocardium are diagnostic for rheumatic fever, which generally presents with mitral or aortic stenosis, not heart failure. Aortic stenosis may be a sequela of rheumatic fever or may present in elderly patients as calcific aortic stenosis. This pathology may, over long periods, lead to left-sided heart failure, but it would not directly insult the right side of the heart.

43. D. A third heart sound (S_3) in a person above age 40 is almost certainly pathological and associated with heart failure. However, a physiological S_3 is often heard in children and is common during the last trimester of pregnancy. The murmur is dull and of low pitch, heard best with the bell of the stethoscope. Pulmonary wheezing, ascites, and orthopnea can all be signs of heart failure but are not as specific as an S_3. A fourth heart sound, S_4, is a dull, low-pitched murmur heard with the bell of the stethoscope. It can be heard occasionally in an apparently normal person, especially in well-trained athletes and older individuals. More commonly, it is due to increased resistance to ventricular filling following atrial contraction.

44. D. Thromboxane A_2 (TXA$_2$) stimulates aggregation and can cause vasoconstriction. This decreased blood flow to the site of a clot can cause ischemia. Aspirin prevents MI by inhibiting cyclooxygenase and thereby preventing the synthesis of TxA$_2$. Bradykinin is part of the kinin pathway, which increases vasodilation, vascular permeability, and pain. It is inhibited ACE. Vasopressin, or antidiuretic hormone (ADH), is secreted by the posterior pituitary. It is stimulated by increased plasma osmolarity and decreased blood volume. Lipoxygenase converts arachidonic acid to various leukotrienes. It is inhibited by zileuton. Phospholipase A_2 is the first enzyme in the arachidonic acid products. It is inhibited by corticosteroids.

45. B. Cardiac output increases by 30 to 50% but systemic vascular resistance decreases, resulting in a fall in arterial blood pressure. This decrease is most likely due to elevated progesterone, leading to smooth muscle relaxation. The systolic blood pressure decreases 5 to 10 mm Hg and the diastolic 10 to 15 mm Hg; these reach their nadirs at week 24. Between 24 weeks' gestation and term, blood pressure slowly returns to pre-pregnancy levels, but it should never exceed them.

46. D. Eisenmenger's syndrome is cardiac failure, with significant right-to-left shunt producing cyanosis due to higher pressure on the right side of the shunt. This condition is usually due to the Eisenmenger complex, a ventricular septal defect with right ventricular hypertrophy and dilatation, severe pulmonary hypertension, and frequent straddling of the defect by a misplaced aortic root. It can also be the result of a PDA. Systemic hypertension, aortic stenosis, mitral insufficiency, and prolapse do not result in right-to-left shunts.

47. B. This history not only provides a general location of the site of the hematoma but also tells us which nerve is adjacent to the vessel. The radial nerve, which supplies the extensor surfaces of the forearm, travels down the posterior aspect of the humerus with the deep artery of the arm (deep brachial artery). In midshaft fractures of the humerus due to the approximation of the nerve and vessel to the bone itself, this nerve and artery are commonly injured. The brachial artery runs along the anteromedial aspect of the arm along with the ulnar, median, and medial cutaneous nerves of the arm. The radial and ulnar arteries are branches of the brachial artery and do not form until the forearm. The posterior circumflex humeral artery also runs adjacent to the humerus but in a more proximal position. The posterior circumflex humeral artery is also adjacent to the axillary nerve, which would exhibit a deficit of the deltoid muscle.

48. A. Aortic stenosis is another common congenital heart defect with a bicuspid aortic valve. Aside from a congenital etiology, aortic stenosis also results from a lifetime of wear and tear, leading to a calcific aortic stenosis in the elderly. This common murmur is heard best along the upper right sternal border. The ECG seen here (Figure 3-7) shows evidence of left ventricular hypertrophy because of pressure load secondary to aortic stenosis. ST-segment depression and T-wave inversion are also seen. VSD is the most common congenital cardiac defect. The size of these defects is often variable; they may decrease in size as the patient grows older. ASD is associated with a left-to-right shunt, which results in late cyanosis. The S_1 heart sound is loud, and there is wide splitting of a fixed S_2. PDA is also associated with a left-to-right shunt and late cyanosis. The PDA can close with indomethacin treatment. Tetralogy of Fallot is the result of a right-to-left shunt and is the most common cause of early cyanosis.

49. C. Mitral regurgitation occurs when the mitral valve fails to close fully during systole. Blood regurgitates from the left ventricle to the left atrium, causing a murmur. The murmur is described as a blowing holosystolic murmur of medium to high pitch that radiates to the axilla (less often to the left sternal border). Mitral valve prolapse is the most common valvular lesion, occurring in approximately 6% of the population. It is characterized by degeneration of the ground substance of the valve and results in a floppy cusp that prolapses in the left atrium during systole.

50. E. The umbilical vein delivers blood from the placenta to the fetus; it is where the highest Po$_2$ level in the fetal circulation will be found. The umbilical artery delivers blood from the fetal circulation to the maternal circulation, so it will have a relatively low Po$_2$. The ductus arteriosus, ductus venosus, and ascending aorta are crucial parts of the fetal cardiovascular system, but the blood in these vessels has a lower Po$_2$ level than the initial blood that comes from the placenta.

51. B. Male patients who present with extreme cold sensitivity in their distal extremities must be asked about smoking history. Cold sensitivity in males is a classic presentation of thromboangiitis obliterans (Buerger's disease). The link between this condition and smoking and males is one of its most consistent features. It can later lead to gangrene of the digits, but if caught in the early stages, patients can get relief and not develop more severe manifestations provided they are able to stop smoking. It is also important to ask about alcohol consumption, but in this case it would not help to explain the patient's condition. Hypothyroidism can present with cold sensitivity, but young males are usually not hypothyroid and cold sensitivity is not the only presenting factor. A family history of poor circulation may be useful in this interview, but it will not contribute much to the diagnosis. In fact, you could miss this diagnosis by assuming that the patient has poor circulation. Any time a patient has what appears to be a neuropathy, asking about diabetes is always important. This patient does not have any other manifestations and peripheral neuropathy is usually a late presentation of diabetes.

52. E. This patient has Turner's syndrome. It can be very obscure at birth, and sometimes these infants just have some mild neck swelling. It is more evident at puberty, when the patients do experience menarche. These patients also have a high incidence of coarctation of the aorta, which is evident by weak pulses in the lower extremities. A continuous machinery-like murmur is diagnostic of PDA. These patients have complications before the age of 11. A carotid bruit is usually appreciated in elderly patients with a history of arteriosclerosis. A late systolic murmur is the murmur of mitral valve prolapse (MVP). Although this is a possibility here, this patient is otherwise healthy and MVP usually presents in young women in their twenties. The stem of this question links the findings at birth to the finding at 11 years of age.

53. A. As underwater depth increases, larger amounts of oxygen dissolve in the blood. Once the ascent begins, the dissolved gases come out of the solution and form minute bubbles in the bloodstream and various tissues. Bubbles formed in the lung cause respiratory difficulty. This also leads to substernal chest pain and difficulty breathing. Fat emboli are associated with long bone fractures. Tumor emboli can result from primary cardiac tumors such as myxoma. Thrombus can originate in the deep veins of the lower extremities.

54. B. This patient has evidence of dilated congestive heart failure, a diagnosis supported by the S_3 heart sound. When the ventricle is stiff and noncompliant, it reaches its physical limits. As a result, you hear an S_3. In children, an S_3 is common and normal. When it is appreciated in adults over 40 years of age, it is almost always indicative of congestive heart failure. Hypertrophic cardiomyopathy is a condition that usually presents in teenagers and young adults and as sudden death in athletes. Elderly patients usually do not present with complications from hypertrophic cardiomyopathy. Mitral regurgitation does not present with an S_3 heart sound but rather with a holosystolic murmur. Right heart failure usually presents with jugular venous distension, and the S_3 is not appreciated in patients with right heart failure. Bacterial endocarditis usually presents with typical findings, but an S_3 will not be heard in a patient with bacterial endocarditis.

55. A. This child is in heart failure. The four classic signs of heart failure in children and infants are tachypnea, tachycardia, hepatomegaly, and cardiomegaly. Heart failure in children usually has an underlying cause such as a ventricular septal defect, coarctation of the aorta, or an ASD. It is important in the treatment of this condition to find the underlying cause and treat it. Peripheral edema does not usually present in children with heart failure; it is a classic finding in adults. Total anomalous venous return and transposition of the great vessels usually presents with cyanosis at birth, and this child appeared normal at birth. Still's murmur is an innocent murmur heard in children; it results from vibration of the chordae tendineae.

56. E. At a P_{O_2} of 25 mm Hg, hemoglobin saturation is approximately 50%. This represents the P_{50}, which means that, on average, two of the four heme groups of each hemoglobin molecule have a bound oxygen molecule. Blood with a low P_{O_2} is purely venous, as mixed venous blood would have a P_{O_2} of approximately 40 mm Hg.

57. A. Immediately following transection of the spinal cord, the limbs become flaccid and reflexes are absent. With time, partial recovery and return of reflexes or even hyperreflexia will occur. If the lesion is at C7, there will be loss of sympathetic tone to the heart and, as a result, the heart rate will slow and arterial pressure will decrease. If the lesion is at C1, death ensues. Decorticate posturing occurs when the lesion is at or above the level of the red nucleus. Loss of sympathetic tone to the heart results in hypotension. If the lesion is at C3, breathing will stop because the muscles of respiration are disconnected from the brainstem control centers.

58. B. This child has the classic murmur of a PDA. Often this condition is found in premature infants. The normal time of PDA closure is 4 to 8 weeks after birth. If a PDA is detected early in the infant's life, indomethacin, a strong-acting nonsteroidal anti-inflammatory drug (NSAID), may be given over a short course to close the PDA. It functions as all NSAIDs do in that it decreases the production of prostaglandins. PGE_2, in particular, is responsible for maintaining the patency of the PDA and may actually be given in the presence of a tricuspid atresia or transposition of the great vessels, where the PDA is needed for proper delivery of oxygenated blood. Hydrocortisone and all glucocorticoids block production of both leukotrienes and prostaglandins by inhibiting phospholipase A_2. However, this would not be effective for the closure of a PDA and would be detrimental to the developing infant. Mifepristone (also known as RU-486) is an abortifacient and functions to inhibit the effects of progestin soon after conception, leading to abortion of the embryo. Misoprostol is a synthetic PGE_1 analog used to protect the gastric mucosa, especially in the prevention of NSAID-induced peptic ulcers. In addition to this function, it also maintains PDAs and is used to induce labor. The chest x-ray (Figure 3-8) reveals enlargement of the pulmonary artery.

59. E. Cardiac output is determined by a formula that relates oxygen consumption to the difference between the oxygen content of the peripheral blood and that of the mixed venous blood. For the present condition, cardiac output = 250 mL/min divided by 0.20 mL/O_2/mL − 0.15 mL/O_2/mL = 5,000 mL/min or 5.0 L/min.

60. C. A common and quick method for differentiating a musculoskeletal from a cardiac issue is the ability to reproduce the pain manually. If the pain can be reproduced, it almost certainly rules out a cardiac cause and is said to be muscular. Having the patient run can often reproduce actual heart ischemia and would not be advisable. Neurological examination or testing of the deep tendon reflexes would have little to no value in distinguishing cardiac from musculoskeletal issues. Heart auscultation may provide evidence of murmurs but no quick information about cardiac status.

61. B. Only three of the above choices are actual types of recognized angina. Prinzmetal's angina is defined as causing intermittent chest pain at rest and is generally believed to be caused by vasospasm. Unstable angina is described as prolonged or recurrent pain at rest and tends to be indicative of a potential myocardial infarction. Stable angina, which is the most common form, is chest pain precipitated by exertion and relieved by rest. Vasodilators can also be used to help relieve stress-induced ischemia. The other choices are distractors and have no bearing on an actual diagnosis.

62. D. A transmural infarction, by definition, crosses all the layers of the cardiac muscle, from the endocardium to the epicardium. Subendocardial infarction is limited to the interior third of the left ventricular wall. Cardiac tamponade is increased pressure and compression of the heart secondary to hemorrhage of blood into the pericardial sack. Ruptured cardiac muscle is an actual rupture of the muscle and not associated with penetration through the muscle.

63. A. Aschoff bodies are classically associated with rheumatic fever, which, based on the above presentation, would be a likely diagnostic sign for this young patient. His prior history of tonsillitis, fevers, mood swings, and joint pain all support the diagnosis of rheumatic fever. Caput medusae are dilated veins around the umbilicus and are related to liver issues. Parotitis is normally associated with mumps, not rheumatic fever. Sialadenitis is caused by blockage of the parotid glands, usually secondary to a stone in the salivary duct. Pinpoint pupils are associated with opioid overdose, and do not mesh with the other symptoms or the patient's age.

64. D. The normal time for development of a gray-white scar is usually 3 to 6 months. In the first 48 hr, serum levels continue to rise, and this lesion is still quite new. After approx-

imately a week, phagocytosis is in full effect, reducing the debris in the lesion. From 6 months to 1 year, no significant cardiac changes are to be noted in the patient.

65. B. The mitral valve is the one most commonly and frequently involved, with a frequency of almost 50%. Possible effects are secondary to stenosis, insufficiency, or a mixture of the two. The aortic valve has a tendency to be affected in conjunction with the mitral valve, but rarely without mitral involvement. The tricuspid valve tends to be affected in only about 5% of cases of rheumatic heart disease. The pulmonary valve is infrequently included among the valves injured by rheumatic heart disease. The myocardial valve is a fictitious valve and therefore not affected either.

66. E. The most likely subject about which this young woman should be educated is that of subacute endocarditis. It is a bacterial infection, usually caused by *Streptococcus viridans*, and has an increased tendency to occur in patients with a history of congenital heart disease or prior valve disease. Acute endocarditis is caused by *Staphylococcus aureus* and is found in conjunction with infection in another part of the body. Pericarditis has a tendency to be associated with rheumatic fever.

67. D. Nonbacterial thrombotic endocarditis is differentiated from the other forms mainly by the sterile emboli that form as a result of the fibrin deposits on the valve leaflets. None of the other forms of endocarditis is associated with cancer or is sterile. Libman-Sacks endocarditis is associated with systemic lupus erythematosus, and it does not produce sterile vegetations.

68. A. A diagnosis of syphilitic aortitis describes an inflammation and dilatation of the aortic valve ring secondary to an untreated syphilis infection. This patient must be treated immediately for her reportable illness and begin taking medication. If the aortic ring were unable to open, she would not be able to sustain life. Calcifications of the aortic valve are related to rheumatic heart disease and infective endocarditis. To estimate the percentage of heart function on the basis of a written diagnosis is not recommended.

69. B. Conduction through the AV node is represented by the PR interval. This area is commonly monitored for AV block, where signal transmission may be slowed and occasionally blocked or completely blocked. These conditions are labeled first-, second-, and third-degree blocks, respectively. The P wave represents atrial depolarization. The QRS wave represents ventricular depolarization. A wide QRS implies abnormal conduction. The QT interval represents the approximate time of ventricular systole. If it is prolonged by drug toxicity or electrolyte disturbances, arrhythmias may ensue. The T wave is the ventricular repolarization phase of the ECG. Spiked or large T waves may indicate hyperkalemia. The ECG here shows features of left ventricular hypertrophy. An area of R- and T-wave inversion is also seen.

70. B. Coarctation of the aorta presents with the clinical symptoms described here. The notching of the ribs, along with the disparity in upper/lower blood pressures, is pathognomonic for coarctation of the aorta. Atrial septal defect usually doesn't present clinically until adulthood. PDA is known for having a "machine gun–like murmur." Tetralogy of Fallot is noted by cyanosis at birth and by ensuing clinical issues, with a tendency to maintain a Valsalva position so as to minimize the right-to-left shunting.

71. D. Beriberi heart, also known as a thiamine-induced cardiomyopathy, is a cause of this clinical presentation shown above. Chronic consumption of alcohol can also produce this presentation, but a night of binge drinking would not be able to create the ventricular dilatation. Intravenous heroin can certainly lead to death, but not with this presentation. Ventricular septal defect could lead to right-sided but not bilateral heart failure.

72. E. Serous pericarditis is the appropriate diagnosis for this fluid. Its production is associated with viral infections, systemic lupus erythematosus, and rheumatic fever. Hemorrhagic pericarditis is recognized by a bloody, inflammatory exudate, not clear exudate. Purulent exudate is characterized by cloudy or purulent fluid. Fibrinous exudate is marked by a high concentration of fibrin. *Infectious exudate* is a fictitious term and therefore not applicable.

73. E. The classic presentation of right-sided heart failure is indicated by renal hypoxia, which in turn causes increased retention of fluids and edema of the extremities. Hepatosplenomegaly is also a common finding in this type of heart failure. Cerebral anoxia and hydrothorax are both symptomatic of left-sided heart failure. Bilateral heart failure is a combination of right- and left-sided components and can ultimately lead to cardiac nonfunction (death).

74. C. Hypertension is the most common cause of left ventricular hypertrophy, along with aortic/mitral valve disease. Asthma and chronic obstructive pulmonary disease have no bearing on the formation of thickened left ventricular muscle. Lack of exercise and smoking can both increase the risk and probability of developing hypertension, but neither one independently will result in a creation of left ventricular hypertrophy.

75. C. The first heart sound (S_1) is first heard at the point produced by the closure of the mitral and tricuspid valve (Figure 3-10), defining the onset of ventricular systole. The first part of this cycle is defined by isovolumetric ventricular contraction, followed by rapid ventricular ejection (indicated by point C) and finally reduced ventricular ejection. The second heart sound is labeled point D and is made by the closure of the aortic and pulmonic valves. It is the beginning of diastole. Point A is the beginning of atrial systole and can be the cause of the fourth heart sound. Point E is the start of rapid ventricular filling from the atria. Rapid blood flow from the atria into the ventricles causes the third heart sound, which is normal in children but associated with disease in adults.

Chapter 4 Central and Peripheral Nervous Systems

Questions

1. A 45-year-old construction worker with complaints of chronic back pain is found to have a herniation of the intervertebral disc between the L4 and L5 vertebrae. With which of the following symptoms is he most likely to present?

A. Bladder distention

B. Fecal incontinence

C. Inability to plantarflex the foot

D. Weakness of muscles innervated by the L4 spinal cord segment

E. Weakness of muscles innervated by the L5 spinal cord segment

2. A 24-year-old woman in her twenty-sixth week of gestation finds out that the fetus she is carrying will be born anencephalic. Which of the following clues led to this diagnosis?

A. Oligohydramnios and decreased alpha-fetoprotein

B. Oligohydramnios and increased alpha-fetoprotein

C. Polyhydramnios and decreased alpha-fetoprotein

D. Polyhydramnios and increased alpha-fetoprotein

3. A 21-year-old man was brought to the emergency department by law enforcement for disorderly conduct and an elevated blood alcohol concentration on the Breathalyzer test. He is displaying ataxia and dysdiadochokinesia. His dysfunction lies in an area of the central nervous system that is derived from which of the following?

A. Diencephalon

B. Mesencephalon

C. Metencephalon

D. Myelencephalon

E. Telencephalon

4. A 27-year-old woman gives birth to a child that has a defect in his lower back demonstrating the protrusion of meninges and spinal cord from the spinal canal. Which of the following actions during pregnancy would have most decreased the risk of this disease?

A. Abstinence from alcohol consumption

B. Avoidance of x-ray imaging

C. Calcium supplementation

D. Close monitoring of fetal growth

E. Maternal diet rich in leafy vegetables and fruits

5. A 10-year-old child is unable to achieve many of the cognitive milestones appropriate for his age group and has impaired overall socioadaptive behavior. His mental age is determined to be 6 years. What is the most common cause of this disorder?

A. Head injury

B. High maternal age at conception

C. Hypoxia during birth

D. Maternal alcohol consumption during pregnancy

E. Perinatal infection

6. An 8-year-old girl is brought to the emergency department after being bitten by a spider. She describes the spider as black, with thin legs and a red design on its abdomen. The toxin from this spider elicits its neurotoxic effect by:

A. Binding presynaptically at the neuromuscular junction, resulting in excessive release of acetylcholine

B. Inhibiting glycine release from the Renshaw cells in the spinal cord

C. Inhibiting the release of acetylcholine at the neuromuscular junction

D. Irreversibly binding nicotinic receptors to prevent acetylcholine action

E. Stimulating the release of GABA at the neuromuscular junction

7. A 30-year-old man undergoes a computed tomography (CT) scan of his abdomen after a motor vehicle accident. No acute abdominal injuries are found, but many cysts are incidentally found on both of his kidneys. The kidneys are also of slightly larger than normal size. Which of the following central nervous system pathologies are most strongly associated with this finding?

A. Cerebellar hemangioma

B. Cysticercosis

C. Embolic infarction

D. Glioblastoma multiforme

E. Subarachnoid hemorrhage

8. A 6-year-old boy is brought to the emergency department 3 hr after being bitten on the hand by a raccoon. Other children that witnessed the event report that the raccoon was walking through the open playground and did not seem afraid of the many children that had gathered to look at it. It seemed to be salivating profusely and behaving strangely. Which of the following histological findings could be found in this child?

A. Councilman bodies

B. Degeneration of the anterior horn cells of the spinal cord

C. Giant cells in the cerebral cortex with eosinophilic inclusions in both the nucleus and cytoplasm

D. Infiltration of neutrophils at the bite site

E. Negri bodies in hippocampus and Purkinje cells

9. A 36-year-old woman presents to her primary care physician with complaints of muscle weakness in her legs and paralysis of her toes. Her disease began as only weakness in her feet and toes. She also has visible fasciculations in her upper and lower extremities as well as her tongue. Vibratory sense is present bilaterally in her lower extremities. Which of the following is true of this disease?

   A. Inherited in an X-linked recessive manner

   B. Long-term glucose dysregulation leads to this disease

   C. Most common motor neuron disease

   D. Only the lateral corticospinal tracts are affected

   E. Patients usually recover with supportive care

10. Magnetic resonance imaging (MRI) of a 49-year-old man reveals degeneration of the mammillary bodies. Physical examination indicates peripheral motor and sensory loss. Which of the following should be suspected in a patient with these findings?

   A. Alcoholism

   B. Amyotrophic lateral sclerosis

   C. *Diphyllobothrium latum* infestation

   D. Pernicious anemia

   E. Subacute sclerosing panencephalitis

11. A 1-year-old child develops bilateral leukocoria. This child's disease can occur as a result of a deletion of the Rb gene. On which chromosome would this deletion be evident if this child were karyotyped?

   A. 3

   B. 4

   C. 13

   D. 19

   E. 21

12. A 72-year-old man has recently had progressive difficulty with word associations and memory. A CT scan and MRI are obtained (see Figure 4-1). What is the most likely explanation for these findings?

   A. Cerebral atrophy

   B. Granovacuolar degeneration

   C. Hirano bodies

   D. Neurofibrillary tangles

   E. Neurotic plaques

13. A 67-year-old man presents to his primary care physician complaining of food not having any taste and suddenly having very sensitive hearing. Physical examination would most likely reveal which of the following clinical deficits?

   A. Flaccid facial paralysis

   B. Heightened corneal reflex

   C. Hypersalivation

   D. Lacrimation while eating

   E. Loss in visual acuity

14. During his yearly physical, a 39-year-old man mentions having taken a blow to the head recently; he has noticed a loss of taste on the back of his tongue. He was drinking at a bar, became involved in an altercation, and doesn't really remember the rest of the circumstances. Which examination would be most beneficial in confirming the suspected lesion?

   A. Alternate eye blinking

   B. Corneal reflex

   C. Opposite finger to the nose

   D. Shoulder shrug

   E. Tongue depressor–induced cough

15. A 48-year-old man presents to the emergency department with twitching head movements, grimacing facial movements, arm fasciculations, and distal jerking movements in the lower extremities. This presentation is classic for what neurological disorder?

   A. Bell's palsy

   B. Cerebral palsy

   C. Delirium tremens

   D. Huntington's disease

   E. Parkinson's disease

16. A recently discharged 51-year-old man who was an inpatient at the psychiatric unit presents to his primary care physician for a general physical examination. He has a long history of taking chlorpromazine. Knowing the hypersensitivity that a dopamine agonist buildup can cause, you expect to find which of the following clinical presentations?

Figure 4-1

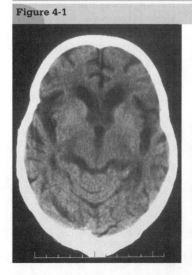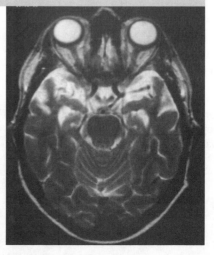

A. Ataxia

B. Nystagmus

C. Priapism

D. Stuttering

E. Tardive dyskinesia

17. You receive a call in your office and are told to expect a new patient who was recently diagnosed with a cerebellar infarct. On exam the patient appears well and in no acute distress. The neurological exam reveals an ataxic gait and another specific cerebellar finding involving alternating movements of the patient's hand against his leg. What is the most likely name of this neurological finding?

A. Dysarthria

B. Dysdiadochokinesia

C. Dysmetria

D. Dyssynergia

E. Nystagmus

18. A 47-year-old man presents to his primary care physician for evaluation of vague neurological symptoms. He informed the doctor that he had been drinking a large amount of alcohol the day before last and had fallen and hit the back of his head on a table. He was very confused after the fall and said he had difficulty walking. He described his gait as feeling as if he were still intoxicated. He was unable to drive owing to his lack of awareness, so his neighbor brought him in. Which area of the brain is most likely affected?

A. Cerebellum

B. Cerebral cortex

C. Medulla

D. Pons

E. Thalamus

19. A 2-year-old infant is brought to the pediatrician for a routine checkup. Upon exam the physician notices many hypopigmented areas on his trunk. There are also areas on his back that resemble keloids. Upon further questioning, it is discovered that the patient's father has a similar condition. What is the most likely diagnosis?

A. Arnold-Chiari malformation

B. Fetal alcohol syndrome

C. Hydrocephalus

D. Neural tube defect

E. Tuberous sclerosis

20. An 18-year-old boy presents to his primary care physician after being involved in a motor vehicle accident. He was in the emergency department the previous evening and was discharged in good condition. He reports that he hit his head on the dashboard and has a contusion on the right side of his temple. He was told that he suffered a contrecoup injury and is asking you to explain what that means. You proceed to tell him that it is a:

A. Nonpenetrating head wound on the right side of the brain

B. Nonpenetrating head wound on the left side of the brain

C. Penetrating head wound on the left side of the brain

D. Penetrating head wound on the right side of the brain

E. Penetrating head wound with minimal hemorrhage

21. An 8-year-old boy is brought to the ambulatory care clinic with fever and a headache that has lasted for 3 days. Physical examination reveals photophobia and nuchal rigidity. Which of the following lab values would most support your suspected diagnosis?

A. Decreased CSF glucose

B. Decreased CSF protein

C. Diplopia

D. Low-grade fevers

E. Low neutrophils

22. A 38-year-old woman presents to her primary care physician with complaints of intermittent periods of heart palpitations, headaches, and sweating. Physical examination reveals that her blood pressure is 160/95 mm Hg. On her previous visits, however, it has been 125/80 mm Hg. Urine metanephrine is positive. An MRI is obtained (Figure 4-2). What is the embryologic origin of the tissue responsible for the production of this condition?

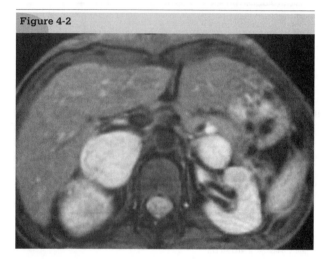

Figure 4-2

A. Endoderm

B. Ectoderm

C. Mesoderm

D. Neural crest

E. Neuroectoderm

23. A newborn baby in the nursery is known to have hydrocephalus. Upon further examination and testing, there are suspected cardiac and lung abnormalities. Periventricular calcifications are identified on radiologic studies. What is the most likely suspected diagnosis for this infant?

A. Escherichia coli

B. Human immunodeficiency virus

C. Kuru

D. Toxoplasmosis

E. Viral meningitis

24. A 28-year-old woman presents to her primary care physician complaining of lower extremity weakness, visual changes, and recent increasing episodes of incontinence. She was fine until the last couple of months and reports that her symptoms seem to be getting worse. She seems really concerned and wonders what other symptoms may present with her disease. What is the most likely explanation for these findings?

A. Excess salivation

B. Hemoptysis

C. Intention tremor

D. Tinnitus

E. Vertigo

25. A 20-year-old woman presents to her primary care physician reporting muscle weakness and paralysis in her toes and legs; she also feels that the weakness is moving up her legs. She has no significant medical history aside from a cold a few weeks earlier, which resolved on its own. Surgical history is limited to a tonsillectomy. What is the best test that can be used to determine the diagnosis?

A. Blood culture

B. Cerebrospinal fluid analysis, glucose

C. Cerebrospinal fluid analysis, protein

D. Gram's stain

E. Urine cytology

26. A 45-year-old man who recently was diagnosed with renal cell carcinoma elects to undergo a kidney transplant. A week before the procedure he is placed on prednisone and tacrolimus. A minute after the transplanted kidney is sewn into place, the surgeon notices a black necrotic area around the cortex. A culture is sent to pathology, where giant cells are found with eosinophilic inclusions in both the nucleus and cytoplasm. Which of the following would be most likely the etiologic agent?

A. Cytomegalovirus

B. Herpes simplex encephalitis

C. Human immunodeficiency virus

D. Poliomyelitis

E. Rabies

27. A 25-year-old primigravida gave birth prematurely to her son 3 days ago. She received no prenatal care and delivered vaginally at her parents' home. She presents to the emergency department, concerned about her son's breathing. She claims that his breathing just doesn't look right. Physical examination reveals respiratory distress in the newborn. Culture reveals a Gram-positive encapsulated coccus. Based on the presentation, what could the mother have been tested and treated for prior to delivery to prevent this?

A. *Chlamydia*

B. Herpes simplex II

C. Human immunodeficiency virus

D. *Streptococcus agalactiae*

E. Syphilis

28. A comatose patient is brought to the emergency department after falling off a ladder. He is suspected of having sustained a severe back injury. The patient is not breathing. He is imme-

diately intubated and oxygen saturation returns to 98%. An MRI of the head is obtained (Figure 4-3). Based on the clinical symptomatology, where is the most likely area of injury in the cervical spine?

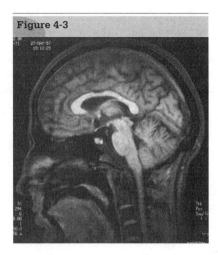

Figure 4-3

A. C1

B. C2

C. C3

D. C4

E. C7

29. A 1-month-old infant is brought to the emergency department by his worried parents. They report that he has been experiencing fever, vomiting, headache, and neck stiffness over the past 48 hr. The child cannot be pacified. Physical examination reveals vasculitic purpura and mild pharyngitis. What is a possible fatal infection that can progress from this condition?

A. Fulminant meningococcemia

B. Guillain-Barré syndrome

C. Jarisch-Herxheimer reaction

D. Lymphogranuloma venereum

E. Pelvic inflammatory disease

30. A 4-day-old neonate is brought to the ambulatory care clinic because of back arching and short, frequent involuntary muscle spasms. Physical examination reveals labored breathing and erythema of the umbilical cord site with purulent discharge. What is the most likely explanation for these findings?

A. *Clostridium tetani*

B. *Escherichia coli*

C. *Haemophilus influenzae*

D. *Neisseria meningitidis*

E. *Streptococcus agalactiae*

31. A 34-year-old woman is being treated for depression. Her symptoms include lethargy, lack of interest in former pleasurable activities, lack of sleep, lack of concentration, and a past attempt of suicide. She has a long-standing history of Valium and cocaine use. Which is the most likely neurotransmitter that has been down-regulated?

A. Acetylcholine
B. Epinephrine
C. Dopamine
D. Glutamate
E. Histidine
F. Histamine

32. A 29-year-old man is brought to the emergency department after attempting to break up a fight between two students. He sustained a laceration to the palmar surface of his hand. Digits 1, 2, 4, and 5 all move normally. However, digit 3 can flex only at the distal interphalangeal joint and not at the metacarpophalangeal joint. Which of the following structures might have been damaged by the laceration?

A. Extensor digitorum
B. Flexor digitorum profundus
C. Flexor digitorum superficialis
D. Flexor pollicis longus
E. Median nerve

33. A 49-year-old man has a deficit of the C5 neurologic level after falling off of a ladder while repairing a leak in his roof. He is brought to the emergency department for further evaluation. He is conscious and has stable vital signs. Which of the following deficits would he be expected to have?

A. Loss of lateral arm sensation
B. Loss of lateral forearm sensation
C. Loss of medial arm sensation
D. Loss of medial forearm sensation

34. A 51-year-old man presents to his primary care physician for an annual checkup. He has a history of diabetes mellitus and has had problems with sensory neuropathic changes in his upper and lower extremities. He is able to walk on his toes and heels but cannot squat. This might suggest which of the following neurological deficits?

A. L4
B. L5
C. S1
D. S2
E. S3
F. S4

35. A 21-year-old man presents to his physician for evaluation of recurrent hoarseness and rhinitis. He has no prior medical history. Physical examination of the oral cavity with a tongue depressor reveals that the pharynx elevates and salivary gland secretion occurs promptly. The tonsils are edematous but without exudate. The most likely explanation for pharyngeal elevation implies that which of the following structures is intact?

A. Abducens nerve
B. Accessory nerve
C. Glossopharyngeal nerve
D. Trigeminal nerve
E. Vestibulocochlear nerve

36. Which of the following structures that carries auditory input from the cochlear nuclei, nuclei of the trapezoid body, and superior olivary nuclei is likely to be involved?

A. Dorsal acoustic striae
B. Intermediate acoustic striae
C. Lateral lemniscus
D. Ventral acoustic striae

37. A 40-year-old man has difficulty turning his head to the right. He is suspected of having an accessory nerve lesion affecting cranial nerve (CN) XI. Based on the assumption of the CN XI lesion, which of the following abnormalities would be expected on physical examination?

A. Inability to fully retract eyelids
B. Left shoulder higher than right
C. Right shoulder higher than left
D. Tongue deviated to the left
E. Tongue deviated to the right

38. A 3-year-old boy has a long history of irritability and self-mutilating behavior. He was the born by spontaneous vaginal delivery at term to a healthy 24-year-old woman. Physical examination of the child is within normal limits. This child's irritability and mutilating behavior may relate to an abundance of

A. adenosine
B. cytosine
C. glycine
D. hypoxanthine
E. inosine

39. A 25-year-old woman presents to the emergency department complaining of decreased vision in both eyes. She also complains of weakness in her lower extremities. Other than diminished reflexes in the lower extremities, weakness of the bulbar muscles, and diminished strength in the lower extremities, her physical examination is unremarkable. She mentioned having had a fever during the past couple of days. An MRI of the head is obtained (Figure 4-4). What is the most likely finding on cerebrospinal fluid (CSF) analysis?

A. Decreased glucose
B. Increased protein
C. Immunoglobulin light chains
D. Oligoclonal bands
E. Pick bodies

40. A 55-year-old man, a retired coal miner, is admitted to the hospital complaining of visual problems. He denies any trauma to his eyes. On exam his extraocular muscles are intact but he has difficulty seeing objects placed in his left visual field. His pupils are equally round and reactive to light and accommodation. There is no conjunctival injection. What is the most likely site of injury?

A. Geniculocalcarine tract
B. Optic tract
C. Optic chiasm
D. Optic nerve
E. Pretectal region

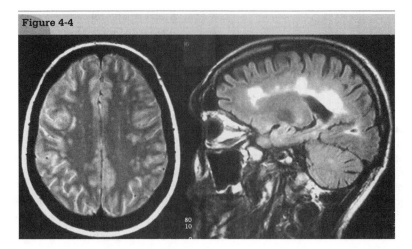

Figure 4-4

41. A 36-year-old man is brought to the emergency department after a motor vehicle accident in which he was a passenger. Wanting to test vestibular/visual integrity, you place three drops of cold water into the patient's right ear canal. Which of the following reactions would then be most indicative of a benign result?

   A. Chills and shivering
   B. Eyes moving to the left
   C. Eyes moving to the right
   D. Pupils constricted
   E. Pupils dilated

42. A 43-year-old man sustains a severe head injury and is now complaining of loss of sweet and salty taste sensations. Which cranial nerve was most likely affected by the head injury?

   A. Cranial nerve II
   B. Cranial nerve IV
   C. Cranial nerve VI
   D. Cranial nerve VII
   E. Cranial nerve IX

43. While driving her car, a 23-year-old woman is struck by another driver. The force of impact drives the temporal area of her skull against the window. She develops a mild headache but does not lose consciousness. Several hours later, she develops a severe headache with nausea and vomiting. Which is the most likely diagnosis?

   A. Bacterial meningitis
   B. Berry aneurysm of the circle of Willis with rupture
   C. Epidural hematoma
   D. Subarachnoid hemorrhage
   E. Subdural hematoma

44. A 65-year-old woman presents to the emergency department complaining of visual difficulties that began while she was working in her garden. Examination reveals ptosis, hemianhidrosis, miosis, and apparent enophthalmos of the left side. Four hours later, her symptoms have resolved completely. An MRI demonstrates no apparent cerebral infarct. What is the most likely explanation for these findings?

   A. Completed stroke
   B. Crescendo transient ischemic attack (TIA)

   C. Reversible ischemic neurologic deficit (RIND)
   D. Stroke in evolution
   E. Transient ischemic attack

45. A 10-year-old girl complains of a rash that began around the ears and spread to her face and trunk, then to her hands. She complains of a cough, runny nose, and itchy eyes, which she has had for a week. Physical examination of the skin reveals red macules and papules on the trunk. Examination of the throat reveals tiny red papules over the soft palate. What is the most likely diagnosis?

   A. Poison ivy dermatitis
   B. Rheumatic fever
   C. Rubeola
   D. Rubella
   E. Toxic shock syndrome

46. A 12-year-old girl complains of a rash that began on her face as single red dots and eventually moved down to her neck and her trunk. She also experienced a low-grade fever. Upon examination of the mouth, the doctor notices some bluish areas on the inside of her mouth. The patient reports that she has a cough and a runny nose as well. She is at increased risk of developing what CNS complication if not treated?

   A. Acute necrotizing hemorrhagic encephalomyelitis
   B. Alzheimer's disease
   C. Creutzfeldt-Jakob disease
   D. Pick's disease
   E. Subacute sclerosing panencephalitis

47. A patient who recently developed severe confusion and lethargy presents with a spike in fever to 102°F (39°C). A CT scan of the head is obtained (Figure 4-5). Of the following choices, which is the most likely to have occurred that led to this patient's meningitis?

   A. Fractured temporal bone secondary to car accident
   B. Recent diagnosis of tuberous sclerosis
   C. Root canal procedure
   D. Sinus infection
   E. Unprotected sex with numerous partners

48. A 58-year-old man has had progressive dementia for some 10 years; over more than 2 years, he has developed behavioral

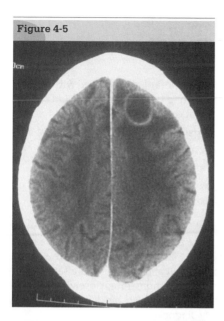

Figure 4-5

changes with alterations in personality as well as language disturbances. A CT scan of the head reveals frontal and temporal lobe atrophy. What is the most likely diagnosis?

A. Alzheimer's disease

B. Ataxia-telangiectasia

C. Huntington's disease

D. Parkinson's disease

E. Pick's disease

49. A 73-year-old man presents to his primary care physician with tremors at rest along with stooped posture. What pathologic involvement is evident in this patient's disease?

A. Decreased dopamine in the corpus striatum

B. Degeneration of the anterior horn of the spinal cord and corticospinal tracts

C. Neurofibrillary tangles

D. Senile (neuritic) plaques with a beta-amyloid core

E. Trinucleotide repeat disorder

50. A 65-year-old man who smokes and has diabetes mellitus type II suffers an ischemic stroke at the anterior cerebral artery. If blood flow is reestablished in as little as 10 min, it will be potentially more damaging than the ischemic episode itself owing to which of the following principles?

A. Blood flow that is reestablished is hypercoagulable and has the propensity to further occlude arteries

B. Blood flow that is reestablished to ischemic areas poses no threat to the stroke patient

C. Reestablishing blood flow after a cerebral vascular accident carries the increased risk of invasion by harmful organisms

D. Generation of oxygen free radicals

E. Increased blood flow to the ischemic areas increases the chance of thromboembolism in the already damaged arteries

51. A 35-year-old man was in his backyard when he began to feel tingling in his lower extremities. He went inside and sat down, then felt as if his legs were numb. He was taken to the

emergency department for further evaluation. Upon arrival his numbness and tingling had ascended up to his knees. His blood pressure was 160/90 mmHg. Papilledema was noted. A spinal tap was performed, revealing elevated CSF protein and a normal cell count. What is the most likely diagnosis?

A. Charcot-Marie-Tooth syndrome

B. Guillain-Barré syndrome

C. Myasthenia gravis

D. Poliomyelitis

E. Spinal cord transection

52. A 25-year-old woman complains of daily throbbing headaches for the past 1 month. She usually experiences six episodes a day, each lasting about 15 min. They are localized to the left orbital region and are accompanied by tearing and rhinorrhea. The patient states that she remembers having had similar episodes about 2 years earlier. What is the most likely diagnosis?

A. Cluster headache

B. Migraine headache

C. Pseudotumor cerebri

D. Tension headache

E. Trigeminal neuralgia

53. A 38-year-old woman who has undergone resection of an intracranial neoplasm has recovered fully from her original symptoms of localized central nervous system (CNS) compression. A CT scan of her head (postcontrast) is shown in Figure 4-6. These clinical findings are characteristic of a specific diagnosis that is most likely to have which of the following features?

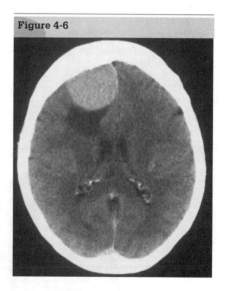

Figure 4-6

A. Amplification of the N-*myc* oncogene

B. Most frequent occurrence in the fourth ventricle

C. Occurs as tumors derived from Schwann cells, characteristically localized to the acoustic nerve

D. Originates in arachnoid cells of the meninges

E. Most likely to originate from metastatic sites of origin

54. A 55-year-old alcoholic man presents to the emergency department with blurry vision. He has a 30-year history of alcohol use, imbibing one case of beer and one fifth of vodka a day. On exam it is found that he has horizontal nystagmus and seems to be very confused. His gait is that of a person who is intoxicated. What is the most likely diagnosis?

A. Cerebral infarction

B. Delirium tremens

C. Korsakoff's syndrome

D. Vitamin B$_{12}$ deficiency

E. Wernicke's syndrome

55. A 45-year-old woman with a history of hypertension and diabetes was working in her basement when she suddenly lost vision in one eye and had difficulty speaking. She was discovered by her husband, who reported that her speech was fuzzy and unclear. When he asked what was wrong, she replied, "I'm having trouble with my words and have difficulty seeing." He then brought her the emergency department for evaluation. What is the most likely explanation for these findings?

A. Delirium

B. Intact speech

C. Intact repetition

D. Intact comprehension

E. Impaired vision

56. An 18-year-old army reservist is brought to the local barracks physician with lethargy, a high-grade fever, and a headache. His mother reports that she had been compliant with prenatal care recommendations and there had been no complications at the time of the patient's birth. A lumbar puncture (LP) is performed and demonstrates increased protein and decreased glucose in the CSF. The neutrophil counts are increased and lymphocyte counts are within normal limits. What is the most likely organism responsible for this patient's condition?

A. Cytomegalovirus

B. *Escherichia coli*

C. Herpes simplex virus

D. *Neisseria meningitidis*

E. *Streptococcus pneumoniae*

57. A 13-month-old infant is diagnosed with bacterial meningitis for the second time. This child should be clinically evaluated for what congenital abnormality?

A. Cytomegalovirus infection

B. Down's syndrome

C. Spina bifida occulta

D. Syphilis infection

E. Toxoplasmosis

58. A 32-year-old man presents to the ambulatory care clinic with new-onset seizures. He also complains of headaches, nausea, and emesis. A CT scan is obtained (Figure 4-7). Surgical resection is performed and specimens are sent to pathology. The resected tumor demonstrates closely packed cells with large round nuclei surrounded by clear cytoplasm. What is the most likely diagnosis?

A. Acoustic neuroma

B. Ependymoma

C. Medulloblastoma multiforme

D. Meningioma

E. Oligodendroglioma

59. An obese 31-year-old woman presents to her primary care physician with new-onset headaches and intermittent visual obscurations. She describes diffuse headaches that are usually worse in the morning. The visual disturbances are described as a general "graying out of vision" usually lasting only a few seconds. Bilateral disc edema is noted on physical exam. What is the most likely diagnosis?

A. Astrocytoma

B. Meningitis

C. Migraine headache

D. Progressive multifocal leukoencephalopathy

E. Pseudotumor cerebri

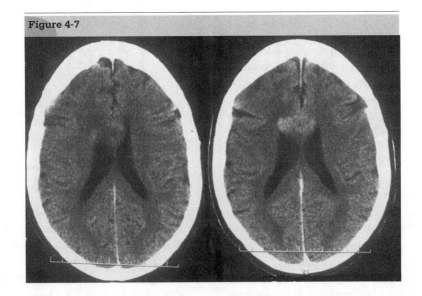

Figure 4-7

60. A 57-year-old woman presents to the emergency department with new-onset lethargy, confusion, and delirium. The treating physician sees the patient experience a mild partial complex seizure. An LP is performed, and testing by polymerase chain reaction (PCR) of the CSF reveals the diagnosis of herpes simplex encephalitis. What is the most common cause of this disease?

   A. *Escherichia coli*

   B. Cytomegalovirus

   C. Herpes simplex type I

   D. Herpes simplex type II

   E. Creutzfeldt-Jakob virus

61. A patient presents with symptoms characteristic of meningitis; therefore a sample of CSF is required for diagnosis. Of the following choices, which best describes the anatomical structures encountered during an LP?

   A. Needle insertion through L4–L5 space, passage order through skin, epidural space, arachnoid, and pia mater, then collection of CSF

   B. Needle insertion through L4–L5 space, passage order through skin, arachnoid, epidural space, and pia mater, then collection of CSF

   C. Needle insertion through L4–L5 space, passage order through skin, epidural space, and arachnoid, then collection of CSF

   D. Needle insertion through L5–S1 space, passage order through skin, epidural space, arachnoid, and pia mater, then collection of CSF

   E. Needle insertion through L5–S1 space, passage order through skin, epidural space, and arachnoid, then collection of CSF

62. A patient presents who has had an insidious onset of progressively worsening confusion, headache, and nausea, always associated with emesis. An MRI of the head demonstrates the development of a cerebral abscess. Of the following choices, which is most likely to be the inciting agent that led to the formation of the abscess?

   A. Bacterial endocarditis

   B. Community acquired infection

   C. Recurrent otitis media

   D. Sinusitis

   E. Temporal bone fracture secondary to a fall down flight of stairs

63. A 45-year-old retired construction worker was doing some work outside his home when his ladder slipped from under him and fell straight onto his back. He got up with no hesitation, only to notice that he had no awareness of painful stimuli in his lower extremities. His muscle strength remained normal. Which of the following neurons were most likely affected?

   A. First-order neurons

   B. Second-order neurons

   C. Third-order neurons

   D. Fourth-order neurons

   E. Fifth-order neurons

64. A 22-year-old woman presents to her primary care physician because of the recent onset of flickering eye movements and trouble with hand-to-eye coordination (for example, inserting the key in and unlocking a door). When asked about other complaints, she says that she has recently been fumbling around with her words, stuttering, or even slurring her speech. Which of the following statements directed to the patient is true?

   A. "I am sorry miss, yours is a terminal condition giving you only 1 year to live."

   B. "Realize that with time these symptoms will resolve, but be prepared for exacerbations that may be worse than the prior episode."

   C. "At some time during your childhood you were probably subject to a persistent infection of measles virus that was never diagnosed."

   D. "These symptoms are due to the progression of your HIV infection, as your CD4 cell count has dropped below 200."

   E. "Your symptoms are treatable with surgical resection followed by a long course of chemotherapy."

65. A 35-year-old homeless man presents to the emergency department after an acute onset of tremors in his fingers, along with muscular rigidity and the development of a shuffling gait. Physical examination reveals an expressionless face as well as numerous needle tracks along both of his arms. What is the etiologic agent suspected in this patient?

   A. Abuse of an intravenous drug containing methyl-phenyl-tetrahydropyridine

   B. Alcohol abuse for numerous years

   C. Cocaine abuse

   D. Long-standing hypertension

   E. Traumatic injury to the skull

66. A mother brings her 2-year-old child to the pediatrician for his regular checkup. She reports that she noticed the child squinting as he is focusing on objects. Physical examination reveals leukocoria of the left eye. Assuming that this child has developed an intracranial neoplasm, what is the etiology of the most likely diagnosis?

   A. Amplification of the N-*myc* oncogene

   B. Homozygous deletion of the Rb gene

   C. Metastasis

   D. Origin in the peripheral nerves

   E. Areas of necrosis that are surrounded by a pseudo-palisading arrangement of tumor cells

67. A 2-day-old neonate is brought to the emergency department because of poor feeding and sucking and a temperature of 103°F (39.4°C). LP is performed, and the CSF demonstrates numerous neutrophils, increased protein, and decreased glucose. What is the most likely causative agent?

   A. *Escherichia coli*

   B. *Haemophilus influenzae*

   C. *Listeria monocytogenes*

   D. *Streptococcus pneumoniae*

   E. *Staphylococcus aureus*

68. A 71-year-old man is evaluated by the medical team an hour after having a stroke. His symptom now is unilateral paralysis of the face and hands. He is also aphasic. Assuming that this cerebrovascular accident is the result of embolism, which vessel is most likely to have been occluded?

A. Anterior cerebral artery

B. Anterior inferior cerebellar artery

C. Middle cerebral artery

D. Posterior cerebral artery

E. Posterior inferior cerebellar artery

69. In your office, you are interviewing a newly expectant couple who have many questions about their pregnancy. They seem particularly concerned about birth defects and tests that can be done to identify potential problems. Neural tube defects are most commonly associated with elevation of which of the following serum levels?

A. Alpha fetoprotein

B. Alanine aminotransferase

C. Aspartate aminotransferase

D. Insulin

E. White blood cells

70. A 73-year-old patient was recently diagnosed as having Alzheimer's disease and his family wants to know about potential ensuing problems that can result from this disease. Owing to the decreased cerebral mass, there is a potential for which of the following?

A. Arnold-Chiari malformation

B. Communicating hydrocephalus

C. External hydrocephalus

D. Hydrocephalus ex vacuo

E. Internal hydrocephalus

71. A 10-month-old infant is brought to the pediatrician; she is suspected of suffering from mental retardation. She has recently had some seizures and is noted to have adenoma sebaceum. A CT scan shows angiomyolipoma of the kidney as well as astrocytes forming tubers in the cerebral cortex and periventricular areas. What is the most likely explanation for these findings?

A. Agenesis of the corpus callosum

B. Arnold-Chiari malformation

C. Fetal alcohol syndrome

D. Hydrocephalus ex vacuo

E. Tuberous sclerosis

72. An 18-year-old man presents to the emergency department following an assault in which he was struck in the abdomen with a baseball bat. He has severe abdominal tenderness, mostly in the left upper quadrant, and complains of left shoulder pain. Which of the following dermatomes is responsible for the left shoulder pain?

A. C1–C2

B. C3–C5

C. C5–C8

D. T1–T3

E. T4–T6

73. After visiting New Guinea, a 52-year-old man, a traveler, returns home to America. He is now complaining of tremors, slurred speech, and a general mental decline. His wife is worried and reports that her husband tried all kinds of meats during their trip. However, she is a vegetarian and therefore did not join him in this. She is very worried and wants to know what he could possibly have. What is the most likely diagnosis?

A. Creutzfeldt-Jakob disease

B. Cytomegalovirus

C. Human immunodeficiency virus

D. Kuru

E. Rabies

74. A 35-year-old woman presents with the acute onset of bilateral lower extremity weakness and pain that have been present for 24 hr. On neurological exam, deep tendon reflexes are minimally decreased, but the sensory exam is normal. On the test of lower extremity strength, she scores 1 bilaterally. Past medical history is significant for a viral infection 2 weeks prior to her presentation. What is the most likely pathophysiological explanation for her condition?

A. Albuminocytologic dissociation of the CSF

B. Lower extremity demyelination

C. Progressive dementia

D. Positive leukocytes in the urinalysis

E. Severe respiratory failure

75. His teacher notes that her 10-year-old student's grades have recently declined. In addition, he seems to "daze off" and often has a blank stare. The child is brought to the physician's office for evaluation. What is the most likely diagnosis?

A. Absence seizures

B. Binswanger's disease

C. Meningioma

D. Pseudotumor cerebri

E. Schwannoma

Answer Key

1. E	**20.** B	**39.** D	**58.** E
2. D	**21.** A	**40.** B	**59.** E
3. C	**22.** D	**41.** B	**60.** C
4. E	**23.** D	**42.** C	**61.** C
5. D	**24.** C	**43.** C	**62.** C
6. A	**25.** C	**44.** E	**63.** B
7. E	**26.** A	**45.** C	**64.** B
8. D	**27.** D	**46.** E	**65.** A
9. C	**28.** C	**47.** E	**66.** B
10. A	**29.** A	**48.** E	**67.** D
11. C	**30.** A	**49.** A	**68.** C
12. D	**31.** D	**50.** A	**69.** A
13. A	**32.** C	**51.** B	**70.** D
14. E	**33.** A	**52.** A	**71.** E
15. D	**34.** A	**53.** D	**72.** B
16. E	**35.** C	**54.** E	**73.** D
17. B	**36.** C	**55.** D	**74.** A
18. A	**37.** C	**56.** D	**75.** A
19. E	**38.** D	**57.** C	

Answers and Explanations

1. E. The L5 spinal cord segment is most likely to be affected in herniation of the intervertebral disc between L4 and L5. L4 passes through the intervertebral foramen between L4 and L5 but passes above the intervertebral disc and would not be impinged during a herniation. The bladder and rectum are under the control of S2, S3, and S4 and would most likely be unaffected. Plantarflexion of the foot is mediated by S1-S2 and would not be affected by herniation of this intervertebral disc.

2. D. Anencephaly is caused by failed closure of the rostral neuropore, which should close by about day 22. The caudal neuropore closes at about day 27; failure of its closure results in spina bifida. Alpha-fetoprotein is elevated with any defect of the neural tube. Because the fetus is anencephalic, it has no swallowing reflex; therefore will not be able to reduce the amount of fluid in the uterus, leading to polyhydramnios. A combination of these two findings suggests that the fetus may be anencephalic.

3. C. This man is exhibiting signs of acute alcohol intoxication. Ataxia and dysdiadochokinesia are cerebellar signs. The cerebellum, along with the pons, is derived from the metencephalon. The telencephalon develops into the cerebral hemispheres, the diencephalons the thalamus, the mesencephalon the midbrain, and the myelencephalon the medulla.

4. E. This child has a meningomyelocele, a severe form of spina bifida. Spina bifida can be caused by low maternal intake of folic acid. Folic acid is found in leafy vegetables and fruits. Alcohol consumption can lead to fetal alcohol syndrome, with characteristic features such as low-set ears, smooth philtrum, and mental retardation. X-ray imaging has no effect on the fetus regarding a meningomyelocele. Close monitoring of fetal growth is accomplished through fetal ultrasound, and this child's condition is due to the mother's low ingestion of folate during pregnancy. Calcium supplementation is useful for developing strong bones and preventing the development of rickets.

5. D. Fetal alcohol syndrome is the most common cause of mental retardation in the United States. All of the other choices can lead to mental retardation, but alcohol is the most common etiology.

6. A. Based on the description provided, this girl was most likely bitten by a black widow spider. Then venom of this spider acts presynaptically at the neuromuscular junction, which results in the massive release of several neurotransmitters, especially acetylcholine. Tetanus toxin acts on Renshaw cells in the spinal cord. Botulinum toxin inhibits the release of acetylcholine at the neuromuscular junction. Bungarotoxin binds irreversibly to nicotinic receptors. Strychnine blocks the glycine receptor in the spinal cord. GABA is not known to be an important neurotransmitter in the peripheral nervous system.

7. E. This man most likely has adult polycystic kidney disease, an autosomal dominant disease. It is the most common inherited disorder of the kidney. Adult polycystic kidney disease is often associated with berry aneurysm in the circle of Willis. These aneurysms are prone to rupture, leading to subarachnoid hemorrhage. Cerebellar hemangioma is associated with von Hippel-Lindau disease, an autosomal dominant disease of chromosome 3. Glioblastoma multiforme is the most common primary intracranial neoplasm in adults. Embolic infarction is made much more likely in the presence of atrial fibrillation due to the potential formation of a mural thrombus, which can shower thrombi into circulation. Cysticercosis is caused by eating vegetation that is contaminated by feces from livestock, usually pigs, infected with *Taenia solium*. Ring-enhancing calcified lesions are evident in the brain and may serve as a focus of seizures.

8. D. Any nocturnal animal that is walking freely in daylight hours and does not shy away from people should raise suspicion for rabies infection. Although the presence of Negri bodies in the cytoplasm of brain cells will be evident eventually, transport of the virus up the axons to the CNS occurs on the order of days and weeks rather than hours. At this time of presentation, only neutrophils at the bite site will be evident, as would be the case in any dirty penetrating injury. Councilman bodies can be found in the liver due to hepatitis or yellow fever. Polio causes degeneration of the cell bodies of motor cells in the anterior horn of the spinal cord. Cytomegalovirus infection is characterized by giant cells and eosinophilic inclusions.

9. C. This patient is presenting with early signs indicative of amyotrophic lateral sclerosis (ALS), the most common motor neuron disease. ALS is believed to be inherited in an autosomal dominant fashion and follows a rapidly fatal course after onset in early middle age. It affects both upper motor neurons and lower motor neurons and results in denervation atrophy of the musculature. Glucose dysregulation can lead to diabetic peripheral neuropathy, which affects sensation only.

10. A. This patient appears to be suffering from thiamine deficiency, which occurs in severe malnutrition, which may be secondary to alcoholism. Thiamine deficiency can lead to Wernicke's encephalopathy, Korsakoff's syndrome, and beriberi. Infestation with the fish tapeworm *Diphyllobothrium latum*, a strict vegetarian diet, and pernicious anemia may lead to vitamin B_{12} deficiency, which is manifest by megaloblastic anemia and peripheral neuropathy. Subacute sclerosing panencephalitis (SSPE) is a fatal sequela of certain measles infections that occurs many years after the initial infection. ALS affects both upper and lower motor neurons but is not associated with the mammillary bodies.

11. C. This child may have the familial form of retinoblastoma, which is caused by a deletion of the Rb gene on chromosome 13. Sporadic retinoblastoma is usually unilateral and monocentric in origin, while the familial type is frequently bilateral and multicentric. Chromosome 3 is associated with von Hippel-Landau disease. Chromosome 4 contains CAG repeats in Huntington's disease. Chromosome 19 contains the ε4 allele of apoprotein E and chromosome 21 contains the APP gene that codes for amyloid precursor protein, both of which are implicated in the suspected etiologies of Alzheimer's disease.

12. D. Neurofibrillary tangles, which are described above, are among the major pathognomonic findings in the diagnosis of Alzheimer's disease. Granovacuolar degeneration is marked by granule vacuoles in the hippocampal pyramidal cells. Cerebral atrophy is most noted in the frontal and hippocampal areas; Hirano bodies are actin-containing bodies in the proximal dendrites. Neuronal plaques contain an amyloid core, which enables their easy identification. The CT scan shows evidence of global atrophy. The MRI scan shows temporal lobe atrophy.

13. A. Flaccid facial paralysis would be expected in a patient presenting with a lesion of CN VII. The corneal reflex would also be absent, not heightened, owing to the damage to the efferent limb. Salivation would not be affected by this lesion. Lacrimation while eating, also known as "crocodile tears," is caused by a very specific lesion of the facial nerve and is not at all indicated by this clinical scenario.

14. E. A lesion of CN IX would produce deficits in the pharyngeal gag reflex (due to injury of the afferent limb), loss of taste on the posterior third of the tongue, and glossopharyngeal neuralgia. The corneal reflex is specific for CN VII. Finger to the nose is not related to CN IX. Shoulder shrug would be useful to test the accessory nerve.

15. D. Huntington's disease presents with the classic symptoms listed here. It is caused by degeneration of the striatal neurons. Bell's palsy is a self-limiting infection of CN VII. Delirium tremens is induced by the sudden withdrawal of alcohol from a chronic alcoholic. Parkinson's disease stems from the degeneration of dopamine neurons in the substantia nigra, and is associated with the classic pill-rolling hand tremor.

16. E. Tardive dyskinesia presents with uncontrollable lip-smacking and chewing motions; these are common in patients with a history of manganese exposure and those who have been taking psychotropic medications on a regular basis for a long time. Stuttering is rarely a noted side effect of psychotropic drugs. Priapism is noted to occur with particular medications, but chlorpromazine is not among the common ones. Ataxia and nystagmus are also possible, but they are not on the common list of medication-induced issues associated with these drugs.

17. B. Dysdiadochokinesia is defined as the inability to perform rapidly alternating hand movements, typically supination and pronation. Constant "to and fro" movements are defined as nystagmus. Inability to arrest muscular movement is known as dysmetria. Loss of coordinated muscle

activity is called dyssynergia. Dysarthria is slurred or scanning speech.

18. A. Cerebellar dysfunction classically presents as the triad of hypotonia, disequilibrium, and dyssynergia. Cerebral dysfunction would be reflected in language, speech, calculation, and spatial perception. Pontine injury can lead to a "locked in" syndrome. Thalamic injury can lead to contralateral hemiparesis/hemianesthesia, elevated pain threshold, and hyperpathia (burning pain).

19. E. Tuberous sclerosis syndrome is characterized by hypopigmented areas on the body and groups of neural deposits known as tubers. It is inherited in an autosomal dominant pattern. Seizures and mental retardation are also features of this disease. Fetal alcohol syndrome is cause by chronic alcohol consumption during pregnancy. The resultant defects include facial abnormalities, developmental defects such as microcephaly, atrial septal defect, and mental and growth retardation. Arnold-Chiari malformation is a downward movement of the cerebellar tonsils secondary to obstruction of the CSF outflow tract. Hydrocephalus is caused by an increased volume of CSF within the cranial cavity. Neural tube defects usually involve the meninges, spinal cord, or brain.

20. B. A contrecoup is a nonpenetrating injury to the brain; it is located on the opposite side of the skull impact. In this case, the patient's impact was located on the right temple, therefore it would be expected that the contrecoup injury would be located on the left side of the brain. Coup injuries are located on the same side as the area of impact.

21. A. On spinal aspiration of CSF, there are certain values that would be indicative of bacterial meningitis. Decreased glucose would support the diagnosis of bacterial meningitis, as the bacteria use glucose as a food supply. Elevated temperatures secondary to infection would be expected, as would increased neutrophils. Diplopia would not be directly supportive of bacterial meningitis.

22. D. Pheochromocytomas are tumors of the adrenal medulla, which is derived embryologically from the neural crest. Tissues derived from the neural crest are located throughout the body because it migrates during development, whereas tissues from the neuroectoderm are directly associated with the brain or spinal cord. The adrenal cortex—which is composed of the zona glomerulosa, zona fasciculata, and zona reticularis—develops from the mesoderm.

23. D. Toxoplasmosis, which is a parasitic infection of the brain, is transmitted transplacentally in utero. Cats are frequently found to be reservoirs. *Escherichia coli* is more commonly causative of pyogenic meningitis, which doesn't present with the clinical issues listed. Kuru is transmitted by cannibalism, or the ingestion of human brain, and is not applicable in this scenario. Viral meningitis presents as nuchal rigidity, fever, and headache.

24. C. Intention tremor is a significant clinical manifestation for the diagnosis of MS. The other two diagnostic presentations—nystagmus and scanning speech, part of the Charcot triad—are also clinical features relevant to MS. Hemoptysis is more relevant to pulmonary infections and not really associated with musculoskeletal issues. Tinnitus and vertigo are neurologically related but not necessarily diagnostic of MS.

25. C. The most likely diagnosis based on the presentation is acute idiopathic polyneuritis, better known as Guillain-Barré syndrome. This is an acute inflammatory demyelinating disease that moves in an ascending pattern from the lower to the upper extremities after a viral infection. CSF analysis for glucose is more likely diagnostic of bacterial meningitis. Blood culture, Gram's stain, and urine cytology will not be beneficial for detecting any viral disease.

26. A. Cytomegalovirus is classically characterized by giant cells with eosinophilic inclusions and usually affects immunosuppressed people (those who undergo transplants). Herpes simplex encephalitis is related to herpes simplex virus infection. Human immunodeficiency virus is characterized by lowered T4 cell counts and reduced immunity. Poliomyelitis is pathologically identifiable by degeneration and necrosis of anterior horn cells of the spinal cord. Identification of Negri bodies is pathognomonic for a diagnosis of rabies.

27. D. *Streptococcus agalactiae* is normally found in the vaginal and oral flora of adult women. Exposure of newborns leads to infection, sepsis, and possibly meningitis. Group B strep tests are done routinely on expectant mothers during their prenatal checkups. *Chlamydia,* herpes simplex II, human immunodeficiency virus, and syphilis affect newborns, but the lab results taken alone point to *Strep. agalactiae.*

28. C. An injury to C3 will likely cause a cessation in breathing secondary to the severing of the respiratory muscles from the control centers in the brainstem. C1 injury results in sudden death, as it is associated with a hangman's fracture or breaking of the neck. C7 injury is noted by a decrease in heart rate as well as arterial pressure due to loss of sympathetic tone. C2 and C4 have no "symptomatic" clinical presentations associated directly with their injury. The MRI shown is normal; there is no evidence of intracerebral bleeding.

29. A. Fulminant meningococcemia occurs when *Neisseria meningitidis* infection is allowed to disseminate to the various tissues of the body (skin, eyes, meninges, lungs) and can lead to death 1 to 5 days after dissemination. Guillain-Barré syndrome is linked to *Campylobacter jejuni* infection. The Jarisch-Herxheimer reaction involves the treatment of secondary syphilis and is indicative of a functional penicillin inflammatory reaction. Lymphogranuloma venereum and pelvic inflammatory disease are due to sexually transmitted infections, which are not relevant to this scenario.

30. A. *Clostridium tetani* is a Gram-positive, spore-forming anaerobe that is transmitted via a laceration/puncture wound and also via infected umbilical cord stump in a neonate.

Death usually occurs after several weeks, secondary to exhaustion and respiratory failure. All the other answer choices are infectious agents but do not present with the clinical symptoms described.

31. D. Glutamate is the most prevalent excitatory neurotransmitter in the brain. The receptors for this agent involve kainate with channels for sodium and potassium. With a history of depression and Valium use, the glutamate receptor most likely has been down-regulated by the inhibitory effects of benzodiazepines. Histidine is present within the neurons of the hypothalamus, while dopamine is present in high concentrations in the midbrain. Acetylcholine is an excitatory neurotransmitter found in the peripheral and central nervous system. Epinephrine is an excitatory transmitter found in the peripheral and central nervous system. Dopamine is prominent in midbrain neurons and is released from the hypothalamus. Histidine is formed from histamine and is present in neurons of the hypothalamus.

32. C. The test for function of the flexor digitorum superficialis is to fix the other digits and have the patient move the metacarpophalangeal joint. If the patient is unable to move that joint with other joints fixed, there is damage to the flexor digitorum superficialis. An injury to the palmar surface would not injure the extensor digitorum. To test for this, however, have the patient extend all fingers. The flexor digitorum profundus is tested by having an assistant hold the patient's metacarpophalangeal joint and asking the patient to flex the distal interphalangeal joint. With a normal examination of the first digit, the flexor pollicis longus would not be damaged. The median nerve has motor function to the thenar muscles (digit 1) and the lumbricals. If the exam of digit 1 is normal, damage to the median nerve is unlikely.

33. A. Neurologic sensation of the C5 level is associated with motor, reflex, and sensory levels. This will result in shoulder abduction, loss of the biceps reflex, and loss of sensation over the lateral arm. The lateral forearm is supplied by the C6 dermatome. The medial arm is supplied by the T1 dermatome. The medial forearm is supplied by the C8 dermatome.

34. A. A patient who is unable to squat might have impairment of the L4 nerve root. The L4 dermatome runs across the knee and is responsible for sensation. The sensory component of the patellar reflex is initiated by the L4 root. The L5 nerve root controls heel walking. The S1 nerve root controls toe walking. The S2 nerve root controls knee flexion.

35. C. The glossopharyngeal nerve exits the skull through the jugular foramen and causes elevation of the pharynx via the stylopharyngeus muscle and secretion of saliva by the parotid gland. This nerve also provides sensation from the external and middle ear and taste from the posterior third of the tongue. The abducens nerve is responsible for eye movement. The accessory nerve is responsible for movement of the head and shoulder. The trigeminal nerve innervates the muscles of mastication. The vestibulocochlear nerve is responsible for equilibrium.

36. C. The lateral lemniscus carries auditory input from the cochlear nuclei, nuclei of the trapezoid body, and superior olivary nuclei to the inferior colliculus of the midbrain. Each lateral lemniscus carries input from both ears. The dorsal acoustic striae send axons that cross in the pontine tegmentum and ascend in the contralateral lateral lemniscus. The intermediate acoustic stria sends axons that cross in the pontine tegmentum and ascend in the contralateral lateral lemniscus. The ventral acoustic stria originates in the ventral cochlear nucleus.

37. C. The right shoulder would be expected to appear higher, as the left shoulder was actually drooping. Tongue deviations are related to CN XII, which is hypoglossal, and not to CN XI. Ipsilateral shoulder droop and contralateral head-turning impingement are commonly found with accessory nerve damage. Eyelid retraction, also known as ptosis, is mediated by lesion to CN III.

38. D. Lesch-Nyhan syndrome is associated with an inborn error of protein metabolism causing hypoxanthine and guanine to accumulate. This occurs because of a deficit in hypoxanthine-guanine phosphoribosyl transferase (HGPRT). These children present with symptoms of hyperirritability and the classic self-mutilating behavior. Adenosine is degraded to hypoxanthine, which is oxidized by xanthine oxidase in the presence of molybdenum. Pyrimidine base salvage still occurs despite the defect in HGPRT. The metabolism of glycine and inosine is unaffected in Lesch-Nyhan syndrome. Inosine is converted to hypoxanthine and then xanthine through the action of xanthine oxidase.

39. D. MS is characterized by destruction of myelin with relative preservation of axons. It is seen mostly in women and presents between the ages of 20 and 30. Viral factors are suspected in its etiology but this is not proven. On CSF analysis, oligoclonal bands are the characteristic finding. Increased protein and decreased glucose levels are characteristic of bacterial meningitis caused by *Streptococcus pneumoniae*. Immunoglobulin light chains are found in the urine in multiple myeloma—a condition known as Bence Jones proteinuria. Pick bodies are not found in CSF analysis. They are characteristic of Pick's disease, leading to a form of atrophy of the cortex similar to that of Alzheimer's disease. The MRI shown reveals periventricular white matter lesions typical of MS.

40. B. Injury to the optic tract would produce homonymous contralateral hemianopia. A cut in the geniculocalcarine tract would result in a homonymous hemianopia with macular sparing. Optic chiasm injury causes heteronymous bitemporal hemianopia. Optic nerve injury leads to blindness in the same-sided eye. Pretectal injury would cause bilateral lateral visual field deficits.

41. B. Eyes moving to the opposite side would be the most appropriate response of an intact system. The mnemonic COWS (cold opposite, warm same) describes the expected change in eye direction as a result of water being placed into the ear canal. Chills and shivering may be an appropriate response, but not neurologically. Constriction and dilation of the pupils should not be affected by water placement in the ear canal.

42. C. CN VII (chorda tympani) functions in the reception of sweet and salty taste receptors and innervates the anterior two-thirds of the tongue. Injury to this nerve would impede the detection of these stimuli. CN II is the optic nerve, which is responsible for vision. CN IV is the trochlear nerve, which serves to control movement of the eyeball. CN VI is the abducens nerve, which helps provide movement of the eyeball. CN IX is the glossopharyngeal nerve, which detects sour and bitter sensation as well as innervating the posterior third of the tongue.

43. C. Epidural hematoma results from hemorrhage into the potential space between the dura and skull. The hemorrhage most likely results from rupture to a meningeal artery that travels within this plane. The middle meningeal artery is the most common source; it branches off the maxillary artery in the temporal area. Normally, the patient experiences a "lucid interval," an asymptomatic period of a few hours following the trauma. A berry aneurysm results from a defect in the media of arteries and is usually located at a bifurcation site. Berry aneurysms are most commonly found in the circle of Willis. Rupture at this location results in bleeding into the subarachnoid space, producing the "worst headache ever" as described by the patient. The source of bleeding due to subdural hematoma is from bridging veins; these often occur in the elderly due to minor trauma, and symptoms usually appear slowly. A diagnosis of bacterial meningitis is confirmed with LP demonstrating increased neutrophils/protein and decreased glucose in the CSF.

44. E. A transient ischemic attack (TIA) consists of neurologic deficits that completely resolve within 24 hr, leaving no infracted tissue on MRI. A completed stroke is defined as a cerebral vascular accident (CVA) consisting of neurologic deficits that have remained stable for 24 to 72 hr. A crescendo TIA is defined as two or more TIAs within a 24-hr period; this type of CVA is highly predictive of an impending stroke and therefore is considered a medical emergency. A reversible ischemic neurologic deficit (RIND) is defined as a CVA with neurologic deficit lasting longer than 24 hr but less than 3 weeks, with progressive improvement to complete or near complete resolution. A stroke in evolution consists of neurologic deficits that fluctuate or increase over time.

45. C. The patient described has the classic presentation of measles, or rubeola: coryza, conjunctivitis, cough, and Koplik's spots (usually located on the buccal mucosa and soft palate). Rash usually occurs after the prodrome of 1 to 7 days. Microscopic examination shows a widespread gliosis with myelin degeneration. Poison ivy rash is an example of contact dermatitis, a type IV hypersensitivity reaction that is cell-mediated and initiated by specific sensitized T lymphocytes. There is nothing in the history to suggest that this child was exposed to poison ivy. Rheumatic fever is an acute, immunologically mediated multisystem inflammatory disease that occurs following an infection with group A (beta hemolytic) streptococcal pharyngitis. Rubella, or German measles, is a milder form of rubeola that is not associated with progression to develop CNS complications. Toxic shock syndrome produces a diffuse, macular, "sunburn"-like rash caused by superantigens that induce systemic inflammatory cytokine cascades similar to those occurring in septic shock.

46. E. Subacute sclerosing panencephalitis (SSPE) is a rare late complication of measles infection that is caused by a hypermutated virus that infects the CNS. Acute necrotizing hemorrhagic encephalitis is a fulminant syndrome of CNS demyelination that is almost always preceded by a recent episode of upper respiratory infection, usually due to *Mycoplasma pneumoniae*. Cases of Alzheimer's disease are mostly sporadic, although at least 5 to 10% are familial. Creutzfeldt-Jakob disease is primarily sporadic; however, iatrogenic occurrences have been documented in cases such as corneal transplantation. Pick's disease is defined as progressive atrophic changes of the cerebral cortex, usually commencing in late middle age.

47. E. The question stem asks which is the most common portal of entry into the CNS that can lead to meningitis. Hematogenous spread is the most common route of passage to the CNS. Unprotected sex with numerous partners is the classic description of a patient who contracts a sexually transmitted disease, perhaps due to *Neisseria gonorrhoeae*. These organisms have the potential to enter the blood circulation, thereby having the greatest access to the CNS. Although all other answers describe routes of infection of the CNS, hematogenous spread is the most common. The CT shown (Figure 4-7) reveals evidence of a brain abscess.

48. E. Although all the listed answers result in dementia, it is important to realize that the behavioral changes and alterations in personality are due to atrophy of the frontal lobe and language disturbances are due to atrophy of the temporal lobe. Pick's disease is a rare, distinct, progressive dementia characterized clinically as stated in the question stem; this disease results from unilateral frontal and/or temporal lobe atrophy. Alzheimer's disease involves diffuse atrophy of the cerebral cortex. Ataxia-telangiectasia is caused by neuronal degeneration predominantly in the cerebellum. Huntington's disease involves atrophy of the caudate and putamen. Parkinson's disease is associated with depigmentation at the substantia nigra and decreased dopamine in the corpus striatum.

49. A. The patient described in the question suffers from a demyelinating disease. The symptoms clearly indicate that the disease is Parkinson's, a clinical syndrome classically described by diminished facial expression, slowness of voluntary movements, festinating gait, stooped posture, cogwheel rigidity, and pill-rolling tremor. The severity of the motor neuron disease is proportional to the deficiency in dopaminergic neurons of the substantia nigra that project to the corpus striatum. Neurofibrillary tangles and senile plaques are key components of Alzheimer's disease. Trinucleotide repeat disorders of CAG nucleotides result in Huntington's disease. The disease associated with degeneration of anterior horn cells and corticospinal tracts is amyotrophic lateral sclerosis.

50. A. Restarting blood flow after more than about 10 min of ischemia is typically more damaging than the ischemia itself because the ischemia sets the stage for oxygen to generate free radicals rather than contribute to cellular energy production; these free radicals contribute to the insult of the already damaged neurons, a phenomenon known as reperfusion injury. None of the remaining answer choices is a true statement.

51. B. Guillain-Barré syndrome (GBS) is characterized by the acute onset of ascending weakness/tingling in the lower extremities, along with autonomic dysfunction. *Campylobacter jejuni* infection is associated with GBS. CSF analysis shows an elevated protein level with normal cell counts. Poliomyelitis is caused by the destruction of the anterior horn cells of the spinal cord; the disease typically presents with lower motor neuron symptoms such as weakness, fasciculations, muscle atrophy, and absent deep tendon reflexes. With a spinal cord transection, there would be muscle weakness and paralysis along with absent sensory components such as vibration, proprioception, and temperature. Myasthenia gravis is a proximal muscle disease characterized by fatigable weakness and ocular symptoms. Charcot-Marie-Tooth syndrome is another muscle disorder characterized by weakness with normal CSF analysis.

52. A. Cluster headaches are characterized by the symptoms stated in the question. Usually a couple of episodes occur in a day, with tearing and rhinorrhea. Migraines are also usually unilateral but have an associated aura, like a certain odor. They also last for about 30 min. Tension headaches occur bilaterally; the patient feels a vise-like pressure on the head. Trigeminal neuralgia is associated with injury to the fifth nerve, characterized by shooting pains in the distribution of the fifth nerve, brought on by cold substances. Pseudotumor cerebri is a headache experienced by obese women around the age of 40. The only neurological sign is papilledema.

53. D. Meningioma is the second most common primary intracranial tumor in adults. It is of benign course and slow growing, occurring more frequently in women. It originates in arachnoid cells of the meninges, and since the tumor is external to the brain, it is often successfully treated by surgical resection. Neuroblastoma is characterized by amplification of the N-*myc* oncogene and has a poor prognosis. Tumors derived from Schwann cells that affect CN VIII are neurilemoma, or acoustic neuroma, and are the third most common primary intracranial tumors behind medulloblastomas and meningiomas. The tumor that most frequently arises in the fourth ventricle is the ependymoma; its incidence is highest in childhood. Although metastatic tumors are more common than primary CNS tumors, they do not carry as good a prognosis as meningiomas. The CT scan (Figure 4-6) shows evidence of a frontal lobe meningioma.

54. E. The question characterizes the classic triad of Wernicke's syndrome: ophthalmoplegia, ataxia, and confusion. If left untreated, it can lead to Korsakoff's syndrome—irreversible confabulation. Delirium tremens is characterized by seizures and hallucinations. Cerebral infarction, usually caused by emboli to the brain, will cause weakness and ocular symptoms. Vitamin B$_{12}$ deficiency is associated with impaired proprioception and vibration sense along with corticospinal tract symptoms.

55. D. Broca's aphasia is characterized by impaired speech and repetition with intact comprehension. Broca's area is found on the left inferior frontal gyrus. The aphasia is usually due to infarction of the middle cerebral artery. Patients with Broca's aphasia do not have delirium. These patients are unable to verbalize, thus, their speech and repetition are not intact. This condition is not associated with visual changes.

56. D. The first question to be answered is whether the source of infection is bacterial or viral. LP from bacterial infections demonstrates increased neutrophils/protein and decreased glucose in the CSF. LP from viral infections demonstrates increased lymphocytes and normal glucose in the CSF. Therefore the source of the infection is bacterial. The next step is to recognize the most common organisms causing meningitis based on age group. In neonates, consider *Escherichia coli* and *Listeria*. In patients 6 months to 6 years of age, *Streptococcus pneumoniae, Neisseria meningitidis,* and *Haemophilus influenzae* type B may be responsible. In those 6 years to 60 years of age, *Neisseria meningitidis,* enterovirus, and *Strep. pneumoniae* should be considered, while *Strep. pneumoniae* is a likely culprit in those over age 60.

57. C. Spina bifida is an abnormal fusion of vertebral arches, most commonly involving the lumbosacral regions. There are several forms of the disorder with varying degrees of severity. The mildest form is spina bifida occulta, in which there is only a defect in vertebral fusion; the neural tube is still retained in its anatomic location and is still covered by skin and dermis. Observation of the skin above the defect demonstrates "dimpling," sometimes covered with hair. Patients with this disorder are potentially at increased risk for developing bacterial meningitis. Other forms are spina bifida with meningocele, characterized by a CSF-filled meningeal sac that protrudes through the defect; spina bifida with myelomeningocele, characterized by spinal cord herniation along the CSF-filled meningeal sac through the defect; and spina bifida aperta, characterized by the incomplete fusion of the caudal end of the neural plate, which results in an open tract through the skin surface. Approximately 1% of all newborns are congenitally infected with CMV, making CMV the most common congenital infection; up to 10% of these will have symptoms at birth, including intrauterine growth retardation, jaundice, hepatosplenomegaly, petechiae or purpura, thrombocytopenia, and pneumonia. Down's syndrome is a genetic defect that results in an extra or irregular chromosome, causing varying levels of mental retardation and physical disability. Some of the symptoms include short stature, decreased muscle tone, transverse palmar crease, and

unusually shorter than normal rib cage, among others. The main features of untreated congenital syphilis during pregnancy are stillbirth, preterm labor, and intrauterine growth restriction; in the newborn, the main features are hepatosplenomegaly, prolonged jaundice, thrombocytopenia, and failure to thrive. Toxoplasmosis is caused by infection with the protozoan parasite *Toxoplasma gondii,* with congenital infections causing severe sequelae in the infant, including mental retardation, blindness, and epilepsy.

58. E. Oligodendroglioma is a slow-growing neoplasm that usually presents in middle age. Patients typically present with new-onset seizures, headache, nausea, and vomiting. The tumors are morphologically characterized by a "fried egg" appearance of the cells and most likely arise in the cerebral hemispheres. Ependymoma is a common neoplasm in childhood that most frequently occurs in the fourth ventricle. Medulloblastoma multiforme is the most common primary intracranial neoplasm in adults and morphologically demonstrates a "pseudopalisading arrangement" of cells. Meningioma originates from arachnoid cells of the meninges and is characterized histologically by laminated calcified psammoma bodies.

59. E. Pseudotumor cerebri, or benign intracranial hypertension, is an abnormal condition characterized by elevated intracranial pressure, headache of varying intensity, and papilledema without any demonstrable intracranial lesion; it tends to occur in overweight women from 20 to 50 years of age. The morbidity of the disease is related mainly to the detrimental effects of papilledema, which can result in an irreversible optic neuropathy. Astrocytomas are CNS neoplasms and present with altered mental status, cognitive impairment, headaches, visual disturbances, motor impairment, seizures, sensory anomalies, or ataxia; these symptoms would indicate further studies, such as CT scan and MRI for diagnosis. Meningitis is an inflammation of the leptomeninges and underlying CSF and may be associated with fever, headache, seizures, nuchal rigidity, and other neurologic symptoms. Migraine headache is a condition marked by recurrent, usually unilateral, severe headache often accompanied by nausea and vomiting; it is of uncertain origin, though attacks appear to be precipitated by dilatation of intracranial blood vessels. Progressive multifocal leukoencephalopathy (PML) is a viral infection of oligodendrocytes characterized by hemianopia, hemiplegia, alterations in mental status, and eventual coma; the disease typically occurs in immunocompromised patients, the causative agent being a papovavirus.

60. C. Herpes simplex encephalitis (HSE) is an acute or subacute illness that causes general and focal signs of cerebral dysfunction. It is sporadic and occurs without seasonal pattern. Although the clinical findings of fever, headache, behavioral changes, confusion, focal neurologic findings, and abnormal CSF findings are suggestive, it is difficult to distinguish herpes simplex encephalitis from other neurologic disorders having similar presentations. Confirmation of the diagnosis depends on identification of herpes simplex virus within the CSF by means of the polymerase chain reaction (PCR) or within brain tissue by means of brain biopsy. HSE in adults is localized to the temporal and frontal lobes and is caused by herpes simplex virus type 1 (HSV-1). In neonates, however, brain involvement is more often diffuse and the usual cause is herpes simplex virus type 2 (HSV-2), which is acquired at the time of delivery. *E. coli* is one of the most common organisms causing meningitis in neonates, along with GBS and *Listeria*. Progressive multifocal leukoencephalopathy (PML) is a viral infection of oligodendrocytes characterized by hemianopia, hemiplegia, alterations in mental status, and eventual coma; the disease typically occurs in immunocompromised patients; the causative agent is a papovavirus. With some viruses, such as varicella zoster virus (VZV) and cytomegalovirus (CMV), an immunocompromised host is a key risk factor.

61. C. In approaching this question, it is best to gather your knowledge of anatomy and construct the answer on your own prior to reviewing the answers below. LP begins by locating the iliac crest bilaterally and drawing an imaginary line connecting the two. This anatomic site aligns with the L4-L5 space. The order of the structures the needle will pass through is as follows: (1) skin; (2) superficial fascia; (3) ligaments: supraspinatus, interspinous, and ligamentum flavum; (4) epidural space; (5) dura mater; (6) subdural space; (7) arachnoid; and (8) subarachnoid space, which harbors the CSF. It is important to note that the pia mater is not punctured, because the subarachnoid space is where the CSF is found.

62. C. All answers are sources of infection for cerebral abscess formation: bronchopulmonary infection (A), infective endocarditis (B), paranasal sinuses (D), and penetrating injuries to the skull (E). However, the most common source of cerebral abscess is the middle ear, as in acute otitis media.

63. B. Second-order neurons receive information in the relay nuclei and transmit it to the thalamus, where sensory information is processed. First-order neurons receive the transduced signals and relay them to the CNS. Third-order neurons send sensory information to the cerebral cortex. Fourth-order neurons are located in the cerebral cortex and result in a conscious awareness of a stimulus.

64. B. This patient presents with the classic Charcot triad of nystagmus, intention tremor, and scanning speech, which is a significant finding in MS, a disease caused by the destruction of myelin with relative preservation of the axons. Although it is of unknown origin, environmental and genetic factors are thought to be involved. MS is a disorder that is confined to the CNS without affecting the PNS. Clinically, the disease is characterized by exacerbations with periods of asymptomatic remission; often there is progressive worsening with each successive episode. Surgical resection is a valid treatment for various types of brain tumors; however, these patients do not classically present with the Charcot triad of symptoms. Subacute sclerosing panencephalitis is caused by an infection with altered measles virus and typically does not become symptomatic until years later; it is marked by intellectual deterioration, convulsions, and paralysis. A nervous system dysfunction known as AIDS dementia complex is characterized by

memory impairment, delayed thinking, depression, behavioral change, and lethargy. Also involved is a loss of balance, coordination, and motor function.

65. A. This individual presents with Parkinson's disease, induced by the dopamine antagonist methyl-phenyl-tetrahydropyridine (MPTP). Parkinson's patients suffer symptoms of resting pill-rolling tremor, expressionless facies, muscular rigidity, and festinating gait. A history of alcohol abuse would add alcoholic encephalopathy to the differential diagnosis. These patients present with the classic triad of confusion, ataxia, and ophthalmoplegia. Cocaine is a strong CNS stimulant that interferes with the reabsorption of dopamine, a chemical messenger associated with pleasure and movement. Physical effects of cocaine use include constricted blood vessels, dilated pupils, and increases in temperature, heart rate, and blood pressure. Long-standing hypertension is associated with numerous medical conditions; however, hypertension itself does not cause any of the described symptoms. A history of traumatic injury to the head should elicit concern regarding possible intracranial hemorrhage.

66. B. Retinoblastoma is a malignant tumor of the eye in children that originates from the retina. It is the most common eye tumor of childhood and results from homozygous deletion of the Rb gene located on chromosome 13. A child can present with a white reflex (leukocoria), squinting eye, crossed eye, painful eye, or proptosis. Neuroblastoma results from amplification of the N-*myc* gene. Retinoblastomas are more common childhood eye tumors than metastatic tumors. Tumors that most frequently arise in peripheral nerves are neurilemomas. The characteristic pseudopalisading arrangement of tumor cells describes glioblastoma multiforme, the most common primary intracranial neoplasm in adults.

67. D. The most likely etiologic agents causing meningitis are based on the age of the patient. In neonates, *Escherichia coli* is most common. In those aged 6 months to 6 years, *Streptococcus pneumoniae* is most common. In patients aged 6 years to 16 years, *Neisseria meningitidis* is most common. And in those above 16 years of age, *Streptococcus pneumoniae* is most common.

68. C. Emboli usually arise from cardiac mural thrombi, vegetation of cardiac valves, clumps of tumor cells, air collections, or fat thrombi. Clinical manifestations depend on the site of vascular occlusion. Arterial obstruction to the middle cerebral artery produces contralateral hemiparesis as well as motor/sensory defects and aphasia. In addition, the middle cerebral artery is the most common site of embolic occlusion. Obstruction to the anterior cerebral artery clinically results in contralateral weakness of the leg or foot, Broca's aphasia, and incontinence. Obstruction to the posterior cerebral artery produces homonymous hemianopia of the contralateral visual field. Occlusion of the posteroinferior cerebellar artery produces nausea, vomiting, vertigo, hoarseness, ataxia, ipsilateral palate and tongue weakness, and contralateral disturbance of pain/temperature sensations. Occlusion to the anterior inferior cerebellar artery produces ipsilateral facial weakness, gaze palsy, deafness, and tinnitus.

69. A. Alpha fetoprotein is typically associated with neural tube defects. An inadequate closure of the neural tube is usually indicated by increased alpha-fetoprotein blood levels. AST and ALT are both liver enzymes that increase during periods of stress or injury to the liver. Insulin levels are monitored in relation to diabetes, and pancreatitis. WBC elevation is more indicative of infection and has no bearing on potential birth defects.

70. D. Hydrocephalus ex vacuo is a noncommunicating hydrocephalus that is not obstructed without increased CSF production. This commonly occurs in Alzheimer's disease and ischemic brain injuries. Communicating hydrocephalus has a free flow of CSF between the ventricles and subarachnoid space but diminished uptake at the arachnoid granulations. External hydrocephalus is associated with an increased volume of CSF limited to the subarachnoid space. Internal hydrocephalus involves increased volume of CSF entirely contained within the ventricles.

71. E. This infant is suffering from tuberous sclerosis. The astrocyte-forming tubers, which represent an autosomal dominant proliferation of multinucleated atypical astrocytes, are indicative of this disease. Arnold-Chiari malformation is a downward displacement of the cerebellar tonsils and medulla through the foramen magnum and usually occurs along with a thoracolumbar meningomyelocele. Fetal alcohol syndrome is caused by maternal ingestion of alcohol during pregnancy and presents with facial and developmental abnormalities.

72. B. During blunt abdominal trauma, the spleen is the most commonly injured organ, followed by the liver, intestines, and kidney. The complaint of left shoulder pain is caused by blood from a ruptured spleen irritating the diaphragm (innervated by C3–C5), which leads to the referral of pain to the left shoulder. This is known as Kehr's sign. C2 innervation is a posterior half of a skull cap. C6 innervation extends along the lateral aspect of the arm to the thumb. C8 innervation extends to the little finger. C7 innervation includes the second and third digits. T4 innervation is at the level of the nipples. T7 innervation is at the xiphoid process. T10 innervation is at the umbilicus. L1 innervation is at the inguinal ligament. L4 innervation is at the knee.

73. D. Based on the location of his recent trip, it is possible that this patient unknowingly ingested human brain and infected himself with kuru, which is prevalent in New Guinea. Though kuru is a rare disease, it is the most likely diagnosis based on presentation and clinical symptoms. Cytomegalovirus usually affects immunosuppressed individuals and there is no indication of compromised status. Human immunodeficiency virus creates the immunocompromised status, of which there is no indication at this time. Rabies presents as muscle contractions and spasms with convulsions, neither of which were in the above presentation.

74. A. In the diagnosis of Guillain-Barré syndrome, the disease directly causes albuminocytologic dissociation of the CSF analysis, with an increased protein concentration and minimal increase in cell count. Lower extremity demyelination and respiratory failure are certainly results of the disease but are not used as a diagnostic pathophysiology. Progressive dementia is related more to other diseases and not specifically Guillain-Barré syndrome. Leukocytes are indicative of an inflammatory reaction and are not related to this diagnosis.

75. A. Absence seizures are a form of generalized seizure associated with 3-Hz spike-and-slow-wave complexes on electroencephalography. Children usually present with a history of "staring spells," frustration on the child's behalf due to lapses of awareness, and a decline in school performance. Binswanger disease, or vascular dementia, refers to a dementia that develops owing to strokes. Typically, these patients do not have "cognitive features" such as anomia, apraxia, agnosia, and neglect, as are seen with cortical lesions. Meningioma is the most common mesodermal CNS tumor and clinically may present as a cranial nerve palsy. Pseudotumor cerebri is a condition characterized by increased intracranial pressure, headaches, and papilledema. Schwannoma is the most common cranial nerve tumor. Any patient who presents with unilateral deafness should be evaluated for a vestibular neuroma, which involves CN VIII.

Chapter 5　Endocrine System

Questions

1. An 18-year-old woman who has suffered a blow to the head in a motor vehicle accident is admitted to the hospital for observation. Radiographic imaging shows that the pituitary stalk has been transected. Which of the following hormones would be expected to increase in this patient?

   A. Adrenocorticotropic hormone

   B. Follicle-stimulating hormone

   C. Luteinizing hormone

   D. Prolactin

   E. Thyroid-stimulating hormone

   F. Growth hormone

2. A 45-year-old woman has a gastrectomy following the discovery of gastric adenocarcinoma. The patient is now to receive nutrition through a feeding tube in her duodenum. Her physician alerts her that her liquid diet will be supplemented with B vitamins, among other nutrients. Which of the following conditions, which occurs secondary to a decrease in gastric parietal cells, will the B vitamins help to prevent?

   A. Autoimmune hemolysis

   B. Beriberi

   C. Cheilosis

   D. Iron-deficiency anemia

   E. Kwashiorkor

   F. Marasmus

   G. Megaloblastic anemia

   H. Night blindness

   I. Pellagra

   J. Scurvy

3. A genotypic female (XX) was born with masculinization of her external genitalia. The cause of her virilization was not determined at birth. At her 1-year checkup, the pediatric nurse records the vital signs and reports to the physician that the child's blood pressure is 70/30 mm Hg. What is the mostly explanation for these findings?

   A. 5-alpha reductase deficiency

   B. 17-alpha hydroxylase deficiency

   C. 11-beta hydroxylase deficiency

   D. 21-beta hydroxylase deficiency

   E. Testicular feminization syndrome

4. A 31-year-old woman, G1P1, gives birth to a baby girl but loses a significant amount of blood during the delivery. After she received intravenous saline and 2 units of packed red blood cells, her blood pressure returned to normal. She had a few episodes of some dizziness but no fainting spells following the delivery. Three months later, she reports decreased libido, failure of the return of her menstrual cycle, slowness of thought, pretibial myxedema, and intolerance to cold temperatures. What is the most likely diagnosis?

   A. Cretinism

   B. Hashimoto's thyroiditis

   C. Iodine deficiency

   D. Sheehan's syndrome

   E. Subacute (de Quervain's) thyroiditis

5. A 55-year-old man has been experiencing severe flushing and diarrhea for 3 weeks. Seven years earlier, he was diagnosed as having irritable bowel syndrome, and he has intermittent diarrhea. He has also recently had some difficulty breathing. His symptoms have been present throughout the week at home and at work. He wonders whether this is an exacerbation of his irritable bowel syndrome. Physical examination shows the patient to be afebrile; his blood pressure is 130/84 mm Hg and his pulse is 76 bpm. Cardiac examination reveals a diastolic rumble, which is louder with inspiration. He does not know whether this murmur was present previously. The patient does not have tenderness or distension of his abdomen. Which of the following medicines could be used to treat this patient's condition?

   A. Albuterol

   B. Bismuth subsalicylate

   C. Cimetidine

   D. Enalapril

   E. Methysergide

6. Microscopic examination of the endometrium following dilatation and curettage of a 33-year-old woman reveals a thick endometrium with glands that have a pronounced corkscrew shape. The appearance of the endometrium seems to be consistent with the secretory phase of the menstrual cycle. Which of the following hormones is responsible for these findings?

   A. Estrogen

   B. Follicle-stimulating hormone

   C. Luteinizing hormone

   D. Testosterone

   E. Progesterone

7. A 32-year-old woman in her second trimester has had palpitations, tachycardia, and hypersensitivity to heat for 2 weeks. She also reports increased sweating, nervousness, and defecation during this time. In addition, she had vaginal bleeding and a sensation of fullness in her lower pelvis. Physical examination reveals no evidence of neck masses. Her total and free T_4 are elevated and her TSH is depressed. Blood work is negative for thyroid-stimulating immunoglobulins. Which of the following hormones is most likely responsible for this patient's symptoms?

   A. Estrogen

   B. Human chorionic gonadotropin (hCG)

   C. Prolactin

   D. Progesterone

   E. Thyroid-stimulating hormone (TSH)

8. For 2 months, a 35-year-old Caucasian man has experienced fatigue, weight loss, and an increase in urination and the amount of liquids consumed. He has had a major depressive episode in the past. He has also noticed some recent darkening of his skin. A blood analysis was performed at his local rotary club. His serum fasting glucose is 98 mg/dL, serum sodium 120 mEq/L, and serum potassium 5.9 mEq/L. What is the most likely explanation of these findings?

A. Addison's disease

B. Conn's disease

C. Diabetes insipidus

D. Insulin-dependent diabetes mellitus

E. Non-insulin-dependent diabetes mellitus

F. Hemochromatosis

G. Psychogenic polydipsia

H. Syndrome of inappropriate antidiuretic hormone (SIADH)

9. A 39-year-old obese diabetic man presents to his primary care physician for a follow-up examination. He complains of new-onset erectile dysfunction and premature ejaculation. Physical examination of the heart, lungs, and abdomen is within normal limits. Urinalysis reveals glucosuria. What is the best indication that he has not been controlling his glucose levels over the past few months?

A. Fasting plasma glucose = 126 on analysis

B. Hemoglobin A1C > 6%

C. Random plasma glucose > 200 with symptoms

D. Two-hour glucose tolerance test > 200 with or without symptoms

E. Unresponsiveness to oral agent such as metformin

10. A 45-year-old Caucasian man who is 5 ft 3 in tall and weighs 250 lb (113 kg) presents to the clinic complaining of increased fatigue, increased urination, and the new onset of tingling in his hands and feet. A random plasma glucose level > 200 mg/dL is determined on serum analysis and the patient is started on a new medication. The patient travels to visit his sister in another city, falls ill, and is hospitalized. The patient cannot remember what medicines he is taking. The hospitalist informs the patient that he has lactic acidosis. Which of the following medicines is likely to cause this condition?

A. Acarbose

B. Glyburide

C. Glipizide

D. Metformin

E. Troglitazone

11. A 30-year-old obese man with diabetes is seen in the emergency department with confusion and an increase in the rate and depth of his breathing. He has hyperglycemia and volume depletion and is treated with insulin and intravenous fluids. Medical records for this man are unavailable, and it is unknown whether he has type I or II diabetes. Which of the following autoantibodies would be most specific for a patient with type I diabetes?

A. Antimitochondrial antibodies

B. Antinuclear antibody

C. Antithyroglobulin antibodies

D. Anti-U1 RNP antibody

E. Glutamic acid decarboxylase antibodies (GAD)

12. A 53-year-old man reports to his physician that he has been extremely fatigued. His wife states that his skin has gradually become more pigmented. Laboratory tests reveal hypocortisolism, with corticotropin levels higher than normal. A picture of this patient's mouth is shown in Figure 5-1. What is the most likely etiology of this condition?

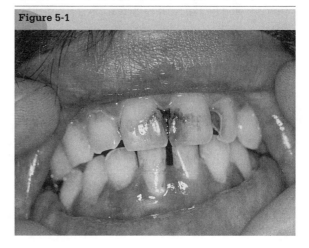

Figure 5-1

A. Alcoholism

B. Autoimmune disease

C. Cancer, primary

D. Cancer, metastasis

E. Drug toxicity

F. Infection

G. Ischemia

H. Trauma

13. A 62-year-old man with type II diabetes and coronary artery disease as well as a previous myocardial infarction is evaluated because of the recent onset of cough. The patient has a 25-pack-year history of smoking. He is currently on metoprolol, enalapril, aspirin, isosorbide mononitrate, metformin, and glyburide. On physical exam, his temperature is 37.0°C (98.6°F), pulse = 74 bpm, blood pressure 135/88 mm Hg, and respirations of 16/min. His heartbeat is regular and without murmurs, and his lungs are clear on auscultation. A transthoracic echocardiogram reveals an ejection fraction of 55 to 60%. Which of the following is the most likely cause of his cough?

A. Aldosterone

B. Bradykinin

C. Lung cancer

D. Pneumonia

E. Pulmonary edema

14. A 32-year-old woman with decreased libido is unable to conceive and seeks medical advice from a fertility expert. Unable to find an anatomical or physiological defect responsible,

the physician prescribes clomiphene. What is the mechanism of action of clomiphene in promoting fertilization?

A. Competitive inhibition of progestins at progesterone receptors

B. Estrogenic analog that increases sexual drive

C. GnRH analog, which stimulates LH and FSH when given in a pulsatile fashion

D. Partial agonist at estrogen receptors in the pituitary, preventing feedback inhibition, which increases LH and FSH and stimulates ovulation

E. Selective estrogenic partial agonist/antagonist

15. A 45-year-old Caucasian man presents to his primary care physician with fatigue and a 10-lb weight gain over recent months. He is worried because his first cousin was diagnosed with thyroid carcinoma the preceding year. Physical examination reveals a nodule in the upper lobe of the right thyroid gland. A fine-needle aspiration and biopsy is scheduled. Serum electrolytes are as follows: sodium 135 mEq/L, potassium 5 mEq/L, chloride 104 mEq/L, and calcium 6.1 mg/dL. What is the most likely diagnosis?

A. Anaplastic carcinoma

B. Follicular carcinoma

C. Hashimoto's thyroiditis

D. Medullary carcinoma

E. Papillary carcinoma

16. A 37-year-old well-proportioned woman who underwent a thyroidectomy for follicular carcinoma of the thyroid 3 months earlier presents with muscle twitching, which began 3 weeks earlier. Physical examination reveals no lymphadenopathy or palpable nodules in the previous location of her thyroid. Tapping the facial nerve produces spasm of the facial muscles. Laboratory studies show serum electrolytes as follows: sodium 135 mEq/L, potassium 5 mEq/L, chloride 104 mEq/L, calcium 5.1 mg/dL, and phosphorus 5.2 mg/dL. What is the most likely etiology of this patient's hypocalcemia?

A. Dietary deficiency

B. Gastrointestinal loss

C. Medullary carcinoma of the thyroid

D. Removal of parathyroid glands at time of thyroidectomy

E. Vitamin D deficiency

17. A 19-year-old woman is worried about an increase in the size of her jaw and forehead over the past 4 years. She is very self-conscious and states that she can notice the difference in pictures of her taken over the past few years. Which of the following hormones is most directly responsible for this patient's condition?

A. Growth hormone

B. Luteinizing hormone

C. Follicle-stimulating hormone

D. Progesterone

E. Thyroid-stimulating hormone

18. A 33-year-old woman presents with complaints of fatigue, dizziness, increased urination, increased skin pigmentation, and nausea and vomiting. She has no significant past medical history. Physical examination reveals her temperature to be 37°C (98.6°F), pulse 86 bpm, blood pressure 90/54 mm Hg, and respiratory rate 16/min. Serum electrolytes show sodium at 120 mEq/L and potassium at 6.1 mEq/L. Which of the following tests is indicated to confirm this patient's diagnosis?

A. Abdominal ultrasound

B. Cosyntropin stimulation test

C. CT scan of the abdomen

D. Free water deprivation

E. Oral captopril test

19. A 32-year-old man with suspected neurofibromatosis had a blood pressure of 175/96 mm Hg at a recent blood pressure screening. Today, he presents to the clinic for a checkup because he has had some abdominal discomfort. His blood pressure is 130/70 mm Hg. Physical examination reveals multiple tumors of his lips, mucous membranes, and skin. Laboratory values reveal a serum sodium 135 mEq/L, potassium 5 mEq/L, chloride 104 mEq/L, calcium 5.1 mg/dL, and phosphorus 5.2 mg/dL. What is the most likely diagnosis?

A. Multiple endocrine neoplasia type I (Wermer's)

B. Multiple endocrine neoplasia type IIa (Sipple's)

C. Multiple endocrine neoplasia type IIb (type III)

D. Laurence-Moon-Biedl syndrome

E. Prader-Willi syndrome

20. A 22-year-old woman is concerned about the palpitations she has been having for 3 months. She reports that she has lost 10 lb over the past year and is excessively nervous. Physical examination reveals slight bulging of her left eye but no other significant findings. Which of the following laboratory values are most consistent with Graves' disease?

A. ↑TSH, ↑T4, ↑T3

B. ↑TSH, ↓T4, ↓T3

C. ↑TSH, ↑T4, ↓T3

D. ↓TSH, ↓T4, ↓T3

E. ↓TSH, ↑T4, ↑T3

21. A 75-year-old man has an infarction in his posterior pituitary because of a severe hemorrhagic stroke. Which of the following actions of a specific pituitary hormone is most likely to be affected in this patient?

A. Contraction of ureteral smooth muscle

B. Reabsorption of free water from the renal collecting ducts

C. Stimulation of the adrenal gland to produce aldosterone and cortisol

D. Stimulation of thyroid hormone production

E. Synthesis of testosterone

22. A 59-year-old woman who has type I diabetes, hypertriglyceridemia, and end-stage renal disease presents to the clinic concerned about weakness and aching in her bones. Physical examination reveals a thin-appearing woman who has crepitus with movement of her joints bilaterally. Serum calcium is decreased. A diagnosis of osteoarthritis is made and the patient is advised to take calcium and avoid falling owing to her high risk of suffering a fracture. What is the most likely cause for this woman's hypocalcemia?

A. Dietary deficiency

B. Hypoparathyroidism

C. Failure of hydroxylation of vitamin D

D. Gastrointestinal losses

E. Pancreatitis

23. A 32-year-old woman who has a history of hypopituitarism presents to the clinic for a general checkup. Which of the following is one way in which her condition would manifest itself?

A. Galactorrhea

B. Hypertension

C. Lack of sexual desire

D. Proptosis

E. Weight loss

24. A 55-year-old obese man with a 10-year history of severe uncontrolled diabetes presents to the clinic for a 3-month follow-up. His serum electrolytes are normal except for an elevation in calcium. Which of the following mechanisms is the most likely cause of his hypercalcemia?

A. Dietary excess

B. Lithium overdose

C. Milk-alkali syndrome

D. Parathyroid adenoma

E. Parathyroid hyperplasia

25. A 45-year-old man with a history of hypertension is brought to the emergency room with complaints of vision changes. His blood pressure is 200/110 mm Hg upon presentation, and he is found to be undergoing a hypertensive crisis. If propranolol is to be given, which of the following single agents should also be given to prevent unrestricted constriction of smooth muscles in blood vessels and a further rise in blood pressure?

A. Atenolol

B. Clonidine

C. Enalapril

D. Labetalol

E. Prazosin

26. A 21-year-old military recruit with a 1-week history of meningitis presents to the emergency department with the new onset of dizziness. Physical examination reveals that his blood pressure is 78/42 mm Hg and he has an abdominal rash. What is the most likely cause of his hypotension?

A. Addison's disease

B. Dehydration due to decreased fluid intake

C. Diarrhea

D. Pituitary infarction

E. Waterhouse-Friderichsen syndrome

27. A 45-year-old patient who previously had a thyroidectomy for follicular carcinoma of the thyroid is brought to the emergency department. Upon examination, her vital signs are as follows: temperature 35.8°C (96.4°F), pulse 60 bpm, blood pressure 70/40 mm Hg, and respiratory rate 8/min. Her daughter reports that she had a viral infection the previous week and had a seizure that morning. Which of the following treatments would most directly treat the underlying cause of this patient's disorder?

A. Amantadine

B. Levothyroxine

C. Methimazole

D. Propylthiouracil.

E. Intravenous fluids

28. A 45-year-old man presents to the clinic reporting an occasionally rapid heartbeat, chest palpitations, and sweating. Looking back through his chart, his physician notices that this patient has had episodic high blood pressure. Which of the following tests or measurements is appropriate in this patient?

A. Captopril stimulation test

B. High-dose dexamethasone suppression test

C. Urinary free cortisol

D. Urinary level of 5-HIAA

E. Serum VMA

29. A 58-year-old woman presents to clinic with new-onset back pain after a fall 2 days earlier. The patient states that she was working in her garden, and when she began to stand up, she lost her balance and fell on her behind. Over the past 2 days she has been experiencing pain in her lower back. At present the patient takes only a diuretic for high blood pressure. She is postmenopausal and does not take any type of hormone replacement. She is a smoker and has smoked a pack of cigarettes every day for the past 35 years. Aside from the back pain, her physical examination is normal. Laboratory studies and radiographs are obtained. Her lab work is normal, and the x-rays of her hip are shown in Figure 5-2. She is then sent for a dual-energy x-ray absorptiometry (DEXA) scan, which gives her a T score of −2. What is the most appropriate treatment for this patient?

A. Alendronate

B. Alendronate and calcium with vitamin D

C. Calcitonin

D. Calcium with vitamin D

E. Hormone replacement therapy

30. A 32-year-old man with AIDS is recovering from intracerebral toxoplasmosis. He has had *Pneumocystis carinii* pneumonia and chronic diarrhea secondary to infection with *Cryptosporidium*. He complains that he has had frequent urination since recovering from toxoplasmosis, although he has not been drinking more fluids. Physical examination reveals vital signs as follows: temperature 37.0°C (98.6°F), pulse 76 bpm, blood pressure 120/74 mm Hg, and respira-

Figure 5-2

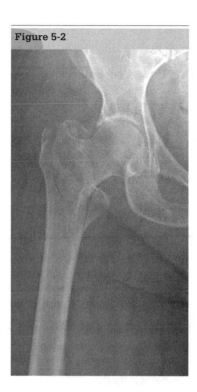

tory rate 16/min. Urine osmolarity is low. What is the next most appropriate step in the evaluation of this patient?

A. Administer ADH and recheck urine osmolarity

B. Blood cultures

C. Urinalysis for leukocytes, hematuria, and proteinuria

D. Urine cultures

E. Urine leukocyte esterase

31. A 52-year-old African American woman presents to her primary care physician with an asymptomatic, cold, nontender nodule of her thyroid gland, firm to palpation. She also has enlarged cervical lymph nodes, hoarseness, and dysphagia. Of the following types of thyroid malignancies, which has the poorest prognosis and which is the patient most likely to have?

A. Anaplastic carcinoma

B. Follicular carcinoma

C. Medullary carcinoma

D. Papillary carcinoma

E. Parathyroid carcinoma

32. A 40-year-old Asian man presents to his primary care physician complaining that he is always thirsty and has to urinate a lot more frequently than he used to. He is also saying that his vision occasionally gets blurry. His body-mass index (BMI) is 32, and a random plasma glucose is 310 mg/dL. What is the proposed pathogenesis of this patient's disease?

A. Anti–islet cell antibody production

B. Anti-insulin antibody production

C. Beta-islet cell ability to produce insulin diminishes and peripheral insulin resistance develops

D. Destruction of pancreatic alpha cells

E. Effacement of aldosterone-producing cells of the adrenal medulla

33. A 40-year-old depressed Asian woman presents to her primary care physician with bone pain, a recent radial fracture, and abdominal pain. She is also noted to have a history of kidney stones. Which of the following lab values would one expect to find in this patient?

A. high PTH, high serum calcium, and low serum phosphate

B. low PTH, high serum calcium, and high serum phosphate

C. high PTH, low serum calcium, and low serum phosphate

D. low PTH, low serum calcium, and low serum phosphate

E. high PTH, low serum calcium, and high serum phosphate

34. The intersection of these two structures is an important landmark in a parathyroidectomy because most parathyroid glands are located within 2 cm of this area. What are these structures?

A. Inferior thyroid artery and middle thyroid vein

B. Inferior thyroid artery and recurrent laryngeal nerve

C. Middle thyroid vein and recurrent laryngeal nerve

D. Superior thyroid artery and middle thyroid vein

E. Superior thyroid artery and recurrent laryngeal nerve

35. A 3-week-old girl is brought to the pediatrician because she has been crying and vomiting. She appears dehydrated and her labs show that she is hyponatremic, hypokalemic, hypotensive, and hypoglycemic. The cosyntropin stimulation test confirms the diagnosis. What other disease should this patient be tested for?

A. Cystic fibrosis

B. Down's syndrome

C. Duchenne muscular dystrophy

D. Pompe's disease

E. Wilms' tumor

36. An asymptomatic 38-year-old woman presents to her primary care physician for a routine health maintenance exam and is noted to have a solitary thyroid nodule. Laboratory studies reveal normal levels of TSH and normal free T_4. Serum electrolytes and calcium, magnesium, and phosphorus are all within normal limits. Fine-needle aspiration of the nodule is indeterminate. Surgical excision of the nodule is most likely to reveal which of the following?

A. Anaplastic carcinoma

B. Follicular carcinoma

C. Lymphatic tissue

D. Medullary carcinoma

E. Papillary carcinoma

37. A 2-week-old girl is brought to the emergency department by her mother, who is concerned about her child's lethargy. Physical examination reveals a temperature of 37°C (98.6°) and blood pressure of 56/32 mm Hg. The anterior fontanelle is sunken, the mucous membranes are dry, the eyes cannot make tears, and the clitoris is enlarged. Laboratory studies show the following: sodium 125 mEq/L, potassium 5.8 mEq/L, chloride 100 mEq/L, HCO_3 20 mEq/L. What is the most likely etiology of this child's symptoms?

A. 11β-Hydroxylase deficiency

B. 21α-Hydroxylase deficiency

C. Congenital syphilis

D. Influenza

E. Pyloric stenosis

38. A 10-year-old girl develops increased thirst, increased urination, and weight loss despite her grandmother's statement that she eats everything that's not nailed down. She has no family history of diabetes. She is at the fiftieth percentile for height and weight. A random blood glucose gives a reading of 284 mg/dL. Which of the following best describes the probable mechanism of her illness?

A. Inadequate release of antidiuretic hormone

B. Inadequately suppressed hepatic gluconeogenesis

C. Immunologically mediated destruction of the pancreatic beta cells

D. Insensitivity of the collecting duct of the kidney to the effects of ADH

E. Peripheral insulin resistance

39. A 32-year-old nulligravida presents to her primary care physician complaining of infertility. She has been trying to conceive for 18 months. Review of systems is significant for polymenorrhea, fatigue, cold intolerance, and a 15-lb weight gain over the same time period despite attempts to diet. Pelvic examination is normal. What is the most likely cause of her infertility?

A. Hypothyroidism

B. Kallmann's syndrome

C. Polycystic ovarian syndrome

D. Prolactinoma

E. Sheehan's syndrome

40. A 38-year-old man undergoes surgical removal of a solitary parathyroid adenoma. While recovering in the hospital, he begins to experience paresthesias of the hands and feet and circumoral region as well as muscle cramps. Physical examination is significant for positive Chvostek's and Trousseau's signs. Total serum calcium is found to be 5.8. Two days later, the serum calcium has normalized. What is the best explanation for these findings?

A. Disruption of blood supply to the remaining parathyroid glands

B. "Hungry bones" syndrome

C. Tumor lysis syndrome

D. Pseudohypoparathyroidism

E. Vitamin D deficiency

41. An 18-year-old man with recently diagnosed type I diabetes mellitus finds that his morning fasting glucose levels are averaging 160 mg/dL. Without consulting his endocrinologist, he increases his dose of NPH insulin at dinner, and wakes up the next morning with a sugar of 275 mg/dL. What best explains this new finding?

A. Dawn phenomenon

B. Eating a sugar snack at bedtime

C. Insulinoma

D. Somogyi effect

E. Type II DM incorrectly diagnosed as type I DM

42. A 54-year-old man is hospitalized after an automobile accident, during which he sustained significant trauma. Two days after the accident, while he is still unconscious and receiving maintenance intravenous fluids, his nurse notices that his routine lab work reveals serum sodium of 122 mEq/L. The patient's vital signs are within normal limits. There is no evidence of jugular venous distension. His heart and lung exams reveal no abnormalities. He has no edema or ascites. Plasma osmolarity is found to be 255 mOsm/kg. Urine osmolarity is then found to be 420 mOsm/kg. What is the best explanation for these findings?

A. Central diabetes insipidus

B. Congestive heart failure

C. Iatrogenic fluid overload

D. Nephrotic syndrome

E. Syndrome of inappropriate antidiuretic hormone secretion

43. A 46-year-old woman undergoes a laparoscopic cholecystectomy. While in the recovery room, she suddenly develops a temperature of 40.3°C (104.5°F), a heart rate of 130 bpm, flushing, sweating, and delirium. Her past medical history is significant for gastroesophageal reflux, for which she takes pantoprazole; hyperthyroidism, for which she takes propylthiouracil; and diabetes mellitus type I, for which she takes insulin. An electrocardiogram (ECG) shows an irregularly irregular rhythm. What is the most likely explanation for these symptoms?

A. Addisonian crisis

B. Anaphylactic reaction to postoperative pain medications

C. Carcinoid syndrome

D. Postoperative infection

E. Thyrotoxic crisis

44. A 40-year-old woman with abdominal obesity, striae, and moon facies is evaluated for hip pain. Vital signs on exam were temperature 37.4°C (99.3°F), pulse 76 bpm, blood pressure 156/94 mm Hg, and respiratory rate 16/min. Figure 5-3 shows the patient during this office visit. What is the most likely cause of her hip pain?

A. Abdominal obesity increases the workload of the hips and legs

B. Cortisol inhibition of osteoblasts and stimulation of osteoclasts

C. Legg-Calvé-Perthes disease

D. Osteomyelitis

E. Previous unreported hip fracture

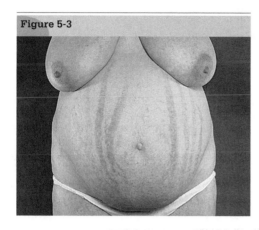

Figure 5-3

	T_3	T_4	Free Thyroxine	TSH
A	↑	↑	↑	↑
B	↑	↑	↑	↓
C	↑	↑	↓	↓
D	↑	↓	↓	↑
E	↓	↓	↓	↓

45. A 39-year-old woman presents to her primary care physician complaining of increased urinary frequency, which she has experienced for 6 months. She is of normal weight for her height. Her medical history is significant for ulcerative colitis, for which she underwent a total colectomy 3 years earlier, and bipolar disorder, for which she currently takes lithium. She also takes two ibuprofen as needed to relieve her menstrual cramps. What is the most likely cause of this woman's polyuria?

A. Diabetes mellitus type II

B. Ibuprofen use

C. Lithium use

D. Postsurgical complications of the colectomy

E. Water intoxication

46. A 57-year-old man presents to his primary care physician complaining of increasing weakness and abdominal pain. He reports some dyspnea on exertion, and his wife says she has noticed that he has an all-season tan, even though he is rarely outdoors. His past history is significant for cirrhosis, diabetes, and atrial fibrillation. Physical examination reveals some mild tenderness in the right upper-abdominal quadrant. What laboratory findings would suggest the most likely diagnosis?

A. Hyperalbuminemia

B. Increased iron-binding capacity

C. Increased testosterone

D. Serum ferritin less than 300 μg/L

E. Transferrin saturation greater than 70%

47. A 42-year-old Caucasian woman is referred for evaluation of a goiter. She takes buspirone for anxiety and metoprolol for hypertension; she has a history of hyperhidrosis, heart palpitations, and insomnia. Physical examination reveals a thin, nervous woman with a warm, palpable goiter. A laboratory workup is completed and indicates hyperthyroidism. Which of the following supports her presentation?

48. A 49-year-old woman undergoes a subtotal thyroidectomy for follicular carcinoma. Which of the following postoperative laboratory tests should be performed shortly after the surgery?

A. Calcium

B. Calcitonin

C. Cortisol

D. Norepinephrine

E. Parathyroid hormone

49. A 49-year-old woman is hospitalized because of seizures. Her history is significant for newly diagnosed diabetes, and she had a lumpectomy for breast cancer 6 months earlier. Her serum calcium is 16.9 mg/dL, phosphorus 2.0 mg/dL, and albumin level is 3.8 g/dL. A chest radiograph reveals some right-lower-lobe masses. Which of the following accounts for this woman's findings?

A. Cancer, metastatic breast

B. Cancer, parathyroid

C. Renal failure

D. Vitamin C toxicity

E. Vitamin D toxicity

50. A 50-year-old man presents with a 2-week history of shortness of breath and hoarseness. He has no significant past medical history and is not a smoker. Physical examination reveals a large, tender, indurated thyroid mass. A fine-needle aspirate shows many spindle-shaped cells. CT reveals that the mass extends into the cervical muscle. Two cervical lymph nodes contain metastases. What is the most likely diagnosis?

A. Anaplastic carcinoma

B. Follicular carcinoma

C. Medullary carcinoma

D. Hürthle cell carcinoma

E. Papillary carcinoma

51. A 29-year-old man presents to his primary care physician with tenderness and enlargement of the breasts, which began 4 months earlier. His laboratory values include a serum total testosterone of 800 ng/dL, estradiol of 96 pg/mL, LH of 3.2 mU/mL, FSH of 1.9 mU/mL, and a human chorionic gonadotropin (hCG) level of 26,000 ng/mL. What type of germ cell tumor does this patient most likely have?

A. Choriocarcinoma

B. Leydig cell tumor

C. Seminoma

D. Testicular cell tumor

E. Yolk sac tumor

52. While playing soccer, a 12-year-old Hispanic boy collapses. He is disoriented and lethargic, hypotensive, tachycardic, and tachypneic on arrival at the emergency room. Laboratory studies reveal sodium of 153 mEq/L, potassium of 4.8 mEq/L, chloride of 100 mEq/L, bicarbonate of 9 mEq/L, and glucose of 510 mg/dL. Ketones are found on urinalysis. What would most likely be found on microscopic examination of his pancreatic islets of Langerhans?

A. Amyloidosis of islet cells

B. Eosinophilic infiltration of islet cells

C. Gangrenous necrosis of islet cells

D. Fat necrosis of islet cells

E. Significantly fewer islet cells

53. A 42-year-old man presents to his primary care physician complaining of weakness and fatigue. His blood pressure is 120/82 mm Hg sitting and 98/60 mm Hg standing. His serum laboratory values are sodium 126 mEq/mL, potassium 5.4 mEq/mL, chloride 100, and bicarbonate 21. Which of the following physical examination findings would be consistent with the most likely diagnosis in this patient?

A. Dark, pigmented spots on his back and shoulders

B. Deviated nasal septum

C. Exophthalmos

D. Macroglossia

E. Pruritic rash of the upper arms

54. A 32-year-old Caucasian woman complains of a milky discharge from her breasts, which she first noticed 2 months earlier. She has not been menstruating since the symptoms began. She does not have any other complaints and is not currently taking any medicines. Laboratory studies reveal hyperprolactinemia. Her MRI is shown in Figure 5-4. A positron emission tomography (PET) scan of here brain is negative. What is the most appropriate treatment for this patient?

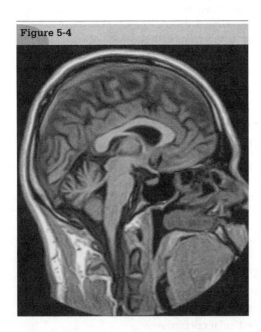

Figure 5-4

A. Bromocriptine

B. Metoclopromide

C. Ondansetron

D. Propranolol

E. Somatostatin

55. A 13-year-old girl is admitted to the pediatrics unit with new-onset diabetic ketoacidosis. After being successfully treated with insulin, intravenous fluids, and potassium, she is discharged and an appointment is made for her to follow up with an endocrinologist. Instead of keeping the appointment, however, her mother decides to treat the girl with her own metformin, which she takes for her diabetes, because she does not want her daughter to be treated with injection therapy. Although the girl does well for a while, she is readmitted to the hospital 8 months later, again with signs and symptoms of diabetic ketoacidosis. What is the best explanation for this course of events?

A. Addison disease

B. "Honeymoon period"

C. Inadequate metformin dosage

D. Inadequate metformin frequency

E. Somogyi effect

56. A healthy 31-year-old woman gives vaginal birth at term to an 8 lb 3 oz boy. Twenty-four hr after his birth, the infant is tachypneic; he has metabolic acidosis and severe hypotension. Laboratory serum findings reveal an elevated testosterone level, low cortisol, low sodium, and elevated potassium. Enlarged adrenal glands are seen on ultrasound. What is the cause of this infant's symptoms?

A. 11β-hydroxylase deficiency

B. 17α-hydroxylase deficiency

C. 21β-hydroxylase deficiency

D. Fabry's disease

E. Gaucher's disease

F. Niemann-Pick disease

G. Tay-Sachs disease

57. During the neck exam of an asymptomatic 52-year-old man, a 2-cm cervical lymph node is palpated and the thyroid seems somewhat enlarged. His chest x-ray is normal. Electrolytes as well as TSH, T_3, and T_4 are within normal limits. A fine-needle aspiration is performed and is positive for cancer. What is the most likely pathology?

A. Anaplastic carcinoma

B. Follicular carcinoma

C. Medullary carcinoma

D. Papillary carcinoma

E. Squamous cell carcinoma

58. At 41 weeks' gestation, a 38-year-old woman delivers a 2,950-g 44-cm neonate with an Apgar score of 6 at 1 and 5 min. The neonate is noted to have an umbilical hernia, macroglossia, enlarged fontanelles, and coarse facial features. Which of the following tests would most likely lead to the correct diagnosis?

A. Antithyroid antibodies

B. Iodine test

C. Radioactive iodine uptake

D. Thyroid-binding globulin

E. Total T_3

F. Total T_4

59. A 23-year-old woman who gave birth to a healthy neonate 3 weeks earlier presents to her primary care physician with anxiety, heat intolerance, and heart palpitations. She has no significant medical history and takes a multivitamin once daily. Her vital signs include a temperature of 37.4°C (99.3°F), blood pressure of 160/90 mm Hg, heart rate of 110 bpm, and respirations of 15/min. The woman's hands are moist and she appears anxious. Physical examination reveals no evidence of thyromegaly. What is the most likely diagnosis?

   A. Anaplastic carcinoma

   B. Follicular carcinoma

   C. Hashimoto's thyroiditis

   D. Graves' disease

   E. Medullary carcinoma

   F. Postpartum thyroiditis

   G. Reidel's thyroiditis

   H. Sheehan's syndrome

   I. Subacute thyroiditis

60. A 62-year-old woman is seen in the clinic with a chief complaint of severe bilateral paresthesias in her feet and ankles, occasionally accompanied by sharp pains in her legs. Her sleep has been minimal due to the severe irritation of the bed sheets touching her feet. The pain is somewhat relieved after she walks for a few minutes. The patient's medical history is significant for osteoporosis, type 2 diabetes, and hypertension. Physical examination reveals diminished bilateral ankle reflexes; patellar and biceps femoris reflexes are normal. Foot vibratory and position sense are lost. What is the most likely diagnosis?

   A. Cauda equina syndrome

   B. Diabetic peripheral neuropathy

   C. Infarction of the spinal cord

   D. L3–L4 herniated disk

   E. L4–L5 herniated disk

61. A couple presents for an evaluation of male infertility. The husband's height is 6 ft 2 in; his weight is 150 lb. His arms and legs are long in comparison with his torso. Genital exam reveals small, firm testicles in the scrotum bilaterally. What is most the likely etiology of this gonadal abnormality?

   A. Bilateral anorchia

   B. Complete androgen insensitivity

   C. Cryptorchidism

   D. Kallmann's syndrome

   E. Klinefelter's syndrome

   F. Panhypopituitarism

   G. Turner's syndrome

62. A 2-year-old girl is brought to the pediatrician for a well-child checkup. On physical exam, the pediatrician notices an irregular abdominal mass. Levels of urinary homovanillic acid and vanillylmandelic acid are markedly elevated. Which of the following is most likely to be noted upon biopsy?

   A. Dense nests of immature small round cells separated by fibrillar bundles, often forming pseudorosettes of cells surrounding a pink fibrillar center

   B. Pleomorphic spindle tumor cells attempting to form an osteoid matrix

   C. Primitive metanephric blastema, dysplastic tubules, and supporting mesenchyme or stroma

   D. Small, round blue cells with evidence of skeletal muscle differentiation

   E. Stromal elements with infiltrates of normal lymphocytes, plasma cells, eosinophils, and Reed-Sternberg cells

63. A 23-year-old man presents with fatigue, weight loss, hypotension, nausea, vomiting, and increased pigmentation of the skin. His physician suspects adrenal insufficiency but wants to perform a confirmatory test. What is the most appropriate hypothalamic or pituitary hormone to be administered to this patient?

   A. Adrenocorticotropic hormone

   B. Gonadotropin-releasing hormone

   C. Growth hormone

   D. Growth hormone-inhibiting hormone

   E. Prolactin

64. A 35-year-old Caucasian woman complains of drainage from her nipples, which she has been noticing for 2 months. She has not been nursing during this time. She also complains of headaches, which have increased over the past 6 months, and some new vision changes. She reports that she has tunnel vision and cannot see anything in her peripheral fields of view. An MRI is obtained (Figure 5-5). What is the most likely diagnosis?

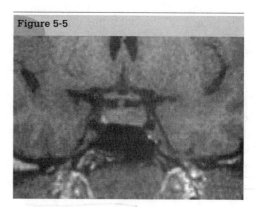

Figure 5-5

   A. Antipsychotic medications

   B. Craniopharyngioma

   C. Meningioma

   D. Prolactinoma

   E. Schizophrenia

65. A 42-year-old woman presents to clinic for her annual checkup. Her only complaint today is some new bone pain. The pain comes and goes and is worse on more active days. She has a long history of moderate persistent asthma that is somewhat controlled with inhaled corticosteroids (budesonide) and salmeterol. She uses a rescue albuterol inhaler as needed. She has several yearly exacerbations, for which she also receives systemic steroids, usually prednisolone. She also has a history of type II diabetes mellitus, for which she currently takes metformin. Her hypertension is semi-controlled with metoprolol and lisinopril. She also takes simvastatin for hyperlipidemia. She has gastroesophageal reflux disease (GERD), which is well controlled with omeprazole. Family history is positive for rheumatoid arthritis. Physical examination of the heart, lungs, and abdomen is normal. Neurological exam is also benign. Musculoskeletal exam is positive for some minor pain with movement. Of all the medications the patient currently takes, which is most likely to be responsible for the bone pain?

A. Albuterol

B. Prednisolone

C. Lisinopril

D. Metformin

E. Metoprolol

F. Salmeterol

G. Omeprazole

H. Simvastatin

66. Which of the following anterior pituitary hormones is a polypeptide dimer?

A. Adrenocorticotropic hormone (ACTH)

B. Growth hormone (GH)

C. Prolactin (PRL)

D. Thyroid-stimulating hormone (TSH)

67. A 35-year-old man presents to his primary care physician complaining of light-headedness on standing and two syncopal events. Physical examination reveals the man to have a suntan, although it is the middle of January in the Northeast. The patient denies sun or other ultraviolet (UV) exposure. A CT scan is ordered and is unremarkable except for bilateral adrenal cortical atrophy. Which two peptide hormones have a similarity that is responsible for this patient's dermatologic change?

A. Thyroid-stimulating hormone and testosterone

B. Follicle-stimulating hormone and prolactin

C. Alpha melanocyte–stimulating hormone and adrenocorticotropic hormone

D. Prolactin and luteinizing hormone

E. Adrenocorticotropic hormone and beta melanocyte–stimulating hormone

68. A 3-year-old child is startled by a jack-in-the-box while waiting in her pediatrician's office. Her heart suddenly begins beating faster, then returns to normal after a short period, when she is reassured that the clown's head is only a toy. What is the amino acid precursor to the substance responsible for her increased heart rate?

A. Glutamic acid

B. Histidine

C. Phenylalanine

D. Valine

E. Urease

69. In the resting state, guanosine diphosphate (GDP) is bound to which subunit of the G protein?

A. Alpha

B. Beta

C. Gamma

D. Delta

E. Chi

70. The binding of which of the following second messengers causes Ca^{2+} to be released from its intracellular store in the sarcoplasmic reticulum?

A. PIP2

B. DAG

C. IP3

D. cAMP

71. A 41-year-old man has been exposed to sunlight both on a tanning bed as well as outdoors. At presentation to his primary care physician, he has areas of extremely black-appearing skin. This finding may relate to the production of which gland's primary hormone that is inhibited by sunlight?

A. Adrenal

B. Anterior pituitary

C. Pineal

D. Posterior pituitary

E. Thyroid

72. Norepinephrine and epinephrine stimulate cellular receptors with which of the following characteristics?

A. They are located on intracellular vesicles.

B. They are bound to DNA regulation sequences.

C. The receptors consist of seven transmembrane helices.

D. The receptors are coupled to cell-surface G proteins.

73. Steroid hormone synthesis takes place in several different intracellular compartments. In which compartment is cholesterol converted to pregnenolone?

A. Golgi apparatus

B. Lysosome

C. Mitochondria

D. Rough endoplasmic reticulum

E. Smooth endoplasmic reticulum

74. A 5-year-old boy is brought to his pediatrician for a well checkup. He has achieved all pertinent milestones for his age. Physical examination of the heart, lungs, and abdomen is within normal limits. His testes are descended bilaterally. The penis is not circumcised and measures 3 cm from pubis to glans. For normal embryonic development of external male genitalia, testosterone alone is insufficient. Which enzyme is responsible for the production of the hormone needed to stimulate growth of the male genitalia?

A. Cytoplasmic 17α-hydroxylase

B. Mitochondrial 18β-hydroxylase

C. 5α-reductase

D. 15-reductase

E. 21-hydroxylase

75. A 24-year-old woman who works as a home health aide presents to her primary care physician with palpitations, nervousness, heat intolerance, and profound fatigue. She indicates that she has also lost 25 lb over 2 months. Vital signs are as follows: heart rate 125 bpm, blood pressure 96/52 mm Hg, temperature 37.3°C, respiratory rate 19/min.

Physical examination reveals a moderately distressed, diaphoretic, thin woman. Her thyroid gland is not tender or enlarged. Lab studies show a TSH of 0.01 µU/mL, total T3 of 300 ng/dL, and free T$_4$ of 15 ng/dL. A radionuclide scan of the thyroid is performed and shows no uptake of radioactive iodine in the gland. What is the most likely cause of her symptoms?

A. Graves' disease

B. Subacute thyroiditis

C. Surreptitious ingestion of thyroxine

D. Toxic adenoma

E. Toxic multinodular goiter

Answer Key

1. D	20. E	39. A	58. F
2. G	21. B	40. B	59. F
3. D	22. C	41. D	60. B
4. D	23. C	42. E	61. E
5. E	24. E	43. E	62. A
6. E	25. E	44. B	63. A
7. B	26. E	45. C	64. D
8. A	27. B	46. E	65. B
9. B	28. E	47. B	66. D
10. D	29. B	48. A	67. C
11. E	30. A	49. A	68. C
12. B	31. A	50. A	69. A
13. B	32. C	51. A	70. C
14. D	33. A	52. E	71. C
15. D	34. B	53. A	72. C
16. D	35. C	54. A	73. C
17. A	36. E	55. B	74. C
18. B	37. B	56. C	75. C
19. C	38. C	57. D	

Answers and Explanations

1. D. Prolactin would be expected to increase in a patient who has suffered a transection of the pituitary stalk. The pituitary stalk connects the hypothalamus to the pituitary gland. The pituitary receives releasing hormones from the hypothalamus, which increase the production of pituitary hormones. Prolactin, however, is regulated by an inhibitory hormone called dopamine. Whenever dopamine is unable to reach the pituitary, as in this patient, prolactin production would be expected to increase. The other pituitary hormones, ACTH, FSH, LH, TSH, and GH, are regulated by stimulating hormones from the hypothalamus. Whenever stimulating hormones fail to stimulate the pituitary for whatever cause, the production of these hormones is reduced.

2. G. Although a few of the above conditions can be caused by a deficiency of B vitamins, only megaloblastic anemia can be caused by destruction in gastric parietal cells. Parietal cells are responsible for producing intrinsic factor, which is involved in the absorption of vitamin B_{12} (cobalamin). Megaloblastic anemia is characterized by a macrocytic anemia (MCV > 100), with hypersegmented neutrophils on peripheral blood smear, typical symptoms of anemia, and neurological dysfunction. Autoimmune hemolysis is not related to nutritional deficiencies and is caused by autoantibodies to red blood cells. Beriberi is caused by a thiamine (vitamin B_1) deficiency. Cheilosis, a periorbital scaling and cracking, can be caused by a deficiency in riboflavin (vitamin B_2). Iron-deficiency anemia is caused by blood loss and rarely a dietary deficiency of iron. Kwashiorkor is caused by protein deficiency and marasmus by severe malnutrition. Night blindness can be caused by a vitamin A deficiency. Pellagra, characterized by diarrhea, dementia, and dermatitis, is due to a deficiency in niacin (vitamin B_3). Scurvy is caused by a vitamin C deficiency.

3. D. A deficiency of 21-beta hydroxylase, an enzyme involved in steroidogenesis by the adrenal gland, is the most common cause of congenital adrenal hyperplasia in children. It is characterized clinically by hypotension and virilization in females. The virilization of the genitalia is due to an increase in adrenal androgens. The hypotension is due mainly to a decrease in aldosterone, which leads to the loss of sodium and consequently water. As children grow older, they will have early acceleration of their height and an early appearance of pubic and axillary hair. A 5-alpha reductase deficiency would lead to a decrease in dihydrotestosterone and would cause male children to have ambiguous genitalia until puberty, when a rise in testosterone would stimulate growth of the testes. A 17-alpha hydroxylase deficiency would present with hypertension in males and females and a failure of the development of secondary sexual characteristics in females. Males and females with 11-beta hydroxylase deficiency would be most likely to have hypertension. Females with the condition would have masculinization of their genitalia, as in 21-beta hydroxylase deficiency. Testicular feminization syndrome would not cause a genotypic female to have genital masculinization. In this condition, males have a defect in their dihydrotestosterone receptor, which prevents their testes from developing.

4. D. Sheehan's syndrome is pituitary necrosis secondary to blood loss during childbirth. The pituitary gland enlarges during pregnancy and requires more blood flow and oxygenation than would exist under normal conditions. Because the gland is enlarged, it becomes more susceptible to necrosis when blood loss and ischemia are present. Patients with Sheehan's syndrome, like this patient, have clinical symptoms that are due to the loss of multiple pituitary hormones. Cretinism is a severe condition of children caused by hypothyroidism; it is characterized by mental retardation and an enlarged tongue and abdomen. Hashimoto's thyroiditis is the most common form of hypothyroidism in patients with adequate iodine intake. Even though this patient presented with multiple symptoms of hypothyroidism, Hashimoto's is not likely in this scenario because of the recent history of blood loss during childbirth. An iodine deficiency would be more likely in third-world countries and is not likely in this patient. Subacute thyroiditis is associated with focal destruction of the thyroid gland and hypothyroidism following a recent viral infection. This patient has no history of viral infection.

5. E. This patient has carcinoid syndrome, which is caused by an increased production of serotonin and is characterized by flushing, diarrhea, right-sided valvular lesions, and bronchospasm. Carcinoid tumors can be malignant and fatal, and a physician must examine and treat the patient for malignancy. Relief of many of the symptoms of carcinoid syndrome can be accomplished with methylsergide, a serotonin antagonist. Albuterol could potentially relieve bronchospasm in this patient but would not alleviate any of his other symptoms. Bismuth subsalicylate is effective in improving a variety of GI symptoms but would also not help this patient's systemic effects of serotonin. Cimetidine is a histamine (H_2) receptor blocker and is used to reduce excess acid production by the gastric parietal cells. Enalapril, an angiotensin-converting enzyme (ACE) inhibitor, is used as an antihypertensive medication and protective agent of the kidneys in patients with diabetes, but it has no role in therapy of this patient.

6. E. Progesterone is responsible for the process whereby the endometrium becomes thickened and edematous, with spiraling of its glands. This stage of the menstrual cycle, called the secretory phase, begins to occur 1 or 2 days after ovulation. Estrogen is responsible for the proliferative phase of the menstrual cycle, which begins at the end of menstruation and continues until day 14 of the 28-day cycle. During this phase, the endometrium is beginning to proliferate and the spiral arteries lengthen but show only slight coiling. Follicle-stimulating hormone is involved in ovarian follicles and estrogen secretion. Luteinizing hormone triggers ovulation and plays a role in the formation of the corpus luteum and in the synthesis of estrogen and progesterone. LH is not directly responsible for the secretory phase of the menstrual cycle. Testosterone is a male sex hormone involved in spermatogenesis and the development of male secondary sexual characteristics.

7. B. By her clinical description, this woman most likely has a hydatidiform mole. hCG is produced by the mole and has structural similarities to TSH. Although hCG has only weak effects on the TSH receptor, it can cause hyperthyroidism when produced in large quantities, as in hydatidiform mole and choriocarcinoma. Often, women with a hydatidiform mole have vaginal bleeding and an increase in uterine size, which can cause discomfort or pain. Estrogen has multiple hormonal roles in the reproductive system in females but does not stimulate the synthesis of thyroid hormone. Prolactin's main role is in the production and secretion of milk; it has no thyroid-stimulating role. Progesterone is another female reproductive hormone involved in breast development and secretory activity during the luteal phase of the menstrual cycle. TSH has the ability to directly increase the thyroid gland's production of T_4 and T_3 but is not the cause of this woman's hyperthyroidism because her TSH levels were low on analysis.

8. A. Addison's disease is characterized by failure of the adrenal glands to produce aldosterone. Aldosterone increases renal absorption of sodium and secretion of potassium. If aldosterone were deficient, sodium and water would be excreted and potassium would increase in the serum. From the information given, the patient clearly has Addison's disease. His weight loss and increase in thirst and urination can be explained by the loss of water, while his increased skin pigmentation is due to increased production of proopiomelanocortin (POMC), a precursor that is cleaved into adrenocorticotropic hormone (ACTH), melanocyte-stimulating hormone (MSH), and lipocortin. MSH is responsible for the increase in skin pigmentation. Conn's disease, or primary hyperaldosteronism, is caused most commonly by an adrenocortical adenoma but can also be caused by adrenal cortical hyperplasia or adrenal carcinoma. Patients with Conn's disease have elevated sodium and decreased potassium, which is the opposite of the case in this patient. Diabetes insipidus is caused by a decrease in the production of antidiuretic hormone (ADH) or renal unresponsiveness to ADH. Patients with this condition have high serum osmolarities and low urine osmolarity owing to the excretion of free water. This patient does not have diabetes mellitus because his

serum fasting glucose level was 96. A serum fasting glucose of 126 or greater on two separate occasions is necessary to make the diagnosis of diabetes mellitus. Hemochromatosis is a condition characterized by the excessive accumulation of iron in the blood and tissues and can present with a multitude of symptoms including cirrhosis, restrictive cardiomyopathy, testicular atrophy, and an increase in skin pigmentation. This patient does not have hemochromatosis because we are told that the only electrolyte abnormalities are in sodium and potassium and not iron. Psychogenic polydipsia is a psychological condition characterized by excess water consumption and a decreased plasma and urinary osmolarity. This patient does have a history of depression, but his increased water intake is caused by an increase in water loss. SIADH, which is caused by pituitary or ectopic production of ADH (common in small cell lung cancer) is characterized by hyponatremia but not an elevation in serum potassium.

9. B. Hemoglobin A1C is a marker of recent glucose control and a serum value ≤ 6% indicates adequate control. Hemoglobin A1C levels are often checked every 3 months, as the normal life span of a red blood cell is 90 to 120 days. Therefore each hemoglobin A1C level is independent of the previous month's value, regardless of how high or low it was. All of the other answer choices can be used to diagnose diabetes but give no true insight into the level of recent glucose control by the patient. Again, diabetes can be diagnosed if symptomatic patients have a random glucose of > 200 mg/dL, asymptomatic patients have a fasting glucose of > 126 mg/dL on two separate occasions, and if a 2-hr 75-g glucose tolerance test shows a glucose of > 200.

10. D. Metformin is an oral agent used in the treatment of type II diabetes and has lactic acidosis as its major side effect. Metformin can also cause GI side effects and should not be given to patients with insufficient renal function because it is excreted by the kidney. Metformin inhibits hepatic gluconeogenesis and increases peripheral tissues' sensitivity to insulin. It does not cause hypoglycemia. All of the other drugs mentioned as choices are used in the treatment of type II diabetes but do not have lactic acidosis as a side effect. Acarbose prevents carbohydrate absorption in the small intestine and can cause diarrhea, nausea, and abdominal pain. Glyburide and glipizide increase insulin secretion from pancreatic beta cells. Their major side effect is hypoglycemia. Troglitazone increases tissue sensitivity to insulin but can cause hepatotoxicity.

11. E. Patients with type I diabetes have antibodies to glutamic acid decarboxylase and to pancreatic beta cells. Although not present in every type 1 diabetic, tests for these antibodies should be ordered whenever there is reasonable doubt as to whether a patient is a type I or type II diabetic. It is not clear which type of diabetes this patient has, but it is not absolutely necessary to know here because the treatment for this patient's emergent condition, whether diabetic ketoacidosis (in type I diabetes) or nonketotic hyperosmolar coma (in type II diabetes), is very similar. Fluids and insulin must be given. It is important to check for ketone bodies, measure serum glucose and electrolytes, and correct any abnormalities. Antimitochondrial antibodies are present in primary biliary cirrhosis, which presents most often in women with the symptoms of jaundice, pruritus, and hypercholesterolemia. Antinuclear antibody is present in many autoimmune conditions and is not specific. Antithyroglobulin or anti–thyroid peroxidase antibodies are present in Hashimoto's thyroiditis. Anti-U1 RNP is an autoantibody specific for mixed connective tissue disease, which presents in young women and has a variety of manifestations.

12. B. This patient has Addison's disease, which most commonly results from an autoimmune condition. Patients with Addison's disease have a higher incidence of other autoimmune diseases, especially those that affect endocrine organs such as the thyroid gland. Addison's disease is associated with pigmentation of skin, scar tissue, and the buccal mucosa. Patients with this condition are educated as to their illness and treated with a specific drug treatment (hydrocortisone) and possibly also an infusion of normal saline. The patient should also be monitored for evidence of a precipitating infection.

13. B. Bradykinin is increased in patients who are taking ACE inhibitors and can lead to a dry cough. It is important to consider other, more serious causes of cough, such as pneumonia, lung cancer, and pulmonary edema before accepting that the ACE inhibitor is the cause of the cough. Even though this patient may have lung cancer because of his smoking history or pulmonary edema because of his coronary artery disease, he is more likely to have a cough because of the ACE inhibitor. Because lung cancer could be possible in this patient, a chest x-ray would be a good option. Pneumonia is unlikely because this patient's lungs were clear to auscultation and he does not have an elevated temperature. Pulmonary edema is not likely because of the clear-sounding lungs and a normal ejection fraction. Aldosterone does not play a direct role in stimulating cough.

14. D. Clomiphene is a partial agonist at estrogen receptors in the pituitary, which prevents feedback inhibition and increases LH and FSH. The increase in LH is necessary for ovulation to occur and fertilization to take place. Mifepristone is a drug that was previously used in abortions; it acts by competitively inhibiting progestins at progesterone receptors. Leuprolide, a GnRH analog, stimulates LH and FSH when given in a pulsatile manner and can be used to treat infertility. Tamoxifen is a mixed estrogen agonist/antagonist that is used to treat breast cancer in patients who have tumors with estrogen receptors. Clomiphene is not an estrogen analog and it does not increase sex drive.

15. D. This patient most likely has medullary carcinoma of the thyroid, because he has a relative with thyroid cancer and a decreased calcium level on laboratory analysis. The medulla of the thyroid produces calcitonin, which inhibits osteoclast destruction of bone and helps to keep blood calcium levels low. This patient's calcium level was 6.1, which is below the normal range of 8.4 to 10.2 and makes a calcitonin-producing tumor of the thyroid most likely. Anaplastic carcinoma presents more commonly in the elderly and has the poorest prognosis of the thyroid can-

cers. Follicular carcinoma also has a poor prognosis and can metastasize through the blood to the lungs and bones, among other locations. Hashimoto's thyroiditis is a noncancerous hypothyroid condition that is more common in females and can be detected by antithyroglobulin or antithyroid peroxidase antibodies. Papillary carcinoma is the most common thyroid cancer; it has a good prognosis, spreads by lymph-node metastasis, and has a ground-glass appearance with psammoma bodies histologically.

16. D. This patient's hypocalcemia was caused by surgical removal of the parathyroids at the time of her thyroidectomy. PTH stimulates renal reabsorption, gastrointestinal absorption, and bone resorption of calcium. Without PTH, patients become hypocalcemic and can present with tetanus. Chvostek's sign, which elicits tetany on flicking the facial nerve, is a physical exam test for hypocalcemia. Dietary deficiencies of calcium or vitamin D are rare and are not likely for this patient, who is described as well-proportioned. Gastrointestinal losses of calcium are possible in a patient with low PTH levels but would not be the most likely etiology of her hypocalcemia. Medullary carcinoma of the thyroid is not possible here, as she had her thyroid gland removed. If a thyroid cancer were to re-appear in part of a gland that was remaining, it would most likely re-present as the previous type of cancer, which was follicular carcinoma.

17. A. This patient has acromegaly, which is caused by an excess of growth hormone, leading to increased bone density after the epiphyseal plates have closed. If an excess of growth hormone is present before the epiphyseal plates close, gigantism occurs. Octreotide, a somatostatin analog, is useful in the treatment of acromegaly because it is an endogenous inhibitor of growth hormone produced by the hypothalamus. Luteinizing hormone is involved in the triggering of ovulation, formation of the corpus luteum, and synthesis of estrogen and progesterone. Follicle-stimulating hormone is involved in the growth of ovarian follicles in females and spermatogenesis in males. Progesterone is a female reproductive hormone that is involved in breast development and secretory activity during the luteal phase of the menstrual cycle. Thyroid-stimulating hormone stimulates the thyroid gland to produce thyroid hormones responsible for maintaining many metabolic functions.

18. B. This patient's electrolyte findings of low sodium and high potassium are consistent with adrenal insufficiency, or Addison's disease. Cosyntropin exhibits full corticosteroidogenic activity of ACTH, stimulating the adrenal cortex to produce and secrete adrenocortical hormones. A cosyntropin-stimulation test measures the adrenal glands' production of cortisol in response to stimulation. Cortisol production should be low in response to cosyntropin administration in Addison's disease. An abdominal ultrasound or CT scan of the abdomen may show atrophic adrenal glands, but these are not the tests of choice in this situation. Free water deprivation is not indicated in this situation. It is a common treatment in hospitalized patients with the syndrome of inappropriate antidiuretic hormone (SIADH). The oral captopril test is sometimes used in the diagnosis of renal artery stenosis.

19. C. The different subtypes of multiple endocrine neoplasia (MEN) syndromes are characterized by small differences. Type IIb (or type III) is associated with pheochromocytomas, medullary carcinoma of the thyroid, and multiple mucocutaneous neuromas. MEN type I (Wermer's syndrome) is associated with tumors of the pituitary, pancreas, and parathyroid. Prolactinomas are the most common pituitary tumor in this condition and in general. The thyroid and adrenal glands may also undergo hyperplasia or have tumors as well. MEN type IIa (Sipple's syndrome) is associated with hyperparathyroidism, medullary carcinoma of the thyroid, and pheochromocytoma. Laurence-Moon-Biedl syndrome is an autosomal recessive condition causing obesity, polydactyly, and often mental retardation in children. Prader-Willi syndrome is inherited from a paternal gene contribution and leads to defects such as mental retardation, short limbs, obesity, and abnormal eye formation.

20. E. Graves' disease is caused by thyroid-stimulating immunoglobulins (TSIs), which bind to receptors on the thyroid gland and increase the production of both T_4 and T_3. Because the levels of the thyroid hormones are high, feedback inhibition on the pituitary leads to a decrease in the production of TSH. This patient had palpitations, weight loss, nervousness, and proptosis. Patients with Graves' disease can also have tachycardia, isolated systolic hypertension, hyperdefecation, tremor, and atrial fibrillation. All of the other lab values are not typically found in Graves' disease. The keys to understanding lab values in conditions with an increase or decrease of a hormone are to know what the primary disorder is and then to understand how negative feedback would respond to the primary disorder.

21. B. The role of antidiuretic hormone produced by the posterior pituitary is to reabsorb free water from the collecting duct in the renal tubules. The stimuli to reabsorb water are an increase in plasma osmolarity and a decrease in fluid volume. Without the action of antidiuretic hormone, a person will lose fluids, the plasma will become more concentrated, and urine will become more diluted. The contraction of uterine smooth muscle is a function of oxytocin, another posterior pituitary hormone. By reading the question carefully, one sees that this patient is a male and does not have any uterine smooth muscle. Stimulating the adrenal gland to produce aldosterone and cortisol is a function of ACTH, an anterior pituitary hormone. The stimulation of thyroid hormone production is a function of TSH, an anterior pituitary hormone. The synthesis of testosterone is stimulated by LH, which is also an anterior pituitary hormone.

22. C. Failure to hydroxylate vitamin D occurs in patients with end-stage renal disease because the kidneys have an enzyme that normally hydroxylates vitamin D at the 1 position. The active form of vitamin D, 1, 25 dihydroxycholecalciferol, increases calcium and phosphorus reabsorption in the kidney, increases calcium and phosphorus absorption in the small intestine, and increases bone resorption. All of these mechanisms increase blood calcium; a deficit in active vitamin D would lead to hypocalcemia. Even though this patient is thin, dietary deficiency is a less likely cause of hypocalcemia than chronic renal failure in this patient. Hypoparathyroidism is often a cause of hypocalcemia following surgical removal of the parathyroid glands after thyroidectomy. This patient has no history of intestinal symptoms, and gastrointestinal losses would not be the cause of his hypocalcemia. Pancreatitis can cause hypocalcemia by producing calcium-absorbing soaps. This patient has hypertriglyceridemia, which is a known risk factor for pancreatitis but is not associated with any signs or symptoms of pancreatitis.

23. C. Lack of sexual desire is one symptom of generalized hypopituitarism, which would produce symptoms secondary to a decrease in FSH, LH, ACTH, GH, and prolactin levels. The other options could be manifestations of an excess of a specific type of pituitary hormone. For example, galactorrhea would be secondary to excess prolactin, and proptosis, weight loss, and hypertension could be associated with excess TSH or hyperthyroidism.

24. E. Renal failure is the most common cause of secondary hyperparathyroidism. This patient, who has had severe uncontrolled diabetes and lab values consistent with diabetes, is most likely to have renal failure as the cause of his hypercalcemia. Whenever the kidney loses its ability to reabsorb calcium and hydroxylate vitamin D for calcium absorption from the gut, hypocalcemia triggers the parathyroid glands to increase their production of parathyroid hormone. In times of increased hormone production, the parathyroid glands enlarge to meet the increased demand of the body's need for calcium. Even though this patient is obese, a dietary excess of calcium is not the likely cause. There are no clues from the history that indicate an extreme excess of meat, cheese, or other dairy products. Milk-alkali syndrome can cause hypercalcemia in patients who eat many antacids or drink an excessive amount of milk. This condition is more commonly found in patients who have gastric ulcers and frequently depend on milk and antacids for relief. Lithium can cause hypercalcemia by leading to hyperparathyroidism. Parathyroid adenomas can cause hypercalcemia by increasing PTH secretion, but they are less likely culprits than hyperplasia secondary to end-stage renal disease in this patient.

25. E. Activation of alpha$_1$ adrenergic receptors leads to smooth muscle contraction in blood vessels. If propranolol, a nonselective beta-blocker, is given as a single agent, alpha$_1$ receptors are left unrestricted to contract blood vessels and increase mean arterial pressures further. Prazosin, an alpha$_1$ receptor blocker, can prevent this effect. The other medications can be used as antihypertensive agents but do not address the specific question being asked. Atenolol is a beta$_1$ receptor blocker. Clonidine, an alpha$_2$ agonist, causes a central decrease in sympathomimetic output. Enalapril, an angiotensin-converting enzyme (ACE) inhibitor, can decrease blood pressure by preventing the conversion of angiotensin I to angiotensin II, which is involved in aldosterone secretion and constriction of arterioles. Labetalol is a beta-blocker that also has some alpha-blocking properties. It is a commonly used intravenous medication in hypertensive crises.

26. E. This patient has Waterhouse-Friderichsen syndrome, which is an adrenal infarction secondary to an infection with *Neisseria meningitidis*. The history gives several clues that this is meningitis caused by the *Neisseria* species. *N. meningitidis* is common in college dormitories and on military bases. It is transmitted via infected respiratory droplets. It often presents with the common symptoms of meningitis, such as fever, stiff neck, headache, and photophobia. In Waterhouse-Friderichsen syndrome, the adrenal glands are destroyed, stopping the production of aldosterone and cortisol, which leads to a decrease in blood pressure. This patient does not have increased urination or increased skin pigmentation, which are found in Addison's disease. He has no history of decreased fluid intake or diarrhea. The meninges line the spinal cord and outer surface of the brain, and meningitis did not cause an infarction of the pituitary, which is located on the base of the brain.

27. B. This patient should be given levothyroxine to replace her inadequate levels of thyroid hormone. She has myxedema coma, which is characterized by coma, seizures, hypoventilation, and hypotension and is caused by a severe deficit in thyroid hormones. Myxedema coma is often precipitated by an infection, drug, or severe illness. Levothyroxine (Synthroid) is used to replace thyroid hormone whenever endogenous production is insufficient. Amantadine is an antiviral agent used to treat the influenza virus. This patient's daughter reports that she had a viral infection a week earlier, but treating her with amantadine would do nothing to replace her need for thyroid hormones. Methimazole and propylthiouracil are used in the treatment of hyperthyroidism. Although they work by slightly different mechanisms, they both act to decrease the synthesis of thyroid hormones. They are used in hyperthyroid conditions such as Graves' disease. Intravenous fluids would be the correct treatment if this patient were volume-depleted or in hypovolemic shock. It is important to assess her volume status and to consider giving intravenous fluids to all patients who may need them.

28. E. VMA, or vanillylmandelic acid, is a metabolite of catecholamines, such as epinephrine and norepinephrine. Blood levels of VMA are elevated whenever excess of catecholamines are present. This patient has a pheochromocytoma, as illustrated by his episodic hypertension and classic symptoms of catecholamine excess. His physician would also want to determine the exact location of the pheochromocytoma, as surgical intervention may be indicated to remove the tumor. Most pheochromocytomas (90%) are found in the adrenal glands, but some (10%) are located in other areas such as the paravertebral ganglia. Performing a high-dose dexamethasone suppression test or measuring urinary free cortisol are methods used in the diagnosis of Cushing's syndrome and Cushing's disease. A positive dexamethasone suppression test causes decreased ACTH and cortisol due to suppression of a pituitary tumor. Urinary cortisol levels are elevated in all causes of Cushing's syndrome. The captopril stimulation test is used to help diagnose renal artery stenosis. In this test, an elevated level of renin following the administration of captopril is suggestive of renal artery stenosis.

29. B. Osteoporosis is a metabolic bone disease involving a decrease in the amount of bone necessary to maintain the structural integrity of the skeleton. The rate of bone formation is often normal, whereas the rate of resorption is increased. Principal areas of demineralization are the spine and pelvis; compression fractures of the vertebrae are very common. Osteoporosis is often found in postmenopausal women and can go undetected until a fracture occurs. Serum calcium, phosphate, and parathyroid hormone are usually normal. Based on this patient's presentation and DEXA score, a bisphosphonate such as alendronate and calcium with vitamin D would be the best first-line treatment to prevent future fractures and progression of the disease. Alendronate alone would not be the best treatment, because current recommendations state that all postmenopausal women should be taking a calcium supplement with vitamin D. Calcitonin is not indicated for the prevention of osteoporosis and is not sufficiently potent to prevent bone loss. Calcium with vitamin D is recommended for all women, especially those who are postmenopausal; however this action alone would not be enough to prevent the progression of this patient's osteoporosis. Hormone replacement therapy is used in the treatment of osteoporosis; however, new guidelines suggest that it be used as a last resort, after all other options have failed. The x-ray shown (Figure 5-2) reveals an intertrochanteric hip fracture.

30. A. This patient has central diabetes insipidus, which is caused by failure of the pituitary to produce antidiuretic hormone. This patient may have acquired this condition secondary to his recent bout with toxoplasmosis. Patients with diabetes insipidus have a low urine osmolarity. To determine whether the condition is caused by a failure of ADH production by the pituitary (central DI) or by renal unresponsiveness (peripheral DI), ADH should be administered and the urine osmolarity rechecked. Patients with central DI will have a high urine osmolarity after ADH is given, while patients with peripheral DI will still have a low urine osmolarity. All of the other choices are options whenever an infection is suspected. An infection was unlikely in this case, as the patient had no systemic signs of infection and was afebrile on examination.

31. A. Anaplastic carcinoma is the least common, most aggressive thyroid carcinoma and has the poorest prognosis. Local invasion often causes hoarseness and dysphagia. Follicular carcinoma has a better prognosis. Medullary carcinoma of the thyroid is often part of the multiple endocrine neoplasia (MEN) syndrome. Parathyroid carcinoma is also part of the MEN syndrome.

32. C. Pancreatic alpha cells are not related to the cause of either type of DM. Type 2 diabetes is characterized by peripheral insulin resistance with an insulin-secretory defect that varies in severity. These defects lead to increased hepatic gluconeogenesis, which produces fasting hyperglycemia. Most patients (90%) who develop type 2 diabetes are obese, and obesity itself is associated with insulin resistance, which worsens the diabetic state. Since patients with type 2 diabetes retain the ability to secrete some endogenous insulin, those who are taking insulin do not develop diabetic ketoacidosis (DKA) if for some reason they stop taking it. Therefore they are considered to require insulin but not to depend on insulin. Aldosterone is produced by cells of zona glomerulosa of the adrenal cortex.

33. A. Increased PTH stimulates the kidneys, intestines, and bones to decrease phosphate reabsorption and increase calcium reabsorption. This causes a decrease in plasma phosphate and an increase in plasma calcium.

34. B. The superior parathyroid glands are located dorsal to the upper two-thirds of the thyroid lobe and posterior to the recurrent laryngeal nerve. The inferior glands, which are less consistent in location, can usually be found inferior to the inferior thyroid artery and ventral to the recurrent laryngeal nerve. They are usually within 1 cm of the inferior lobe of the thyroid gland.

35. C. This patient has congenital adrenal hypoplasia, an X-linked disorder caused by a mutation or deletion of the DAX1 gene, which is on the same chromosome as the gene for Duchenne muscular dystrophy (DMD). Therefore an extension of the chromosomal deletion can cause DMD. The other choices are unrelated. Cystic fibrosis is associated with recurrent sinopulmonary infections. Down's syndrome is associated with characteristic facies and mental retardation.

36. E. This question paints a typical scenario of a patient with a malignant thyroid nodule. These patients are usually euthyroid and present with a painless single nodule. Diagnosis of thyroid carcinoma cannot be made based on the FNA results, so surgical excision to obtain a tissue sample must be done. Without any more information in the question stem, you need to know, in order to determine the right answer, that papillary carcinoma is by far the most common type of thyroid carcinoma. It constitutes 60% of thyroid carcinomas, while follicular is 20%, anaplastic is 14%, medullary is 5%, and lymphoma is 1%.

37. B. This disorder classically presents with signs and symptoms of adrenal crisis in the first 2 weeks of life. The symptoms in girls include masculinization of the genitalia, while both sexes can have hyponatremic, hyperkalemic dehydration as well as hypotension and acidosis. 21α-hydroxylase deficiency accounts for 95% of the cases of congenital adrenal hyperplasia (CAH). 11β-hydroxylase deficiency may present similarly but it only accounts for 5% of CAH cases. Not only would influenza present without virilization, but July is not influenza season. Pyloric stenosis presents within the first few months of life, with vomiting (often projectile) and hypokalemic, hypochloremic metabolic alkalosis. There is often a firm palpable mass in the abdomen, as well. Congenital syphilis in a newborn would present with irritability, failure to thrive, watery discharge from the nose, a rash on the hands and feet, and an absent nasal bridge.

38. C. This pediatric patient is most likely to have type I diabetes mellitus, the mechanism of which is an immunologically mediated destruction of the beta cells of the pancreas. Peripheral insulin resistance and inadequately suppressed

hepatic gluconeogenesis are both features associated with type II diabetes. Answer A describes central diabetes insipidus. Insensitivity of the collecting duct of the kidney to the effects of ADH describes the mechanism of nephrogenic diabetes insipidus.

39. A. Polymenorrhea (frequent periods with a cycle length of less than 21 days) and infertility along with the other mentioned symptoms are typical of hypothyroidism. Kallmann's syndrome would have revealed signs of hypogonadism (loss of secondary sexual characteristics) along with anosmia. If the patient had polycystic ovarian syndrome, amenorrhea rather than polymenorrhea would have been expected, as well as hirsutism or other signs of increased androgen levels. A prolactinoma would present with suppressed ovulation and amenorrhea as well as possible galactorrhea. Sheehan syndrome is hypopituitarism due to pituitary necrosis caused by hypotension during the delivery of a baby. This patient has never been pregnant.

40. B. The phenomenon of transient hypocalcemia after removal of a solitary parathyroid adenoma is attributed to the rapid movement of calcium and phosphate back into the bones because the serum levels of PTH have rapidly dropped. If the blood supply to the remaining parathyroid glands had been disrupted, the hypocalcemia would not have been transient. Tumor lysis syndrome is seen after administration of chemotherapy for treatment of malignancies and is accompanied by hyperphosphatemia, hypocalcemia, hyperkalemia, and hyperuricemia. In pseudohypoparathyroidism, PTH levels are elevated in hypocalcemic patients due to end-organ resistance to PTH. This would not develop suddenly after the described surgery in a previously hypercalcemic patient. Vitamin D deficiency is a cause of hypocalcemia but would not be likely to cause the sudden transient dip in calcium seen here.

41. D. Somogyi effect is a phenomenon of reactive hyperglycemia following a period of relative hypoglycemia. This causes the release of hyperglycemic agents (epinephrine, norepinephrine, cortisol, glucagon, and growth hormone), as seen when diabetic patients are given too much insulin in the evening. The resulting early-morning hyperglycemia sometimes prompts an increase in the evening insulin dose, thus aggravating the problem. By contrast, the dawn phenomenon is early-morning hyperglycemia, due to increased morning cortisol levels, that does not follow a period of relative hypoglycemia. Raising the evening insulin dose here would not have exacerbated the morning hyperglycemia. Eating a sugary snack before bedtime could cause morning hyperglycemia, but the increased insulin dose would have led to a lower morning glucose reading the following day. Not only is an insulinoma, by definition, unheard of in a type I diabetic, it would cause extremely low blood glucose levels with no periods of the hyperglycemia seen here. If the patient has type II diabetes instead of type I, the worsened morning hyperglycemia after increasing the evening insulin dose would still not be explained.

42. E. The syndrome of inappropriate antidiuretic hormone (SIADH) secretion is diagnosed when a hyponatremic patient is found to have low plasma osmolarity in conjunction with high urine osmolarity in the absence of hypervolemia. This patient's heart and lung exams are normal, and he has no jugular venous distension (JVD), edema, or ascites. Therefore he is not hypervolemic. The question stem alludes to a history of trauma, and although it does not explicitly say head trauma, the patient is still unconscious. He most likely has SIADH secondary to head trauma. Central diabetes insipidus would have opposite plasma and urine osmolarity findings, i.e., urine osmolarity that is much less than that of plasma osmolarity because it is an inappropriate diuresis. Congestive heart failure, iatrogenic fluid overload, and the nephrotic syndrome would have signs of volume overload, but the patient has no edema, no ascites, and no JVD. The heart exam is normal, so he has no extra heart sounds, which would also have been expected in congestive heart failure.

43. E. This condition, also known as "thyroid storm," is a life-threatening complication of hyperthyroidism that can be precipitated by surgery, radioactive iodine therapy, or severe stress, including uncontrolled diabetes mellitus. The syndrome presents acutely with excessive adrenergic symptoms of thyrotoxicosis. The patient can have, in addition to the above symptoms, cardiac failure and coma. The hallmark is the elevated fever out of proportion to the other clinical findings. An addisonian crisis, or acute adrenocortical insufficiency, is brought on by illness or other stress but presents with hypotension, nausea, vomiting, hyperthermia, hyponatremia, hyperkalemia, and hypoglycemia. Anaphylaxis would be associated with flushing, but the patient would be in respiratory distress as well as hypotensive. Carcinoid syndrome can also involve irregular mottled blushing, but other symptoms would include diarrhea, bronchospasm, and acquired pulmonary and tricuspid stenosis. This syndrome is due to the release of serotonin from carcinoid tumors in the GI tract that have metastasized to the liver. A postoperative infection would usually take a few days to develop and would not present acutely.

44. B. This patient's multiple symptoms are characteristic of Cushing's syndrome, which is caused by an increase in cortisol. Cortisol causes bone destruction and osteoarthritis by inhibiting osteoblasts and stimulating osteoclasts. Osteoarthritis can be caused by excessive wear and tear on the joints and is more common in hips and knees of obese people. In most instances, it is a condition that presents in the elderly. Even though this woman is obese, she is much below the age at which people usually have osteoarthritis. Legg-Calvé-Perthes disease is avascular necrosis of the hip. It is most commonly caused by steroid-induced vascular compression but can be due to a variety of emboli. This patient does not have osteomyelitis, as is suggested by her history of being afebrile. A previously unreported hip fracture cannot be considered as it was not suggested by the history.

45. C. This patient has nephrogenic diabetes insipidus due to lithium use. Lithium causes the collecting tubule of the kidney to be unresponsive to ADH, therefore causing the symptoms of polyuria. Diabetes mellitus is not likely to be seen in this patient because of lack of hyperglycemia symptoms and normal weight. A colectomy may cause gastrointestinal complications but is not likely to cause urinary symptoms. Although interstitial nephritis may be caused by ibuprofen, it is not likely to be seen, especially in low dosages.

46. E. This patient has hemochromatosis, a hereditary disorder in which the small intestine absorbs excessive iron. Since the body lacks any way to excrete iron, the excess is stored in glands and muscle, such as the liver, pancreas, and heart. These organs fail over time. Transferrin saturation greater than 70% is diagnostic of iron overload (it is the serum iron concentration divided by total iron-binding capacity × 100). Serum ferritin would be greater than 300 µg/L. Iron-binding capacity would be decreased. Hypoalbuminemia and decreased testosterone may be seen.

47. B. This patient's symptoms of anxiety/nervousness, hypertension, hyperhidrosis, heart palpitations, and insomnia, along with the goiter, support a diagnosis of hyperthyroidism, most likely caused by an active goiter. TSH would be decreased due to negative feedback inhibition. Some possible causes include Graves' disease, toxic goiter, and Hashimoto's thyroiditis. The functions of T_3 include brain maturation, bone growth, adrenergic effects, and increase in basal metabolic rate. T_3 also functions to provide negative feedback to the anterior pituitary gland, which will decrease sensitivity to TSH.

48. A. Parathyroid removal or damage is a common complication of thyroid surgery. This is the most common cause of hypoparathyroidism, which in turn causes hypocalcemia. Measurement of calcitonin does not give information on the status of calcium metabolism. Calcium is a better immediate test than parathyroid hormone for hypoparathyroidism. Cortisol and norepinephrine have no role in evaluating parathyroid function.

49. A. Cancer is the most common cause of significant hypercalcemia seen in adults. Breast, lung, and kidney metastatic disease is much more common than parathyroid malignancy. Renal failure is not likely to cause a significant amount of hypercalcemia, and the vignette points to a malignant etiology. Vitamin C toxicity does not lead to hypercalcemia. Vitamin D can lead to hypercalcemia, but this is very uncommon.

50. A. The vignette portrays an aggressive neoplasm. The most aggressive thyroid carcinoma is anaplastic. The spindle-shaped cells support this diagnosis. Although the other thyroid malignancies are more common, they do not include spindle cells and are not nearly as aggressive. Follicular carcinoma is less aggressive than anaplastic carcinoma. Medullary carcinoma is associated with multiple endocrine neoplasia (MEN) syndromes.

51. A. When painful breast enlargement occurs in a young man, a hormonal cause is likely. hCG activates the aromatase gene, which allows for increased conversion of testosterone to estradiol, causing gynecomastia. Human chorionic gonadotropin is usually absent in men, and high levels usually indicate choriocarcinoma. This is a highly malignant tumor known for widespread metastasis, often to the lungs and liver. A Leydig cell tumor can cause gynecomastia but will not be associated with significant levels of hCG and is a sex cord stromal tumor, not a germ cell tumor. Although seminoma is the most common germ cell tumor in adults between the ages of 15 and 35, the tumor marker is placental alkaline phosphatase (PLAP). This tumor has an excellent prognosis, unlike choriocarcinoma. Testicular lymphoma is the most common testicular tumor in men over the age of 50. Yolk sac tumor is the most common germ cell tumor in children. Its tumor marker is alpha fetoprotein (AFP).

52. E. This patient is in ketoacidosis, which occurs in type I diabetes after the insulin level is markedly reduced. This signifies that a large number of beta islet cells are absent. Amyloidosis of islet cells is a characteristic of a type II diabetic, who would not have ketoacidosis. Although inflammatory cells could be seen in the early stages of type I diabetes, eosinophilic infiltration, gangrenous necrosis, or fat necrosis of the islet cells is not likely.

53. A. Addison's disease is a lack of adrenal cortical hormones, mainly aldosterone. The laboratory findings indicate hyponatremia and hyperkalemia, which is seen with hypoaldosteronism. This disease causes hyperpigmentation due to increased production of melanocyte stimulating hormone (MSH) due to an excess ACTH production in the anterior pituitary. Macroglossia is associated with Wilms' tumor syndromes. Pruritic rash of the arms is uncommon with Addison's disease. Exophthalmos is commonly seen with hyperthyroidism.

54. A. Bromocriptine is a dopamine agonist that acts to inhibit the production of prolactin. This patient is found to have isolated hyperprolactinemia without evidence of malignancy or other pituitary hormone elevations. It is much more likely that this patient would present with symptoms of a generalized hyperpituitarism, having elevated FSH, LH, ACTH, TSH, and GH as well. However, given the history, one must answer the question and not become distracted at the unusual presentation of the patient's condition. Metoclopramide is a dopamine antagonist that is used as an antiemetic and antihiccup medication. It could possibly increase prolactin levels even further because it inhibits endogenous dopamine production. Ondansetron is a serotonin $5HT_3$ receptor antagonist used to prevent nausea and vomiting. Propranolol is a nonselective beta-blocker used to reduce blood pressure, heart rate, and mortality in patients with cardiovascular disease. It is also used in the long-term treatment of esophageal varices. Somatostatin is a hormone produced in the hypothalamus and pancreas that has inhibitory functions.

55. B. To answer this question appropriately, one must recognize that only type I diabetes mellitus presents with diabetic ketoacidosis (DKA), while also being aware of the "honeymoon" period, where patients with type I DM are transiently able to secrete endogenous insulin. This period can last up to 1 year before the ability to secrete insulin is lost forever. Addison's disease, or chronic adrenocortical insufficiency, can present with nausea, vomiting, and hypotension; without proper treatment, it can lead to hyperthermia, hyponatremia, hyperkalemia, and hypoglycemia. The dosage and frequency of metformin administration are basically irrelevant here. Metformin is used in the treatment of type II DM, as it decreases hepatic glucose production and may increase the response of tissues to insulin. The Somogyi effect is a rebound phenomenon described in diabetic patients who are given too much insulin. This causes them to develop unrecognized nocturnal hypoglycemia and leads to compensatory morning hyperglycemia.

56. C. This patient has 21β-hydroxylase deficiency, blocking the formation of aldosterone and cortisol and leading to the presented symptoms and labs. This is the most common cause of ambiguous genitalia in the newborn. 11β and 17α deficiency would not present with these symptoms. Fabry's disease is a deficiency of alpha-galactosidase, resulting in accumulation of ceramide trihexoside and leading to renal failure. Gaucher's disease is caused by deficiency of beta glucocerebrosidase, leading to accumulation of glucocerebroside in the brain, liver, spleen, and bone marrow. In Niemann-Pick disease, deficiency of sphingomyelinase leads to accumulation of sphingomyelin; findings include a cherry-red spot on the macula and hepatosplenomegaly. Tay-Sachs disease is a deficiency of hexoaminidase, leading to GM_2 ganglioside accumulation, also with a cherry-red spot on the macula.

57. D. Papillary carcinoma is the most common thyroid cancer; it often presents with metastases to lymph nodes. Pathological findings include "ground glass" nuclei and psammoma bodies. Anaplastic carcinoma typically presents in older patients and has a very poor prognosis. Follicular cell carcinoma forms uniform follicles and spreads hematogenously. Medullary carcinoma produces calcitonin and associated symptoms (hypocalcemia) and also spreads hematogenously.

58. F. This neonate has congenital hypothyroidism, as indicated by the symptoms at birth; total T_4 is the best test for this condition. The Apgar score, which ranges from 1 to 10, indicates the health of the neonate. It is decreased in congenital hypothyroidism. The other symptoms of umbilical hernia, macroglossia, enlarged fontanelles, and coarse facial features also indicate that this neonate has hypothyroidism. The physiology of the thyroid hormones is as follows: T_3 functions include brain maturation, bone growth, and increase in basal metabolic rate. Thyroid-releasing hormone stimulates TSH release, which stimulates thyroid follicular cells. Negative feedback is provided by T_3 to the anterior pituitary gland.

59. F. The hyperthyroid symptoms and the clinical picture of 3 weeks postpartum fit best with the diagnosis of post-partum thyroiditis, which is a common, usually self-limited condition. It is believed be an autoimmune phenomenon. Cancer is not indicated in this vignette. Hashimoto's thyroiditis results from autoantibodies against thyroid antigens and produces nodules and/or swelling of the thyroid. In Graves' disease, TSH antibodies are produced, which stimulate the thyroid and cause it to become enlarged and warm. Riedel's thyroiditis causes sclerosis and hypothyroidism. A hard thyroid would be palpated. Sheehan's syndrome is a result of ischemic necrosis of the pituitary gland due to a complicated delivery. It causes panhypopituitarism and secondary hypothyroidism. Sub-acute thyroiditis causes painful swelling of the thyroid gland and can produce dysphagia. It usually resolves on its own.

60. B. Peripheral neuropathy is commonly caused by diabetes. It presents with the sensation described by this patient and is usually worse at night. It often affects the ankle reflexes and position and vibratory sense of the feet. In cauda equina syndrome, the patient will have bilateral pain, loss of the stretch reflexes, loss of sensation around the perineum, and diminished sphincter tone. An L3–L4 herniated disk compresses L4 and will result in diminished patellar reflex and weakness in extension of the great toe. L4–L5 disk herniation compresses L5, causing diminished biceps femoris reflex.

61. E. Klinefelter's syndrome is the most common congenital cause of primary testicular failure. It is found in 1 in 1,000 live male births and is associated with an XXY geno-type (secondary to maternal meiotic chromosomal non-disjunction). These males often present with infertility and the other features described above. In testicular feminization, the androgen receptors are absent. During embryogenesis, this interferes with the fusion of the labial-scrotal folds, resulting in the presence of a short vagina. Anorchia is not plausible given the fact that the husband has testicles palpable on examination. Cryp-torchidism is unlikely given that no information regarding the husband's prior surgical history was provided.

62. A. This patient likely has neuroblastoma. Some 90 to 95% of these tumors secrete the catecholamine metabolites mentioned in the question stem because the cells lack the enzyme to produce epinephrine from norepinephrine and dopamine, instead converting them to HVA and VMA. The pathology described would be seen on light microscopy. Pleomorphic spindle tumor cells attempting to form an osteoid matrix would be expected if the patient had osteosarcoma. Primitive metanephric blastema, dys-plastic tubules, and supporting mesenchyma or stroma describes the pathology of a Wilms' tumor. Small round blue cells with evidence of skeletal muscle differentiation describes the biopsy results of rhabdomyosarcoma. Stromal elements with infiltrates of normal lympho-cytes, plasma cells, eosinophils, and Reed-Sternberg cells describes Hodgkin's lymphoma.

63. A. Adrenocorticotropic hormone (ACTH), also known as corticotropin or cosyntropin, is an anterior pituitary hor-mone whose target organ is the adrenal cortex. Its pres-ence is important in the synthesis and release of the adrenocorticosteroids and the adrenal androgens. To diagnose acute adrenal insufficiency, a 1-hr cosyntropin test should be performed. In this test, ACTH is adminis-tered intravenously and plasma cortisol is drawn at 0, 30, and 60 min. A normal response would be a plasma corti-sol level > 20 μg/dL at any time during the test. If the patient's morning plasma cortisol level is < 12 μg/dL and a stimulated cortisol level is < 18 μg/dL, he most likely has adrenal insufficiency and would require treatment.

64. D. This patient has a prolactinoma, which is the most com-mon tumor of the pituitary. Prolactinomas, because they secrete an excess of prolactin, cause milk secretion in females as well as infertility. The mass effect of the tumor produces headaches due to increased intracranial pres-sure. Tunnel vision or bitemporal hemianopsia is caused by compression of the optic chiasm. Craniopharyngiomas are cystic tumors of the pituitary gland that form from Rathke's pouch. They may produce headache and bitem-poral hemianopsia if large enough but would not produce milk secretion. Meningiomas can cause headache but not this patient's other symptoms. They are often resectable. Finally, if this patient had schizophrenia, which is believed to be caused by an excess of dopamine, her excess milk production could come from taking antipsychotic med-ications such as haloperidol or chlorpromazine, which decrease dopamine production. Dopamine is the inhibitory hormone for prolactin. This patient reports no history of schizophrenia or usage of dopamine-inhibiting drugs.

65. B. Chronic glucocorticoid therapy can result in severe bone loss or osteopenia. These drugs induce changes in bone density through suppression of intestinal calcium absorption, with a subsequent induction of secondary hyperparathyroidism. Also, corticosteroid administration increases bone turnover by altering osteoblast differentia-tion and inhibiting collagen synthesis. Albuterol is a beta$_2$ agonist that has very few side effects when inhaled. How-ever, chronic use can sometimes result in nervousness, tremor, tachycardia, palpitations, headache, nausea, vom-iting, and sweating. Lisinopril is an ACE inhibitor used in the treatment of myocardial insufficiency and congestive heart failure. The most common side effect is a persistent dry cough. Metformin is an oral hypoglycemic agent clas-sified as a biguanide. Its most common side effects include nausea, vomiting, anorexia, metallic taste, abdominal discomfort and diarrhea. Salmeterol is a selective β_2-adrenoceptor agonist that can cause a muscle tremor when orally administered. Omeprazole is a proton pump inhibitor commonly used for the treatment of GERD. It has very few reported side effects. Simvastatin is an HMG-CoA reductase inhibitor used in the treatment of hyperlipi-demia. Side effects include myositis.

66. D. Thyroid-stimulating hormone (TSH) as well as FSH and LH are all anterior pituitary polypeptide hormone dimers that share an identical alpha subunit. The remaining anterior pituitary hormones (alpha and beta melanocyte-stimulating hormone [MSH], GH, PRL, ACTH, beta lipotropin, beta endorphin, and corticotrophin-like intermediary peptide [CLIP]) are all single polypeptides. CLIP, alpha and beta MSH, and beta endorphins are all secreted from pars intermedia–like cells. FSH, LH, ACTH, and TSH are secreted by basophilic cells of the anterior pituitary. PRL and GH are secreted by acidophilic cells.

67. C. The first 13 amino acids of ACTH contain the alpha-MSH sequence. In Addison's disease, there is a primary deficiency of aldosterone and cortisol due to adrenocortical atrophy. Without negative feedback from adrenocortical hormones, the anterior pituitary produces excess ACTH, which, owing to the shared amino acid sequence between ACTH and alpha MSH, leads to increased skin pigmentation. Testosterone is not a peptide hormone.

68. C. Phenylalanine and tyrosine are precursors to epinephrine. Secretion of epinephrine is signaled by a neuronal stress response via preganglionic acetylcholinergic neurons to the adrenal medulla. Acetylcholine release causes increased availability of intracellular calcium, which promotes exocytosis of epinephrine stored in chromaffin granules. Once epinephrine reaches the heart via the bloodstream, it acts on beta-receptors to increase heart rate. Histidine can be converted to histamine. Glutamate can be converted to glutamic acid. Valine is not converted from phenylalanine, tryptophan, histidine, glycine, or arginine. Urease is an enzyme that hydrolyzes uric acid.

69. A. In the resting state, GDP is bound to the alpha subunit of the G protein. When a hormone is bound to the receptor, a conformational change takes place, causing GDP to be released and GTP to be bound. The alpha subunit then dissociates from the beta and gamma subunits. The alpha subunit linked to GTP then binds to adenylate cyclase, which transforms ATP into cAMP. Adenylate cyclase is deactivated when GTP is hydrolyzed back to GDP.

70. C. Inositol triphosphate (IP3) is one of the resulting products from phospatidylinositol-4,5-bisphosphate (PIP2) hydrolysis by phospholipase C. When a peptide hormone binds a cell membrane receptor that is linked to an intermembrane G protein, phospholipase C is ultimately activated by the G protein. When phospholipase C hydrolyzes PIP2 into DAG (diacylglycerol) and IP3, IP3 binds to receptors on the sarcoplasmic reticulum and causes stored Ca^{2+} to be released. Calcium ions are important in exocytosis by aiding fusion of secretory granules with the cytoplasmic side of the plasma membrane. DAG activates a protein called protein kinase C.

71. C. Light entering the eyes is transmitted to the pineal gland via the CNS. Pinealocytes are innervated by adrenergic neurons, which are inhibited by light entering the eyes.

Norepinephrine released during darkness stimulates cAMP formation via a beta-receptor and causes increased synthesis of *N*-acetyltransferase. This enzyme catalyzes the first step of serotonin transformation into melatonin. The posterior pituitary receives input from the hypothalamus and produces antidiuretic hormone (ADH) and oxytocin. The anterior pituitary receives input from the hypothalamus and produces follicle-stimulating hormone, growth hormone, thyroid-stimulating hormone, and luteinizing hormone. The pineal gland is involved in light-dark adaptation.

72. C. Beta$_1$ and beta$_2$ receptors consist of seven transmembrane amino acid helices. When these receptors are stimulated, there is intrareceptor phosphorylation, which ultimately leads to activation of cytoplasmic adenylate cyclase. Steroid hormone receptors are bound to DNA transcription regulation sequences. Peptide hormone receptors are coupled to cell-surface G proteins.

73. C. Cholesterol is transported into the mitochondrion by a protein. Once inside, side chain cleavage enzyme converts cholesterol to pregnenolone. Most of the remaining steps of steroid hormone synthesis are carried out in the cytoplasm. The Golgi apparatus functions to move proteins from the endoplasmic reticulum to the plasma membrane. This organelle also functions to modify certain oligosaccharides and assemble proteoglycans. The rough endoplasmic reticulum is the site of synthesis of secretory proteins. The smooth endoplasmic reticulum is the site of steroid synthesis and detoxification of toxins (drugs or poisons).

74. C. Testosterone is the main secretory product of testicular Leydig cells. In some androgen target cells, testosterone undergoes conversion to dihydrotestosterone via the enzyme 5α-reductase, located in the endoplasmic reticulum (ER). The other choices are enzymes located on the pathway to production of aldosterone and DHEA.

75. C. This is a factitious disorder that can be seen in patients wanting to lose weight, and they often work in the medical field. This patient has symptoms of hyperthyroidism as well as suppressed TSH and elevated total T$_3$ and free T$_4$. However, her scan shows no uptake of radioactive iodine. In Graves' disease, patients typically have one or more of the following features: goiter, thyrotoxicosis, eye disease, and pretibial myxedema. In addition, the radionuclide scan would show increased uptake. For toxic multinodular goiter, physical exam would have revealed a multinodular goiter, and the radioactive scan would have shown multiple functioning nodules. For subacute thyroiditis, the thyroid gland would have been enlarged and exquisitely tender. Lab values fluctuate with the course of the disease, but radioactive uptake would also be low. In toxic adenoma, the scan would have shown a single functioning "hot nodule," with the rest of the gland suppressed.

Chapter 6   Gastrointestinal System

Questions

1. A 5-year-old boy with a long history of chronic diarrhea has pale, bulky, frothy, foul-smelling stools. He undergoes a small bowel biopsy, which reveals a flat mucosal surface with increased lymphocytes and plasma cells in the lamina propria. There is villous atrophy and flattening of the mucosal surface. Which of the following foodstuffs would be safe for ingestion by this patient?

   A. Oats
   B. Pretzels
   C. Rye bread
   D. Salted rice cakes
   E. Stone-ground corn tortilla chips

2. A 2-day-old neonate is hospitalized and has not yet passed meconium. After a consult with the gastroenterologist, the neonate is diagnosed with Hirschsprung's disease. Which comorbid illness is this neonate at increased risk of having?

   A. Chagas' disease
   B. Colonic adenocarcinoma
   C. Crohn's disease
   D. Down's syndrome
   E. Ventricular septal defect

3. An 11-year-old child who has had bloody diarrhea for 3 weeks is brought to ambulatory care clinic for evaluation. After examination and diagnostic testing, colonoscopy is performed. Biopsies are taken. On histological section, in the crypts of the colonic glands, there are flask-shaped ulcers with narrow necks and broad bases. Which of the following is the child at risk of having?

   A. Acquired megacolon
   B. Colonic adenocarcinoma
   C. Hepatic abscess
   D. Necrotizing enterocolitis
   E. Ulcerative colitis

4. A 32-year-old woman presents to the clinic with symptoms of diarrhea, flatulence, weight loss, and fatigue. A biopsy of her small bowel reveals marked atrophy and total loss of villi. The number of intraepithelial lymphocytes is increased. What HLA typing is likely to be found in this patient?

   A. DQ w2
   B. DR 2
   C. DR 3
   D. DR 4
   E. DR 7

5. A 34-year-old man presents to the ambulatory care clinic with a 4-month history of diarrhea, polyarthralgias, and mild pleuritic chest pain. A biopsy of the small intestine reveals intestinal mucosa with macrophages laden with periodic acid–Schiff (PAS)–positive granules. What is the most appropriate treatment for this patient?

   A. Antibiotics
   B. Corticosteroids
   C. Mesalamine enema
   D. Reassurance
   E. Reassurance, then check serum CEA levels in 1 month

6. A 46-year-old woman presents to her primary care physician with a history of progressive dysphagia. Laboratory testing reveals iron-deficiency anemia. Upper gastrointestinal endoscopy reveals an esophageal web. What is the most likely sequela of this syndrome?

   A. Carcinoid tumor
   B. Lymphoma
   C. Peptic ulcer disease
   D. Postcricoid carcinoma
   E. Rheumatoid arthritis

7. A 54-year-old Brazilian man complains of progressive dysphagia. After barium swallow, he is found to have a positive bird-beak sign; microscopically, he is found to have loss of ganglion cells in the myenteric plexus. What is the most likely cause of his illness?

   A. Barrett's esophagus
   B. Congenital achalasia
   C. Chagas' disease
   D. Esophageal carcinoma
   E. Plummer-Vinson syndrome

8. A 52-year-old alcoholic man presents to the emergency department with a 2-hr history of hematemesis. He had been vomiting the evening before for many hours. He has no history of any other illnesses or symptoms. What is the most likely explanation for these findings?

   A. Esophageal varices
   B. Gastric carcinoma
   C. Mallory-Weiss syndrome
   D. Peptic ulcer disease
   E. Zollinger-Ellison syndrome

9. A 2-week-old infant presents to the emergency department with a 1-day history of projectile vomiting and regurgitation. Physical examination reveals visible peristalsis and a palpable oval abdominal mass. What other syndrome might be suspected in a neonate with this presentation?

   A. Down's syndrome
   B. Hirschsprung's disease
   C. Necrotizing enterocolitis
   D. Turner's syndrome
   E. Zollinger-Ellison syndrome

10. A 52-year-old man presents to his primary care physician with a 2-month history of diffuse abdominal pain and anorexia. He has lost 30 lb during this period, which he feels is because of his loss of appetite. He has a 40-pack-year history of smoking. Based on the history and histological section (Figure 6-1), what is the most likely diagnosis?

Figure 6-1

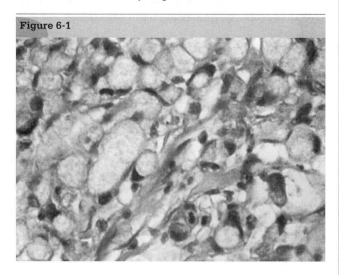

A. Adenocarcinoma

B. Gastric carcinoma, signet-ring type

C. Pancreatic carcinoma

D. Ulcerative colitis

E. Zollinger-Ellison syndrome

11. A 56-year-old man presents to his primary care physician with abdominal pain and currant jelly stools. Colon x-rays reveal telescoping of the large bowel. What is the most likely explanation for these findings?

A. Carcinoma

B. Hirschsprung's disease

C. Necrotizing enterocolitis

D. Ulcerative colitis

12. An entire community in Central America is stricken with profuse watery diarrhea up to 20 L/day. Approximately 30 patients (age range 4 years to 40 years) are brought to the local emergency department for evaluation. Stool samples reveal organism growth on thiosulfate-citrate-bile-salts-sucrose (TCBS) agar. What is the most likely diagnosis?

A. *Campylobacter enteritis*

B. *Campylobacter jejuni*

C. *Escherichia coli*

D. *Vibrio cholerae*

E. *Yersinia enterocolitica*

13. A 52-year-old woman returns to her primary care physician with diarrhea, fever, and abdominal cramping. She was recently treated with ampicillin for a sinus infection. *Clostridium difficile* toxin is present in the stool. What is the most appropriate therapy for this patient?

A. Azithromycin

B. Clindamycin

C. Erythromycin

D. Metronidazole

E. Oral rehydration therapy

14. A 32-year-old patient is found to have multiple osteomas. He has a history of multiple colonic adenomatous polyps that he has had removed. A mutation in the APC gene on chromosome 5 is suspected. What is the most likely diagnosis?

A. Gardner's syndrome

B. Lynch's syndrome

C. Peutz-Jeghers syndrome

D. Turcot's syndrome

E. Ulcerative colitis

15. A 54-year-old man has had a partial colostomy owing to a history of colonic carcinoma. What is a possible way to monitor for disease recurrence?

A. CEA levels

B. CA 19-9

C. CA 27-29

D. β-hCG

E. Prostate-specific antigen

16. A 53-year-old woman is diagnosed with a tumor of the appendix. Small, uniform cells are noted on hematoxylin-and-eosin (H&E) stain under high power. What would be the most appropriate modality to confirm this diagnosis?

A. Appendectomy

B. CT scan of the abdomen

C. MRI of the abdomen

D. Urinary 5-hydroxyindoleacetic acid (5-HIAA)

E. Urinary vanillylmandelic acid

17. A 14-year-old boy presents with mucocutaneous pigmentation on the vermilion border, inside his mouth, and on the palmar surfaces of his hands. A colonoscopy reveals multiple hamartomatous polyps. What is the most likely mutation causing this disorder?

A. SKT-11

B. S-100

C. p53

D. RET

E. t (8, 14)

18. A 50-year-old alcoholic man presents to the emergency department with stabbing epigastric pain radiating to the back. He has a prior medical history of recurrent pancreatitis. Physical examination of the heart and lungs is normal. Abdominal examination reveals epigastric tenderness and mild rigidity. His serum amylase and lipase are elevated. What is a possible sequela of this disease?

A. Acute respiratory distress syndrome

B. Diabetes mellitus

C. Esophageal varices

D. Myocardial infarction

E. Pancreatic carcinoma

19. A 42-year-old obese man is diagnosed with diabetes mellitus because he has a fasting glucose of 272 mg/dL. He also has a history of hypertension, asthma, erectile dysfunction, and seasonal allergies. His current medications include an antihistamine, sildenafil, and a calcium channel blocker. Physical examination of the heart, lungs, and abdomen are within normal limits. What would be the best measurement of his blood sugar regulation over the last few months?

A. Amylase and lipase
B. Cardiac stress test
C. Hemoglobin A1c
D. Insulin level
E. Liver function tests

20. A 45-year-old African American man with a history of sickle cell anemia presents to the emergency department with severe right-upper-quadrant pain radiating to the right shoulder. His vital signs are blood pressure 150/90 mm Hg and pulse of 90 bpm. Physical examination of the abdomen reveals right-upper-quadrant tenderness and inspiratory arrest with deep palpation in the right upper quadrant. Ultrasonography reveals a thickened gallbladder wall, pericholecystic fluid, and gallstones. What are the stones most likely composed of?

A. Calcium bilirubinate
B. Calcium oxalate
C. Cholesterol
D. Cystine
E. Serine

21. A 52-year-old man with a history of coronary artery disease and diabetes mellitus presents to the emergency department with severe watery diarrhea and vesicular lesions on his arms and legs. He had been fishing in Louisiana, where he consumed many raw oysters. Physical examination reveals right- and left-lower-quadrant tenderness to deep palpation, with mild rigidity. Bowel sounds are present and are hyperactive. What is the most likely causative agent for his illness?

A. *Campylobacter jejuni*
B. *Salmonella*
C. *Shigella*
D. *Vibrio cholerae*
E. *Vibrio vulnificus*

22. A 41-year-old woman from China who recently came to the United States to visit her family presents to the emergency department. She had been feeling ill, with fever, rigors, and malaise. She then developed jaundice with vomiting, abdominal pain, and clay-colored stools. She has also had generalized itching. What is the most likely explanation for these findings?

A. *Entamoeba histolytica*
B. *Enterobius vermicularis*
C. *Clonorchis sinensis*
D. *Plasmodium ovale*
E. *Trypanosoma cruzi*

23. A 42-year-old woman with a history of polycythemia vera develops progressive ascites and tender hepatomegaly. She presents to her primary care physician for further evaluation. Physical examination confirms the presence of an ascites wave and tenderness in the right upper quadrant. The liver span is 16 cm in the midclavicular line. Liver function tests are normal. What is the most likely diagnosis?

A. Budd-Chiari syndrome
B. Cirrhosis
C. Obstructive cholangitis
D. Pancreatic carcinoma
E. Wilson's disease

24. A 42-year-old Caucasian woman presents to her primary care physician with a 6-week history of pruritus, jaundice, and xanthomas. After lab testing, she is found to have elevated conjugated bilirubin and elevated alkaline phosphatase. Primary biliary cirrhosis is the suspected diagnosis. What other lab test would lead to this diagnosis?

A. Antimitochondrial antibodies
B. Anti-GBM antibodies
C. Auto-IgG antibodies
D. Perinuclear antineutrophil cytoplasmic autoantibodies
E. SCL-70

25. The abdominal viscera in a neonate are found to be protruding through an opening in the abdominal wall. What is the most likely defect causing this presentation?

A. Failure of the intestinal loop to retract from the umbilical cord
B. Failure of peritoneal fusion
C. Failure of the yolk stalk to degenerate
D. Incomplete fusion of the lateral body folds
E. Umbilical herniation

26. Recent reports from a small community in southern Mexico have noted an outbreak of hepatitis. A large percentage of the patients affected have been pregnant women. What is the most likely agent causing this outbreak?

A. Cytomegalovirus
B. Hepatitis A virus
C. Hepatitis B virus
D. Hepatitis C virus
E. Hepatitis D virus
F. Hepatitis E virus
G. Hepatitis G virus
H. Herpes simplex virus

27. A 51-year-old man presents with crampy abdominal pain that becomes worse with eating. He has a 35-pack-year history of smoking and often takes ibuprofen for arthritis. His prior surgical history is notable for the repair of bilateral inguinal hernias and a circumcision. Physical examination of the heart, lungs, and abdomen is unremarkable. Bowel sounds are noted in all four quadrants. What would be the best treatment for this patient?

A. Cimetidine
B. Calcium carbonate
C. Mesalamine
D. Omeprazole and antibiotics
E. Penicillin and ciprofloxacin

28. Two days after a large picnic, many attendees show up at the ambulatory care clinic complaining of watery diarrhea. Some had blood in their stools and some had cramping and fever. Stool cultures at 42°C (107.6°F) grew microaerophilic Gram-negative curved rods with polar flagella. What was the most likely source of this infection?

A. Carrier food handlers
B. Milk and cream products — *listeria*
C. Poorly canned vegetables — *clostridia*
D. Poorly cooked beef dishes
E. Poorly washed vegetables — *E. coli*
F. Potato salad — *S. aureus*
G. Poultry dishes — *campylobacter*
H. Rice dishes — *B. cereus*
I. Uncooked fish

29. A 34-year-old man with a long history of HIV infection has recently developed AIDS; he has now had severe diarrhea for 2 months. Physical examination of the heart and lungs is normal. Gastrointestinal examination reveals mild tenderness in all four quadrants. Bowel sounds are hyperactive. Peritoneal signs are absent. Digital rectal examination reveals external hemorrhoids. A stool sample demonstrates acid-fast oocysts. What is the most likely offending agent?

A. Ascariasis
B. Cryptosporidiosis
C. Cytomegalovirus
D. Toxocariasis
E. Toxoplasmosis
F. Trichinellosis

30. A 41-year-old woman recently visited Haiti for 2 weeks. While still in Haiti, she had chills and a fever. It has been just over a week since her illness began and she now has a rash, severe abdominal pain, and enlarged lymph nodes. She still has a high fever. Physical examination of the heart and lungs is normal. The spleen tip is palpable and tender. There is no evidence of hepatomegaly. What is the most likely diagnosis?

A. *Campylobacter jejuni*
B. *Salmonella enteritidis*
C. *Salmonella typhimurium*
D. *Shigella*
E. *Vibrio cholerae*
F. *Yersinia enterocolitica*

31. A 40-year-old man presents to his primary care physician with a history of bloody diarrhea. After biopsy, in the distal ileum and colon microabscesses rimmed by activated macrophages are found. After the patient recovers, he has symptoms of arthritis and a rash consistent with the diagnosis of erythema nodosum. What is the most likely diagnosis?

A. *Campylobacter pylori*
B. *Salmonella enteritidis*
C. *Salmonella typhimurium*
D. *Shigella sonnei*
E. *Vibrio cholerae*
F. *Yersinia enterocolitica*

32. A family reunion was recently held at the local park. Half of the people who attended the picnic developed bloody diarrhea. A stool sample of one of the patients had Gram-negative facultative anaerobes. What is the most likely diagnosis?

A. *Campylobacter jejuni*
B. *Salmonella enteritidis*
C. *Salmonella typhimurium*
D. *Shigella*
E. *Vibrio cholerae*
F. *Yersinia enterocolitica*

33. A 71-year-old man complains of a sudden onset of left-lower abdominal pain associated with an urge to defecate. The patient's pain is not relieved by passing stools, and within 3 hr, the patient begins to pass bright red stools per rectum. The patient is evaluated in the emergency department after the fourth bloody bowel movement in 15 hr. Physical exam reveals normal vital signs. His abdomen is markedly tender with left-lower-quadrant pain associated with guarding and rebound tenderness. Laboratory studies reveal a white blood cell count of 20,000/mm³. Sigmoidoscopy is normal. What is the most likely diagnosis?

A. Acute colonic ischemia
B. Acute diverticulitis
C. Adenocarcinoma
D. Polyposis coli
E. Pseudomembranous colitis

34. Which of the following will stimulate contraction of the gallbladder and simultaneously causes relaxation of the sphincter of Oddi for secretion of bile?

A. Cholecystokinin
B. Creatine kinase
C. Gastrin
D. Secretin
E. Vasoactive intestinal peptide

35. A 76-year-old man presents to the emergency department with severe left-sided abdominal pain. Physical examination reveals diffuse guarding and rebound tenderness in all four quadrants. Peritoneal signs are suspected. The patient is taken for exploratory laparotomy. Surgical findings include an area of infarcted bowel in the shaded area shown in Figure 6-2. Which artery provides circulation to the area denoted with an X on the figure?

A. Celiac artery
B. Gastroepiploic artery
C. Inferior mesenteric artery
D. Splenic artery
E. Superior mesenteric artery

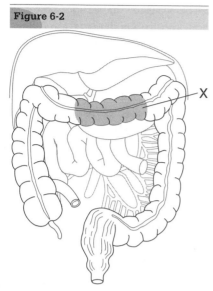

Figure 6-2

X

36. A 39-year-old man complains of chronic irritable bowel syndrome. He has tried numerous anticholinergic and antimuscarinic agents. Physical examination of the heart, lungs, and abdomen is within normal limits. He has no guarding or peritoneal signs. He does have some tenderness along the course of the sigmoid colon. Which of the following is released from neurons in the mucosa and smooth muscle of the GI tract that may produce a beneficial response in this patient, denoted by improved symptoms?

A. Cholecystokinin

B. Creatine phosphate

C. Gastrin

D. Secretin

E. Vasoactive intestinal peptide

37. A pH probe is placed to monitor gastric acid output in a 39-year-old man with chronic gastroesophageal reflux disorder. In the past he has been treated with an H_2 blocker and a proton-pump inhibitor. Which of the following will be found in increased concentrations because of the low pH in the local environment surrounding the pH probe?

A. Creatine kinase (BB fraction)

B. Creatine kinase (MB fraction)

C. Creatine kinase (MM fraction)

D. Secretin

E. Vasoactive intestinal peptide

38. A pH probe placed in the stomach of a 40-year-old woman reveals a pH of 4. She has a history of peptic ulcer disease and currently takes an H_2 blocker and an antacid. Based on this information, which of the following will be inhibited in terms of release?

A. Cholecystokinin

B. Creatine kinase

C. Gastrin

D. Secretin

E. Vasoactive intestinal peptide

39. A 45-year-old woman presents to her primary care physician with periodic facial flushing, watery diarrhea, and chronic abdominal cramps. Physical exam reveals bilateral wheezes and hepatomegaly. CT scan reveals several masses within the liver and a large mass in the small intestine. Which of the following substances is likely to be elevated in the urine of this individual because of her disease?

A. Aminolevulinic acid (ALA)

B. 5-Hydroxyindoleacetic acid (5-HIAA)

C. N-Formiminoglutamate (FIGlu)

D. Normetanephrine

E. Vanillylmandelic acid (VMA)

40. A 39-year-old woman with a perforated gastric ulcer complains of sharp pain in her epigastrium. Radiograph reveals that the gastric contents have spilled into the lesser sac. The abdominal surgeon who opens the gastrosplenic ligament to reach the lesser sac accidentally cuts an artery. Which of the following vessels is the most likely one injured?

A. Gastroduodenal artery

B. Left gastric artery

C. Left gastroepiploic artery

D. Right gastric artery

E. Splenic artery

41. A 32-year-old woman presents to her primary care physician for evaluation of yellow sclerae and yellowish pallor. She has a history of hepatitis. She is an alcoholic and an intravenous drug abuser. Physical examination of the head, neck, heart, lungs, and abdomen is within normal limits. Complete blood count reveals a hematocrit of 25%. Which is the most likely diagnosis?

A. Cirrhosis

B. Hemolytic jaundice

C. Type II diabetes mellitus

D. Viral hepatitis A

E. Viral hepatitis B

42. An 81-year-old woman being treated for typical pneumonia with clindamycin progressively develops worsening diarrhea. Physical examination of the heart and lungs is within normal limits. Abdominal examination reveals mild diffuse tenderness without peritoneal signs. Laboratory studies reveal white blood cell count of 20,000/mm³. What is the most likely explanation for these findings?

A. *Clostridium difficile*

B. *E. coli* O157:H7

C. Rotavirus

D. *Salmonella*

E. *Shigella*

43. A 22-month-old child has had severe, watery diarrhea for 2 days. She is brought to her pediatrician for further evaluation. She is a healthy infant who goes to a day care while her parents are at work. Physical examination of the heart, lungs, and abdomen is within normal limits. Examination of the female genitalia examination is within normal limits. The spine is grossly normal. What is the most likely diagnosis?

A. *Entamoeba histolytica* infection

B. Enterotoxigenic *E. coli* infection

C. Lactase deficiency

D. Rotavirus infection

E. *Vibrio cholerae* infection

44. A 39-year-old man presents to his primary care physician with abdominal pain, which he has had for 3 months. He does not exercise, works at a desk, smokes 1 and 1/2 packs of cigarettes a day, and takes five or six tablets of nonsteroidal anti-inflammatory drugs (NSAIDs) a day for his normal aches and pains. Upper GI endoscopy is performed (Figure 6-3). Which of the following factors would most likely elicit abdominal pain and help to determine whether this patient has a gastric versus a duodenal ulcer?

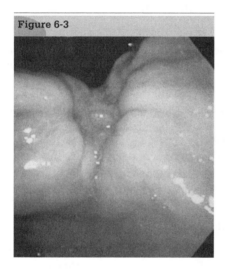

Figure 6-3

A. Deep breathing

B. Exercise

C. Food

D. Position

E. Size of an inguinal hernia

45. A 68-year-old man with a 20-year history of heartburn presents to his primary care physician with progressively worsening dysphagia and heartburn with reflux. He claims never to have taken any medications for this other than occasional over-the-counter antacids. He also complains of a chronic cough. He denies fever, chills, and recent weight loss. He also has no history of allergies. Based on the history and physical findings, the histology of an esophageal biopsy would most likely show which of the following?

A. Columnar epithelium in the distal esophagus

B. Decreased ganglion cells in the myenteric plexus

C. Dilated blood vessels in the submucosa

D. Mucosal diverticula in the distal esophagus

E. Numerous neutrophils with scattered eosinophils

46. A 45-year-old man presents to his primary care physician with a 4-month history of dysphagia, substernal pain, and melena. The patient's substernal pain is worse when he eats large meals and/or goes to sleep. Physical examination of the head, neck, heart and lungs is within normal limits. Dysfunction of which of the following sphincters is causing these symptoms?

A. Ileocecal

B. Lower esophageal

C. Pyloric

D. Sphincter of Oddi

E. Upper esophageal

47. A 15-month-old child is brought to the emergency department because of several episodes of rectal bleeding. A technetium-99m perfusion scan reveals a 3-cm ileal outpouching located 50 cm from the ileocecal valve. Which of the following types of ectopic tissue does this structure most likely contain?

A. Duodenal

B. Esophageal

C. Gastric

D. Hepatic

E. Jejunal

48. A 50-year-old woman presents to a gastroenterologist for a colonoscopy. She has a family history of colon cancer. She currently denies any bloody stools, but she is anxious to have a colonoscopy because of her family history. A colonoscopy is performed and multiple polyps are found. One of the biopsies reveals a benign hamartoma. Physical examination reveals dark pigmentation of the buccal mucosa and lips. What is the most likely diagnosis?

A. Gardner's syndrome

B. Peutz-Jeghers syndrome

C. Polyposis coli

D. Turcot's syndrome

E. Uremia

49. An 18-year-old woman went to dinner with her boyfriend at a local Chinese restaurant. They both ate sweet-and-sour chicken with rice. Within 4 hr of eating dinner, they both experienced nausea, vomiting, diarrhea, and abdominal pain. Which pathogen is the most likely cause of these symptoms?

A. *Bacillus cereus*

B. *Campylobacter jejuni*

C. *Clostridium botulinum*

D. *Clostridium perfringens*

E. Enterohemorrhagic *Escherichia coli*

F. *Salmonella*

G. *Staphylococcus aureus*

H. *Vibrio cholerae*

50. A healthy infant is born but fails to pass meconium until 48 hr after birth. Several weeks later, his mother brings him in to his pediatrician worried as to why he has not been passing stools regularly. The infant has also begun to show some abdominal distension. This condition is caused by an absence of which of the following kinds of neural cell bodies?

A. Parasympathetic postganglionic neuron cell bodies

B. Parasympathetic preganglionic neuron cell bodies

C. Sensory neuron cell bodies

D. Sympathetic postganglionic neuron cell bodies

E. Sympathetic preganglionic neuron cell bodies

51. A 75-year-old man presents to his primary care physician with excruciating abdominal pain that is out of proportion to the physical exam. He claims to have had similar abdominal pain before, especially after eating. He has a history of atrial fibrillation and is currently taking digoxin. What is the best study to obtain to arrive at a diagnosis for this patient?

A. Angiography

B. CT without contrast

C. Intravenous pyelography

D. Magnetic resonance imaging

E. Ultrasound

52. A 40-year-old man presents to his primary care physician because of burning epigastric pain, vomiting, and diarrhea. The pain is relieved by food, antacids, or antisecretory agents. He claims to be belching a lot as well, which is causing him some embarrassment. Laboratory studies reveal lipase of 130 U/L and amylase of 1.1. What is the most likely cause of this patient's discomfort?

A. *H. pylori*–associated duodenal ulcer

B. Gastric carcinoma

C. Gastric ulcer

D. Gastroesophageal reflux

E. Pancreatitis

53. Which of the following specialized epithelial cells in the small intestine serve as a host defense against foreign bodies?

A. Enterocytes

B. Oligomucous cells

C. Paneth cells

D. Stem sells

E. Urachal cells

54. An 18-year-old man is brought to the emergency department with sudden excruciating abdominal pain localized to the right lower quadrant, nausea and vomiting, mild fever, and slight tachycardia. Physical exam reveals marked right-lower rebound tenderness and guarding. A CT scan is obtained; it is shown in Figure 6-4. Serum white blood cell count is 18,000/mm³. What is the most likely diagnosis?

A. Acute appendicitis

B. Acute pancreatitis

C. Crohn's disease

D. Diverticulitis

E. Gastritis

F. Ulcerative colitis

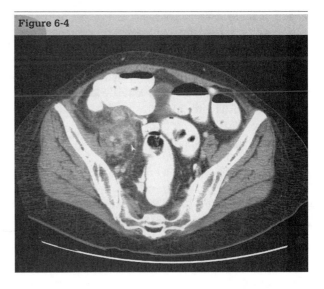

Figure 6-4

55. A medical student is engaged in a summer research project that involves determination of the pancreatic exocrine products. Utilizing dog pancreatic cells, secretory products and their concentrations are determined. Which of the following secretory products is produced from the central acinar portion of the pancreas?

A. Amylase

B. Carboxypeptidase

C. Sodium bicarbonate

D. Trypsin

E. Trypsinogen

56. The cleavage of a zymogen into an active enzyme requires hydrolysis of a peptide bond. Where is the site of the protease cleavage in relation to the peptide bond?

A. Amine

B. Carboxyl

C. Hydroxyl

D. Nitrite

57. A 24-year-old college student presents to the emergency department with complaints of vomiting, severe abdominal cramps, and diarrhea. She reports having had leftover Chinese food for dinner some hours earlier and had felt fine all day. Physical examination reveals mild diffuse abdominal tenderness. Bowel sounds are hyperactive. Peritoneal signs are absent. What is the most likely etiology of this illness?

A. *Bacillus cereus*

B. *Clostridium botulinum*

C. *Salmonella*

D. *Shigella*

E. *Staphylococcus aureus*

58. A 63-year-old blind man presents to his primary care physician with the assistance of his daughter. He reports having had no visual issues until his recent trip to the Congo. While he was on this trip, a local medic gave him an antidiarrheal medication to take during his stay. Blindness soon followed. What prophylactic medication was this patient given?

A. Clioquinol (Enterovioform)

B. Doxycycline

C. Loperamide (Imodium)

D. Lomotil

E. Isoniazid

59. A 45-year-old man is found to have bacillary dysentery, also known as shigellosis. He was born in the United States and has never left the country. Which serologic group is most likely to be the cause of his symptoms?

A. Group A

B. Group B

C. Group C

D. Group D

E. Group E

60. A 52-year-old woman presents to the emergency department with vomiting, diarrhea, and generalized malaise. She reports having eaten at a local seafood restaurant the previous evening. Physical examination reveals right- and left-lower-quadrant tenderness. Guarding is present in the left lower quadrant. Bowel sounds are present in all four quadrants. Which of the following pathogens is most likely to be producing those symptoms?

A. *Clostridium perfringens*

B. *Staphylococcus aureus*

C. *Streptococcus pyogenes*

D. *Vibrio parahaemolyticus*

E. *Yersinia enterocolitica*

61. A 27-year-old graduate archaeology student who recently spent a month in Mexico complains of malaise, anorexia, abdominal cramps, and watery diarrhea, which she has had for 3 weeks. Physical examination of her abdomen reveals diffuse tenderness without guarding or rebound. Bowel sounds are present in all four quadrants. What is the most likely explanation for these findings?

A. *Entamoeba histolytica*

B. Enterotoxigenic *E. coli* (toxigenic *E. coli*)

C. Enterohemorrhagic *E. coli* (hemorrhagic *E. coli*)

D. Enterovirus

E. Rotavirus

62. A 47-year-old woman presents to the ambulatory care clinic complaining of chronic diarrhea, weight loss, and abdominal cramping that she has had for 2 months. A colonoscopy is performed, and friable, inflamed mucosa as well as crypt abscesses and continuous lesions are found throughout the colon. Barium enema is obtained (Figure 6-5). Based on the symptoms and clinical findings presented, what is the most likely diagnosis?

A. Colorectal carcinoma

B. Crohn's disease

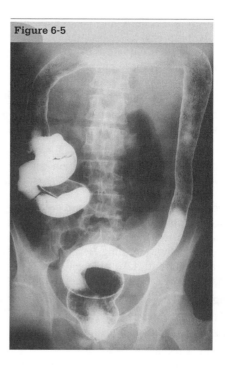

Figure 6-5

C. Diverticulosis

D. Mesenteric adenitis

E. Ulcerative colitis

63. A 3-year-old girl is brought to the emergency department with fever and abdominal pain; she has been producing bloody mucus with diarrheal stools. Physical examination reveals bilateral lower-quadrant tenderness. Bowel sounds are present in all four quadrants. What would be the most appropriate and definitive diagnostic test for this patient to undergo?

A. Breath analysis

B. Colon biopsy

C. Gastric lavage

D. Sputum sample

E. Stool sample

64. Working in a low-income neighborhood in Haiti, you notice poor sanitation and overflowing garbage and debris in the streets. A local patient presents to the clinic with diarrhea, lower abdominal pain, and changes in bowel habits. Physical examination reveals hepatomegaly, and the patient reports moderate abdominal pain to palpation. How is this condition most likely to be transmitted?

A. By contaminated food and drink

B. By intravenous drug use

C. By kissing

D. By the oral-fecal route

E. By sexual intercourse

65. A local health department is interested in controlling the incidence of salmonellosis in the county. This initiative is due to a recent significant outbreak in surrounding counties. Which of the following patient subtypes should be targeted to potentially decrease the incidence of this condition?

A. 3-year-old boy in day care

B. 14-year-old girl at summer camp

C. 23-year-old male camper

D. 77-year-old woman in nursing facility

E. 80-year-old man in nursing facility

66. A 9-year-old boy is brought to the emergency department; he has had persistent diarrhea for 4 weeks. Several other children who live on the same block also have diarrhea. Physical examination of the heart, lungs, and abdomen is within normal limits. Stool fluid reveals cysts and trophozoites. What is the most likely diagnosis?

A. *Giardia lamblia*

B. *Trichomonas hominis*

C. *Trichomonas vaginalis*

D. *Trypanosoma cruzi*

E. *Wuchereria bancrofti*

67. A 41-year-old obese woman presents to her primary care physician complaining of pain in her lower rib cage and points to the area of her twelfth rib. She has had fever over the last 3 days. What is the most plausible explanation for these findings?

A. Acute pancreatitis

B. Appendicitis

C. Gallstones

D. Hepatocellular carcinoma

E. Urinary tract infection

68. A 34-year-old man reports being told that he is unable to relax his lower esophageal sphincter. He has a history of dyspepsia after meals. His current medications include calcium carbonate (Tums) as needed. Physical examination of the heart, lungs, and abdomen is within normal limits. Which of the following is the deficient product causing his problem?

A. Acetylcholine

B. Gastrin

C. Nitrous oxide

D. Secretin

E. Thrombin

69. A 23-year-old woman complaining of greasy and odorous stools, generalized weakness, and hair loss presents to her primary care physician for evaluation. Physical examination of the heart, lungs, and abdomen is unremarkable. She has no guarding or rebound tenderness. Bowel sounds are present in all quadrants. Female pelvic examination is deferred at the patient's request. What is the most likely explanation of these findings?

A. Gastric ulcer with bleeding

B. Glucose malabsorption

C. Menstruation

D. Pancreatic insufficiency

E. Pituitary tumor

70. These are commonly found along the brush border of the intestine and represent the rate-limiting step during carbohydrate digestion, responsible for the making of glucose, galactose, and fructose. Which of the following is being described?

A. Oligosaccharide hydrolases

B. Pancreatic amylase

C. Salivary amylase

D. Sandostatin

E. Somatostatin

71. A 49-year-old man with diabetes mellitus, hypertension, and chronic renal failure who is on dialysis is hospitalized with dehydration, cachexia, and a 40-lb weight loss. He is currently unable to tolerate solid foods. Enteral feeding products are suggested for this patient. Which of the following would be the best source of protein for this individual?

A. Casein

B. Crystalline amino acids

C. Essential amino acids

D. Hydrolyzed protein

E. Whole protein with arginine supplemented

72. A 39-year-old man with a known LDL-receptor deficiency is treated with lovastatin. As a consequence of the action of this agent, which of the following is most plausible?

A. Fewer LDL receptors in cell membranes

B. Higher blood triacylglycerol levels

C. Lower blood cholesterol levels

D. Increased ACAT activity

E. Increased de novo cholesterol synthesis

73. A 19-year-old prisoner has been denied parole. He has expressed anger with this decision and wants to begin a hunger strike. He has no prior medical or surgical history. He is now 6 hr into his hunger strike. Which of the following sources are least likely to be used for gluconeogenesis?

A. Acetyl CoA

B. Amino acids

C. Glycerol

D. Lactate

E. Propionate

74. A medical student is conducting a research project using two substances and a semipermeable membrane. Substance A is fat-soluble whereas substance B is water-soluble. Which of the following factors will facilitate the passage of a solute through a membrane?

A. Decreased oil/water partition coefficient of the solute

B. Increased membrane thickness

C. Reduction in the size of the solute

D. Utilization of hydrophilic substrates for lipid membranes

75. A 39-year-old man is participating in a triathlon. He will run 6 mi, swim 1 mi, and bicycle 20 mi. Regarding potential sources of energy, adenosine triphosphate is synthesized and heat is generated. Which of the following fuels would produce the greatest amount of energy for this individual during the meet?

A. Alcohol

B. Carbohydrates

C. Fats

D. Protein

E. Trypsinogen

Answer Key

1. A	**20.** A	**39.** B	**58.** A
2. D	**21.** E	**40.** C	**59.** D
3. C	**22.** C	**41.** B	**60.** D
4. A	**23.** A	**42.** A	**61.** B
5. A	**24.** A	**43.** D	**62.** E
6. D	**25.** D	**44.** C	**63.** E
7. C	**26.** F	**45.** A	**64.** A
8. C	**27.** D	**46.** B	**65.** A
9. D	**28.** G	**47.** C	**66.** A
10. B	**29.** B	**48.** B	**67.** C
11. A	**30.** C	**49.** A	**68.** C
12. D	**31.** F	**50.** B	**69.** D
13. D	**32.** D	**51.** A	**70.** A
14. A	**33.** A	**52.** A	**71.** C
15. A	**34.** A	**53.** C	**72.** C
16. D	**35.** E	**54.** A	**73.** A
17. A	**36.** E	**55.** C	**74.** C
18. A	**37.** D	**56.** B	**75.** C
19. C	**38.** C	**57.** A	

Answers and Explanations

1. A. Treatment of gluten-sensitive enteropathy involves a life-long, strict gluten-free diet. All wheat, rye, and barley products must be eliminated from the diet. Many children are able to tolerate oats; thus, this foodstuff provides the building blocks for a good diet.

2. D. Ten percent of neonates with Hirschsprung's disease have Down's syndrome. Down's syndrome is caused by trisomy 21. Increased risk is associated with increasing maternal age. Signs and symptoms include cardiac defects, psychomotor retardation, and classic Down's facies. An increased risk of leukemia is also associated with this condition. Chagas' disease is an infectious agent that can be a cause of acquired megacolon. Hirschsprung's is not associated with later development of cancer or Crohn's disease. A ventricular septal defect can be seen less commonly with Down's syndrome.

3. C. This patient likely has a hepatic abscess. The agent involved is *Entamoeba histolytica,* which has a propensity to invade the portal vessels and embolize to produce liver abscesses. Ulcerative colitis is not associated with infectious agents. Acquired megacolon is caused by Chagas' disease. Colonic adenocarcinoma is not associated with a previous infection. Necrotizing enterocolitis develops in the first 2 months of life most frequently when neonates start on oral food.

4. A. The correct answer is DQ w2. Some 95% of patients with celiac sprue have this HLA typing; more specifically, the patients have an alpha/beta heterodimer of the DQ w2. For this reason, familial clustering of this disease is common. DR 2 is associated with hay fever and multiple sclerosis. DR 3 is associated with diabetes mellitus type I. DR 4 is associated with rheumatoid arthritis. DR 7 is associated with steroid-responsive nephritic syndrome.

5. A. This patient has Whipple's disease, and the agent is *Tropheryma whippelii,* a Gram-positive bacillus. The appropriate treatment is antibiotics. PAS-positive macrophages are diagnostic of this disease. This is not cancer, so it is not necessary to test for CEA. Prednisone would be used to treat Crohn's disease. Mesalamine derivatives would be used for ulcerative colitis. Finally, if left untreated, this patient will not improve.

6. D. This patient has postcricoid carcinoma, which is a sequelae of Plummer-Vinson syndrome. Dysphagia is nearly always a symptom of organic disease rather than a functional complaint. The other answer choices are not associated sequelae of Plummer-Vinson syndrome. Lymphoma is rarely associated with iron-deficiency anemia. Peptic ulcer disease is associated with gastric pain related to meals but is not associated with progressive dysphagia. Rheumatoid arthritis is associated with arthralgias of joints of the hands. Iron-deficiency anemia is uncommon with this condition.

7. C. This patient likely has Chagas' disease. The etiologic agent is *Trypanosoma cruzi,* which is transmitted by the tsetse fly. Diagnosis is by blood smear. Treatment includes suramin for blood-borne disease. Melarsoprol is indicated for CNS disease. This patient probably acquired the disease during his recent stay in South America and after his diagnosis of achalasia. Esophageal carcinoma is a sequela of Chagas' disease, not a cause. Cardiomyopathy is an associated condition. Plummer-Vinson disease and Barrett's esophagus do not cause achalasia. Congenital illness would not present at age 54.

8. C. Because of his recent history of vomiting and his alcoholism, this patient likely has Mallory-Weiss syndrome. Esophageal varices would be in the differential diagnosis if he had a history of liver disease. Peptic ulcer disease, gastric carcinoma, and Zollinger-Ellison syndrome would most likely present with other associated symptoms. Peptic ulcer disease can be due to increased acid production and is associated with *Helicobacter pylori* in 90% of cases of duodenal ulcers. Diagnosis is by endoscopy or by barium swallow if endoscopy is not available.

9. D. The correct answer is Turner's syndrome. Pyloric stenosis is associated with Turner's and Edwards' syndromes. It has no association with the other diseases listed. Down's syndrome is caused by trisomy 21. Increased risk is associated with increasing maternal age. Signs and symptoms include cardiac defects, psychomotor retardation, Down's facies (epicanthal folds, flattened occiput, and upslanted palpebral fissures). Necrotizing enterocolitis is a disease of newborns. Hirschsprung's disease is a congenital megacolon and is characterized by lack of enteric nervous plexus on intestinal biopsy. The condition presents as chronic constipation early in life. Zollinger-Ellison syndrome is due to a gastrin-secreting tumor that is usually located in the pancreas. It is associated with recurrent ulcers and MEN I.

10. B. The histological section suggests the diagnosis of gastric carcinoma (signet-ring type). Mucin formation causes the nucleus of the cells to be pushed to the periphery, forming the signet-ring cell. Ulcerative colitis would be associated with a characteristic bloody diarrhea. Colon and pancreatic cancer would be in the differential diagnosis of the clinical scenario; however, the histology would not favor this diagnosis. Pancreatic cancer may also present in the context of obstructive jaundice. Zollinger-Ellison syndrome would present as multiple ulcers due to excess gastrin production.

11. A. The correct answer is carcinoma. Risk factors for colon cancer include chronic villous adenomas and inflammatory bowel disease. In addition, a high-fat diet, increased age, and familial polyposis coli are also risk factors. Patients over the age of 50, like this patient, should be screened with fecal occult blood testing at the minimum. Intussusception in adults is often associated with a mass lesion in the affected area. Hirschsprung's disease, or necrotizing enterocolitis, is most often present in neonates. Ulcerative colitis is not associated with intussusception. Necrotizing enterocolitis is a disease of newborns.

12. D. *Vibrio cholerae* has been long recognized as the major cause of acute diarrheal disease in Asia, North Africa, the Middle East, and Central and South America. The disease can occur where socioeconomic conditions are poor, and it can be endemic to communities. Stool microbiology may reveal vibrios. Culture on TCBS medium is helpful. *Campylobacter enteritis* is commonly associated with ingestion of raw milk, specifically in Los Angeles and Colorado. *Yersinia enterocolitica* mainly affects animals and can cause human infection as a result of contact with them. It is also found in lakes and streams in the United States and Europe. *Escherichia coli* is common worldwide but is not the most common cause of acute diarrheal disease in Japan.

13. D. The correct answer is a course of metronidazole. *Clostridium difficile* produces an exotoxin. This kills enteric cells and causes pseudomembranous colitis. Antibiotic use is often the culprit, particularly clindamycin and ampicillin. Erythromycin, clindamycin, and azithromycin would not treat the condition and might exacerbate it. Oral rehydration therapy is not sufficient treatment for pseudomembranous colitis.

14. A. The correct answer is Gardner's syndrome, which a variant of familial adenomatous polyposis with osteomas. These patients are at risk for colon cancer and must be screened with periodic colonoscopic examination. Close follow-up is required. Turcot's syndrome is familial adenomatous polyposis with CNS gliomas. Peutz-Jeghers syndrome is multiple hamartomatous polyps. Lynch's syndrome is hereditary nonpolyposis colorectal cancer. Ulcerative colitis is associated with pseudopolyps. However, these patients with inflammatory bowel disease are also at risk for the development of colon cancer and should be followed up frequently.

15. A. The correct answer is to measure the levels of carcinogenic embryonic antigen (CEA). This agent is very nonspecific but is produced by 70% of colorectal carcinomas and pancreatic cancers. In addition, it may be produced by breast and gastric carcinomas. CA 19-9 would be used for pancreatic cancer. CA 27-29 would be used for breast cancer. Beta hCG would be used for choriocarcinoma. PSA stands for prostate-specific antigen and would be used for monitoring patients with prostate cancer; it can suggest which patients should undergo prostatic needle biopsy for diagnostic purposes.

16. D. The correct answer is urinary 5-hydroxyindoleacetic acid. Serotonin is converted to 5-HIAA. CT and MRI would diagnose the tumor but would not tell what kind of tumor it was. Carcinoid tumor can produce carcinoid syndrome, which is characterized by flushing, diarrhea, wheezing, and salivation. Treatment for bronchial carcinoid may include methysergide, which is a serotonin antagonist. Urinary vanillylmandelic acid would be used to diagnose pheochromocytoma. Appendectomy would not be the best way to diagnose a carcinoid tumor.

17. A. The correct answer is SKT-11, serine threonine kinase. This is located on chromosome 19. This patient has Peutz-Jeghers syndrome. S-100 is a tumor marker associated with melanoma. p53 is a tumor suppresser gene; a mutation in p53 is the cause of many cancers. RET mutations are associated with the MEN syndromes. A translocation in chromosomes 8, 14 would be associated with Burkitt's lymphoma.

18. A. The correct answer is acute respiratory distress syndrome, which is a sequela of acute pancreatitis and can lead to death. Signs and symptoms include dyspnea, tachycardia, resistant hypoxia, and diffuse alveolar infiltrate on chest x-ray. Treatment involves oxygen, diuretics, and positive end-expiratory pressure (PEEP). This will prevent airway collapse in a failing lung and expand alveoli for better diffusion. Diabetes mellitus is a sequela of long-standing chronic pancreatitis. Esophageal varices are associated with cirrhosis. Myocardial infarction and pancreatic carcinoma are not associated with acute pancreatitis.

19. C. The correct answer is hemoglobin A1c, a measurement of the glycosylated hemoglobin. It indicates the degree of blood sugar control over the preceding 3 months. The other tests would not assess blood sugar control. Amylase and lipase would be a better measure of pancreatic function, particularly for patients with pancreatitis. Insulin level is not the best test for this patient. Liver function tests would be nonspecific in patients with diabetes mellitus.

20. A. The correct answer is calcium bilirubinate. This is because of the patient's history of sickle cell anemia. Hemolytic anemias are associated with excessive bilirubin, causing pigment stones. The other products are not associated with gallstones in patients with sickle cell anemia. Gallstones have a higher incidence in women, especially those who are 40, fertile, and fat. Patients with gallstones who are below age 20 should also be evaluated for the possibility of congenital spherocytosis. Diagnosis of gallstones is with ultrasound or CT scan. Approximately 15% of gallstones are visible on plain abdominal x-ray films.

21. E. The correct answer is *Vibrio vulnificus,* which is known to cause a severe diarrhea and cellulitis in individuals cleaning and consuming raw shellfish. *Shigella* and *Salmonella* are known to cause dysentery and are not acquired from raw oysters. *Vibrio cholerae,* a comma-shaped organism, would not be obtained from shellfish. *Campylobacter jejuni,* which is comma- or S-shaped, can cause bloody diarrhea. *Salmonella* is a motile organism that does not ferment lactose and can cause bloody diarrhea.

22. C. The correct answer is *Clonorchis sinensis,* a protozoan responsible for infectious cholangitis. It is transmitted through undercooked fish. Inflammation of the biliary tract can result. Treatment is praziquantel. *Plasmodium ovale* causes malaria. *Trypanosoma cruzi* causes Chagas' disease. *Entamoeba histolytica* causes dysentery and liver abscess. *Enterobius vermicularis* causes pinworm. It is transmitted through food that is contaminated with eggs. Anal pruritus results. Treatment is with mebendazole or pyrantel pamoate.

23. A. The correct answer is Budd-Chiari syndrome. Patients with thrombogenic disorders are at increased risk for hepatic vein obstruction (Budd-Chiari). Cirrhosis would most likely present with jaundice and abnormalities on liver function tests. Obstructive cholangitis and pancreatic carcinoma often present with jaundice. Wilson's disease would present with Kayser-Fleischer rings and increased levels of ceruloplasmin.

24. A. The correct answer is antimitochondrial antibodies. This patient has primary biliary cirrhosis. Anti-GBM antibodies are present in Goodpasture's disease. Perinuclear antineutrophil cytoplasmic autoantibodies are present in polyarteritis nodosum and other vasculitis syndromes. SCL-70 is present in scleroderma. Auto-IGM antibodies are present in rheumatoid arthritis.

25. D. The correct answer is incomplete fusion of the lateral body folds. This should take place during the fourth week of development. The lateral body folds fuse ventrally to form the anterior body wall. Failure of peritoneal fusion results in an omphalocele. Failure of yolk sac degeneration results in Meckel's diverticulum. An umbilical herniation would be covered with subcutaneous fascia and skin.

26. F. The correct answer is hepatitis E virus, which is a waterborne infection with a propensity to affect pregnant women. Epidemics have been reported in Asia, Africa, and Mexico. The other hepatitis viruses do not have a propensity for causing severe disease in pregnant women. Herpes simplex virus does not cause hepatitis. Cytomegalovirus has a propensity to affect immunocompromised individuals.

27. D. The correct answer is a proton-pump inhibitor plus proper choice of two antibiotics. This patient has a peptic ulcer. A proton-pump inhibitor is necessary to decrease gastric acid secretion and the antibiotics are necessary to eradicate the *Helicobacter pylori* infection that is present in nearly 100% of ulcers. The other medication choices would not be sufficient to help with healing while also eradicating the infection.

28. G. The correct answer is poultry dishes. The agent responsible for this outbreak is *Campylobacter jejuni*. It is most commonly found in chicken or other poultry products. *Staphylococcus aureus* is most likely in potato salad or custard. Carriers are usually the cause of *Salmonella typhi*. *Clostridium botulinum* is often acquired from poorly canned vegetables. *Escherichia coli* or *Entamoeba histolytica* can be acquired from poorly washed vegetables. *Escherichia coli* can also be acquired from rare meat. *Bacillus cereus* is acquired from rice dishes. Milk and cream products can carry *Listeria*.

29. B. The correct answer is cryptosporidiosis. This protozoan infects the brush border of the small intestine. Cytomegalovirus does not produce acid-fast oocysts. Ascariasis is caused by an intestinal roundworm and is not associated with increased incidence in AIDS patients. Toxoplasmosis would present in this manner. *Toxocara* causes larva migrans and is not associated with an increased incidence in AIDS patients. Trichinellosis is an infection that invades muscle tissue.

30. C. The correct answer is *Salmonella typhimurium*. This is an example of typhoid fever. The patient's recent travel to Haiti and associated fever during the first week with worsening symptoms the second week is consistent with typhoid fever. *Yersinia enterocolitica* has a propensity to involve the distal ileum and colon, forming microabscesses. It is also associated with postinfectious autoimmune arthritis and erythema nodosum. *Campylobacter jejuni* is associated with infectious diarrheal syndromes and can produce bloody diarrhea. *Vibrio cholerae* is associated with an infected water supply in underdeveloped countries. Such infections usually result in mass outbreaks, affecting entire communities.

31. F. The correct answer is *Yersinia enterocolitica*. It has a propensity to involve the distal ileum and colon, forming microabscesses. It is also associated with postinfectious autoimmune arthritis and erythema nodosum. *Campylobacter pylori* causes infection in the upper GI tract and is not usually associated with microabscess formation. *Salmonella* enteritis is associated with bloody diarrhea. This organism is motile but is unable to ferment lactose. *Shigella* causes bloody diarrhea and is neither motile nor able to ferment lactose. *Vibrio cholerae* causes watery diarrhea without blood. This organism is comma-shaped.

32. D. The correct answer is *Shigella*. The high percentage of people infected leads to the conclusion that it must be an organism that has a low index of infection. Since it takes only 10 organisms of *Shigella* to cause infection, this is the most likely agent. In addition, *Shigella* is a Gram-negative facultative anaerobe. *Yersinia enterocolitica* has a propensity to involve the distal ileum and colon, forming microabscesses. It is also associated with postinfectious autoimmune arthritis and erythema nodosum.

33. A. The correct answer is acute colonic ischemia. This condition usually presents in the seventh decade of life or beyond, with a sudden onset of abdominal pain, usually in the left lower quadrant. Shortly after the pain presents, there is passage of blood per rectum. This indicates ischemic damage to the mucosa. The disease most commonly affects the watershed area involving the splenic flexure, where anastomotic connections of the superior mesenteric and inferior mesenteric circulations supply blood. The bleeding found with acute diverticulitis is usually painless. Adenocarcinoma normally does not present in such an acute manner. Multiple polyps would not present with this much pain or an increased leukocyte count. *Clostridium difficile* infections cause pseudomembranous colitis, but this rarely involves bleeding. Also, the absence of fever and previous antibiotics make this diagnosis less likely.

34. A. Cholecystokinin (CCK) is released from the I cells of the duodenal and jejunal mucosa owing to the presence of small peptides, amino acids, fatty acids, and monoglycerides. The main actions of CCK are to stimulate contraction of the gallbladder and simultaneously cause relaxation of the sphincter of Oddi; to stimulate the secretion of bile and pancreatic enzymes; to potentiate secretin-induced secretion of pancreatic HCO_3; to stimulate growth of the exocrine pancreas; and to inhibit gastric emptying.

35. E. The correct answer is the superior mesenteric artery. The left side of the transverse colon is supplied by the middle colic artery, a branch of the superior mesenteric artery. The celiac artery is the first branch off the abdominal aorta and gives rise to branches supplying the stomach, liver, and spleen. The inferior mesenteric supplies the descending colon and rectum. The splenic artery supplies the spleen. The gastroepiploic artery supplies parts of the stomach and pancreas.

36. E. Vasoactive intestinal peptide is a GI neurocrine that causes relaxation of GI smooth muscle. It also stimulates pancreatic HCO_3 secretion and inhibits gastric acid secretion. In these actions, it resembles secretin. Cholecystokinin causes gallbladder contraction and pancreatic enzyme secretion and also increases gastric emptying. Creatine phosphate is released from muscles. Gastrin is secreted in response to gastric distension and vagal stimulation. Secretin is secreted in response to acid and fatty acid that enters the duodenum. Bicarbonate secretion results and inhibits gastric acid secretion.

37. D. Secretin is released by the S cells of the duodenum in response to acid and fatty acids in the lumen of the duodenum. It stimulates HCO_3 secretion and increases the secretions of the exocrine pancreas. It also inhibits acid secretion by the gastric parietal cells. Alkaline pancreatic juices from the duodenum cause a neutralization reaction with gastric acid. This augments the function of pancreatic enzymes. Creatine kinase has three fractions; they are MM, which is found in muscle; BB, which is found in the brain; and MB, which is found in both.

38. C. Gastrin is secreted by the G cells of the gastric antrum in response to the following: small peptides, amino acids, distension of the stomach, and gastrin-releasing peptide. Gastrin's principal physiologic action is to increase H^+ secretion. This decreases the pH and, in turn, inhibits further secretion of gastrin's negative feedback. Cholecystokinin is released in response to amino acids and fatty acids entering the duodenum. This causes contraction of the gallbladder and relaxation of the sphincter of Oddi. Vasoactive intestinal peptide is secreted by the smooth muscles and nerves of the intestines.

39. B. This patient is presenting with flushing, diarrhea, and bronchoconstriction, which are all signs of the carcinoid syndrome. This syndrome results from excess serotonin secretion by either a primary carcinoid tumor in the lungs or ovary or from hepatic metastases from a primary carcinoid tumor in the GI tract. Diagnosis is based on finding increased 5-HIAA in the urine from the metabolism of excess serotonin. Increased levels of ALA are seen with lead toxicity, increased normetanephrine, or VMA with tumors of the adrenal medulla such as pheochromocytoma in adults and neuroblastoma in children, and increased FIGlu is seen with folate deficiency.

40. C. The left gastroepiploic artery runs through the gastrosplenic ligament to reach the greater omentum. The gastroduodenal artery and the right gastric artery branch off of the common hepatic artery. The gastroduodenal artery descends behind the first part of the duodenum. The right gastric artery runs to the pylorus and then along the lesser curvature of the stomach. The left gastric artery and the splenic artery arise from the celiac trunk. The left gastric artery runs upward and to the left toward the cardia, giving rise to esophageal and hepatic branches, and then turns right and runs along the lesser curvature within the lesser omentum to anastomose with the right gastric artery.

41. B. Yellow skin color and yellow sclerae are indicative of jaundice. The low red blood cell count along with jaundice is diagnostic for hemolytic jaundice. Cirrhosis presents with jaundice, but not usually a low red blood cell count. Type II diabetes is a disease of hyperglycemia and glucose intolerance due to defects in insulin secretion and peripheral insulin action. It does not present with jaundice or low red blood cells. Hepatitis A and B are systemic infections involving the liver. Both infections can cause jaundice but do not cause a low red blood cell count.

42. A. Pseudomembranous colitis is an inflammatory bowel infection caused by *Clostridium difficile* toxin arising from antibiotic use, particularly clindamycin, lincomycin, ampicillin, and cephalosporins. Exudates and plaques are noted on the colonic mucosa. Microscopy reveals epithelial cell necrosis and goblet cells distended with mucus. It also typically affects the elderly. The other pathogens can cause diarrhea but are not specifically associated with antibiotic use. *E. coli* O157:H7, *Salmonella,* and *Shigella* typically present with bloody diarrhea due to bacterial invasion of the colon. Rotavirus is a possibility but is more likely to be seen in children.

43. D. Rotavirus is the number one cause of diarrhea in children between the ages of 6 and 24 months. Bacterial colitis may be related to production of preformed toxins, as in infections with *Vibrio cholerae* and enterotoxigenic *E. coli*. *E. histolytica* is a cause of amebiasis and is endemic in underdeveloped countries. It characteristically produces flask-shaped ulcers in the colon and may also cause amebic liver abscesses. Lactase deficiency commonly presents as an acquired disorder in adults that results in malabsorption of milk and milk products.

44. C. The classic presentation for a gastric ulcer is burning epigastric pain, which worsens with eating. In contrast, a duodenal ulcer typically presents with burning epigastric pain 1 to 3 hr after eating, which is relieved by food. Deep breathing, exercise, and position do not normally elicit pain in these patients. The endoscopic image (Figure 6-3) reveals a gastric ulcer at the pylorus near the bottom of the image.

45. A. This patient is presenting with Barrett's esophagus due to his long-standing untreated gastroesophageal reflux disorder (GERD). The esophagus is normally a stratified squamous nonkeratinized epithelium, but when exposed to acid for a long period of time, it can change to the columnar epithelium, which is seen in Barrett's. Barrett's esophagus is associated with an increased risk of adenocarcinoma. In contrast, decreased ganglion cells in the myenteric plexus are seen in achalasia, which is characterized by incomplete relaxation of the lower esophageal sphincter (LES) with swallowing and increased resting tone of the LES. This leads to esophageal dilatation and symptoms of progressive dysphagia. Dilated blood vessels in the submucosa suggest esophageal varices due to portal hypertension. In the majority of patients with esophageal varices, the etiology is alcoholic cirrhosis. Mucosal diverticula in the distal esophagus would not cause such severe dysphagia. Numerous neutrophils are seen in GERD, which our patient likely has, but do not explain the new onset of worsening dysphagia and cough which is typical of the metaplastic change to Barrett's esophagus.

46. B. This patient is presenting with GERD. The lower esophageal sphincter separates the esophagus from the stomach. GERD is due to an incompetent lower esophageal sphincter. The patient's symptoms arise from the reflux of the acidic gastric contents back into the esophagus, leading to inflammation of the esophageal mucosa. His symptoms are exacerbated by large meals, which lead to increased gastric H+ secretion. Also, by lying in bed, he is in a position that allows more of the gastric contents to pass back through the incompetent lower esophageal sphincter. The ileocecal sphincter separates the small intestine from the large intestine. The presence of food in the stomach stimulates the relaxation of this sphincter, which facilitates the transfer of the contents of the small intestine into the large intestine. The pyloric sphincter separates the stomach from the duodenum. Pyloric stenosis results in a palpable mass that obstructs gastric outflow and leads to projectile vomiting. The sphincter of Oddi is a muscular band that surrounds the opening of the bile duct and the main pancreatic duct into the duodenum. CCK stimulates the relaxation of this sphincter. The upper esophageal sphincter separates the pharynx from the esophagus. This sphincter is under voluntary control, so that it relaxes to allow swallowing and the passage of food into the esophagus.

47. C. This child has a Meckel's diverticulum, which is a congenital anomaly resulting from an unobliterated yolk stalk. More specifically, it is a vestigial remnant of the omphalomesenteric duct. It presents as an ileal outpocketing typically located close to the ileocecal valve. The presence of inflammation, ulceration, and GI bleeding due to the presence of ectopic acid-secreting gastric epithelium is seen in approximately half of these patients. Remember the rule of twos with Meckel's diverticulum: it occurs in about 2% of children, occurs within approximately 2 ft of the ileocecal valve, contains two types of ectopic mucosa (gastric and pancreatic), and usually causes symptoms by age 2.

48. B. All of the choices are familial polyposes. However, the answer is Peutz-Jeghers syndrome owing to the diagnostic clue of darkened pigmentation of buccal mucosa and lips. Peutz-Jeghers syndrome presents with polyps that are hamartomas and not premalignant. These hamartomas are found throughout the colon, with the small intestine usually being the most affected. Gardner's syndrome is an autosomal dominant disease that presents with multiple polyps along with other neoplasms of the bone or skin as well as desmoid tumors. The risk of colon cancer in these patients is close to 100%. Polyposis coli, or familial multiple polyposis, is an autosomal dominant disease that spreads from the rectosigmoid area to the entire colon. Colectomy is the standard treatment right after diagnosis because of the almost 100% risk of developing cancer. Turcot's syndrome presents with multiple polyps along with brain tumors, such as medulloblastomas and gliomas.

49. A. Fried rice and seafood can be contaminated with the *Bacillus cereus* preformed enterotoxin. The incubation period is around 4 hr. This bacteria causes a self-limited diarrhea, vomiting, and abdominal pain. *Campylobacter jejuni* typically causes illness 1 to 7 days after ingestion. *Clostridium botulinum* produces a neurotoxin that blocks the release of acetylcholine, resulting in a symmetrical descending paralysis that may lead to death due to paralysis of the diaphragm. Most cases are associated with the ingestion of contaminated home-canned food. *Clostridium perfringens* has an incubation period of 8 to 24 hr after ingesting contaminated meat or poultry. The meats have usually been cooked, cooled, and then warmed, which causes germination of the clostridial spores. It presents as abdominal pain and severe diarrhea. Enterohemorrhagic *Escherichia coli* produces a bloody, noninvasive diarrhea due to the ingestion of the toxin found in undercooked hamburgers. *Staphylococcus aureus* has a 1- to 6-hr incubation period after ingestion of the enterotoxin. The organism is found in foods such as mayonnaise, potato salad, and custards. The classic presentation for *Vibrio cholerae* is a watery, nonbloody diarrhea with flecks of mucus, often known as rice-water stools. Abdominal pain is not a symptom. It is associated with poorly cooked crabs, shrimps, or oysters.

50. B. Congenital aganglionic megacolon (Hirschsprung's disease) is caused by failure of the neural crest cells to migrate all the way to the anus, resulting in a portion of the distal colon that lacks ganglion cells and both Meissner's submucosal and Auerbach's myenteric plexuses. This results in a functional obstruction and dilatation proximal to the affected portion of the colon. The classic presentation of Hirschsprung's disease includes failure to pass meconium soon after birth followed by constipation and possible abdominal distension.

51. A. This is a typical scenario of mesenteric ischemia. The ischemia is caused by a compromised mesenteric blood supply to the small bowel. This can be due to atherosclerosis, an embolus from the atrial fibrillation, mesenteric venous thrombosis, hypercoagulability, and/or a low-flow state such as hypotension of poor cardiac output. The "gold standard" for diagnosis is angiography. Spiral CT scan with oral and intravenous contrast can also be helpful. Treatment is to maintain tissue perfusion and arrange for early surgical involvement. Intravenous pyelography is used in evaluating the urinary system. Angiography is more precise than MRI, ultrasound, or CT scan would be at identifying the ischemic bowel.

52. A. Duodenal ulcers typically present with a gnawing or burning epigastric pain 1 to 3 hr after meals; they are relieved by food, antacids, or antisecreting agents. Epigastric pain is seen in 60 to 90% of these patients. Nonspecific dyspeptic complaints (belching, bloating, abdominal distension) are seen in 40 to 70%. The etiology of duodenal ulcer is multifactorial. *Helicobacter pylori* gastritis is present in > 80% of duodenal ulcers. Gastric carcinoma would have associated weight loss and tends to occur in patients over the age of 55. Gastric ulcer is exacerbated by food, not relieved by food, as in duodenal ulcer. GERD is reflux disease caused by relaxation or incompetence of the lower esophageal sphincter. Pancreatitis is typically an acute inflammatory process that tends to present with epigastric pain along with radiation to the back. It also tends to be associated with elevated lipase and amylase.

53. C. Paneth cells, which are found at the base of the crypt, are classified as serous cells with the function of host defense. Enterocytes are columnar absorptive cells, with long microvilli, containing digestive bound enzymes. Oligomucous cells are immature mucous cells. Stem cells, which are also found in the crypt, give rise to all epithelial cell layers aside from Paneth cells.

54. A. Acute appendicitis is predominantly seen in young adults. It causes right-lower-quadrant pain, nausea, vomiting, mild fever, and leukocytosis. The inflamed appendix may become gangrenous and perforate in 24 to 48 hr. The CT scan shows nonfilling of a dilated appendix and inflammation of the periappendiceal fat. Therefore immediate appendectomy is standard treatment. Acute pancreatitis typically presents with epigastric pain radiating into the back, nausea, vomiting, and fever. Crohn's disease and ulcerative colitis are inflammatory bowel diseases that typically present with long-standing diarrhea. They do not typically present in an acute fashion, as in the above patient. Diverticulitis is predominantly found in the elderly and typically presents with left-lower-quadrant pain. Gastritis typically presents with epigastric pain often aggravated by eating.

55. C. Sodium bicarbonate is the only product of the central acinar portion of the pancreas. Amylase, trypsinogen, carboxypeptidase are all produced in the acinar pancreas. Amylase is a pancreatic enzyme that is responsible for starch digestion. Trypsinogen is converted to active

enzyme trypsin by enterokinase, an enzyme located on the brush border of the duodenum.

56. B. The site of hydrolysis of a zymogen to an active enzyme is always on the carboxyl end of the peptide bond. The other choices are incorrect. The amine site is not cleaved by protease in relation to the peptide bond. The amine site is not cleaved by the protease in relation to the nitrate group.

57. A. The most common association for *Bacillus cereus* infection is the ingestion of "reheated" rice. The symptoms are general, but again, attributing to the leftover food, they point to the answer. *Staphylococcus aureus* is the other highly common etiologic cause for nausea and vomiting within 6 hr of ingestion, its effects are due to preformed enterotoxins. *Clostridium botulinum* is associated with improperly sealed cans and jars, not reheated foods. *Salmonella* is caused by a milk- or other dairy-based pathogen.

58. A. Clioquinol (Enterovioform), also known as iodochlorhydroxyquin, is not prescribed in the United States owing to the possibility of a subacute myelooptic neuropathy (SMON) reaction, including blindness and neurologic dysfunction. Lomotil may worsen the symptoms of a shigellosis but causes no associated SMON side effects. Doxycycline is currently used in the Peace Corps, with no reported major adverse reactions. Loperamide (Imodium) is also widely used without any major issues.

59. D. Group D, also known as *Shigella sonnei*, is the single stereotype in group D, and is the most common cause of shigellosis in the United States. Group A consists of *S. dysenteriae*, which is rarely found in the United States, and is characterized by its inability to ferment mannitol. Group B includes *S. flexneri*, which is commonly found in the United States but is not the *most* common. Group C includes *S. boydii* and is biochemically indistinguishable from group B but serologically unique.

60. D. *Vibrio parahaemolyticus* is most commonly associated with ingestion of bivalve mollusks and crustaceans. *Clostridium perfringens* is linked with gravies, spices, and dried potatoes. *Yersinia enterocolitica* in the United States is mainly caused by contaminated milk. *Staphylococcus aureus* is commonly associated with ham, poultry, potato/egg salads, and cream-filled pastries.

61. B. ETEC, also known as toxigenic *E. coli*, is the most common cause of "traveler's diarrhea," occurring at a rate of 40 to 70%. *E. histolytica* occurs at a rate of 0 to 2%. EHEC, which is known for producing bloody stools, has an occurrence of 0 to 4%, and enterovirus is virtually nonexistent.

62. E. Ulcerative colitis presents with friable and inflamed mucosa. Continuous inflammation and pseudopolyps are common findings, along with crypt abscesses, severe stenosis, and the possible occurrence of a toxic megacolon. Higher risk of colorectal carcinoma and sclerosing cholangitis are commonly associated with this diagnosis. Barium enema shows subtotal disease with superficial ulceration and loss of haustrations extending from the rectum to the hepatic flexure. Crohn's disease is not confined to the colon but comprises the entire length of the GI tract. Skip lesions are pathognomonic, as well as cobblestone mucosa and "string" sign on x-ray. Diverticulosis is identified by the presence of "outpouchings" of the colon, especially in the sigmoid. It is commonly associated with low-fiber diets, and a vague discomfort.

63. E. Stool sample is the most direct and effective method of detecting the pathogen. *Shigella* must penetrate the epithelial lining of the large intestine to induce dysentery; a biopsy is not only excessively invasive but uninformative as well. Gastric lavage would also be of no use, as the pathogen is mainly found in the colon, or the lower GI tract.

64. A. During the cystic stage, which is the latter growth stage of *Entamoeba histolytica,* intestinal infections occur via ingestion of contaminated food and drink as well as hand-to-hand contact. In many tropical countries, over 40% of the population is infected. Intravenous drug abuse and sexual intercourse do not utilize the proper vectors for cystic transmission. Oral-fecal transmission may be possible, but this is not the most likely route.

65. A. Children under 5 years of age are the most prevalent population infected by salmonellosis. The main route of transmission is via ingestion of contaminated food and drink. The pathogen is mainly a disease of lower animals and occurs in greatest frequency from July through November.

66. A. *Giardia lamblia* is the most common and leading cause of diarrhea in the United States. *Homo sapiens* is the only host and only reservoir for this flagellate. The other choices are prevalent in much lesser degrees. Acute infections are characterized by watery small bowel diarrhea. The clinical features are not always self-limiting and can be persistent. Diagnosis is made by identifying cysts and trophozoites by microscopy of the stool sample.

67. C. Charcot's triad of right-upper-quadrant pain, fever, and jaundice is indicative of gallstones. In association with the classic risk factors for gallstones (female, fat, fertile, and forty), this would point to a primary differential of stones. Acute pancreatitis can be caused by gallstones, but this would not be a primary assumption. Hepatocellular carcinoma has no relation to above the presentation. Appendicitis is indicated by right-lower-quadrant pain, not pain in the right upper quadrant.

68. C. Nitrous oxide causes smooth muscle relaxation in the body, including the sphincters. Acetylcholine is a parasympathetic that increases production of saliva and gastric acid secretion and also plays a minor role in sphincter relaxation. Gastrin is secreted in response to gastric distension and vagal stimulation. Secretin is secreted by the pancreas in response to the entrance of H^+ and fatty acids into the duodenum.

69. D. Pancreatic insufficiency, which is commonly seen in patients with cystic fibrosis, presents with malabsorptive issues and severe steatorrhea. Proper advice is to limit fat intake as well as to increase ingestion of fat-soluble vitamins. Glucose malabsorption would not have such effects on stooling. Menstrual loss could lead to an anemic condi-

tion but not odorous stools. Bleeding ulcers can also cause anemia and black tarry stools but without the odor issues.

70. A. The chief function of oligosaccharide amylases is the production of monosaccharides. Pancreatic amylase is found primarily in the lumen of the duodenum and breaks down starches. Somatostatin aids in the inhibition of secretin and gastrin. Salivary amylase is responsible for the breakdown and creation of maltose and other products.

71. C. Patients with renal failure who need enteral feedings should be placed on particular renal-sparing products. These products will utilize essential amino acids as a protein source and provide a fat content of 45%. Casein is a whole protein and is the most common protein in enteral feeding products. Crystalline amino acids are found in elemental enteral feedings, which are useful in patients with conditions such as inflammatory bowel disease. Hydrolyzed protein is in the peptide class of enteral feedings and is useful in patients who are hypoalbuminemic. Whole protein with amino acid supplements are useful in patients with acute stress such as trauma or burns and are thought to decrease infectious complications.

72. C. HMG-CoA reductase inhibitors cause cells to decrease the rate of cholesterol synthesis, which causes decreased conversion of cholesterol to cholesterol esters for storage and increased production of LDL receptors. An increased number of receptors will cause more LDL to be taken up by cells and degraded by lysosomes. Blood cholesterol levels subsequently decrease. LDL receptor production increases. Blood triacylglycerol levels decrease slightly. ACAT activity decreases. De novo cholesterol synthesis decreases.

73. A. Acetyl CoA is used by the liver for the production of ketone bodies such as acetoacetate and beta-hydroxybutyrate. The liver will release ketone bodies into the blood but is unable to oxidize them. Amino acids such as alanine can be used as carbon sources for gluconeogenesis. Glycerol is a product of degradation of triacylglycerol and can be used as a carbon source for gluconeogenesis. Lactate is produced by red blood cells and can be used as a carbon source for gluconeogenesis. Propionate is produced by fatty acid oxidation and can be used as a carbon source for gluconeogenesis.

74. C. Permeability describes the ease with which a solute will diffuse through a membrane. The permeability will increase when the radius (size) of the solute decreases. Small hydrophobic solutes have the highest permeabilities in lipid membranes. Increase of the oil-water partition coefficient of the solute increases solubility in the lipid of the membrane. Decrease in membrane thickness decreases the diffusion distance. Hydrophilic substances must cross cell membranes through water-gated pores.

75. C. When fuels are metabolized in the body, adenosine triphosphate is synthesized and heat generated. The oxidation of fats will produce 9 kcal/g. This heat that is produced by fuel oxidation is used to maintain core body temperature. Alcohol when present as a dietary substance will produce 7 kcal/g. The oxidation of carbohydrates to carbon dioxide and water produces 4 kcal/g. Protein oxidation produces 4 kcal/g of energy.

Chapter 7   Hematopoietic and Lymphoreticular Systems

Questions

1. A 22-year-old woman presents to her primary care physician complaining of swollen lymph nodes in her neck, which have been present for 1 and 1/2 months. She reports that she has not had a cough, cold, or sore throat during this time. Physical examination reveals bilateral lymphadenopathy in the posterior cervical nodes. Biopsy of the nodes reveals binucleated giant cells with eosinophilic inclusion-like nuclei. A CT scan of the abdomen is obtained (Figure 7-1). What type of cells does the pathology report describe?

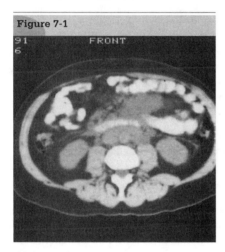

Figure 7-1

A. Auer rods
B. Burr cells
C. Reed-Sternberg cells
D. Teardrop cells
E. Smudge cells

2. A 12-year-old African American girl presents to her primary care physician complaining of pain in her fingers, which began 2 days ago. She reports that she had some numbness and tingling following the pain. However, her symptoms have resolved. She reports that she has a family history of sickle cell anemia. Which of the following options is a beneficial treatment for this disease?

A. Dialysis
B. Hydroxyurea
C. Lamivudine
D. Liver transplant
E. Quinidine

3. A 22-year-old man presents to his primary care physician complaining of hemoptysis and hematuria, which began 3 months earlier. Renal biopsy is performed; under immunofluorescence, this reveals linear staining of IgG to the glomerular basement membranes. In which of the following groups is this young man's disease classified?

A. Acute rejection
B. Type I hypersensitivity
C. Type II hypersensitivity
D. Type III hypersensitivity
E. Type IV hypersensitivity

4. A 68-year-old man is found unconscious in the street by paramedics. He is wearing a MedicAlert bracelet with the following information: "blood disorder and valve replacement." The medics are able to draw a tube of blood, which shows evidence of RBC membrane destruction on peripheral smear. What is the most likely explanation for these findings?

A. Beta thalassemia
B. Hemophilia A
C. Idiopathic thrombocytopenic purpura
D. Prosthetic valves
E. Von Willebrand's disease

5. A physician wishes to get preoperative tests and labs on a 65-year-old man who is to undergo an elective hemicolectomy to remove his sigmoid colon after three episodes of diverticulitis. The patient has been taking aspirin for osteoarthritis. Physical examination of the heart, lungs, and abdomen is unremarkable. There is no evidence of guarding or rebound tenderness. Peritoneal signs are absent. Bowel sounds are present in all four quadrants. Rectal examination reveals external hemorrhoids. Which of the following tests would most likely be affected?

A. Bleeding time
B. Hemoglobin
C. Hematocrit
D. Prothrombin time
E. Partial thromboplastin time

6. The oxygen dissociation curve illustrates the relationship of oxygen binding to hemoglobin under certain conditions. As the partial pressure of oxygen increases, hemoglobin becomes more saturated with oxygen. In which of the following conditions would a patient's oxygen dissociation curve be expected to shift to the right?

A. Decrease in altitude
B. Decrease in temperature
C. Exercise (such as weight lifting)
D. Hyperventilation
E. Metabolic alkalosis

7. A 19-year-old college tennis player presents to the university health center with the chief complaint of itchiness. She reports a family history of hemolytic anemia. Physical examination reveals scleral icterus and her skin appears jaundiced. She also has an enlarged spleen. Laboratory studies reveal a total bilirubin of 6 and an indirect bilirubin of 4.9. Hematocrit is 28%. Which positive test result would confirm the diagnosis in this patient?

   A. Coombs' test

   B. Electrophoresis

   C. Hamm's test

   D. Osmotic fragility test

   E. Urine observation test

8. A 52-year-old man is undergoing a coronary artery bypass graft procedure for significant coronary artery disease. Preoperatively, he had normal coagulation studies and no family or prior history of a bleeding disorder. The procedure was complicated by a moderate amount of blood loss. The patient received 5 Us of packed RBCs over the next 24 hr. Early the next day, the patient accidentally cut himself while shaving, causing him to bleed excessively. What is the most likely explanation for these findings?

   A. Acquired factor VIII inhibitor from transfused blood

   B. Dilutional coagulopathy

   C. Hemophilia A

   D. Hemophilia B

   E. Von Willebrand's disease

9. A 12-year-old boy presents to the pediatrics clinic with a deep thigh abscess and eczema on his skin. His mother reports that he has previously had eczema and that this is his second time with an abscess. She is worried that he may have an immunodeficiency. The physician incises and drains the abscess and sends the exudate for culture. He also sends away for several laboratory studies, including immunoglobulin assays. These lab tests show high levels of IgE. What is the most likely explanation for these findings?

   A. Ataxia-telangectasia

   B. Chediak-Higashi syndrome

   C. DiGeorge's syndrome

   D. IL-12 deficiency

   E. Job's syndrome

10. A 62-year-old man presents to his primary care physician complaining of increasing abdominal size in his right and left upper quadrants. He also reports that he had an increased white blood cell count at his local rotary club screening 3 weeks earlier. Physical examination reveals hepatosplenomegaly, which is confirmed by ultrasound. Laboratory studies reveal a decreased level of leukocyte alkaline phosphatase. Which of the following chromosomal translocations could confirm the most likely diagnosis in this patient?

   A. t(9:22)

   B. t(11:14)

   C. t(11:18)

   D. t(14:18)

   E. t(14:21)

11. A 45-year-old woman presents to her primary care physician with the chief complaint of extreme fatigue and dizziness. Her past medical history is significant for back pain for the previous 2 years due to a herniated lumbar disc. On physical examination, her face appears pale. Her mucous membranes are moist and she has good capillary refill. Laboratory studies reveal a decreased hemoglobin and hematocrit. Mean corpuscular volume (MCV) is 95. Total iron-binding capacity (TIBC) and serum iron are low. What is the most likely explanation for these findings?

   A. Anemia of chronic disease

   B. Iron deficiency

   C. Lead poisoning

   D. Megaloblastic anemia

   E. Thalassemia

12. A 32-year-old woman is brought into the emergency department complaining of fever and extreme lethargy. Blood work reveals a preponderance of lymphocytes, which leads to the suspicion of lymphoma. The pathologist notes that the blood specimen under the microscope reveals tumor cells being engulfed by macrophages. This particular lymphoma has been linked to which of the following viruses?

   A. Cytomegalovirus

   B. Epstein-Barr virus

   C. Human immunodeficiency virus

   D. Human papillomavirus

   E. Human T-cell lymphoma virus

13. A 32-year-old black woman presents to the ambulatory care clinic complaining of fatigue and a recent sore throat. Physical examination reveals that the patient has extremely red cheeks and petechiae on her trunk. Her peripheral smear is shown in Figure 7-2. Which of the following complications of her sickle cell disease can explain her symptoms?

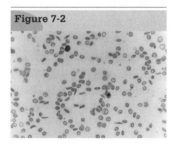

Figure 7-2

   A. Aplastic crisis

   B. Autosplenectomy

   C. Hemolytic anemia

   D. Osteomyelitis

   E. Vasoocclusive crises

14. A 31-year-old man with hypertension undergoes a renal biopsy for further evaluation. Which of the following features would be found on the lymphatic vessels exiting the superficial inguinal nodes but not on the efferent arteriole exiting a glomerulus in the kidney?

   A. Fenestrations to facilitate the exit of fluid from the vessel

   B. Postsynaptic innervation from parasympathetic neurons

C. Postsynaptic innervation from sympathetic neurons

D. Three cell layers of smooth muscle comprising the wall

E. Valves preventing the retrograde flow of fluid

15. A 33-year-old man with a history of lymphoma presents for follow-up. He has some palpable anterior cervical lymph nodes and undergoes lymph node biopsy. The lymph node and germinal center is sectioned by the pathologist and stained with hematoxylin and eosin. The germinal center of a lymph node has which of the following characteristics?

A. Degranulates upon IgE entering the lymph node and binding to the cell surface

B. Phagocytoses bacteria and uses NADPH oxidase

C. Possesses CD40L on its surface

D. Recognizes MHC II on certain antigen-presenting cells

E. Will eventually produce antibody

16. A 58-year-old woman with metastatic breast cancer and a chest wall abscess is hospitalized in the intensive care unit. She has recurrent epistaxis. Blood and urine cultures are positive for Gram-negative cocci. Which of the following findings is consistent with this condition?

A. Decreased fibrinogen

B. Decreased fibrin split products

C. Decreased D-dimer

D. Thrombocytosis

E. Decreased PTT

17. A 40-year-old man presents to his primary care physician complaining of fatigue. For the past 4 months he has noticed he cannot complete his usual exercise regimen. Review of systems is unremarkable. Physical exam reveals a pale man, older-appearing than his age. Heart rate is 103 bpm, blood pressure is 113/65 mm Hg. The remainder of the physical examination is within normal limits. Laboratory studies reveal a hematocrit of 27%, mean corpuscular volume (MCV) 69, ferritin 27. What is the next most appropriate step in the management of this patient?

A. Admit to the hospital for transfusions

B. Colonoscopy

C. Iron therapy

D. Increase red meats in his diet and follow up in 1 month

E. Vitamin B_{12} and folate therapy

18. A 39-year-old woman with a history of Crohn's disease is seen for a follow-up examination by her primary care physician. Review of her recent laboratory studies shows an increase in her erythrocyte sedimentation rate (ESR) from 10 to 45 mm/hr. Which of the following most contributes to an elevated ESR?

A. Albumin

B. Ceruloplasmin

C. Ferritin

D. Fibrinogen

E. Transferrin

19. A 64-year-old woman comes to the emergency department with a 3-day history of swelling and tenderness in her right calf following an overseas airplane flight. She has a 50-pack-year history of smoking. Duplex ultrasound reveals a left popliteal deep venous thrombus. What is the next step in the management of this patient?

A. Physical examination and chest x-ray

B. Physical examination and MRI of chest/abdomen

C. Physical examination and upper GI follow-through radiographs

D. Physical examination and serum PSA

E. Follow-up in clinic in 2 weeks

20. A 38-year-old man presents to his primary care physician after being discharged from the hospital following an admission for idiopathic thrombocytopenic purpura. Prior to discharge, he was started on prednisone and was to taper the dose as his platelet count permitted. Recently his dose was tapered to 20 mg daily and the platelet count dropped to 20,000. He now has mask-like facies and a buffalo hump. His hemoglobin is 12.6 mg/dL. Which of the following is the best option for long-term management?

A. High-dose steroids

B. Methotrexate

C. Plasma exchange

D. Splenectomy

E. Thymectomy

21. A 5-year-old boy presents with his parents who are concerned about possible lead poisoning. Their son has been exposed to lead through the home of a friend. His medical history is unremarkable. Which of the following symptoms is atypical for lead poisoning?

A. Ataxia

B. Abdominal pain

C. Cyanosis

D. Headaches

E. Nausea and vomiting

22. A 35-year-old man with AIDS is hospitalized for fever of unknown origin. He has a prior history of splenectomy at age 21 due to a stab wound to the flank. Which of the following pathogens is the most common cause of sepsis in splenectomized patients?

A. *Haemophilus influenzae*

B. *Neisseria meningitidis*

C. *Pseudomonas aeruginosa*

D. *Staphylococcus aureus*

E. *Streptococcus pneumoniae*

23. A 31-year-old primigravida is 25 weeks pregnant. She complains of recurrent nosebleeds and is concerned that she may have a bleeding disorder. She is reassured that she probably has an alteration in the levels of blood clotting factors. Which coagulation factor changes the most during pregnancy?

A. Factor I

B. Factor V

C. Factor VII

D. Factor XII

E. Fibrinogen

24. A 62-year-old Caucasian man is scheduled for an elective arthroscopy of the knee. He has no complaints except some epigastric discomfort, which is relieved with antacids. His medical history is significant for asthma and chronic knee pain. Physical examination and vital signs are within normal limits. Results of his laboratory studies are as follows: Hgb, 9.2 mg/dL; MCV, 68; MCHC, 26; WBCs 4,800 mm³; platelets, 500,000 mm³. What is the next diagnostic step?

    A. Colonoscopy
    B. Hemoglobin electrophoresis
    C. Protoporphyrin levels
    D. Reticulocyte count
    E. Vitamin B_{12} level

25. A 47-year-old man presents to his primary care physician for an annual checkup. His medical history is significant for hypertension. He has a 40-pack-year history and has consumed five to seven beers per day for approximately 20 years. He has been experiencing numbness and pain in his lower extremities. Physical examination is unremarkable except for diminished sensation to light touch distally. Which of the following is the most likely cause of his symptoms?

    A. Alcohol abuse
    B. Asbestosis
    C. Diabetes
    D. Hypothyroidism
    E. Tobacco abuse

26. An 82-year-old woman complains of fatigue and shortness of breath. Lab findings are as follows: HCT, 22%; MCV, 85; white blood cell count, 5,000/mm³; BUN, 60; creatinine, 4.1 mg/dL. Urinary dipstick for protein is negative, with a total urine protein of 2.8g/24 hr. A radiograph of the head is shown in Figure 7-3. What is the most likely diagnosis?

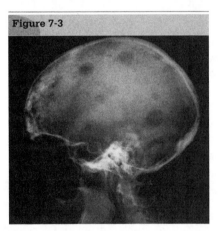

Figure 7-3

    A. Adrenal insufficiency
    B. Anemia of chronic disease
    C. Anemia of chronic renal disease
    D. Hemolysis
    E. Multiple myeloma

27. A 41-year-old woman with a history of gallstones is scheduled for laparoscopic cholecystectomy. She has a history of easy bruising and bleeds easily during dental procedures.

She is sent to the laboratory for preoperative studies, including a bleeding time, which is a measure of:

    A. Extrinsic clotting pathway
    B. Intrinsic clotting pathway
    C. Liver function
    D. Platelet function
    E. Factor VIII

28. A 30-year-old presents to the emergency department with shortness of breath. Her medical history is unremarkable, though she does complain of heavy menstrual periods. She also has a craving for ice. The patient denies cold intolerance, weight gain, or constipation. She lives in a home that is 10 years old. Her social history is not significant. The patient mentions that there is a family history of low blood counts. Physical examination reveals a woman who is thin and pale. Her vital signs are stable. Slight cheilosis is noticed. The results of her laboratory studies are as follows: Hgb, 7 g/dL; MCV, 65; leukocytes, 9,300/mm³; reticulocytes, 1.6%; platelets, 630,000/mm³. What is the most likely diagnosis?

    A. Glucose-6 phosphatase deficiency
    B. Hypothyroidism
    C. Iron deficiency
    D. Lead poisoning
    E. Thalassemia

29. A 7-year-old girl is admitted to the pediatrics ward and diagnosed with hemolytic uremic syndrome. What are the most likely laboratory findings compatible with this condition?

Platelets	Schistocytes	Prothrombin Time	Partial Thromboplastin Time
A. Low	+	Normal	Normal
B. Low	–	Normal	Normal
C. Low	+	Increased	Increased
D. Low	+	Increased	Normal
E. Low	+	Normal	Increased

30. A 60-year-old Caucasian woman was recently diagnosed with a deep venous thrombus. She presented to the emergency department with a 2-day history of swelling of the right leg. She has no injuries of recent date nor been immobilized. Which of the following conditions is the most likely risk factor?

    A. Antithrombin deficiency
    B. Factor V Leiden mutation
    C. Hemophilia B
    D. Protein C deficiency
    E. Protein S deficiency

31. A 46-year-old woman has undergone resection of a leiomyosarcoma and the distal ileum (due to compression, resulting in small bowel obstruction). Five months later she presents with fatigue. Her HCT is 25%. Which of the following is most likely to be seen on peripheral smear?

    A. Hypersegmented neutrophils
    B. Microcytosis

C. Schistocytes

D. Spherocytosis

E. Thrombocytosis

32. A 61-year-old man with a history of radiation therapy for colon cancer presents to his primary care physician for evaluation of progressive weakness. His physical examination is unremarkable except for abdominal fullness. His spun hematocrit is 25%. What is the most likely explanation for these findings?

A. Bone marrow fibrosis ⟶ *replacement of bone marrow c̄ tumor cells by fibrosis*

B. Damage to stem cells

C. Destruction of marrow stem cells

D. Intoxication syndrome (alcohol induced)

E. Tuberculosis

33. A 31-year-old athlete collapses after a track meet. She is brought to the hospital for evaluation. Review of prior medical records indicates a history of anorexia nervosa and easy bruising. She undergoes a complete workup including peripheral smear and bone marrow biopsy. What would be the most likely finding?

A. Aplastic anemia

B. Bone marrow myelofibrosis

C. Cellular bone marrow with substrate deficiency

D. Hypocellular bone marrow

E. Myelofibrosis with myeloid metaplasia

34. An 18-year-old African American man presents to the emergency department complaining of severe pain in his joints and back. Physical examination reveals an ulcer on his left lateral malleolus (Figure 7-4). Which of the following suggestions would help this patient to prevent future attacks?

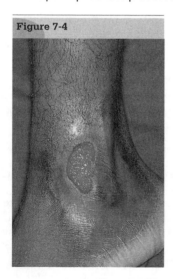

Figure 7-4

A. Avoid tobacco

B. Maintain hydration

C. Get regular exercise

D. Practice safer sex

35. A 50-year-old man presents to the emergency department with a 1-month history of midepigastric pain, and he has just vomited bright red blood. He is ataxic. Physical examination reveals an ill-appearing man who is oriented to person and place but not time. He has diffuse abdominal tenderness. Rectal examination reveals tarry-black stool in the vault, which is positive for occult blood. Lab testing shows his blood alcohol level to be elevated. What is his complete blood count most likely to show?

A. Macrocytic anemia

B. Microcytic anemia

C. Normocytic anemia

D. Leukopenia

E. Thrombocytopenia

36. A 45-year-old man recently diagnosed with acute myelogenous leukemia (AML) presents to the emergency department with a nosebleed that will not stop. Lab work is done, which notes the following:

Prothrombin time = elevated

Activated partial thromboplastin time = elevated

Platelets = decreased

Fibrin split products = present

Based on these data, the most likely form of acute myelogenous leukemia that this patient has is:

A. M1

B. M2

C. M3

D. M4

E. M5

37. A 24-year-old woman presents to her primary care physician for a routine checkup. Examination proceeds without any major issues or findings. During the interview, she mentions having been a proud vegetarian for 3 years but complains of recent bouts of fatigue, labored breathing, and feeling winded while walking up stairs. She denies any drug or tobacco history. The most likely lab result that would confirm your suspected diagnosis is which of the following:

A. Increased hemoglobin

B. Increased serum iron

C. Increased TIBC (total iron-binding capacity)

D. Increased body iron storage

E. Increased serum ferritin

38. A 56-year-old man presents to his primary care physician and reports having a blood problem, mentioning a recent diagnosis of myelophthisic anemia. He does not seem to understand his diagnosis and wants to know what causes this disorder. His physician immediately orders labs and films and explains that this condition is usually caused by a problem located in the:

A. Bone marrow

B. Kidneys

C. Liver

D. Pancreas

E. Spleen

39. A 44-year-old man presents to his primary care physician with a history of alcoholism; he is currently an active drinker. Physical examination reveals a yellowish tinge to his skin. Laboratory studies reveal hypersegmented neutrophils. What is the most likely explanation for these findings?

    A. Aplastic anemia
    B. Erythroblastosis fetalis
    C. Folate-deficiency anemia
    D. Glucose-6 phosphate deficiency
    E. Pernicious anemia

40. A 28-year-old man presents to his primary care physician for follow-up on routine bloodwork. The report reveals spherocytes, and he also had a positive direct Coombs' test. In thinking of this diagnosis, which of the following diseases would be immediately considered?

    A. ABO incompatibility
    B. Hodgkin's disease
    C. Kernicterus
    D. Mycoplasmal pneumonia
    E. Raynaud's phenomenon

41. A 34-year-old African-American woman presents to the emergency department complaining of shortness of breath while exercising. She normally exercises daily without difficulty. Bloodwork reveals hemolytic anemia. What is the most relevant question to ask this patient pertaining to her clinical presentation and laboratory findings?

    A. Employment status
    B. General mood
    C. Recent diet
    D. Recent vacations
    E. Sexual activity

42. A 36-year-old woman presents to her primary care physician for follow-up on her diagnosis of polycythemia vera. This condition can be differentiated from all the other forms of polycythemia by which of the following characteristics?

    A. Adult polycystic kidney disease
    B. Chronic hypoxia
    C. Decreased erythropoietin
    D. Increased erythropoietin
    E. Increased levels of transferrin

43. A 17-year-old girl presents to her primary care physician reporting sore throat, fever, and generalized malaise over the preceding 4 days; on physical exam, severe lymphadenopathy is noted. Laboratory studies reveal reactive CD8+ T lymphocytes and heterophil antibodies. Based on the presentation, which of the following comorbidities is of the greatest concern?

    A. Aplastic anemia
    B. Elevated creatinine
    C. Febrile-induced seizures
    D. Splenic rupture
    E. Tongue swallowing

44. A 22-year-old man presents to his primary care physician complaining of constant pruritus as well as ongoing fever, shallow breathing, and fatigue. Blood analysis reveals binucleated giant cells with eosinophilic inclusion–like nuclei. What is the name of the cell that has revealed this pathology?

    A. Bence Jones
    B. Beriberi
    C. Kwashiorkor
    D. Reed-Sternberg
    E. Rouleaux formation

45. A 3-year-old child has a significant history of easy bruising, which has never been worked up. He seems to have bleeding into his muscles, subcutaneous tissues, and joints. Which of the following is the causative etiology?

    A. Factor II
    B. Factor VII
    C. Factor VIII
    D. Factor IX
    E. Vitamin K

46. A 23-year-old woman presents to the emergency department because of recurrent nosebleeds that are difficult to control. Her mother has the same problem. Hematologic studies reveal a skin bleeding time of 15 min and an abnormal response to ristocetin. What is the most likely explanation for these findings?

    A. Failure of the blood to coagulate
    B. Failure of the marrow to produce blood cells
    C. Failure of platelet adhesion
    D. Inability of the blood to transport oxygen
    E. Sickling of the RBCs

47. An infant delivered at 37 weeks' gestation has severe megaloblastic anemia. Treatment with vitamin B$_{12}$ and folic acid has not reversed her anemia. Urinalysis reveals crystals of orotic acid. Which of the following enzymes is deficient?

    A. Glucose phosphatase
    B. Glucose phosphorylase
    C. Orotidylic pyrophosphorylase orotidylic decarboxylase
    D. Phosphoribosyl transferase
    E. Urease dehydrogenase

48. A 65-year-old man presents to his primary care physician; he complains of having had generalized swollen glands and malaise for some 10 days. He denies any recent changes or issues aside from those mentioned. Laboratory studies reveal WBCs at 150,000/mm^3 and a peripheral smear as shown in Figure 7-5. Based on these results, what is the most likely explanation?

    A. Acute lymphoblastic leukemia
    B. Acute myelogenous leukemia
    C. Chronic lymphocytic leukemia
    D. Chronic myelogenous leukemia

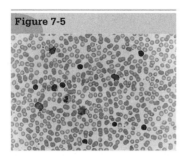

Figure 7-5

49. A 29-year-old man with male-factor infertility has a left-sided varicocele and will be scheduled for elective repair. He has no prior medical history and currently takes no medications. Physical examination reveals a young man in no acute distress. Cardiac and pulmonary examinations are within normal limits. Abdominal examination is unremarkable. The testes are descended bilaterally and the presence of a grade II varicocele is noted on the left side. Anorectal examination was not performed. Laboratory studies indicate a prolonged bleeding time. Which of the following substances might have been ingested by the patient to produce such a result?

A. Aspirin

B. Enalapril

C. Furosemide

D. Prednisone

E. Tetracycline

50. Research on the ultrastructure and function of IgG indicates that:

A. Disulfide bonds link the H and J chains

B. The entire molecule is shaped in the letter L configuration

C. This is the most abundant immunoglobulin in blood

D. The composition includes two heavy and two light chains

E. This molecule is an exocrine secretion into mucus and milk

51. A cadaver kidney becomes available for transplantation into a 39-year-old man with end-stage renal disease. Which of the following would be an absolute contraindication to the use of this organ for transplantation?

A. AB incompatibility

B. Cold ischemia lasting more than 36 hr

C. HLA tissue typing with a poor match

D. Positive T-cell cross-match

E. Prior positive T-cell match but currently negative

52. A 4-year-old boy is brought to the emergency department for evaluation of failure to thrive and lethargy. Several other children living in the same apartment complex have been diagnosed with lead poisoning. Which of the following findings would be the most compelling reason to suggest this diagnosis?

A. Basophilic stippling

B. Gingival discoloration

C. Gastrointestinal complaints

D. Peripheral neuropathy

E. Lead lines in the eyes

53. A 66-year-old man with insulin-dependent diabetes mellitus, hypertension, and congestive heart failure presents to a vascular surgeon for examination of ulceration on his left lower leg. Physical examination reveals an ulceration measuring 1.5 by 1.0 cm just proximal to the medial malleolus. The most likely inciting event in the pathogenesis of this condition is which of the following?

A. Calf muscle pump dysfunction

B. Creation of the ulcer cavity

C. Peripheral neuropathy

D. Ulceration and denervation hypersensitivity

E. Venous valvular injury

54. A 61-year-old woman complains of the presence of spider and dilated veins on her lower legs. She presents to her primary care physician for evaluation. Physical examination reveals superficial varicose veins of the legs. Which of the following situations would predispose a patient to this condition?

A. Anorexia

B. Bulimia

C. Daily exercise

D. Obesity

E. Pregnancy termination

55. A 53-year-old African American man presents to his primary care physician complaining of back pain, generalized weakness, constipation, and weight loss. He also reports three bone fractures during the past year, which he had never had before. Labs show Bence Jones proteinuria. X-ray studies are shown in Figure 7-6. What is the most likely diagnosis?

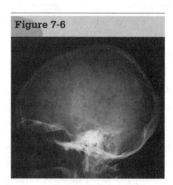

Figure 7-6

A. Acute lymphocytic leukemia

B. Acute myelogenous leukemia

C. Chronic myelogenous leukemia

D. Lymphoma

E. Multiple myeloma

56. A first-time mother presents to the pediatrician with her newborn son. She is concerned because he has a skin lesion—a red-purple shaded area on his face and neck. What is the most likely diagnosis?

A. Angiosarcoma

B. Cystic hygroma

C. Glomangioma

D. Hemangioma

E. Hemangiopericytoma

57. A 34-year-old woman is brought to the emergency department complaining of fever, weight loss, abdominal pain, joint pain, and nausea, which she has experienced for some 2 months. Medical history is positive for hepatitis B. Blood pressure is 180/100 mm Hg, with the remainder of her vitals stable. Arterial biopsy shows necrotizing immune complex inflammation of various small and medium-sized arteries. Aneurysmal nodules are also noted on the pathology report. What is the most likely explanation for these findings?

   A. Angiosarcoma
   B. Kaposi's sarcoma
   C. Leukocytoclastic vasculitis
   D. Polyarteritis nodosa
   E. Wegener's granulomatosis

58. An 83-year-old man is brought to the emergency department complaining of severe headaches and changes in his vision over the past few days. He also mentions feelings of stiffness on rising in the mornings and a general feeling of malaise. Blood testing reveals an elevated ESR. Which of the following findings would also support the suspected diagnosis?

   A. Diaphoresis
   B. Hemangioma
   C. Palpable nodules
   D. Pruritus
   E. Xerostomia

59. A 72-year-old woman is brought to the emergency department complaining of generalized malaise, fever, painful skin bumps, arthritis, and visual changes. Upon physical exam, pulses are noted to be absent in the carotid, radial, and ulnar arteries. What is the most likely explanation for these findings?

   A. Glomus tumor
   B. Henoch-Schönlein purpura
   C. Serum sickness
   D. Takayasu's arteritis
   E. Wegener's granulomatosis

60. A 41-year-old African American man presents to his primary care physician for a well checkup. He has no prior medical history. His family history is positive for hypertension and diabetes mellitus. Physical examination reveals a blood pressure of 160/100 mm Hg. Which of the following would be the most significant determinant in the development of hypertension in this patient?

   A. African-American race
   B. Cigarette smoking
   C. Lack of physical activity
   D. Obesity
   E. Positive family history

61. A 40-year-old African-American man presents to his primary care physician complaining of visual changes, headaches, facial flushing, and dyspnea on exertion. Physical examination shows upper and lower extremity +3 pitting edema, with a blood pressure of 170/120 mm Hg. What pathological finding would be expected in relation to this presentation and the clinical findings?

   A. Coarctation of the aorta
   B. Cushing's syndrome
   C. Malignant nephrosclerosis
   D. Pheochromocytoma
   E. Unilateral renal artery stenosis

62. A 34-year-old woman presents to her primary care physician complaining of fever, excessive bleeding when cut, headaches, and reported mental status changes. Physical exam reveals elevated temperature of 102°F (38.8°C), abdominal and upper extremity petechiae, and marked splenomegaly. What is the most likely diagnosis?

   A. Glucose-6 phosphate deficiency
   B. Idiopathic thrombocytopenic purpura
   C. Polycythemia vera
   D. Thrombotic thrombocytopenic purpura
   E. Transfusion reaction

63. A 16-year-old girl is brought to the emergency department complaining of fever, chills, uncontrollable bleeding, a cold feeling in her fingertips, and trouble breathing. She reluctantly admits to having had an illegal abortion in Mexico 2 days earlier. Physical exam reveals distal extremity cyanosis, tachycardia, and hypotension. Which of the following lab values would be most in line with the clinical presentation of this patient?

   A. Decreased D-dimer
   B. Decreased PT/PTT
   C. Elevated fibrin spilt products
   D. Elevated platelets
   E. Elevated hematocrit

64. A 65-year-old man presents to his primary care physician complaining of back pain, which he has now had for a year. He attributes his pain to having lifted a crate at home while doing yard work. He lost 20 lb over the past year and had pneumonia twice during that time. He has no prior history of back pain. Past medical history is significant for cardiovascular disease. Physical examination is normal and the patient does not have a positive straight leg-raising test. Laboratory studies show an elevated calcium and LDH. His blood film is shown in Figure 7-7. What is the most likely diagnosis?

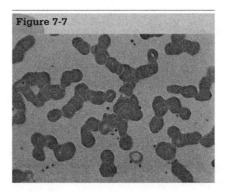

Figure 7-7

   A. Hyperparathyroidism
   B. Hypervitaminosis D
   C. Milk-alkali syndrome

D. Multiple myeloma

E. Spinal stenosis

65. A young couple (man age 29 and woman age 26) with hemophilia present for consultation. They are interested in having a child. What is the best genetic predictor of transmission of hemophilia to a male child?

A. Father is a carrier of hemophilia

B. Father is positive for hemophilia

C. Maternal environmental exposure during pregnancy

D. Mother is a carrier of hemophilia

E. Mother is a negative carrier of hemophilia

66. A 2-year-old child is brought to the emergency department with a temperature of 104°F (40°C). On physical exam, tachypnea and dyspnea are noted, as well as an oxygen saturation of 93%. The child's hands and feet appear to be edematous and painful to the touch. What would be a logical test to diagnose this child's condition?

A. Complete blood count

B. CT abdomen/pelvis

C. Chest x-ray

D. Hemoglobin electrophoresis

E. Urinalysis

67. A 73-year-old man presents to his primary care physician complaining of systemic pruritus over the previous month. He denies any changes in laundry or diet. He admits to night sweats, weight loss, and generalized body pains. Physical exam notes hepatosplenomegaly and regional adenopathy. Biopsy reveals a mixed cell infiltrate. What is the most likely diagnosis for this patient?

A. Hodgkin's lymphoma

B. Human immunodeficiency virus

C. Non-Hodgkin's lymphoma

D. Sepsis

E. Tertiary syphilis

68. A 23-year-old man presents to the emergency department complaining of abdominal pain, cough with blood, urticaria, and fever over the previous 3 days. He claims the symptoms are not resolving and is apprehensive because of the hemoptysis. He also reports a recent onset of increasingly severe dyspnea. Which of the following issues in his history would further support your potential diagnosis?

A. Allergy to environmental allergens

B. Hepatitis B

C. Human immunodeficiency virus

D. Recent unprotected sexual encounter

E. Streptococcal pharyngitis

69. A 44-year-old woman presents to her primary care physician complaining of rapidly progressing symptoms of xerostomia, keratoconjunctivitis, and bilaterally swollen parotid glands. Past medical history is positive only for rheumatoid arthritis, for which she takes no medication. Laboratory tests are positive for hypergammaglobulinemia. What is the most likely explanation for these findings?

A. Amyloidosis

B. Polymyositis

C. Raynaud's phenomenon

D. Sjögren's syndrome

E. Systemic lupus erythematosus

70. A patient planning on going to Kenya was placed on prophylactic medications prior to his trip, including antimalarial and antiviral treatment. The patient should be informed of what potential side effect/disorder due to the medicinal regimen?

A. Aplastic anemia

B. Folate-deficiency anemia

C. Iron-deficiency anemia

D. Pernicious anemia

E. Sprue

71. A 32-year-old man presents to the emergency department and is diagnosed with a *Diphyllobothrium latum* infestation. What is the main associated abnormality that would be expected in his laboratory results?

A. Abnormal Schilling test

B. Decreased serum ferritin

C. Megaloblastic anemia

D. Polychromatophilia

E. Reticulocytosis

72. A 77-year-old man who is a survivor of World War II was exposed to ionizing radiation and benzene as a serviceman. He complains of weight loss, anorexia, and sweats. Physical examination reveals hepatosplenomegaly. Laboratory studies reveal low levels of neutrophil alkaline phosphatase. A translocation between which chromosomes is probably present within this patient's leukocytes?

A. 9 and 22

B. 8 and 14

C. 15 and 17

D. 14 and 18

E. 14 and 21

73. Alpha thalassemia has varying degrees of expression and penetrance. What is the minimum number of deletions required to produce intrauterine death in a fetus affected with this condition?

A. One

B. Two

C. Three

D. Four

E. Five

74. A 23-year-old man was recently diagnosed with "chronic cold agglutinin disease" and understands the implications of this. He mentions that he was also told of another concomitant disease but cannot recall what it is. You proceed to tell him that he was thinking of:

A. Hydrops fetalis

B. Kernicterus

C. Mycoplasmal pneumonia

D. Raynaud's phenomenon

E. Spherocytosis

75. A 5-year-old boy is admitted to the hospital with a 3-day history of bloody diarrhea, which began hours after a picnic. The patient has been lethargic since and has been unable to eat because of vomiting. Physical examination reveals an ill-appearing child who is difficult to arouse. Vital signs are: temperature 39.2°C (102.2°F), blood pressure 89/74 mm Hg, heart rate 131 bpm, respiratory rate 23/min. Numerous petechiae are noted on his legs. The abdomen is diffusely tender, with decreased bowel sounds. Laboratory studies reveal the following: BUN, 72; creatinine, 8.1; WBCs, 11,000/mm³; Hgb, 5 mg/dL; platelet count, 10,000/mm³; PT, normal; PTT, normal. The peripheral smear demonstrates numerous schistocytes. What is the most likely diagnosis?

A. Crohn's disease

B. Disseminated intravascular coagulopathy

C. Hemolytic uremic syndrome

D. Idiopathic thrombocytopenic purpura

E. Ulcerative colitis

Answer Key

1. C	**20.** D	**39.** C	**58.** C
2. B	**21.** C	**40.** B	**59.** D
3. C	**22.** E	**41.** C	**60.** E
4. D	**23.** E	**42.** C	**61.** C
5. A	**24.** A	**43.** D	**62.** D
6. C	**25.** A	**44.** D	**63.** C
7. D	**26.** E	**45.** B	**64.** D
8. B	**27.** D	**46.** C	**65.** D
9. E	**28.** C	**47.** C	**66.** D
10. A	**29.** A	**48.** C	**67.** A
11. A	**30.** B	**49.** A	**68.** B
12. B	**31.** A	**50.** D	**69.** D
13. A	**32.** A	**51.** D	**70.** A
14. E	**33.** C	**52.** A	**71.** C
15. E	**34.** B	**53.** E	**72.** A
16. A	**35.** B	**54.** D	**73.** D
17. B	**36.** C	**55.** E	**74.** D
18. D	**37.** C	**56.** D	**75.** C
19. A	**38.** A	**57.** D	

Answers and Explanations

1. C. The description of the cells in the pathology report is pathognomonic for Reed-Sternberg cells, which are present in Hodgkin's disease. Be able to identify these cells from a picture and from their description. Because it is a common disease, Hodgkin's lymphoma is a likely test subject on step 1. Patients often complain of night sweats and swollen lymph nodes that have been present for more than a few days. Imaging studies may show a mediastinal mass as well. Auer rods appear as intracytoplasmic rods inside leukocytes and are present in acute myelogenous leukemia. Burr cells are present in some renal diseases. Teardrop cells are present when the bone marrow is fibrotic and is trying to squeeze out cells, as in primary myelofibrosis. Smudge cells are lymphocytes that are easily destroyed when the coverslip is placed over the slide in chronic lymphocytic leukemia. The CT scan reveals enlarged mesenteric, retroperitoneal, and paraortic lymph nodes.

2. B. Hydroxyurea is an agent that increases fetal hemoglobin (HbF) production and slightly raises the total hemoglobin concentration in the body. HbF reduces the chance that RBCs will sickle in a person with sickle cell disease. Increased production of HbF can therefore reduce the occurrence of sickling-related complications. Lamivudine is an antiviral agent; it is not used in the direct treatment of sickle cell disease. Patients with sickle cell disease are susceptible to aplastic crises from viral infections, but it is not known whether lamivudine can prevent this. Dialysis is used in patients who have kidney failure, such as patients with late-stage diabetes. A splenectomy is a curative treatment option for patients with hereditary spherocytosis but not sickle cell disease. Quinidine is an antiarrhythmic drug that has many side effects including hemolytic anemia and agranulocytosis. There are no indications for giving quinidine to this patient. In fact, administering this drug may cause hemolytic anemia, which is one of the undesirable complications of the disease.

3. C. This patient has Goodpasture's syndrome. His symptoms and pathological description are classic for a patient with this disease. Patients with Goodpasture's syndrome are often described as young men in their twenties who present with the chief complaint of hemoptysis and hematuria. Goodpasture's syndrome is characterized as a type II (or cytotoxic) hypersensitivity, in which antibodies are produced against certain cell-surface antigens. Some other examples of type II hypersensitivities are myasthenia gravis and Rh incompatibility. A type I (or anaphylactic) hypersensitivity reaction occurs when antigens cross-link IgE antibodies bound to mast cells or basophils, which leads to the release of histamine or other specific factors that can cause an allergic reaction. The histamine release produces a characteristic wheal and flare around the site of its release. A type III (or immune complex) hypersensitivity reaction occurs when antigen-antibody complexes deposited in tissue cause an inflammatory reaction. Examples of a type III reaction are serum sickness and the Arthus reaction. A type IV (or cell-mediated) hypersensitivity reaction is caused when helper T cells mediate an inflammatory response that occurs hours to days after activation. Examples are purified protein derivative (PPD) testing and a poison ivy reaction. An acute rejection reaction, which occurs when host cells attack a transplanted graft, can be classified as a type IV hypersensitivity reaction because it is often mediated by T lymphocytes (it is cell mediated).

4. D. Prosthetic valves can cause schistocytes to be visualized on peripheral smear secondary to trauma to the red blood cell (RBC) membrane. Idiopathic thrombocytopenic purpura is not associated with RBC abnormalities. However, thrombotic thrombocytopenic purpura and disseminated intravascular coagulopathy are. Hemophilia A will not cause damage to the RBC. Von Willebrand's disease involves poor adhesion of platelets, not RBC destruction. Thalassemia will cause a microcytic anemia with normal-shaped RBCs.

5. A. In addition to having anti-inflammatory, analgesic, and vasodynamic properties, aspirin has the ability to irreversibly inhibit platelets. It does this by inhibiting cyclooxygenase and thromboxane A2. This effect increases the bleeding time, as platelets are needed in forming the platelet plug that is required in the earliest stage of clotting. Hemoglobin and hematocrit are laboratory indicators of the concentration of cells in blood. Hematocrit is the proportion of blood that is occupied by RBCs. These values will not be decreased in acute episodes of bleeding but will be decreased whenever a patient has bled for a significant amount of time and has replaced the blood with fluids. Prothrombin time (PT) is a measure of the extrinsic pathway of the clotting cascade. Factor VII is the factor that influences the extrinsic pathway the most, as it has the shortest half-life of all the clotting factors. PT will be elevated in patients taking warfarin (Coumadin). Partial thromboplastin time (PTT) is a measure of the intrinsic pathway and measures factors such as XII, XI, IX, and VIII. It will be elevated in a patient with a decrease in the intrinsic pathway factors, as in hemophilia A or B (factors VIII and IX, respectively) and also in a patient taking heparin.

6. C. Exercise would be expected to shift the oxygen dissociation curve to the right, unloading oxygen molecules from hemoglobin to the tissues. During exercise, the metabolic needs of skeletal muscle increase significantly and the release of oxygen from hemoglobin helps to meet these needs. Some other factors that cause a shift of the curve to the right are an increase in Pco_2, a decrease in pH, an increase in temperature, an increase in altitude, and an increase in 2,3 DPG. In a leftward shift of the curve, oxygen is bound to hemoglobin without being released to the tissues. This occurs under certain conditions such as a decrease in Pco_2, an increase in pH, a decrease in temperature, and a decrease in 2,3 DPG. Hyperventilation would decrease the partial pressure of carbon dioxide and increase the pH, thus shifting the curve to the left.

7. D. This patient has hereditary spherocytosis, an autosomal dominant hemolytic anemia characterized by sphere-shaped RBCs that are sequestered in the spleen. In addition to ordering a peripheral blood smear to look for spherocytes, an osmotic fragility test with hypotonic saline would cause lysis of erythrocytes in patients with the disease. Coombs' test is used in determining autoimmune hemolytic anemias. Hereditary spherocytosis has a negative Coombs' test. Electrophoresis is an effective test in diagnosing thalassemia and sickle cell anemia. It is not used in making the diagnosis of hereditary spherocytosis. Hamm's test is sometimes used for diagnosing paroxysmal nocturnal hemoglobinuria, a disease that presents with dark urine on awakening. A urine observation test can be used in alkaptonuria. In alkaptonuria, urine turns dark on standing.

8. B. This is an example of a dilutional coagulopathy. Stored blood is deficient in clotting factors V and VIII and the transfusion of a large amount of blood can significantly reduce the concentration of these factors. Factor VIII inhibitors, which are antibodies to factor VIII, can be acquired during life and can cause hemophilia at a late age. In theory, it is possible that an inhibitor could have been present in the transfused blood and could have caused this patient to bleed excessively when cut. Although possible, this is extremely rare and is not likely in this case. Hemophilia A and B are characterized by deficiencies in clotting factories VIII and IX, respectively, and are transmitted as X-linked recessive diseases that would have likely presented at an earlier age. Von Willebrand's disease is characterized by impaired platelet adhesion, prolonged bleeding time, and a deficiency of factor VIII. Patients with Von Willebrand's disease also have an elevated PTT. This man had normal coagulation studies, thus eliminating the possibility of hemophilia or Von Willebrand's disease.

9. E. This patient has Job's syndrome, which is characterized by elevated levels of IgE, repeated staphylococcal abscesses, and eczema. Patients with ataxia-telangiectasia have a defect in DNA repair processes and have symptoms that explain the name of the condition. They have balance problems and telangiectasias on their bodies. Patients with DiGeorge's syndrome have tetany and T-cell immune deficiencies due to failure of development of the third and fourth pharyngeal pouches, which mature into the parathyroid glands and thymus. Patients with Chediak-Higashi syndrome have defective phagocytes due to impaired microtubules, leading to repeated staphylococcal and streptococcal infections. A deficiency of interleukin-2 (IL-2) has been associated with mycobacterial infections that spread throughout the body.

10. A. This patient has chronic myelogenous leukemia, which is characterized by hepatosplenomegaly, leukocytosis, a decreased leukocyte alkaline phosphatase, and an end-stage blastic crisis. The disease presents initially at 40 to 55 years of age. The case vignette depicts several of these disease associations. The Philadelphia chromosome, which is a (9:22) translocation, confirms the diagnosis and is pathognomonic for the disease. An (11:14) translocation is associated with mantle cell lymphoma. An (11:18) lymphoma is associated with marginal zone lymphoma. A (14:18) translocation is associated with follicular lymphoma, and a (14:21) translocation is the robertsonian translocation, which leads to Down's syndrome.

11. A. This patient has an anemia of chronic disease, which is due to a persistent inflammatory state caused by her herniated lumbar disc and chronic back pain. This diagnosis is made by knowing that the TIBC and serum iron are decreased in anemias of chronic disease. This pattern of lab values is unique for anemias of chronic disease. Iron-deficiency anemias, thalassemias, and lead poisoning are all types of microcytic, hypochromic anemias. They have an increased TIBC, a decreased serum iron and an MCV < 80. Megaloblastic anemias are also called macrocytic anemias because they have MCV values > 100. Examples of causes of megaloblastic anemias are vitamin B_{12} and folate deficiencies and medications that block DNA synthesis.

12. B. This is most likely Burkitt's lymphoma, which has been extensively linked to the Epstein-Barr virus. The histological specimen shows a unique pattern where macrophages ingest the tumor cells, producing the "starry sky" appearance. Cytomegalovirus is implicated in causing various systemic diseases in infants and immunocompromised patients. The human immunodeficiency virus (HIV) is linked to AIDS. The human papillomavirus is linked to warts as well as cervical cancer. The human T-cell lymphoma virus (HTLV-1) is linked to a unique T-cell lymphoma.

13. A. Aplastic crises occur most frequently with sickle cell disease and the B19 parvovirus. The B19 parvovirus causes fifth disease, or a "slapped cheek" syndrome that is described in this scenario. The B19 parvovirus has a predilection for bone marrow and has been known to cause aplastic crises in patients with sickle cell disease. Symptoms of aplastic crises are specific to each type of cell that is insufficient. This patient had an infection due to decreased leukocytes and petechiae due to decreased platelets. The other options are all complications of sickle cell disease. Autosplenectomy can occur in patients as a consequence of defective RBCs, which become sickled and occlude the blood supply to the spleen. This process is referred to as a vasoocclusive crisis. Sickle cell patients are also susceptible to hemolytic anemia, as the RBCs are more easily destroyed due to their shape. These patients are also more susceptible to osteomyelitis due to *Salmonella*. The peripheral smear shows many sickle-shaped cells, polychromasia, and target cells.

14. E. Lymphatic vessels (also called lymphatic capillaries) have valves to prevent the retrograde flow of fluid. Arterioles do not have valves, as retrograde flow of blood is prevented via a blood pressure gradient. There are no fenestrations, or small gaps, on lymphatic vessels or arterioles. They are, however, present in capillaries on certain organs such as the liver. Lymphatic vessels are not innervated by any branch of the autonomic nervous system. In contrast, arterioles are innervated mainly by the sympathetic nervous system. The parasympathetic nervous system has a very insignificant role in regulating arteriolar tone. The wall of a lymphatic vessel usually consists of an endothelial lining and a small amount of connective tissue. In contrast, arterioles consist of a single layer of smooth muscle, allowing them to change tone periodically.

15. E. The germinal center of a lymph node has maturing B cells, which will eventually mature to memory B cells and antibody-producing plasma cells. Cells that would degranulate upon IgE exposure are mast cells and are not found in lymph node germinal centers. Polymorphonuclear neutrophils (PMNs) and macrophages phagocytose bacteria use NADPH oxidase. They are not found in significant numbers compared to B cells in lymph node germinal centers. T cells have CD40L on their surfaces and also will bind MHC II on APCs if they are CD4-positive. They are found surrounding the germinal centers.

16. A. This patient likely has disseminated intravascular coagulation (DIC). DIC is associated with laboratory findings of increased PT, increased PTT, increased D-dimer, decreased fibrinogen, increased split products, and usually thrombocytopenia.

17. B. This patient's symptoms and laboratory findings are consistent with iron-deficiency anemia. With his age in mind, gastrointestinal bleeding is most likely and colon cancer most worrisome. Admission to hospital for transfusions is not required for this patient. Iron therapy may be required but colonoscopy should be performed to rule out colon cancer. Dietary changes and folate supplementation should not be considered until colonoscopy is completed.

18. D. Fibrinogen has the greatest effect on the elevation of the ESR, since fibrinogen is the most abundant acute-phase reactant. Albumin is a protein. Ferritin synthesis is controlled by the amount of iron in the body. Transferrin is a transport molecule that is an indicator of iron status in the body. In iron-deficiency states, serum iron and ferritin are low.

19. A. Deep venous thrombus (DVT) without significant risk factors in the elderly should raise concern of a possible malignancy. However, an extensive and expensive workup is not warranted for reasons of cost-effectiveness. Since this patient has an extensive smoking history, a chest film is adequate at this time. MRI examination is not likely to find evidence of a DVT. Upper GI follow-through radiography is unlikely to provide evidence of a DVT. PSA testing is unnecessary in women. This patient must be diagnosed immediately; thus, follow-up examination in 2 weeks is not an appropriate option for this patient.

20. D. Splenectomy is reserved for those who failed to respond to steroids or require high-dose steroids in order to obtain a normal platelet count. For these two scenarios, splenectomy is the most definitive treatment for chronic ITP. This patient was already treated with steroids at a high dose and was tapered. The taper led to worsening of symptoms. Plasma exchange is not an appropriate treatment for this patient. Thymectomy is not an appropriate treatment for this patient.

21. C. Lead affects the brain, peripheral nervous system, bone marrow, and the kidneys. Some general signs of lead poisoning include anorexia, nausea and vomiting, constipation, diarrhea, irritability, ataxia, headaches, abdominal pain, convulsions, and peripheral neuropathy. Cyanosis is not a feature.

22. E. *Streptococcus pneumoniae* is the most common agent, followed by *Haemophilus influenzae*, *Neisseria meningitidis*, and *Pseudomonas*. In this case, the fever might suggest a pulmonary source secondary to AIDS. In considering a fever of unknown origin, one must look at the following sources: respiratory infection, deep venous thrombosis, urinary tract infection, wound infection in postoperative patients, and drug fever.

23. E. During pregnancy, the coagulation factors undergo great change. However, fibrinogen increases by more than 50%. Factors 7, 8, and 10 also increase significantly, but not as much as fibrinogen. Factors 11 and 13 will decrease mildly.

24. A. The patient has microcytic, hypochromic anemia, which is most likely iron-deficiency anemia. In a man of this age, the most likely cause is blood loss from the GI tract, and an evaluation with colonoscopy is mandatory. The rest of the choices provide no useful information. There is no reason to suspect sickle cell anemia in this patient on the basis of clinical presentation and race. This patient is Caucasian and sickle cell anemia typically occurs in African-Americans. Protoporphyrin levels are likely to be normal in this patient. Reticulocyte count may be increased in this patient; however, this will not provide the diagnosis. Vitamin B_{12} levels are likely to be normal in this patient.

25. A. This patient has signs and symptoms consistent with peripheral neuropathy. Given this patient's history, the symptoms are most likely due to alcoholism. Diabetic polyneuropathy is uncommon at the time of diabetes diagnosis. It usually begins with sensory loss in the feet. The patient has no symptoms of hypothyroidism. Tobacco abuse and asbestos exposure are not well-known causes of peripheral neuropathy.

26. E. This patient presents with a constellation of anemia, renal failure, and proteinuria on 24-hr collection but a negative dipstick for protein. Knowing that the dipstick displays only albuminuria and that the 24-hr analysis determines total protein, one can make the diagnosis of multiple myeloma. The head radiograph shows multiple small punched-out osteolytic lesions in the skull. Adrenal insufficiency is associated with hypotension and hypo-aldosteronism, neither of which is present in this patient. In anemia of chronic disease, the peripheral smear will show hypochromic, microcytic anemia. Anemia of chronic renal disease will also show hypochromic, microcytic anemia. Hemolysis will be associated with hyperkalemia and evidence of destruction of RBCs on peripheral smear.

27. D. The bleeding time is a test of platelet–vessel wall interaction. This test involves making a small incision over the forearm and measuring the time to cessation of bleeding. The bleeding time is prolonged in thrombocytopenia, qualitative platelet deficiencies, Von Willebrand's disease, and primary vascular disorders, but not in factor deficiency.

28. C. This patient has a microcytic anemia, most likely iron deficiency secondary to an increased menstrual flow. The history of pica (abnormal cravings for nonfoods or non-nutritive substances), low MCV, low hemoglobin, the patient's age, and an increase in menstrual flow is diagnostic. Hypothyroidism is not correct because the patient denies any symptoms consistent with the diagnosis. Also, the MCV would be normal or increased as hypothyroidism would present as normocytic or macrocytic. Although there is some family history of low blood, the patient's previously normal hemoglobin level rules out any hereditary disorder. Lead poisoning is unlikely in this patient, given her current living situation. No lead lines were noticed and no comment of basophilic stippling was mentioned on the peripheral smear.

29. A. Hemolytic uremic syndrome (HUS) classically presents with a triad of renal failure, anemia, and thrombocytopenia. In terms of laboratory values, one expects to see decreased platelets, schistocytes on peripheral smear, and normal coagulation studies. Disseminated intravascular coagulopathy is consistent with the parameters in choice C. Idiopathic thrombocytopenic purpura is consistent with choice B. Answer choices D and E are not usually encountered clinically.

30. B. Factor V Leiden, a common disorder, is carried by about 15% of Caucasians. Conditions such as protein C and S deficiency and antithrombin III deficiency are much less common, affecting about 0.5% of the population. Affected patients with factor V Leiden mutation usually present with the first thromboembolic event at an age older than 50. Antithrombin deficiency is unlikely to be associated with these findings. Hemophilia B is associated with increase in PTT due to factor IX deficiency. PT, bleeding time, and platelet count will be normal in this situation.

31. A. The ileum plays a critical role in the absorption of vitamin B_{12}. With removal of this patient's ileum, the intrinsic factor–B_{12} complex cannot be absorbed and is lost in the stool. Thus, vitamin B_{12} stores are diminished and clinical deficiency results. A decrease in vitamin B_{12} is a macrocytic anemia, which classically demonstrates hypersegmented neutrophils on blood smear. Since iron is absorbed in the proximal bowel, no iron deficiency would be seen in this patient. Thus, no microcytosis would be identified. Schistocytes are not present in this condition. Spherocytosis is an intrinsic extravascular hemolysis due to a spectrin or ankyrin defect. Coombs' testing is negative in this patient. No laboratory value for platelets is provided in this question; thus, one is not able to suggest the diagnosis of thrombocytosis in this patient. The platelets are likely to be normal in this patient.

32. A. This patient has myelophthisic anemia. The likely etiology is his history of radiation therapy for colon cancer. This can lead to bone marrow fibrosis (replacement of normal cells and disturbance of the blood–bone marrow barrier). Cells released are premature and abnormally shaped. Damage to stem cells occurs with myelodysplastic syndrome. Damage to marrow stem cells occurs with aplastic anemia. There is no evidence by history to suggest either intoxication syndrome or tuberculosis.

33. C. This patient has a history of anorexia nervosa, which can be associated with the presence of a cellular bone marrow with substrate deficiency. Aplastic anemia is associated with a hypocellular bone marrow. Primary myelofibrosis can be associated with myeloid metaplasia. Aplastic anemia is a pancytopenia characterized by anemia, neutropenia, and thrombocytopenia. It can be caused by radiation, benzene, or antibiotics. Bone marrow myelofibrosis can be chronic and progressive. The bone marrow space is infiltrated by fibrosis. The bone marrow will not be hypocellular.

34. B. Although all of the answers are correct in living a healthy and happy lifestyle, maintaining proper fluid hydration is crucial to minimizing recurrence of sickle cell crisis. Sickle cell disease is associated with sickling of the RBCs under oxidative stress. This is associated with sludging in the venous system and development of ulceration and venous stasis changes. Safer sex, daily vitamins, regular exercise, and avoiding tobacco should all be encouraged and will certainly be better for your patient's general health, but again, these are not germane to the prevention of future sickle cell attacks.

35. B. This patient's history is consistent with chronic gastrointestinal bleeding with a coexisting acute process. Patients with acute GI bleeding may have a normocytic anemia because the red cells are produced normally until they are rapidly lost. However, this patient more likely has an anemia that is more chronic in nature and thus microcytic.

36. C. The patient is presenting with signs and symptoms of disseminated intravascular coagulation, a known complication of the M3 (promyelocytic) form of AML. The other forms of AML are associated with different complications, but none has DIC as a likely complication. M1 is associated with chronic myelogenous leukemia and myelofibrosis. M2 is associated with chronic myelogenous leukemia. M4 is associated with chronic myelomonocytic leukemia. M5 is associated with chronic monocytic leukemia.

37. C. Increased TIBC is indicative of an iron-deficiency anemia. Because of the "low" levels of iron present in the body, the iron storage capacity is increased. All of the other answer choices are incorrect in the sense that the choices are presented in the opposite value. Decreased hemoglobin, serum iron, body iron storage, and ferritin are presentations of iron-deficient anemia.

38. A. Myelophthisic anemia is predominantly caused by a replacement of the normal bone marrow by malignant tumor, hence the need to draw labs and order films. Kidney function can affect the production of erythropoietin, but does not play a role in this disease process. The liver and pancreas have vital functions but are not involved in the pathology of this diagnosis. The spleen can destroy RBCs and cause anemia, but again, this is not germane to the indicated illness.

39. C. Folate deficiency is the most probable diagnosis based on the history of alcohol abuse. The yellowish tinge and neutrophils are indicative of a megaloblastic anemia, but the alcohol history narrows it down. Pernicious anemia is related to intrinsic factor deficiency, not alcohol. Aplastic anemia is induced by toxic chemical exposure. Glucose-6 phosphate deficiency has to do with the hexose monophosphate shunt mechanism, and erythroblastosis fetalis is an Rh incompatibility during infancy and would in no way affect a grown man.

40. B. Hodgkin's, non-Hodgkin's, and systemic lupus erythematosus are all primary potential causes of this particular form of anemia. ABO incompatibility is manifest in newborn Rh-positive babies, with Rh-negative mothers, and those with prior blood exposure. Kernicterus is also associated with ABO incompatibility and red cell destruction. Mycoplasmal pneumonia would show as a positive acute "cold agglutinin" disease, whereas Raynaud's would show as a chronic cold agglutinin disease.

41. C. Recent diet would be an appropriate area to investigate, since the presentation seems to be pointing to a deficiency in glucose-6 phosphate dehydrogenase (G6PD). This is an X-linked disorder that occurs in 10% of African Americans. In particular, you would want to ask about the ingestion of fava beans, which are a likely culprit. Mood, vacations, and sexual activity can all play a role in various health changes, but in this scenario, with the lab report, they would all be secondary to changes in diet.

42. C. Decreased erythropoietin is the sole distinguishing factor in polycythemia vera from the rest of the polycythemias. In all of the other polycythemias, there is an increased level of erythropoietin. All of the other characteristics are pertinent to polycythemia vera but do not in any way enable the differentiation of vera from the other forms of the disease.

43. D. This presentation is indicative of infectious mononucleosis, and an area of major concern is that of traumatic splenic rupture secondary to the ensuing hepatosplenomegaly. Elevated creatinine is always an issue of concern with decreasing kidney function but is not a pertinent issue secondary to this diagnosis. Febrile seizures are not associated with this presentation and need to reach temps of > 104°F (40°C). Tongue swallowing is associated, and falsely so, with epilepsy, which is not germane to this case presentation.

44. D. Reed-Sternberg cells, as described above, are thought to be the actual malignant cells of Hodgkin's lymphoma. Beriberi is associated with thiamine deficiency. Kwashiorkor is a protein deficiency related to a starch-laden, protein-deficient diet. Rouleaux are formations associated with the congregation of RBCs in multiple myeloma.

45. B. In the diagnosis of classic hemophilia, factor VII dysfunction is the classical culprit. The degree and severity of the hemophilia are based upon the functional level of factor VII. Factors II, VII, IX, and X are all dependent on vitamin K for their synthesis, but are not all directly associated with the indicated issue of classic hemophilia. Exogenous administration of factor VII would be helpful for this patient.

46. C. Von Willebrand's disease is a deficiency of vWF (von Willebrand factor), which functions as an adjunct to factor VIII and enables platelet adhesion. Coagulation of blood would impede circulation and would be pathological. Aplastic anemia would lead to a failure to produce cells and be indicative of marrow tumor. Sickling of the RBCs would point to sickle cell anemia and has no relation to von Willebrand's disease.

47. C. This child has evidence of orotic acidemia. This condition is caused by an autosomal recessive mutation in the pyrimidine synthesis pathway. The enzyme orotidylic pyrophosphorylase orotidylic decarboxylase is deficient. Glucose phosphatase is unaffected by this condition. Glucose phosphorylase levels as well as those of phosphoribosyl transferase and urease dehydrogenase are normal in this condition.

48. C. Chronic lymphocytic leukemia (CLL) would be the most appropriate diagnosis based on the presentation given. The mechanical breakdown of the cells creates the "smudge cells." Acute lymphoblastic leukemia (ALL) is usually limited to children and would be unusual in a 65-year-old man. Acute myelogenous leukemia (AML) is a non-lymphoblastic leukemia and not indicated by smudge cells. Chronic myelogenous leukemia (CML) is noted by the presence of the Philadelphia chromosome (9:22 translocation); it has a peak incidence in 35- to 50-year-olds.

49. A. The bleeding time cannot be used to reliably identify patients who may have recently ingested aspirin or other nonsteroidal anti-inflammatory drugs (NSAIDs) or who have a platelet defect attributable to these drugs. Thus the patient's bleeding time may be prolonged or normal. Beta-blockers, calcium channel blockers, and NSAIDs can prolong the bleeding time. Furosemide does not prolong bleeding time. Tetracycline has not been shown to have an effect on the bleeding time.

50. D. The most abundant immunoglobulin in plasma is IgG. It is composed of two heavy and two light chains with a total molecular weight of 150,000 daltons. Disulfide bonds are found between the heavy and light chains and also between the heavy chains. IgA, on the other hand, is an immunoglobulin abundant in mucus and milk secretions. IgG is the main antibody in the secondary response. It can fix complement and crosses the placenta. It neutralizes bacterial toxins and viruses.

51. D. A current positive T-cell cross-match indicates the presence of circulating antibodies against class I antigens and the certainty of a hyperacute rejection reaction. This represents an absolute contraindication to transplantation. ABO incompatibility may preclude transplantation, not AB incompatibility. Cold ischemia can last for up to 72 hr. HLA typing with a poor match can still be used for transplantation; however, there may be a higher risk of rejection.

52. A. Lead poisoning is associated with basophilic stippling. Chronic toxicity can lead to peripheral neuropathy. Abdominal pain is an associated finding, as is gingival discoloration. These findings can be confused with mercury poisoning. However, mercury poisoning does not affect the hematopoietic system. Dilantin use is associated with the side effect of gingival hyperplasia. Gastrointestinal complaints are common with many pharmacologic agents. Lead lines are commonly found in bone, not in the eyes.

53. E. The initial step in the pathogenesis of lower leg venous ulceration is a prior history of deep venous thrombosis or varicose veins. This can lead to venous valvular injury, which causes venous reflux and venous hypertension. Capillary pressure increases, which leads to increased endothelial permeability and edema formation. Eventually, dysfunction of the calf muscle pump results, which precedes the final step, formation of the ulcer cavity.

54. D. Varicosity is caused by increased venous pressure, which can be caused by obesity. Anorexia and bulimia are both eating disorders, neither of which is directly related to varicose veins. Termination of pregnancy would have no bearing on this disease, whereas pregnancy is known to increase the risk of developing varicose veins. Daily exercise will actually help to prevent the development of this condition, not cause it.

55. E. This presentation is classic for multiple myeloma. African Americans > 50 years of age are most often affected. Multiple-agent chemotherapy is used to treat this disease, but the prognosis remains poor. Acute lymphocytic leukemia is predominantly a malignancy of childhood and rarely affects adults. Acute myelogenous leukemia affects both children and adults and presents with fatigue, dyspnea, and fever. Chronic lymphocytic leukemia usually strikes adults > 65 years of age and presents with isolated lymphocytosis. Chronic myelogenous leukemia will present with a significantly elevated white blood cell count as well as a blast crisis later in the progression of the disease.

56. D. This baby most likely has been diagnosed with a simple hemangioma. This is usually caused by a malformation of a larger vessel and blood filled channels. Cystic hygroma occurs in the neck and axilla, and does not present with the skin discoloration. A glomangioma or glomus tumor is a painful nodule usually located in the finger or toe. Hemangiopericytomas arise from pericytes and can be either benign or malignant.

57. D. Polyarteritis nodosa is characterized by aneurysmal nodules and has a 25 to 30% association with hepatitis B infection. Findings are usually in the kidney, coronary artery, musculoskeletal system, GI tract, and central nervous system. The majority of deaths are due to renal lesions and hypertension. Kaposi's sarcoma is a malignant vascular disorder often occurring with AIDS. Leukocytoclastic vasculitis is characterized by acute inflammation of arterioles, capillaries, and venules along with palpable purpura on the skin. Wegener's granulomatosis is an inflammatory disease of the respiratory tract and kidneys associated with clinical signs of respiratory distress.

58. C. Palpable nodules along the involved artery would help to support a suspected diagnosis of temporal arteritis. This is a systemic vasculitis that affects the branches of the carotid artery. Diaphoresis is a possible effect but does not serve to solidify this diagnosis. Hemangioma would be more indicative of a blood disorder. Idiopathic pruritus is usually linked with a diagnosis of malignancy. Xerostomia is not related to this case at all.

59. D. Takayasu's arteritis is caused by inflammation and stenotic changes of medium and large-sized arteries, which has a propensity to involve the aortic arch and hence produces the aortic arch syndrome. Glomus tumor is a small purple nodule in a finger or toe and not really relevant to the presentation at hand. Henoch-Schönlein purpura presents as hemorrhagic hives and similar clinical issues. Wegener's granulomatosis is an inflammatory disease of the respiratory tract and kidneys associated with clinical signs of respiratory distress.

60. E. A positive family history in 75% of patients is an accurate predictor of the future development of essential hypertension. Issues such as smoking, obesity, lack of exercise, and African American ethnicity are all known and accepted as being linked with the development of essential hypertension, but none is as strongly linked as a positive reported family history.

61. C. Malignant nephrosclerosis, which is the end product of renal damage, manifests itself as an arteriolar–glomerular capillary rupture, causing the "flea-bitten" kidney appearance. Malignant hypertension occurs in < 5% of hypertensive patients, but in that 5% it has predominance in the young African American population. Coarctation of the aorta, pheochromocytoma, and unilateral renal artery stenosis are all causative agents of secondary hypertension but not necessarily malignant hypertension.

62. D. Thrombotic thrombocytopenic purpura is the best diagnosis for this clinical presentation. Splenomegaly is a differentiating factor between idiopathic thrombocytopenic purpura and thrombotic thrombocytopenic purpura. Associated risk factors include pregnancy, use of oral contraceptives, and HIV infection. G6PD deficiency is identifiable by the presence of Heinz bodies and bite cells. Idiopathic thrombocytopenic purpura is an autoimmune platelet disorder with a female-to-male ratio of 2:1. Polycythemia vera presents with a surge in RBC production. It is more common in men > 60 years of age. Transfusion reaction is caused by blood-product incompatibility and presents with chills, high fever, and hemoglobinuria.

63. C. This patient appears to be suffering from disseminated intravascular coagulation (DIC) secondary to a potentially septic illegal abortion. Elevated fibrin split products, D-dimer, and potentially elevated PT/PTT are expected lab values. Decreased fibrinogen, platelets, and hematocrit would all be in line with this presentation of DIC.

64. D. This patient has multiple myeloma. It is important for all physicians to consider this diagnosis in an elderly patient with back pain, even if he or she reports having some other reason for the pain. Multiple myeloma produces lytic bone lesions, causing pain and increasing the serum calcium level. The diagnosis can be confirmed by finding Bence-Jones proteins, which are immunoglobulin light chains in the urine, by electrophoresis. Patients with multiple myeloma are at increased risk for infection even though their total immunoglobulins are high. This is because multiple myeloma is a monoclonal gammopathy with an abnormal proliferation of plasma cells but a decreased number of the remaining immunoglobulins. Hyperparathyroidism, hypervitaminosis D, and the milk-alkali syndrome are causes of hypercalcemia but are not involved in this patient's condition. Milk-alkali syndrome is found in patients drinking too much milk, a good source of calcium, and taking antacids. Spinal stenosis is another cause of back pain that often arises when walking or exercising, but it is relieved whenever the patient bends forward or sits down to ride an exercise bike. This relief is caused because both of these actions increase the spaces between the vertebrae and decrease pressure on the spinal cord. The blood smear shown indicated rouleaux formation, which is a common finding in multiple myeloma.

65. D. A positive maternal carrier would ensure that any male children would be born as hemophiliacs. Hemophilia is an X-linked recessive disease, and since the father donates only the Y chromosome, his status has no bearing on the hemophilia inheritance of his male offspring. Maternal exposure has not been shown to have any causative effect on development of this hematologic disorder.

66. D. Hemoglobin electrophoresis would be the most effective way of diagnosing sickle cell anemia. A complete blood count would potentially show a normocytic anemia with a high reticulocyte count. A chest x-ray may potentially show widening of the intervertebral spaces in the lumbar spine, which is associated with this disease. CT or MRI would not be diagnostic or cost-effective in this situation. There are no metabolites or abnormalities that would be found in the urine to diagnose sickle cell anemia.

67. A. Hodgkin's lymphoma presents with systemic pruritus and regional adenopathy. Reed-Sternberg cells are also pathognomonic for this type of lymphoma. Human immunodeficiency virus would present with generalized flu-like symptoms and a compromised immune system. Non-Hodgkin's lymphoma presents with painless systemic adenopathy, fever, malaise, night sweats, and fever. Sepsis is usually secondary to an infection that has spread systemically via the blood. There is no relation between sepsis and pruritus. Tertiary syphilis presents with gummas and neurological involvement such as tabes dorsalis and the Argyll-Robertson pupil.

68. B. There is an implication of the hepatitis B antigen in 30% of reported cases of polyarteritis nodosa. This is an immune complex–mediated vasculitis affecting small and medium arteries, with a much higher occurrence in men. Environmental allergens would not cause the symptoms described here, especially fever and hemoptysis. Human immunodeficiency virus is a systemic immunocompromised state and would present as flu-like symptoms. Recent unprotected sex and strep throat can cause generalized malaise but not hemoptysis.

69. D. This patient is exhibiting the "sicca syndrome," which is characterized by dry mouth and dry eyes. Sicca syndrome is directly attributable to Sjögren's syndrome. Her connective tissue disorder, rheumatoid arthritis, as well as the elevation in her serum gamma globulins are also possible features of her disorder. Polymyositis is a chronic inflammatory process involving the proximal muscles of the upper and lower extremities. Raynaud's phenomenon is caused by vasospasm in the small arteries and arterioles and often occurs after chills. Systemic lupus erythematosus is an autoimmune disease marked by joint pain and the pathognomonic malar butterfly rash.

70. A. A potential side effect of antimalarial therapy is aplastic anemia, which occurs with some anti-inflammatory medications. Folate-deficiency anemia usually occurs in one of three ways: dietary imbalance, pregnancy, and intestinal malabsorption. Iron-deficiency anemia is induced by pregnancy, growth, dietary lack, or chronic blood loss. Pernicious anemia is usually caused by type A gastritis, which leads to a marked decrease in the production of intrinsic factor.

71. C. Megaloblastic anemia would be a likely result of *Diphyllobothrium latum* infection and results in B_{12} depletion. An abnormal Schilling test indicates poor B_{12} absorption but is secondary to an intrinsic factor issue. Decreased serum ferritin levels would be indicative of an iron-deficiency anemia, which is not related to this patient's infestation. Polychromatophilia is equivocal to an increased reticulocyte count as well as reticulocytosis, both of which would be in line with a hemolytic anemia.

72. A. Over 75% of the cases of chronic myelogenous leukemia are characterized by a translocation of chromosomes 9 and 22, producing a hybrid gene called the *bcr-abl* gene. This gene causes an overproduction of mature polymorphonuclear leukocytes. The 9:22 translocation is referred to as the Philadelphia chromosome. The 8:14 translocation is implicated in Burkitt's lymphoma. The 15:17 translocation is implicated in the promyelocytic variety of acute myelogenous leukemia. The 14:18 translocation is implicated in mantle cell lymphoma. The 14:21 translocation, also called the robertsonian translocation, is implicated in hereditary Down's syndrome.

73. D. With four deletions, it is accepted that intrauterine death is a likely event. One deletion tends to be without clinical abnormality. Two to three deletions can produce a mild to moderate clinical presentation with thalassemic effects. Zero deletions would have none of the mentioned effects.

74. D. Raynaud's phenomenon is marked by pallor and cyanosis in the fingers and toes secondary to arterial vasospasm. It is commonly seen with scleroderma and systemic lupus erythematosus. Hydrops fetalis and kernicterus are both diseases of childhood and have no association with adult disease processes. Mycoplasmal pneumonia is linked to acute cold agglutinin disease, not chronic. Spherocytosis is a finding in immune hemolytic anemias and has to do with lack of RBC membrane stability.

75. C. This patient has hemolytic uremic syndrome (HUS), which is usually associated with *E. coli* infection and begins with bloody diarrhea and abdominal pain. The classic triad is thrombocytopenia, anemia, and renal failure. Disseminated intravascular coagulopathy (DIC) can be confused with HUS, but coagulation studies are normal with HUS and increased in DIC. Idiopathic thrombocytopenic purpura (ITP) shows isolated thrombocytopenia without anemia or renal failure. Ulcerative colitis and Crohn's disease are not supported by the lab findings or peripheral smear.

Chapter 8   Musculoskeletal System

Questions

1. A 28-year-old woman comes to see her primary care physician with nonspecific complaints of weakness and severe muscle and joint pain. She has no other symptoms and cannot pinpoint the pain. She mentions that she just returned from vacationing in Cancún, where she got sunburned and ate the local food and water. She also describes her numerous adventures, including a parasailing trip, a helicopter ride, and her first scuba diving venture. Physical exam is unremarkable. She is afebrile. What is the most likely diagnosis?

   A. Caisson disease
   B. Disseminated intravascular coagulation
   C. Osteomalacia
   D. Pyogenic osteomyelitis
   E. Scurvy

2. A sexually active 20-year-old college student who is a cross-country runner at a Connecticut college makes an appointment with her primary care physician because of a large skin rash that keeps spreading. She also complains of fatigue, fever, and muscle and joint aches. Physical examination reveals an erythematous rash with central clearing. What is the most likely diagnosis?

   A. Gonococcal septic arthritis
   B. Leptospirosis
   C. Lyme disease
   D. Relapsing fever
   E. Rocky Mountain spotted fever

3. A mother brings her 2-year-old child to the emergency department for evaluation. The boy has had a fever of 101 to 103°F (38.2 to 39.4°C) for 2 days and has been refusing to walk. There is no history of trauma. The child appears ill and exhibits pain with palpation of his left thigh. Lab work reveals a leukocytosis. What is the most likely diagnosis?

   A. Chondrosarcoma
   B. Ewing's sarcoma
   C. Osteochondroma
   D. Osteoclastoma
   E. Osteoid osteoma
   F. Osteomyelitis
   G. Osteosarcoma

4. The first event in osteogenesis is the formation of a stacked cell layer. Osteoid is then secreted by:

   A. Capillaries
   B. Cartilage
   C. Osteoblasts
   D. Osteoclasts
   E. Osteocytes

5. A 33-year-old African American woman presents to her primary care physician with extreme fatigue and a rash on her cheeks. She says that she has had this rash for a while, but she was working outside in her yard all the previous day and the rash suddenly got much worse. Her history reveals a large intake of over-the-counter pain medications for achy joints. She is afebrile. Physical examination reveals ulcers in her mouth, and her legs are edematous. Which test might help with the diagnosis?

   A. ALP-isoenzyme test
   B. Anti-Sm blood test
   C. Direct Coombs' test
   D. Thyroid function test
   E. Uric acid test

6. A 19-year-old female track runner who collapsed during a recent event is brought to the emergency department. Physical examination reveals ketotic breath, bradycardia, and hypotension. There is parotid gland hypertrophy, peripheral edema, dry skin, and decreased muscle mass. Lab findings reveal normochromic normocytic anemia, hypothyroidism, and decreased estrogen. This illness is best characterized by which of the following?

   A. Begins around 13 years of age and mortality is found in industrialized societies
   B. Damage to mammillary bodies and loss of rhythmic eye movements
   C. Equally prevalent in both sexes, prognosis worsens with each episode
   D. Guilt and shame with good response to drug treatment
   E. Most common cause of high use of medical services and commonly presents with headaches or backaches

7. A 34-year-old woman in a monogamous relationship presents to her primary care physician with pain in the joints of her hands, which are stiff in the morning. She also complains of fatigue, malaise, anorexia, and weight loss. She has not been dieting and takes a multivitamin daily. She is febrile and, on physical exam, is found to have subcutaneous nodules. HLA-typing reveals that she is DR4-positive. Figure 8-1 shows an x-ray of her hand. What is the most likely diagnosis?

   A. Gout
   B. Gonococcal arthritis
   C. Hypertrophic osteoarthropathy
   D. Rheumatoid arthritis
   E. Tuberculosis

Figure 8-1

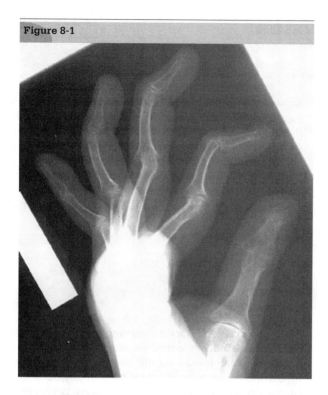

8. A 13-month-old infant is brought to the pediatrician by his parents, who complain that he is not moving around as often and is not as strong as he had been previously. Although he began walking at 10 months, he has not walked now for 2 weeks. Furthermore, he no longer grabs objects well. Physical examination reveals that he cannot stand, although he appears to have large calf muscles. What is the most likely diagnosis?

A. Central core disease

B. Disuse atrophy

C. Duchenne muscular dystrophy

D. Metachromic leukodystrophy

E. Niemann-Pick disease

9. A 35-year-old man presents to clinic with complaints of pain and swelling of his shoulder blade. He first noticed this last month but did not think anything of it at the time. Since then, the swelling has significantly increased in size and become very painful. X-ray reveals the lesion to be lobular, with mottled calcification of the cartilaginous matrix. What is the most likely diagnosis?

A. Chondrosarcoma

B. Ewing's sarcoma

C. Osteoclastoma

D. Osteoid osteoma

E. Osteomyelitis

10. The final number of skeletal muscle fibers is reached before birth. Therefore, growth of the muscle takes place by _____ and increases in muscle length take place by _____ respectively.

A. increases in sarcomere numbers, increases in muscle thickness

B. increases in muscle thickness, increases in sarcomere numbers

C. increases in myoblasts, increases in sarcomere numbers

D. increases in muscle thickness, increases in myoblasts

11. A 45-year-old man presents to his primary care physician with fatigue and occasional blind spells. He states that there are no triggers for his blind spells but that every few days, for a few seconds, everything goes black. His fatigue has been bothering him for several months. An MRI is performed, which reveals a marked density of the skull. What is the most likely diagnosis?

A. Avascular necrosis

B. Osteogenesis imperfecta

C. Osteomalacia

D. Osteopetrosis

E. Rickets

12. A 23-year-old woman who is in graduate school for a master's degree in music presents to the ambulatory care clinic with a tingling numbness in her fingers and difficulty playing the piano. She states that she has been clumsy of late and that she often drops things. When asked how much time she spends practicing the piano, she reports anywhere between 4 and 6 hr a day. She is not pregnant, obese, or diabetic. She has never had this problem before. What test might be done to aid in diagnosis?

A. ACTH stimulation test

B. Bilirubin test

C. Gallium scan

D. Phalen test

E. Toxicology screen

13. A 43-year-old obese Caucasian man complains of difficulty exercising because of pain in his leg. He presents to his primary care physician for evaluation. He also suffers from fatigue. His past medical history reveals kidney stones, which were treated with percutaneous nephrolithotripsy. His wife mentions that he has recently had difficulty hearing. An x-ray of his skull is shown in Figure 8-2. Laboratory studies reveal a serum alkaline phosphatase of 580 IU/L. What is the most likely diagnosis?

Figure 8-2

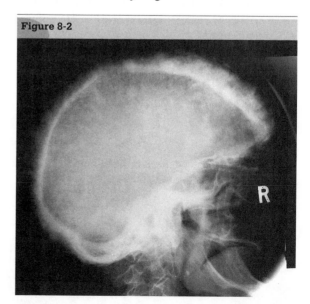

A. Achondroplasia
B. Osteitis fibrosa cystica
C. Osteogenesis imperfecta
D. Osteopetrosis
E. Paget's disease

14. A 25-year-old woman patient presents to the emergency department and is found to have hemarthrosis of the right knee. Physical examination reveals a positive Lachman test. What is her most likely occupation?

A. Body builder
B. Car salesperson
C. Durable goods factory worker
D. Elementary school teacher
E. Loan officer
F. Physician
G. Sign language interpreter
H. Soccer player

15. A 63-year-old woman presents to her primary care physician with stiffness and pain in her neck as well as her hips. She states that she is more tired than usual, explaining that it is worst in the morning and especially after the long train ride to her daughter's house. Physical examination reveals significant pain when her muscles are palpated. What is the most likely diagnosis?

A. Ankylosing spondylitis
B. Dermatomyositis
C. Polymyalgia rheumatica
D. Poliomyositis
E. Sjögren's syndrome
F. Systemic lupus erythematosus

16. A 43-year-old woman presents to her primary care physician with dry eyes and a dry mouth. She also complains of pain in her joints, especially the fingers, which is worst in the morning. She states that her mother and grandmother both had rheumatoid arthritis and tests positive HLA-DR4. What is the most likely diagnosis?

A. Polyarteritis nodosa
B. Poliomyositis
C. Rheumatoid arthritis
D. Sjögren's syndrome
E. Systemic lupus erythematosus

17. A 35-year-old primigravida presents to her primary care physician with generalized tenderness of her muscles. She attributes this pain to her pregnancy, which she also claims is causing her extreme fatigue and restless nights. She gets up in the morning and feels as though she had not gotten any sleep at all. All this sounds a little strange to her physician, as she is only 7 weeks pregnant. She also complains of emotional disturbances and poor memory. Physical exami-

nation reveals significant pain when her muscles are palpated, and her reactions seem wildly out of proportion to the touch. What is the most likely explanation for these findings?

A. Fibromyalgia
B. Hepatitis
C. Hypercalcemia
D. Hypothyroidism
E. Polymyositis

18. A 35-year-old painter presents to his primary care physician complaining of pain in his elbow. Since the weather has finally turned nice enough to paint outdoors, he has been working 85 hr a week, much more than his typical 45-hr workweek. He complains that the outer part of his elbow is painful and tender to the touch. Physical examination reveals that the pain gets worse when the patient extends his wrist against resistance. What is the most likely diagnosis?

A. Acute gout
B. Carpal tunnel syndrome
C. Lateral epicondylitis
D. Medial epicondylitis
E. Tenosynovitis

19. A 23-year-old woman who cleans houses for a living presents to her primary care physician complaining of tenderness in her right knee. The pain is constant and has been present for 3 weeks. She is in a monogamous relationship. Physical examination reveals that her knee is slightly swollen and tender. A synovial aspiration is performed. Neither crystals nor bacteria are found. What is the most likely diagnosis?

A. Bursitis
B. Gonoccocal arthritis
C. Rheumatoid arthritis
D. Septic bursitis
E. Trauma

20. A mother brings her 11-year-old boy to the emergency department. He has been running a fever of 103°F (39.4°C) and has not been feeling like doing anything, not even going outside to play with his buddies. He complains of pain in the area of his tibia but cannot recall any trauma to his shin. A complete blood count reveals an elevated white cell count; the erythrocyte sedimentation rate (ESR) and C-reactive protein are both elevated. X-ray shows tibial bone destruction and soft tissue swelling. What is the most likely diagnosis?

A. Asbestosis
B. Inflammatory arthritis
C. Neuropathic osteoarthropathy
D. Osteomyelitis
E. Stress fracture

21. A 25-year-old man presents to his family physician with joint pain. Physical examination reveals that his knees and wrists are painful to palpation. He also has ulcers in his mouth and on his genitals. His eyes are inflamed and irritated. What is the most likely explanation for these findings?

    A. Behçet's disease

    B. Lyme disease

    C. Multiple sclerosis

    D. Sarcoidosis

    E. Sjögren's syndrome

22. Exercise requiring significant effort, either from high-energy demands (low resistance, rapid contraction rate) or substantial muscle effort (high resistance, low contraction rate) is often associated with muscle pain or discomfort. What is the most likely substance causing a burning sensation in the muscles?

    A. Ammonia

    B. Lactic acid

    C. Low calcium levels

    D. Pyruvic acid

    E. Sodium bicarbonate

23. A 33-year-old professional golfer presents to his primary care physician with elbow pain. He recently spent a lot of time refinishing some old golf clubs, as his busy seasonal tour has just ended. He admits to consuming three glasses of wine daily. Physical examination reveals tenderness over the inner elbow and pain on wrist flexion. What is the most likely diagnosis?

    A. Acute gout

    B. Carpal tunnel syndrome

    C. Lateral epicondylitis

    D. Medial epicondylitis

    E. Tenosynovitis

24. A 55-year-old man presents to the emergency department complaining of severe pain in his left great toe. He admits to having drank himself into a semistupor earlier in the evening, but is relatively coherent in the examining room. He says he has had similar occurrences before, but not quite so painful. Fluid is aspirated from the metatarsophalangeal joint of his great toe; under polarized light, negatively bire-fringent crystals are found. Microscopy is shown in Figure 8-3. What is the most likely explanation for his pain?

    A. Chondrocalcinosis

    B. Lesch-Nyhan syndrome

    C. Primary gout

    D. Pseudogout

    E. Tuberculosis

25. An enzyme deficiency leading to an accumulation of homog-enate that is cleared by the kidneys will result in which of the following patient appearances?

    A. Abnormal dilations of capillary vessels in mucosa, skin, and GI tract

    B. Coarse facies, crouched posture, thick stubby fingers, enlarged tongue, and joint stiffness

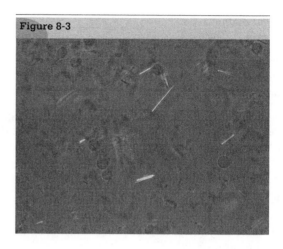
Figure 8-3

    C. Gray-blue cartilage on ear and dark-appearing urine

    D. Doll-like facies, protuberant abdomen, short stature, thin extremities, fat cheeks, poorly developed musculature

    E. Pregnant-looking child who also looks young for age

26. A 22-year-old baseball player presents to the ambulatory care clinic with pain in his knee. He cannot recall any trauma to his knee, but he admits to a possible overuse injury. His knee has been tender for a couple of weeks. He recalls being feverish a few weeks earlier. He admits to having an active sex life and using no protection. Physical examination reveals that his knee is swollen, tender, and warm. Synovial aspiration reveals Gram-negative cocci. What is the most likely diagnosis?

    A. Gonoccocal arthritis

    B. Nonseptic bursitis

    C. Rheumatoid arthritis

    D. Septic bursitis

    E. Staphylococcus aureus–induced bursitis

27. A 29-year-old man presents to his primary care physician with pain in his sacroiliac region. He also has tenderness and swelling in his knees and ankles. His eyes are red, puffy, and irritated. He also complains of burning on urination. A blood test reveals presence of HLA-B27. What is the most likely explanation for these findings?

    A. Fibrosarcoma

    B. Infectious arthritis

    C. Osteoarthritis

    D. Pseudogout

    E. Reiter's syndrome

28. A 45-year-old Filipino man presents to his primary care physician with severe kyphosis, and he appears stiff in his movements. His past medical history is nonrevealing. How-ever, at age 21, he had a positive TB test. He takes a multivi-tamin daily and eats regularly. He wants to know why he is getting shorter. What is the most likely explanation for these findings?

    A. Ankylosing spondyloarthritis

    B. Degenerative joint disease

C. Lyme arthritis

D. Pott's disease

E. Reiter's syndrome

29. A 25-year-old man presents to the emergency department with sudden severe pain and swelling in his left knee. Physical examination of the left knee reveals that it is red, full of effusion, and radiating heat. The joint is aspirated, and basophilic-staining rhomboid crystals are found. What is the most likely diagnosis?

A. Chondrocalcinosis

B. Gout

C. Infectious arthritis

D. Reiter's syndrome

E. Suppurative arthritis

30. A 30-year-old woman makes an appointment with a high-risk obstetrician because she has had four miscarriages in the last 3 years. She claims that she was told by one of her previous doctors that she had a form of arthritis. She also has a visible rash across her face and cheeks. She takes over-the-counter anti-inflammatory medications for her muscle and joint pains. She tests positive to the antinuclear antibody (ANA) test. What is the most likely diagnosis?

A. Discoid lupus

B. Drug-induced lupus

C. Dermatitis

D. Rheumatoid arthritis

E. Systemic lupus

31. A 21-year-old woman is rushed to the emergency department after a car accident. Although she is rattled, she is able to answer questions and describe the incident. She was in the passenger seat, reading, with her knees on the dashboard. On impact, her femur went forward and her tibia was forced into her body. What ligament is most likely torn?

A. Anterior cruciate ligament

B. Lateral collateral ligament

C. Medial collateral ligament

D. Posterior cruciate ligament

E. Posterior tibial ligament

32. A 21-year-old tennis player presents to the clinic with complaints of pain in the lateral aspect of her left elbow. She has been training hard for an upcoming tennis tournament, and other than practicing three times per day, she denies any type of trauma. She rates the pain as a 5 to 6 out of 10 and describes it as a sharp feeling that radiates into her forearm and the back of her wrist. It is generally worse after practice. Physical examination of the heart, lungs, and abdomen is within normal limits. Her musculoskeletal exam is significant for tenderness to palpation of the lateral aspect of her left elbow. No ecchymosis or gross swelling is noted. She has +2 brachial, brachioradialis, and triceps reflexes, and normal strength throughout. The patient is advised to rest the affected joint, use ibuprofen for pain, and ice the affected area frequently. In the office, she receives an injection of a glucocorticoid using a small-gauge needle. How do glucocorticoids help to alleviate this condition?

A. These drugs are reversible inhibitors of the cyclooxygenases and thus inhibit the synthesis of prostaglandins but not that of leukotrienes.

B. They irreversibly block the conversion of arachidonic acid into PGG2, thereby reducing the inflammatory effect.

C. They enter cells via active transport, bind to dihydrofolate reductase, and inhibit the enzyme. Glucocorticoids therefore block folate reduction, which is necessary for cell function.

D. They increase the concentration of neutrophils while decreasing the concentration of lymphocytes, basophils, eosinophils, and monocytes. They also reduce the amount of histamine released from basophils and inhibit the activity of kinins. They also block the conversion of phospholipid into arachidonic acid, thereby reducing both leukotriene and prostaglandin production.

E. They inhibit prostaglandin synthesis in the CNS and thus have antipyretic and analgesic properties.

33. A 41-year-old woman presents with erythema on the extensor surfaces of her extremity joints (see Figure 8-4). She also complains of weakness in her upper extremity. She is positive for the anti-Jo-1 antibody test. What is the most likely diagnosis?

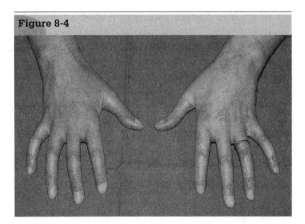

Figure 8-4

A. Dermatomyositis

B. Polyarteritis nodosa

C. Poliomyositis

D. Sjögren's syndrome

E. Systemic lupus erythematosus

34. An 88-year-old woman presents to the emergency department after falling in her bathroom. She is in pain and is having difficulty ambulating. Her prior medical history is notable for hypertension and osteoporosis. She takes a bisphosphonate once a week for this condition. Physical examination of the heart, lungs, and abdomen is normal. However, a thorough musculoskeletal exam reveals an apparently shortened and externally rotated left leg. This clinical presentation and x-ray of the affected leg would most likely reveal a fracture of which part of the femur?

A. Greater trochanter

B. Lateral epicondyle

C. Medial epicondyle

D. Metaphysis

E. Neck

35. An 8-year-old boy is brought to the emergency department after falling on his right arm while sliding into home base in his Little League baseball game. He is experiencing some pain with obvious swelling and bruising in the area of the injury. Physical examination reveals that he cannot move his arm without discomfort. He is sent for an x-ray, which shows a distal spiral fracture of the right humerus. Given this information, what type of bone would one initially find at the fracture site in the early stages of the healing process?

    A. Cancellous
    B. Compact
    C. Spongy
    D. Trabecular
    E. Woven

36. A 28-year-old man is brought to the emergency department after a head-on collision in which he was the unrestrained driver of an SUV. His airway was open and his O_2 saturation was 95% on room air. His heart rate was 88 bpm and blood pressure 142/84 mm Hg. Physical examination reveals periorbital ecchymosis and otorrhea; heart, lung, neurological, and abdominal examinations were all within normal limits. X-rays of the cervical spine showed no gross deformity or fracture. The patient began to complain of a persistent clear nasal discharge. He was then sent for a CT scan, which revealed a basilar skull fracture with extension into the cribriform plate. Which cranial nerve is most likely to be injured?

    A. Cranial nerve I
    B. Cranial nerve III
    C. Cranial nerve VII
    D. Cranial nerve X
    E. Cranial nerve XII

37. A 36-year-old white woman presents to her primary care physician with a 2-week history of blurry vision and fatigue that is generally worse at the end of the day. She works as a third-grade teacher and is generally fine at work. However, when she arrives at home and is attempting to do chores or watch television, her vision becomes blurry. Also, depending on the activity, she has been fatiguing easily. For instance, she was jogging the previous day and had to cut her workout short because she just could not run anymore. Physical examination of the heart, lungs, and abdomen is within normal limits. Her neurological exam is significant only for a positive curtain sign; reflexes and muscle strength are normal. Given the patient's symptoms, the physician suspects a certain diagnosis and performs an edrophonium test, which results in resolution of the positive curtain sign. What is the process by which this disease causes fatigability and weakness?

    A. Obviously, based on the clinical findings and test results, the condition is drug-induced.
    B. This condition is caused by an autoimmune process in which the TSH receptor of the thyroid gland is overstimulated by an autoantibody. This overstimulation results in excess thyroid hormone production, thyroid cell growth, and ultimately fatigue and weakness.
    C. This disease is a result of autoantibodies against P/Q type calcium channels at the motor nerve terminals.

    D. This disease is acquired through the ingestion of a toxin, which binds to presynaptic nerve cells and prevents the release of neurotransmitters.
    E. This disease is an acquired autoimmune process in which the body produces antibodies to acetylcholine receptors. These antibodies reduce the number of available ACh receptors available at any neuromuscular junction, which leads to fatigue and weakness.

38. A 42-year-old woman presents to her primary care physician with the complaint of rubbery legs. She first noticed this weird feeling 2 days earlier at work, when she almost fell while filing some papers. Since then, she has also been experiencing tingling dysesthesias in her feet and legs. All in all, she just feels weak. She denies any trauma or back pain and has never had a feeling like this before. She did mention that she had an upper respiratory infection approximately 3 weeks earlier, but it resolved on its own. She denies any bladder or bowel dysfunction. Physical examination reveals that vital signs are stable and her heart, lung, and abdominal exams are all within normal limits. Her lower extremity deep tendon reflexes are absent, and upper extremity reflexes are +1. Strength is greatly diminished throughout, but more so in the lower extremities. A lumbar puncture is preformed and reveals an elevated protein level of 850 mg/dL. What is the most likely diagnosis?

    A. Botulism
    B. Charcot-Marie-Tooth disease
    C. Guillain-Barré syndrome
    D. HIV Infection
    E. Multiple sclerosis

39. A 12-year-old boy is brought to the pediatrician with complaints of pain in his right leg, which began 4 weeks earlier. The pain is localized to the lower anterior aspect of his right thigh. It is a constant pain that does not radiate anywhere and is generally worse at night. Use typically aggravates the pain, and ibuprofen provides some relief. He is very active and participates in football, baseball, and basketball. However, he denies any history of trauma. Physical examination of the heart, lung, and abdomen is within normal limits. On examining the affected thigh, there is localized tenderness with palpation, but no erythema or swelling is noted. There is some mild atrophy of the affected thigh. An x-ray of the femur reveals a radiolucent nidus with surrounding reactive, sclerotic bone. What is the most likely diagnosis?

    A. Ewing's sarcoma
    B. Osteoclastoma
    C. Osteosarcoma
    D. Osteoid osteoma
    E. Stress fracture

40. A 14-year-old boy presents to the pediatric clinic for a sports participation physical. He has no health issues to date, has met all developmental milestones on time, and is up to date on all of his vaccinations. Review of systems was negative. Physical examinations of the heart, lungs, and abdomen as well as neurological exams were all within normal limits. It is noted that the patient's right shoulder is slightly higher than and posterior to the left. What would be the next step in the evaluation of this patient?

A. Adam's test

B. Lachman's test

C. McMurray's test

D. Radiographs

E. Straight-leg-raising test

41. A healthy 30-year-old G1P0 presents to labor and delivery with contractions every 2 min and gives birth to a 6 lb 9 oz baby girl shortly thereafter. The infant's Apgar scores at 1 and 5 min are 7 and 9, respectively. Physical examination reveals that the child's limbs are very short, especially the proximal portions. The trunk appears normal but has an exaggerated lumbar lordosis. What is the most common genetic mutation or anomaly responsible for this condition?

A. A single DNA base change leads to an amino acid substitution of valine for glutamine in the sixth position on the beta-globin chain.

B. An arginine is substituted for glycine in the transmembrane domain of fibroblast growth factor receptor 3 (FGFR3), which results in a gain-of-function and abnormal proliferation at the growth plate.

C. The condition represents a phenotypic spectrum of disorders caused by activating mutation in the GNAS1 gene, which encodes the $G_{s\alpha}$ protein.

D. The patient's genotype is most likely 45,XO.

E. The patient's genotype is most likely 47,XXY.

42. A 50-year-old man presents to his primary care physician with complaints of intermittent fever, muscle soreness, headaches, and malaise for the preceding month or so. Also, he claims to have lost about 15 lb over the past month and recently noticed painful red bumps on his shins. He finally decided to see a doctor when he noticed blood in his urine three days earlier. His only medications are a daily multivitamin and an 81-mg aspirin tablet. His vital signs are as follows: blood pressure 150/96 mm Hg, pulse 80 bpm, respiratory rate of 16/min, and temperature (oral) 99.1°F (37.2°C). The remainder of the physical examination is within normal limits. Urinalysis reveals 2+ protein and 2+ blood. Blood testing reveals leukocytosis, an elevated ESR, mild anemia, and positive p-ANCA titers. Renal angiography is then performed and reveals aneurysms, stenotic segments, and obliteration of vessels in both kidneys. What is the most likely diagnosis?

A. Buerger's disease

B. Kawasaki disease

C. Polyarteritis nodosa

D. Takayasu's arteritis

E. Wegener's granulomatosis

43. A 48-year-old woman presents to the clinic with complaints of low back pain. While walking her dog 2 days earlier, she became tangled in the leash and fell on her behind. Since then, her low back pain has gotten progressively worse. She is premenopausal and has a long-standing history of a seizure disorder, for which she takes phenytoin. She also takes Lasix and a beta-blocker for hypertension, metformin for diabetes mellitus type II, simvastatin for hyperlipidemia, and rofecoxib for occasional joint pain. She also takes a daily

multivitamin and uses antacids for heartburn. She exercises three times a week by walking and eats a healthy diet. All physical exam findings are normal except for localized tenderness with palpation at the T12-L1 levels. X-rays of the area are taken and show osteopenia with compression fractures at those levels. What is the most likely explanation for this patient's osteopenia?

A. Low estrogen state

B. Malnutrition

C. Metformin

D. Phenytoin

E. Renal osteodystrophy

F. Rofecoxib

G. Simvastatin

44. A 55-year-old woman presents to the emergency department with a sudden onset of severe lower back pain. She says that the pain began when she picked up a box while she was helping her daughter to move. She states that she takes a multivitamin daily and supplements that with combined calcium/vitamin D tablets. She exercises regularly and has never had any health problems. An x-ray of her spine reveals widespread radiolucency. She agrees to have her blood drawn for lab tests and is found to have high serum calcium, low phosphorus, and high alkaline phosphatase. What is the most likely diagnosis?

A. Osteitis fibrosa cystica

B. Osteomalacia

C. Paget's disease

D. Rickets

E. Scurvy

45. A 56-year-old woman presents to her primary care physician with a 1-month history of pain and stiffness in the shoulder and hip areas. She has recently been experiencing intermittent low-grade fevers, malaise, and a 5-lb weight loss. She denies any headaches or changes in appetite. She reports having trouble combing her hair in the morning because of her shoulder pain. She denies any recent trauma. She has been fairly healthy and takes only a daily multivitamin. Physical examination is normal. Laboratory studies reveal an elevated ESR, an elevated C-reactive protein, and a mild normochromic, normocytic anemia. What is the most likely diagnosis?

A. Behçet's syndrome

B. Buerger's disease

C. Polyarteritis nodosa

D. Polymyalgia rheumatica

E. Takayasu's arteritis

F. Temporal arteritis

G. Wegener's granulomatosis

46. A 43-year-old woman who runs marathons has had a painful right ankle on and off for 7 months and acute left knee pain for 4 days. She has a positive family history of skin disorders. Examination of the scalp reveals dry, white, scaly skin. Laboratory studies show an increased white blood cell count and mildly increased sedimentation rate. What pathologic features are seen in this disease?

    A. Complication of infectious invasion, which forms abscesses in soft tissue

    B. Early lymphocytic infiltrate of synovium, onionskin arteritis, and accompanying myocarditis, which may progress to severe damage of joints

    C. Synovial fluid containing neutrophilic infiltrate and macrophage phagocytosis of crystals

    D. Thickening of the epidermis, bleeding occurring when scraped, and bright pink, scaly, new eruptions after trauma

47. A 65-year-old man presents to clinic with complaints of fatigue, bone pain, especially of the lower back, and intermittent dizziness. His symptoms have gotten progressively worse over the course of a month. He has also had an upper respiratory infection that has been intermittent over the same time period. Physical examination of the heart, lungs, and abdomen is normal. Pain is elicited with palpation of the lower back. He appears pale, and some soft tissue masses are noted in his quadriceps bilaterally. Laboratory studies show anemia with marked rouleau formation of the red blood cells. A monoclonal spike is visible in the beta globulin region of a protein electrophoresis study. What is the most likely diagnosis?

    A. Metastatic bone disease

    B. Multiple myeloma

    C. Osteoporosis

    D. Osteosarcoma

    E. Paget's disease

    F. Stress fracture of the vertebrae

48. A morbidly obese 41-year-old man who lives a sedentary lifestyle complains of debilitating knee joint pain. He presents to his primary care physician for evaluation. He is not sexually active, does not use illicit drugs, and rarely leaves the house. A picture of this patient's hands is shown in Figure 8-5. What is the most likely finding on aspiration of the affected joint?

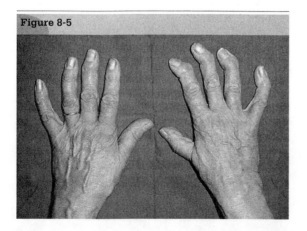

Figure 8-5

A. Anti IgG antibody

B. Antistreptolysin O, anti-DNase, and antihyaluronidase Abs

C. Extrusion of wear particles into synovial fluid

D. Gram-negative rods, oxidase-positive

E. Presence of IgM antibodies

49. A 52-year-old man presents to the primary care clinic with complaints of morning stiffness that lasts approximately 15 min. He has also been experiencing knee pain that is made worse with use, as in walking. Examination reveals coarse crepitus of the knee joint. Radiographs show a narrowing of the joint space of the knee with osteophyte formation. What is the most likely diagnosis?

    A. Ankle sprain

    B. Ankylosing spondylitis

    C. Charcot joint

    D. Osteoarthritis

    E. Reiter's syndrome

50. A 23-year-old man presents to the emergency department with complaints of a fever, right knee pain, and conjunctivitis. He was recently treated for a chlamydial infection. What is the most likely diagnosis?

    A. Ankylosing spondylitis

    B. Charcot joint

    C. Osteoarthritis

    D. Reiter's syndrome

    E. Rheumatoid arthritis

51. A 12-year-old boy presents to the emergency department with complaints of left thigh pain. He is very active in sports but denies any recent trauma. There is no obvious bruising or swelling. He is sent for radiographs of the affected area, which show an onion peel periosteal reaction accompanied by a soft tissue mass. What is the most likely diagnosis?

    A. Chondrosarcoma

    B. Ewing's sarcoma

    C. Osteochondroma

    D. Osteoclastoma

    E. Osteoid osteoma

52. A 70-year-old woman presents to the clinic for evaluation of persistent back pain, difficulty moving, and mild depression. She fractured a vertebra while sick with a severe cough and cold. What would be the best overall preventive measure for this patient?

    A. Abstaining from alcohol

    B. Eating broccoli and kale

    C. Estrogen replacement

    D. Installing railings on both sides of the stairs

    E. Swimming regularly

53. A female patient with 10-year history of rheumatoid arthritis says, "My family doesn't understand how painful some days can be. They think I'm faking this just to get attention. I'm tired all the time and can't even get out of bed sometimes because I'm in so much pain. Why is this happening to me?" Your best response is:

A. Have your family come speak to me about your illness.

B. Rheumatoid arthritis is a challenging chronic disease and you cannot let it interfere with things you need to do. You need to keep pushing yourself a little more.

C. We probably should increase the dosage for your pain medications.

D. Your disease will never go away.

54. A 13-year-old girl recently diagnosed with scoliosis has been given a thoracolumbosacral orthosis to prevent the curve from progressing. Compliance is best achieved by which of the following?

A. Counseling

B. Prohibiting exercise while wearing the brace

C. Reprimand

D. Switching to the cervicothoracolumbosacral orthosis (Milwaukee brace)

E. The mother's neutral attitude

55. A 7-year-old child presents to her primary care physician with a distal forearm fracture but does not remember any traumatic event that might have caused it. Past medical history indicates 10 previous fractured bones. In addition, she is shorter than expected for her age. What is the most likely diagnosis?

A. Achondroplasia

B. Osteitis fibrosa cystica

C. Osteitis deformans

D. Osteogenesis imperfecta

E. Osteopetrosis

56. A 43-year-old man who is a chronic alcoholic presents to the emergency department after another drinking binge. He also has a history of HIV, hepatitis C, and recurrent pneumonia. Physical examination reveals wheezes in both lung bases. The remainder of the physical examination is within normal limits. His underlying condition (alcoholism) may be characterized by

A. Decreased tolerance for alcohol

B. Collapse of bone due to loss of blood supply

C. Hypochromic microcytic anemia

D. Recurrent sinopulmonary infections

57. A 71-year-old man who had a lacunar infarct is returned home after a short stay in a rehabilitation unit to regain his strength. He is able to ambulate at 60% of his prior baseline. His speech and language are within normal limits. He plans to begin an exercise program so that he can try to return to a more normal lifestyle. Which of the following activities will put him at greatest risk for injury?

A. Cycling on a daily basis

B. Daily long brisk walks

C. Shoveling snow

D. Walking near a roadway

E. Yoga

58. A 17-year-old boy with Down's syndrome has graduated from his special-needs school and is being introduced to more mainstream activities. He has intelligible speech and language. His motor defects are minimal. He has been warned to be careful in engaging in physical activity because of

A. Bronchoconstriction

B. Improved cardiac function and decreased risk of obesity

C. Increased susceptibility to falls

D. Joint instability

E. Shortness of breath, increased coughing

59. A 26-year-old man presents to his primary care physician for evaluation. Physical examination reveals a positive chair-raise test. Wrist extension or supination against resistance provokes symptoms similar to the patient's complaints. Passive flexion of the fingers causes pain. X-ray studies reveal calcification in the degenerated tissue of the extensor carpi radialis muscle. What is the most likely profession of this patient?

A. Body builder

B. Car salesman

C. Durable goods factory worker

D. Elementary school teacher

E. Loan officer

F. Physician

G. Sign language interpreter

H. Soccer player

I. Tennis player

J. Violinist

60. An 82-year-old man presents to his primary care physician because of nonspecific back pain. Physical examination reveals severe kyphosis and a bone density scan uncovers a loss in bone mass. An x-ray reveals a compression fracture of L4. Laboratory levels of serum calcium, phosphorus, alkaline phosphatase, parathyroid hormone, and potassium are all within the normal ranges. What is the most likely diagnosis?

A. Osteitis deformans

B. Osteitis fibrosa cystica

C. Osteomyelitis (pyogenic type)

D. Osteoporosis

E. Scurvy

61. A 14-year-old child of divorced parents who is active in cheerleading and is president of her class appears malnourished during a physical examination at school. Her working mother gets home late in the evening but does not know of any eating problems that her child might be having. She feels that her daughter does spend a lot of time exercising. What is a likely finding on physical examination and laboratory analysis of this patient?

A. Bradycardia and hypothermia

B. Hyperalbuminemia and hypocholesterolemia

C. Hyperkalemia

D. High gonadotropin levels

E. Hypertension

62. A 37-year-old man with full-blown AIDS and Kaposi's sarcoma presents to his primary care physician for a follow-up examination. Which of the following is the main cytokine to be involved in the pathogenesis of this patient's problem?

A. Gamma interferon

B. IL-1

C. IL-2

D. IL-3

E. IL-4

F. IL-5

G. Tumor necrosis factor alpha

63. A wife brings her 57-year-old husband to his primary care physician. He has difficulty standing up and slurs his speech. He had worked as a truck driver but was fired after a drug screening found his alcohol level to be above the legal limit. During your interview of the patient, you obtain a history of progressively worsening hip pain, which now persists at rest. What is the most likely explanation for these findings?

A. Type I hyperlipoproteinemia

B. Type II hyperbetalipoproteinemia

C. Type III familial broad beta disease

D. Type IV hypertriglyceridimia, hyperbetalipoproteinemia

E. Type V mixed hyperlipidemia

64. Muscles contract by shortening each sarcomere. The sliding-filament model of muscle contraction has thin filaments on each side of the sarcomere sliding past each other until they meet in the middle. The myosin heads swivel toward the center of the sarcomere, detach, and then reattach to the nearest active site of the actin filament. The energy for this muscle contraction comes from _____, and _____ is required for each cycle of myosin-actin interaction.

A. ATP, potassium

B. ATP, sodium

C. ATP, calcium

D. ADP, potassium

E. ADP, calcium

65. A 58-year-old obese woman with type II diabetes and gout has severe pain in her left knee, which becomes sore after use. Physical examination reveals warm, erythematous, and tender swelling of the knee. The most effective form of primary prevention of this disease is which of the following?

A. Aggressive treatment of type II diabetes

B. Environmentally based strategy that addresses societal contributors

C. Follow-up of obese children annually

D. Providing access to physical activity

E. Reduction of alcohol consumption

66. A 54-year-old man presents to his primary care physician with back pain and stiffness that has lasted for 4 months (see Figure 8-6). He complains that he is stiff in the morning, but after a hot shower, this stiffness usually subsides. He also complains of muscle spasms that occur randomly but often at night. He has not had a sound night's sleep for several weeks. Genetic testing reveals that he is positive for HLA-B27. What is the most likely diagnosis?

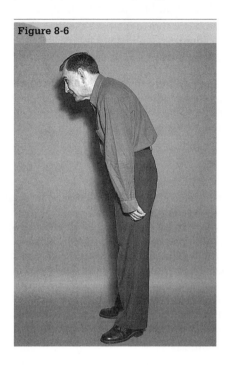

Figure 8-6

A. Ankylosing spondylitis

B. Dermatomyositis

C. Polymyalgia rheumatica

D. Polymyositis

E. Systemic lupus erythematosus

F. Tuberculosis

G. Tularemia

67. A 59-year-old obese woman who is a type II diabetic presents to her primary care physician for a follow-up examination. She is concerned about the possibility of lower extremity vascular disease because her sister, a type I diabetic, just underwent surgery for a left below-knee amputation. Which of the following statements of primary prevention should be made to this patient at this time?

A. Don't change your shoes or you may get blisters.

B. I need to check your finger for oxygen saturation.

C. Look at your feet once a week and use a mirror to look at the bottoms.

D. Shape your toenails so that they are pointed.

E. Wash your feet with warm water and soap. Pat gently to dry.

68. A 50-year-old tennis player, who has had meniscal surgery on his right knee presents to his primary care physician with a 6-month history of pain in the knee that has gradually increased, limiting his mobility and decreasing range of motion. Aspirin does not relieve his pain. What process is involved in this patient's pain?

A. Bacterial proliferation causing an acute inflammatory response and ensuing cell death

B. Cells dissecting along the length of trabeculae with a concurrent increase in anabolic cell activity

C. Hematoma-filled gap stimulates anabolic and catabolic processes, providing a foundation for future remodeling

D. Round to oval gritty tan hemorrhagic tissue, well-defined margins, and small, round, lucent area that may be mineralized

E. Slow deposition of new bone through resorption of necrotic tissue, resulting in collapse

69. A retired 74-year-old man of Swedish descent who has diabetes has noticed, over the past year, that his fingers are slowly bending. They became painful only recently. There are no clicking noises. He can no longer hold a coffee mug or throw a baseball. What are the physical examination findings and/or characteristics of this man's problem?

A. Cyanotic, ischemic fingers from vascular spasms, more common in colder climates and in women than men. *Raynaud's*

B. Finger is flexed and cannot be extended, but when pulled hard it extends and then cannot be flexed. *Trigger finger*

C. Nerve entrapment, causing tingling and inability to make a fist. Hurts when wrist is flexed. *Tinel test*

D. Palmar nodule, flexion contracture of ring finger, cannot extend, more difficult to control if concurrent systemic disease present, such as HIV, alcoholism, or diabetes.

E. Symmetrical involvement of MCP and PIP joints, nodules over bony prominences. *RA*

70. A 72-year-old man who is a retired foundry worker presents to his primary care physician with painless hard nodules on his left palm that have grown over the past year. Physical examination reveals that there are no distinct borders. Palm lines appear thickened and the patient cannot extend his fourth and fifth fingers. Which of the following is most closely associated with this disorder?

A. Glycosaminoglycan deposition on the palmar fascia

B. Increased expression of IL-6 and TNF-α

C. Myxoid stroma with lymphocytes, red blood cells, and random spindle cells expressing lots of mitotic figures; no recurrence after treatment

D. Stellate fibroblasts

71. Prior to injuring his hip, a 53-year-old man had been experiencing headache and pain in the back and hips. Physical examination reveals decreased hearing and abnormal-looking tibias. Laboratory studies reveal an elevated alkaline phosphatase. Which of the following appropriately characterizes this disease?

A. At high risk of a pleomorphic spindle cell disorder that destroys bone cortex *osteosarcoma*

B. Failure of osteoclasts to resorb bone, islands of calcified cartilage within mature bone marrow *osteopetrosis*

C. Musculoskeletal radiographic findings of undermineralized bone *osteomalacia*

D. IL-1 and IL-6 activation of osteoclasts, blue droplets in the cytoplasm of cells *multiple myeloma*

E. Result of a prolonged negative calcium balance due to alcoholism, decreased gonadal function, or prolonged heparin therapy *osteoporosis*

72. A 46-year-old man undergoes an x-ray of his painful hip, which shows small, irregular bony outgrowths from the edges of the joint. What other findings may be present with this disease?

A. Abnormal curvature of the spine and a previous hand fracture *osteoporosis*

B. An acutely hot, tender, inflamed metatarsophalangeal joint; severe back pain *Gout*

C. Fibroblast-like synovial cells produce enzymes that degrade bone; anti-IgG Ab; stiff, weak, painful muscles *RA*

D. High serum calcium, which may result in confusion and lethargy; renal disease

E. Metastatic osteoblastic disease due to hematogenous spread *Prostate CA*

F. Overweight, difficulty walking, swollen, tender nodes on fingers

73. A 64-year-old man with poorly controlled non-insulin-dependent diabetes mellitus was experiencing renal failure and was put on dialysis a year earlier. He presents to his primary care physician with bilateral ankle, foot, and elbow pain that he has had for a month and which has not subsided. Which of the following findings is present?

A. Aluminum interfering with calcium deposition, amyloid deposits in bone

B. Chief cell hyperplasia in a multinodular pattern with mobilization of calcium salts *Primary hyperparathyroidism*

C. Deficiency of G protein, leading to diminished cAMP response

D. Increased presence of IL-2, IL-5, and gamma interferon *involved in infection*

E. Hormone-related peptide secretion

74. A 13-year-old boy who plays basketball on the junior high school team presents to his primary care physician with a history of a dislocated lens, scoliosis, and a valvular disorder; he also complains of shortness of breath and tiredness. This patient, with a family history of the disease, may:

A. Be treated with steroids and sex hormones, inducing precocious puberty

B. Be treated with testosterone injections

C. Have difficulty with wound healing and be at increased risk for joint dislocation

D. Have unusually large calves

E. Have self-inflicted injuries and engage in self-biting

75. Osteogenesis imperfecta is a disorder characterized by multiple fractures occurring with little trauma. It is also called brittle-bone disease and may be confused with child abuse. Sometimes fractures occur during the birth process. The most common form is autosomal dominant with an abnormal synthesis of which type of collagen?

A. Type I

B. Type II

C. Type III

D. Type IV

E. Type V

Answer Key

1. A	20. D	39. D	58. D
2. C	21. A	40. A	59. I
3. F	22. B	41. B	60. D
4. C	23. E	42. C	61. A
5. B	24. C	43. D	62. G
6. A	25. C	44. A	63. D
7. D	26. A	45. D	64. C
8. C	27. E	46. D	65. D
9. A	28. D	47. B	66. A
10. B	29. A	48. C	67. C
11. D	30. E	49. D	68. E
12. D	31. D	50. D	69. D
13. E	32. D	51. B	70. A
14. H	33. A	52. B	71. A
15. C	34. E	53. B	72. F
16. D	35. E	54. A	73. A
17. A	36. A	55. D	74. C
18. C	37. E	56. B	75. A
19. A	38. C	57. C	

Answers and Explanations

1. A. Caisson disease (also known as dysbaric osteonecrosis or compressed-air illness) is a decompression sickness that occurs on exposure to high-pressure environments. When one is exposed to increased air pressure, the blood and other tissues (especially fat) become supersaturated with nitrogen. If the air pressure is reduced too quickly, the nitrogen is released as bubbles, which cause local tissue damage and generalized embolic phenomena. This is apt to be followed by disagreeable and even dangerous physiological effects. The symptoms may include pain in the muscles and joints ("the bends"), deafness, labored breathing, vomiting, paralysis (diver's palsy), fainting, and sometimes even sudden death. This patient does not have the classic findings of disseminated intravascular coagulopathy, as shown clinically and by the lack of abnormal laboratory blood findings. Osteomalacia is vitamin D deficiency in adults. Bone scan and CT scan findings do indicate pyogenic osteomyelitis. Scurvy is a deficiency of vitamin C. This vitamin is necessary for hydroxylation of proline and lysine in collagen synthesis.

2. C. *Borrelia burgdorferi,* a spirochete, is the causative agent of Lyme disease, the most common tick-borne disease in the United States. Transmission is via the bite of an infected deer tick, usually in the northeastern United States. Contact with the tick usually occurs in areas of brush and tall grass, a likely exposure for a cross-country runner from Connecticut (the disease is named after the town of Lyme, CT). The disease is usually recognized by a distinctive skin lesion, erythema migrans, and may be accompanied by headache, stiff neck, myalgias, arthralgias, fatigue, and possible swelling of the lymph nodes. No sexual history that would suggest the presence of gonococcal arthritis is given. There is no travel history consistent with Rocky Mountain spotted fever. In this situation, the rash is located on the palms of the hands and soles of the feet.

3. F. Osteomyelitis is an acute bacterial infection of bone. In children, the spread is hematogenous, the source of bacteremia is often inapparent, and the long bones are most often affected. On presentation, the child usually appears ill, with a high fever, chills, localized pain and tenderness, and leukocytosis. Radiographs often show nothing in the acute phase of the infection; however, a periosteal reaction will be apparent approximately 10 days after the infection. Lytic changes can be detected after 2 to 6 weeks. Chondrosarcoma is a tumor that most often affects flat bones and has a peak incidence in the fourth to sixth decades of life. This tumor can arise de novo or as a malignant transformation of an enchondroma or as a cartilaginous cap of an osteochondroma. Ewing's sarcoma is common in adolescence and typically involves the diaphyseal region of long bones and/or flat bones. Radi-

ographs show a characteristic "onion peel" appearance with a soft tissue mass. The mass is composed of sheets of monotonous small round blue cells.

4. C. The stacked cell layer produces osteoblasts, which are of mesodermal origin and secrete osteoid. Osteoid is unmineralized bone containing type I collagen and ground substance. Osteoblasts eventually differentiate into osteocytes. Bone formation occurs in two processes. The first is endochondral, which involves ossification of cartilaginous molds. Long bones form by this type of ossification at primary and secondary centers. The second process involves intramembranous ossification, which is spontaneous bone formation without preexisting cartilage.

5. B. This woman most likely has systemic lupus erythematosus (SLE or lupus), a chronic autoimmune disorder that can affect virtually any organ of the body. In lupus, the body's immune system, which normally functions to protect against foreign invaders, becomes hyperactive, forming antibodies that attack normal tissues and organs, including the skin, joints, kidneys, brain, heart, lungs, and blood. Lupus is characterized by periods of illness, called flares, and periods of wellness, or remission. No single test can determine whether a person has lupus, but several laboratory tests may help to make a diagnosis. The most useful tests identify certain autoantibodies often present in the blood of people with lupus. For example, most people with lupus test positive on the antinuclear antibody (ANA) test. However, there are a number of other causes of a positive ANA besides lupus, including infections and other autoimmune diseases. Occasionally too, healthy people will test positive. In addition, there are blood tests for individual types of autoantibodies that are more specific to people with lupus, although not all of them test positive for these and not all people with these antibodies have lupus. These antibodies include anti-DNA, anti-Sm, anti-RNP, anti-Ro (SSA), and anti-La (SSB). Thyroid-function testing and uric acid testing are unlikely to be of value in this patient.

6. A. This is a typical presentation of severe anorexia. The illness begins in the early teens, is more common in females, and is found in industrialized societies. Thiamine deficiency will cause damage to the mammillary bodies and loss of rhythmic eye movement. This patient has no history of alcohol abuse. Schizophrenia is equally prevalent and worsens with time. Bulimics respond well to treatment, unlike those with anorexia, who tend to deny their illness vigorously. Patients with major depressive disorder make the highest use of medical services.

7. D. Rheumatoid arthritis (RA) is a chronic inflammatory disorder primarily affecting synovial joints; it is most commonly seen in women between 20 and 50 years of age. RA is likely of autoimmune origin, with interplay of genetic and environmental factors. It is often characterized by the presence of serum rheumatoid factor, an immunoglobulin with anti-IgG Fc specificity. It occurs most often in HLA-DR4–positive individuals. Clinically, patients are often fatigued, anorexic, and febrile. Swelling of the joints can be seen, as well as stiffness, especially in the morning. The proximal interphalangeal and metacarpophalangeal joints are frequently affected sites. This patient's x-ray (Figure 8-1) reveals the classic swan-neck deformity of the hands. There is hyperextension of the PIP joint and hyperflexion of the DIP joint. There are no Gram-negative diplococci seen on joint aspiration to suggest the diagnosis of gonococcal arthritis. There is no indication to suggest tuberculosis such as an exposure history or a positive PPD.

8. C. Duchenne muscular dystrophy is the most common and most severe of the muscular dystrophies and occurs almost entirely in male children. It begins with weakness around 1 year of age and progresses to immobilization, wasting, muscle contracture, and death in the early teens, usually due to pneumonia caused by weak respiratory muscles. It exhibits X-linked inheritance and is caused by a deficiency of dystrophin. Labs reveal increased serum creatinine phosphokinase, and physical examination shows hypertrophy of distal muscles (such as the calf muscles). Disuse atrophy occurs with advanced age. Metachromic leukodystrophy is associated with deficiency of arylsulfatase A and results in sulfate accumulation in the brain. Niemann-Pick disease is a deficiency of sphingomyelinase and causes buildup of sphingomyelin and cholesterol in the reticuloendothelial and parenchymal cells.

9. A. Chondrosarcoma is a tumor that most often affects flat bones and has a peak incidence in the fourth to sixth decades of life. This tumor can arise de novo or as a malignant transformation of an enchondroma or as a cartilaginous cap of an osteochondroma. Radiographically, the tumor appears lobular with mottled, punctate, or annular calcification of the cartilaginous matrix. One should be highly suspicious of this diagnosis if a patient presents with the new onset of pain, inflammation, and progressive increase in the size of the mass in a short period of time. Ewing's sarcoma is common in adolescence and typically involves the diaphyseal region of long bones and/or flat bones. Radiographs show a characteristic "onion peel" appearance with a soft tissue mass. The mass is composed of sheets of monotonous small round blue cells. Osteomyelitis is a bone infection. It can be diagnosed with CT scan or radiolabeled bone scan.

10. B. Growth of the muscle takes place by increases in muscle thickness due to an increase in fiber thickness. Increases in muscle length take place by increases in the number of sarcomeres.

11. D. Osteopetrosis, also known as marble bone disease or Albers-Schonberg disease, is a rare inherited disease marked by the abnormal, decreased functioning of osteoclasts. This abnormality results in reduced bone resorption and abnormally thickened bone. In these patients, multiple fractures are frequent, as the bones are structurally weak and abnormally brittle. This disease is also associated with anemia as a result of decreased marrow space. Patients can present with blindness, deafness, and cranial nerve involvement due to narrowing and impingement of neural foramina. Osteomalacia is vitamin D deficiency in adults, while rickets is vitamin D deficiency in children. Osteogenesis imperfecta, also known as brittle bone disease, is characterized by multiple fractures occurring with minimal trauma. This disease is caused by defective collagen synthesis, which results in generalized connective tissue abnormalities affecting the teeth, skin, eyes, and bones.

12. D. Carpal tunnel syndrome occurs when tendons or ligaments in the wrist become enlarged, often from inflammation and after being aggravated. In this patient's case, the 6 hr of practicing each day is the source of the problem. The narrowed tunnel of bones and ligaments in the wrist pinches the nerves that reach the fingers and the muscles at the base of the thumb. The first symptoms usually appear at night. Symptoms range from a burning, tingling numbness in the fingers, especially the thumb and the index and middle fingers, to difficulty gripping or making a fist, to dropping things. Some cases of carpal tunnel syndrome are due to cumulative trauma of the wrist. Physicians can use specific tests to try to produce the symptoms of carpal tunnel syndrome. In the Tinel test, the doctor taps on or presses on the median nerve in the patient's wrist. The test is positive when tingling in the fingers or a resultant shock-like sensation occurs. The Phalen, or wrist-flexion, test involves having the patient hold his or her forearms upright by pointing the fingers down and pressing the backs of the hands together. The presence of carpal tunnel syndrome is suggested if one or more symptoms, such as tingling or increasing numbness, are felt in the fingers within 1 min. Toxicology screen is unlikely to be positive on this patient. ACTH stimulation testing would be indicated if hypoadrenalism were suggested by physical examination findings of hypotension and sluggishness.

13. E. Paget's disease, also known as osteitis deformans, is a chronic disorder characterized by excessive bone loss. It affects men more than women, usually those over the age of 40. It most frequently occurs in the bones of the spine, skull, pelvis, thighs, and lower legs. Complications include fractures, neoplasia, nerve compression, and high-output cardiac failure. The difficulty hearing is caused by skull enlargement and subsequent nerve compression. There is an increase in osteoclastic and osteoblastic activity, resulting in an elevated alkaline phosphatase. The skull x-ray shown (Figure 8-2) reveals thickening of the skull vault and regions of lucency with sclerosis. Achondroplasia is an autosomal dominant cell-signaling defect of fibroblast growth factor receptor 3. It results in dwarfism. Osteitis fibrosa cystica is a result of renally induced hypercalciuria. Osteogenesis imperfecta is characterized by multiple fractures occurring with minimal trauma, such as may occur during the birth process. It is due to genetic defects that result in abnormal collagen synthesis.

14. H. This patient is suffering from an anterior cruciate ligament (ACL) injury. The ACL, which prevents anterior movement, is injured in twisting motions or hyperextension of the knee. Thus, a soccer player who is constantly running may suffer such an injury. The Lachman test assesses the grade of laxity by stabilizing the knee and pulling forward on the tibia. When injury occurs, there is usually a loud pop followed by swelling since the ACL is well vascularized.

15. C. Polymyalgia rheumatica (PMR) is a disease that causes stiffness and pain in the neck, shoulders, and hips. The stiffness is usually worse in the morning. Without treatment, the stiffness and pain can grow worse over time. PMR is most common in people above age 50. Women are affected more often than men, and it is more common among Caucasians than people of other races. Poliomyelitis is caused by poliovirus, which is transmitted by the fecal-to-oral route; it causes malaise, headache, fever, nausea, and abdominal pain. Sjögren's syndrome is associated with the triad of dry eyes, dry mouth, and arthritis. Systemic lupus erythematosus is associated with fever, fatigue, weight loss, joint pain, malar rash, and photosensitivity.

16. D. Xerostomia, keratoconjunctivitis sicca, and rheumatoid arthritis make up the triad of Sjögren's syndrome. Another important finding includes enlargement of the parotid glands. Progressive systemic sclerosis (scleroderma) can occur in the skin as well as other structures such as the esophagus. Rheumatoid arthritis is a multisystemic disorder resulting in symmetrical joint inflammation, articular erosions, and extra-articular complications. Polyarteritis nodosa is characterized by necrotizing immune complex inflammation of small or medium-sized muscular arteries. Poliomyelitis is caused by poliovirus, which is transmitted by the fecal-to-oral route. It causes malaise, headache, fever, nausea, and abdominal pain. Sjögren's syndrome is associated with the triad of dry eyes, dry mouth, and arthritis. Systemic lupus erythematosus is associated with fever, fatigue, weight loss, joint pain, malar rash, and photosensitivity.

17. A. Fibromyalgia is a chronic condition causing pain, stiffness, and tenderness of the muscles, tendons, and joints. Fibromyalgia is also characterized by restless sleep, awakening feeling tired, fatigue, anxiety, depression, and disturbances in bowel function. Fibromyalgia was formerly known as fibrositis. Patients with fibromyalgia have an impaired non–rapid-eye-movement (non-REM) sleep phase (which likely explains the common feature of waking up fatigued and unrefreshed). The onset of fibromyalgia has been associated with psychological distress, trauma, and infection. This patient's pregnancy may have triggered this condition. There is no reason to suspect hepatitis in this patient, who has no history of transfusions or intravenous drug abuse. Hypercalcemia is associated with renal stones, abdominal pain, and psychiatric symptoms. Thyroid function tests are not pro-

vided for this patient; thus, there is no reason to suspect hypothyroidism.

18. C. Lateral epicondylitis, also known as tennis elbow, is commonly seen in people who overuse their arm(s). The most common cause is overuse of the wrist extensors. All the extensor muscles of the hand attach to the lateral epicondyle; if they are strained or overused, they become inflamed. Carpal tunnel syndrome occurs at the wrist due to entrapment of the median nerve in the carpal tunnel. Acute gouty attacks often involve the great toe. Medial epicondylitis is inflammation of the medial epicondyle. Carpal tunnel syndrome is entrapment of the median nerve in the carpal tunnel of the wrist. This can cause difficulty with abduction of the thumb and atrophy of the thenar eminence.

19. A. Bursae are fluid-filled sacs that cushion areas of friction between tendon and bone or skin. Bursae are lined with special cells called synovial cells, which secrete a fluid rich in collagen and proteins. This fluid acts as a lubricant when parts of the body move. When the synovium becomes inflamed secondary to too much movement, the painful condition known as bursitis results. Rheumatoid arthritis is a multisystemic disorder that results in symmetrical joint inflammation, articular erosions, and extra-articular complications. Gonococcal arthritis is unlikely in the absence of joint fluid aspiration that reveals Gram-negative diplococci. Rheumatoid arthritis is an autoimmune disease that affects the synovial joints, with pannus formation in the joints (such as the metacarpophalangeal [MCP] and proximal interphalangeal [PIP] joints), subcutaneous rheumatoid nodules, ulnar deviation, and subluxation. Septic bursitis is unlikely in the absence of a joint fluid aspiration that reveals organisms on Gram's stain. Trauma is unlikely given this patient's history.

20. D. Osteomyelitis is an acute or chronic bone infection usually caused by bacteria. In children, osteomyelitis usually affects the metaphysis of the tibia or femur as well as growing bones with a rich blood supply. Patients with acute osteomyelitis of peripheral bones are usually febrile, have had weight loss and suffer from fatigue, and have localized warmth, swelling, erythema, and tenderness. X-rays become abnormal after 3 to 4 weeks, showing bone destruction, soft tissue swelling, periosteal elevation, loss of vertebral body height or narrowing of the adjacent infected intervertebral disk space, and destruction of the endplates above and below the disk. Asbestosis is associated with diffuse pulmonary interstitial fibrosis caused by inhaled asbestos fibers. Inflammatory arthritis would be associated with the presence of inflammatory cells in joint fluid aspirate. Stress fracture is unlikely given the presentation of this patient.

21. A. Behçet's disease is a rare chronic inflammatory disorder. Its cause is unknown, although there have been reports of a virus found in some individuals with the disease. Behçet's generally begins when individuals are in their 20s or 30s, although it can occur at any age. It tends to occur more often in men than in women. Symptoms of Behçet's disease include recurrent ulcers (resembling canker sores) in the mouth and on the genitals as well as eye inflammation. The disorder may also cause various types of skin lesions, arthritis, bowel inflammation, meningitis, and cranial nerve palsies. Behçet's is a multisystemic disease; it may involve all organs and affect the central nervous system, causing memory loss and impaired speech, balance, and movement. Lyme disease is associated with a tick bite and produces arthralgia and skin lesions. Multiple sclerosis is an immune-mediated disease associated with neurologic findings such as weakness and incontinence. Sarcoidosis is an immune-mediated disease associated with subcutaneous granuloma formation. Sjögren's syndrome is associated with the triad of dry eyes, dry mouth, and arthritis.

22. B. Lactic acid is a by-product of anaerobic glycolysis. If enough oxygen is not available, lactic acid is produced and begins to accumulate in the muscles. Lactic acid causes the burning sensation felt in muscles during high-intensity exercise and also prevents muscles from working at their best. This burning sensation is the result of a change in muscular acidity.

23. E. Medial epicondylitis, also known as golfer's elbow, is commonly seen in people who overuse their arm(s). The most common cause is overuse of the wrist flexors. The hand flexors attach to the medial epicondyle, and if they are strained or overused, they become inflamed, causing pain. Carpal tunnel syndrome occurs when tendons or ligaments in the wrist become enlarged, often from inflammation and after being aggravated by overuse. The narrowed tunnel of bones and ligaments in the wrist pinches the nerves that reach the fingers and the muscles at the base of the thumb. Lateral epicondylitis is known as tennis elbow and is associated with inflammation of the lateral epicondyle. Medial epicondylitis is inflammation of the medial epicondyle. Acute gout often affects the great toe.

24. C. This patient has primary gout, which is often precipitated by a large meal or alcohol intake, both of which may aggravate hyperuricemia. Gout is characterized by deposition of urate crystals in a number of tissues, especially the joints. It is marked by an intense inflammatory reaction beginning with opsonization of crystals by IgG, followed by phagocytosis by neutrophils and eventuating in the release of proteolytic enzymes and inflammatory mediators from the phagocytic cells. This patient has painful, acute arthritis and bursitis in the metatarsophalangeal joint of the great toe, which is known specifically as podagra. The histologic slide shows needle-shaped negatively birefringent urate crystals. Chondrocalcinosis is an abnormal proliferation of cartilage. Pseudogout is caused by deposition of calcium pyrophosphate crystals within the joint space. Tuberculosis can affect the spine but rarely occurs in the toe.

25. C. Alkaptonuria is caused by a deficiency in homogentisic acid. The accumulation of alkapton bodies from failure of tyrosine degradation causes dark urine, dark cartilage, and possible arthralgias. In Osler-Weber-Rendu disease, a mutated protein involved in angiogenesis causes abnormal dilation of the mucosal capillaries as well as vessels in mucosa, gastrointestinal tract, retina, and skin, affecting the lungs, brain, and liver. This condition may also cause osteolysis of the metacarpals and metatarsals. Gaucher's disease, due to beta-glucocerebrosidase deficiency, has a characteristic crinkled-paper look on bone marrow smear owing to elongated glucocerebroside-filled lysosomes in the cytoplasm. In type I, the most common form of Gaucher's disease, patients experience growth retardation until their teens (they then catch up) and develop anemia, hepatosplenomegaly, Erlenmeyer flask–like thigh bones, and erosion of the femoral head. In Von Gierke's disease, which is due to a deficiency in G6P, an enzyme involved in gluconeogenesis, glycogen accumulation in the liver leads to hepatomegaly. Patients fail to maintain blood glucose levels, causing an increase in hormones in an attempt to raise blood sugar. Adult patients tend to develop renal disease, osteopenia, and fractures. Hurler's disease, caused by deficient alpha-L-iduronidase in the glycosaminoglycan (GAG) degradation pathway, is an autosomal recessive trait causing mental retardation and corneal clouding from the accumulation of GAG in connective tissue. Patients appear gargoyle-like.

26. A. There are two forms of gonococcal arthritis: one with skin rashes and multiple joint involvement and a second, less common, form in which disseminated gonococcemia leads to infection of a single joint (monoarticular) and joint fluid cultures are positive. Single-joint arthritis follows generalized spread (dissemination) of the gonococcal infection. Dissemination is associated with symptoms of fever, chills, multiple joint aches (arthralgia), and rashes (1-mm to 2-cm red macules). This episode may end as a single joint becomes infected. The most commonly involved joints are the large joints, such as the knee, wrist, and ankle. Nonseptic bursitis would not produce a joint aspirate that shows organisms on Gram's stain. Rheumatoid arthritis is an inflammatory disorder that affects the synovial joints, particularly the MCP and PIP joints. Subcutaneous nodules, ulnar deviation, and subluxation are also common. *Staphylococcus aureus* would show Gram-positive cocci in clusters.

27. E. Reiter's syndrome consists of arthritis, nongonococcal urethritis or cervicitis, and conjunctivitis. It is a form of arthritis that produces pain, swelling, redness, and heat in the joints and is one of a family of arthritic disorders affecting the spine. Reiter's commonly involves the joints of the spine and the sacroiliac joints, areas where the spine attaches to the pelvis. Men are most often affected in their twenties or thirties, and most are positive for HLA-B27. The lack of organisms on joint fluid aspiration makes the diagnosis of infectious arthritis unlikely. Osteoarthritis is associated with wear and tear on the joints, which leads to destruction of the articular cartilage. Pseudogout is caused by deposition of calcium pyrophosphate crystals within the joint space.

28. D. Pott's disease, also known as tuberculous spondylitis or tuberculosis of the spine, is characterized by softening and collapse of the vertebrae, often resulting in kyphosis, a hunchback deformity (Pott's curvature). Occasionally, the spinal nerves are affected, and a rigid paralysis (Pott's paraplegia) may result. Affected persons complain of pain on movement and tend to assume a protective, upright, stiff position. The course of the disease is slow, lasting months or years. Ankylosing spondylitis is a chronic inflammatory disease of the spine and sacroiliac joints that leads to stiffness, uveitis, and aortic regurgitation. Osteoarthritis is a degenerative joint disease associated with destruction of articular cartilage, subchondral bone formation, and osteophytes. Reiter's syndrome is associated with urethritis, arthritis, and conjunctivitis.

29. A. Calcium pyrophosphate dihydrate crystal deposition disease, also known as pseudogout or chondrocalcinosis, is a condition that causes pain, redness, heat, and swelling in one or more joints. It is caused by deposits of calcium pyrophosphate dihydrate crystals in a joint, which weakens the cartilage and causes it to break down more easily. The presence of crystals in the joints and the body's reaction to these crystals create inflammation as the crystals are attacked. This condition is diagnosed by finding basophilic-staining rhomboid crystals in the synovial fluid. Gout is precipitation of monosodium urate crystals in joints due to hyperuricemia. Reiter's syndrome is associated with urethritis, arthritis, and conjunctivitis. Suppurative arthritis is associated with the presence of infectious cells (neutrophils) on joint aspiration.

30. E. This woman has systemic lupus erythematosus (SLE), a chronic autoimmune disorder that can affect virtually any organ of the body. In lupus, the body's immune system, which normally functions to protect against foreign invaders, becomes hyperactive, forming antibodies that attack normal tissues and organs, including the skin, joints, kidneys, brain, heart, lungs, and blood. Recurrent miscarriage is often a problem with these patients. Lupus is characterized by periods of illness, called flares, and periods of wellness, or remission. Ninety percent of lupus victims are women, and the onset of the disease usually occurs between the ages of 15 and 44. Most people with lupus test positive to the antinuclear antibody (ANA) test. Discoid lupus typically affects only the skin. Systemic lupus is associated with fever, fatigue, weight loss, and joint pain. Malar rash and photosensitivity are also common. Lab testing may reveal a positive antinuclear antibody test. Dermatitis comprises a group of inflammatory pruritic skin disorders. The typical etiology is allergic.

31. D. The most common mechanism of injury of the posterior cruciate ligament (PCL) is the "dashboard injury." When the knee is bent, and an object forcefully hits the tibia and forces it backwards; this motion can push the tibia back and cause a PCL tear. The anterior drawer sign indicates tearing of the anterior cruciate ligament (ACL). Abnormal passive abduction indicates a torn medial collateral ligament (MCL).

32. D. Glucocorticoids function to dramatically reduce the manifestations of inflammation by affecting the distribution, concentration, and function of leukocytes. They increase the concentration of neutrophils while decreasing the concentration of lymphocytes, basophils, eosinophils, and monocytes. They also inhibit the ability of leukocytes and macrophages to respond to mitogens and antigens, reduce the amount of histamine released from basophils, and inhibit the activity of kinins. Finally, they block the conversion of phospholipid into arachidonic acid, thereby reducing both leukotriene and prostaglandin production. Ibuprofen is a nonsteroidal anti-inflammatory drug (NSAID) that is a reversible inhibitor of cyclooxygenases and thus inhibits the synthesis of prostaglandins but not that of leukotrienes. Aspirin and other salicylates are unique among the NSAIDs in that they irreversibly inhibit cyclooxygenase. This, in turn, prevents the production of prostaglandins, thereby inhibiting the inflammatory process. Methotrexate functions to bind dihydrofolate reductase and prevent the reduction of folate, which is necessary for cell propagation. When used for inflammatory purposes, as in severe rheumatoid arthritis, lower doses are required than that for cancer chemotherapy. Acetaminophen acts by inhibiting prostaglandin synthesis in the CNS and thus has antipyretic and analgesic properties. It has less effect on cyclooxygenase in peripheral tissues and therefore has a weak anti-inflammatory effect.

33. A. Dermatomyositis is an idiopathic disorder that includes an inflammatory myopathy and characteristic skin manifestations. Polymyositis includes the inflammatory myopathy without the cutaneous findings. The average age at diagnosis is 40, and almost twice as many women are affected as men. There is usually proximal muscle weakness (upper or lower extremity and trunk). The pathognomonic cutaneous manifestation of dermatomyositis is Gottron's sign: violaceous or erythematous plaques over the extensor surfaces of the joints, especially of the hands. Laboratory findings may reveal an elevated level of serum creatine kinase or aldolase. A helpful diagnostic indicator includes a positive anti-Jo-1 antibody test (histidyl-tRNA synthetase). Polyarteritis nodosa is characterized by necrotizing immune complex inflammation of small or medium-sized muscular arteries. Poliomyelitis is caused by poliovirus, which is transmitted by the fecal-to-oral route; it causes malaise, headache, fever, nausea, and abdominal pain. Sjögren's syndrome is associated with the triad of dry eyes, dry mouth, and arthritis. Systemic lupus erythematosus is associated with fever, fatigue, weight loss, joint pain, malar rash, and photosensitivity.

34. E. This patient's clinical presentation is typical of a fracture of the neck of the femur. The shortening and external rotation occurs secondary to contraction of the gluteal muscles, which attach to the femur in the area of the fracture. This fracture is very common in postmenopausal women, especially those with osteoporosis. A dislocation of the head of the femur will mimic this fracture; however, based on the patient's history, the femur is most likely fractured. A fracture of the greater trochanter would not result in significant shortening or external rotation because only the gluteus medius and gluteus minimus attach to it. Fractures of the lower femur, including the lateral epicondyle, medial epicondyle, and metaphysis, would not result in an external rotation of the entire leg.

35. E. Bone is composed of type I collagen fibers, ground substance, and hydroxyapatite crystals. The collagen itself is organized in a lamellar or layered fashion. The layers may be organized in a parallel fashion, as in trabecular bone and periosteum, or concentric, as in the haversian system. When bone is formed quickly, the collagen is randomly organized and called woven bone. Woven bone is the predominant type of bone in a healing fracture site, metabolic bone disease, and/or tumors. Cancellous, spongy, and trabecular bone are all synonyms for the thinner type of bone found in the cortex. These types of bone are also lamellar bone. Compact bone is lamellar bone and is the calcified external part of the bone.

36. A. Cranial nerve I, or the olfactory nerve, passes through the cribriform plate on the way to the olfactory bulb. Any damage or fracture to the cribriform plate could potentially injure or sever CN I, resulting in hyposmia or anosmia. Cranial nerve III, the oculomotor nerve, courses through the cavernous sinus before emerging through the superior orbital fissure. Deficits to this nerve generally result from pressure or compression at any point along its course; damage would present as a deficit in medial, superior, and inferior eye movements. CN VII, the facial nerve, travels with CN VIII through the internal auditory meatus within the temporal bone and exits the skull via the stylomastoid foramen. Damage would result in facial paralysis or deficits in salivation and lacrimation. CN X, the vagus nerve, exits the skull via the jugular foramen. Lesions to this nerve are not common; however, injury would result in paralysis of the soft palate, causing the uvula to tilt to the intact side, impaired swallowing, and paralysis of the vocal cords. CN XII, or the hypoglossal nerve, leaves the skull through the hypoglossal canal to innervate the ipsilateral tongue. Damage to this nerve results in paralysis of the tongue. On examination, the tongue will deviate to the affected side.

37. E. Myasthenia gravis is an acquired autoimmune disease in which the body produces antibodies against acetylcholine receptors located postsynaptically in the neuromuscular junction. The disease occurs most commonly in females (6:4) and has an average onset in the twenties and thirties. MG can involve either the external ocular muscles selectively or the general voluntary muscle system. The symptoms fluctuate and are exacerbated by exertion, extremes of temperature, viral or other infections, menses, and excitement. On examination, fatigue is most reliably demonstrated in the eyes. A positive curtain sign entails worsening ptosis with sustained upward gaze. The diagnosis can be made several different ways, including the edrophonium test, in which 2 mg of edrophonium is given intravenously; shortly thereafter, the symptoms of weakness and fatigue resolve. One can also perform electromyographic (EMG) testing and check for titers of the AchR antibody. Several drugs—including aminoglycoside antibiotics, antiarrhythmic agents, propranolol, phenothiazines, lithium, trimethaphan, methoxyflurane, and magnesium—can exacerbate MG or cause similar symptoms in patients without MG. Option B is a description of the pathology of Graves' disease. Graves' disease is the most common cause of thyrotoxicosis, with a peak age incidence between 20 and 40 years of age. Signs and symptoms include goiter, nervousness, increased sweating, fatigue, lid lag or eye signs, tachycardia, and palpitations. Lambert-Eaton myasthenic syndrome is a presynaptic disorder of the neuromuscular junction that can cause weakness similar to that of MG. This disease is a result of autoantibodies against P/Q-type calcium channels at the motor nerve terminals. However, patients with LEMS have depressed or absent reflexes, show autonomic changes such as dry mouth, and show incremental responses on repetitive nerve stimulation. Botulism is a paralytic disease that begins with cranial nerve involvement and progresses caudally to involve the extremities. Essentially, the *C. botulinum* toxin binds to presynaptic nerve terminals and prevents the release of neurotransmitter. This results in the paralysis described above.

38. C. Guillain-Barré syndrome (GBS) is an acute, frequently severe, and fulminant polyradiculoneuropathy that is autoimmune in nature. It manifests as a rapidly evolving ascending areflexic motor paralysis with or without sensory deficits. The lower extremities are most often affected. Once clinical worsening stops, the crisis is usually over. However, a patient may require ventilatory support. Seventy-five percent of cases of GBS begin 1 to 3 weeks earlier with an acute infectious process, usually respiratory or gastrointestinal. The condition has been linked to infection with *Campylobacter jejuni*. Cerebrospinal fluid (CSF) findings are distinctive, showing elevated protein without accompanying pleocytosis. Treatment with high-dose intravenous immune globulin (IVIg) or plasmapheresis can be initiated. Approximately, 85% of patients will have a full functional recovery within several months to a year. The mortality is less than 5%. Botulism is a paralytic disease that begins with cranial nerve involvement and progresses caudally to involve the extremities. Essentially, the *C. botulinum* toxin binds to presynaptic nerve terminals and prevents the release of neurotransmitter. This results in the paralysis described above. Charcot-Marie Tooth neuropathy consists of a heterogeneous group of inherited peripheral nerve diseases. Transmission is most often autosomal dominant but can also be recessive or X-linked. Onset is usually in the first or second decade of life. Patients present with a variety of clinical findings ranging from pes cavus and minimal weakness to severe distal atrophy and marked hand and foot deformity. HIV infection that has spread into the nervous system can present very much like GBS. However, CSF findings will reveal an elevated white cell count (10 to 100 mg/dL), along with increased protein levels. Multiple sclerosis is defined clinically by typical symptoms, signs, and disease progression separated by time and space. Onset usually occurs between the ages of 15 and 50. Individual bouts of inflammatory demyelination may be accompanied by clinical symptoms termed relapses, followed in most cases by some degree of recovery, producing the typical relapsing-remitting course. Diagnosis requires intermittent or progressive CNS symptoms supported by evidence of two or more CNS white matter lesions occurring in an appropriately aged patient who lacks an alternative explanation.

39. D. Osteoid osteoma generally affects patients between the ages of 5 and 25. It is a benign tumor that arises from osteoblastic connective tissue. The tumor can occur in any bone but is most common in the lower extremities. Patients usually present with localized pain that is worse at night and relieved by ibuprofen or naproxen. X-rays of the affected area will generally show a sclerotic lesion with or without a localized lytic nidus within the sclerotic bone. Histologically, the nidus consists of immature woven bone and osteoblasts surrounded by dense sclerotic bone. Treatment involves surgical excision. Ewing's sarcoma is a malignant tumor that arises in medullary tissue and usually affects long bones. A patient will present with pain, fever, and leukocytosis; x-rays show an onionskin appearance of the affected area. Osteoclastoma or giant cell tumors of bone arise from osteoclasts and are benign approximately 50% of the time. Treatment includes surgical excision, but the lesions often return. Osteosarcoma is the most common malignancy of bone and typically presents with pain and swelling in a bone or joint (especially the knee). Radiographs reveal bone destruction and production as well as periosteal elevation. Stress fractures often mimic the symptoms of osteoid osteoma; however, they may not be detectable on x-ray. A bone scan will show increased uptake in the affected area of a stress fracture and is more useful in the diagnosis.

40. A. An Adam's test or forward-bend test will allow one to evaluate the patient's spine for scoliosis. Scoliosis is an asymmetry of the spine that causes both a lateral deviation and rotational abnormality of the spine. The forward-bend test allows one to see any lateral curvature or signs of asymmetry in the levels of the shoulders, scapulae, and hips. Scoliosis can affect anyone at any age, but it is most common in late childhood and adolescence. Often, previously insignificant curves become evident during the adolescent growth spurt. Lachman's test is used to evaluate for ACL tears. It is performed by placing the knee in 15 degrees of flexion and external rotation. Then the examiner, with the distal femur in one hand and the upper tibia in the other, moves the tibia forward and the femur back. Significant forward excursion suggests an ACL tear. McMurray's test is used to evaluate for meniscal tears. One hand grasps the heel while the other is placed over the knee, with the fingers and thumb along the medial and lateral joint line. From the heel, the lower leg is rotated internally and externally. The feeling of a click or pop with applied stress implies a meniscal tear. Radiographs are necessary only if a curvature is detected after the forward-bend test is performed. If curvature is detected, the extent of the curve can be evaluated by determining the Cobb angle from the radiograph. A straight-leg raise is used to evaluate low back pain and disk herniation. A test is positive if one elicits pain that shoots down the leg below the knee. Pain should be elicited between 30 and 70 degrees of hip flexion.

41. B. Achondroplasia, a type of dwarfism, is inherited as an autosomal dominant trait, although most cases are sporadic and due to new mutations in fibroblast growth factor receptor 3 (FGFR3). The appearance of short limbs with a normal trunk is characteristically accompanied by a large head, a saddle nose, and an exaggerated lumbar lordosis. The length of the spine is usually normal, and these characteristics are recognizable at birth. The most common mutation responsible for achondroplasia substitutes an arginine for glycine in the transmembrane domain of FGFR3 and causes a dysfunction in the FGFR3 receptor. Essentially, fibroblast growth factor normally acts via the FGFR3 to inhibit chondrocyte proliferation in the growth plate. With the mutation in the receptor, inhibition is prevented, leading to the abnormal proliferation of chondrocytes at the growth plate and resulting in the production of short, thick bones. Sickle cell anemia is an autosomal recessive disorder in which abnormal hemoglobin leads to chronic hemolytic anemia. Change in a single DNA base leads to an amino acid substitution of valine for glutamine in the sixth position on the beta-globin chain, which results in the production of hemoglobin S. McCune-Albright syndrome or fibrous dysplasia manifests clinically as localized pain, deformities, or fractures. It can also present with headaches, seizures, cranial nerve abnormalities, and hearing loss. It represents a phenotypic spectrum of disorders caused by activating mutation in the GNAS1 gene, which encodes the $G_{s\alpha}$ protein. Turner's syndrome (45,XO) generally becomes manifest in adulthood and is characterized by short stature, hypogonadism, webbed neck, high-arched palate, wide-spaced nipples, hypertension, and renal abnormalities. 45,XO is the most common major chromosomal abnormality in humans. Klinefelter's syndrome (47,XXY) occurs in males and manifests after puberty, at which time the patient develops disproportionately long legs and arms, a female escutcheon, gynecomastia, and small testes.

42. C. Polyarteritis nodosa is a multisystemic necrotizing vasculitis of small and medium-sized muscular arteries in which renal and visceral artery involvement is characteristic. The mean age of onset of polyarteritis nodosa is 50 years, and it is more common in males than females. Patients generally present with nonspecific symptoms such as weakness, malaise, headache, abdominal pain, and myalgias. Complaints specific to the organ affected may also be the presenting complaint. Painful, subcutaneous nodules are also a common finding. Bloodwork generally shows a leukocytosis, elevated ESR, and positive pANCA titers. Angiography of the affected organ generally shows aneurysms, stenotic segments, and obliteration of vessels. Biopsy of affected areas shows infiltration of polymorphonuclear neutrophils (PMNs) into all layers of the vascular wall and perivascular areas, which results in intimal proliferation and degeneration of the vessel wall. Buerger's disease or thromboangiitis obliterans is an inflammatory occlusive peripheral vascular disease that affects arteries and veins in the distal upper and lower extremities. This disorder often develops in men under the age of 40 and is prevalent in Asians and individuals of eastern European descent. The cause is unknown. The disease presents as claudication of the affected extremity, Raynaud's phenomenon, and migratory superficial vein thrombophlebitis. Kawasaki disease is an acute febrile multisystemic disease of children. It is characterized by a fever of unknown origin, cervical adenitis, conjunctivitis, erythema of the oral cavity, lips, and palms, and desquamation of the palms. Although the disease is generally benign, it is associated with coronary artery aneurysms in approximately 25% of cases. Treatment involves aspirin and high-dose gamma globulin. Takayasu's arteritis is an inflammatory and stenotic disease of medium-sized and large arteries characterized by a strong predilection for the aorta. It occurs most often in young Asian women and presents as fever, malaise, night sweats, arthralgias, anorexia, weight loss, and loss of peripheral pulses. Wegener's granulomatosis is characterized by granulomatous vasculitis of the upper and lower respiratory tracts together with glomerulonephritis. Patients present with severe upper respiratory tract findings such as paranasal sinus pain and drainage, cough, conjunctivitis, skin lesions such as subcutaneous nodules, and glomerulonephritis. Laboratory findings include an elevated ESR, anemia, leukocytosis, hypergammaglobulinemia, and a mildly elevated rheumatoid factor.

43. D. Chronic administration of phenytoin is known to cause decreases in bone density and osteomalacia. It induces changes in bone density through suppression of intestinal calcium absorption, with a subsequent induction of secondary hyperparathyroidism. This decrease in bone density resulted in the patient's compression fracture from a seemingly harmless fall. Since she is premenopausal, she should not be in a low-estrogen state. Malnutrition is an unlikely cause of this patient's fracture, since she takes a multivitamin and eats a healthy diet. Metformin is a biguanide used in the treatment of DM II; it has no known side effect of bone demineralization. The patient does not have any signs of renal insufficiency, thus renal osteodystrophy is not a likely cause. Rofecoxib is a cyclooxygenase-2 inhibitor used to treat osteoarthritis and is not a cause of bone demineralization. Simvastatin is an HMG-CoA reductase inhibitor used to treat hyperlipidemia and is not a likely cause of her fracture.

44. A. Osteitis fibrosa cystica, also known as Von Recklinghausen's disease of bone, is caused by primary or secondary hyperparathyroidism. It is characterized by widespread osteolytic lesions and may manifest by diffuse radiolucency of bone, mimicking osteoporosis. Laboratory values reveal manifestations of hyperparathyroidism (high calcium, low phosphorus, and high alkaline phosphatase). Osteomalacia is vitamin D deficiency in adults. Rickets is vitamin D deficiency in children. Scurvy is a deficiency of vitamin C. This vitamin is necessary for hydroxylation of proline and lysine in collagen synthesis.

45. D. Polymyalgia rheumatica is a clinical diagnosis based on pain and stiffness of the shoulder and pelvic girdle areas, frequently in association with fever, malaise, and weight loss. It is essentially the same disease as temporal arteritis, but it does not cause blindness and responds to low-dose prednisone therapy. Patients often complain of having trouble combing their hair, putting on a coat, or rising from a chair. They can present with joint swelling, but that is not usually the primary complaint. Behçet's syndrome is characterized by recurrent episodes of oral and genital ulcers, iritis, and cutaneous lesions. The underlying pathology is a leukocytoclastic venulitis. Buerger's disease or thromboangiitis obliterans is an inflammatory occlusive peripheral vascular disease that affects arteries and veins in the distal upper and lower extremities. This disorder often develops in men under the age of 40 and is prevalent in Asians and individuals of eastern European descent. Polyarteritis nodosa is a multisystem, necrotizing vasculitis of small and medium-sized muscular arteries in which renal and visceral artery involvement is characteristic. The mean age of onset of polyarteritis nodosa is 50 years, and it is more common in males than females. Patients generally present with nonspecific symptoms such as weakness, malaise, headache, abdominal pain, and myalgias. Takayasu's arteritis is an inflammatory and stenotic disease of medium-sized and large arteries characterized by a strong predilection for the aorta. It occurs most often in young Asian women and presents as fever, malaise, night sweats, arthralgias, anorexia, weight loss, and loss of peripheral pulses. Temporal arteritis is a systemic panarteritis affecting medium-sized and large vessels in patients over the age of 50. The temporal artery is frequently involved, and the condition can result in blindness if not treated with high-dose steroids. Headaches and blurry vision are common presenting complaints. Wegener's granulomatosis is characterized by granulomatous vasculitis of the upper and lower respiratory tracts together with glomerulonephritis. Patients present with severe upper respiratory tract findings such as paranasal sinus pain and drainage, cough, conjunctivitis, skin lesions such as subcutaneous nodules, and glomerulonephritis.

46. D. Men and women, typically between the ages of 20 and 50, are equally affected with psoriatic arthritis. Remissions are common, and the condition is less severe than other arthritides. Joint involvement normally begins asymmetrically with the DIP joints of the hands and feet; conjunctivitis and iritis may also occur and the sedimentation rate is mildly elevated. Punctate bleeding upon scraping may be seen, and the arthritis is thought to be a deep version of the Koebner reaction, where new eruptions occur after trauma to the skin. In tuberculous arthritis, hips are affected more frequently and granulomas form in the joint spaces. Lyme arthritis may develop within weeks to 2 years after infection with *Borrelia burgdorferi*; the arthritis may be migratory in nature, and it can evolve into chronic arthritis, frequently affecting the knee. Gouty arthritis, which typically affects older males, contains needle-shaped crystals of monosodium urate; it can be treated with indomethacin and prevented with decreased intake of alcohol, cholesterol, and fat.

47. B. Multiple myeloma is a malignancy of plasma cells that is characterized by replacement of the bone marrow, bone destruction, and paraprotein formation. Older adults are usually affected, with a mean age at presentation of 65. A patient will typically present with bone pain, anemia, and infection. Bone pain is most common in the back or ribs, or it may present as a pathologic fracture, especially of the femoral neck. Patients may also have symptoms of hyperviscosity syndrome. These include mucosal bleeding, vertigo, nausea, visual disturbances, and altered mental status. Laboratory studies show anemia and normal RBC morphology; however, rouleaux formation is very common. The hallmark of myeloma is the finding of a paraprotein on serum protein electrophoresis. Most patients will have a monoclonal spike visible in the beta- or gamma-globulin region. Metastatic tumors to bone are more common than primary bone tumors and often present with bone pain that is localized, develops gradually over weeks, and is severe at night. Bone is a common site of metastasis for carcinomas of the prostate, breast, lung, kidney, bladder, and thyroid. Metastatic tumors usually spread to bone hematogenously, but local invasion from soft tissue can occur. This patient's laboratory profile fits multiple myeloma, a metastatic cancer that was not the most likely cause of his pain. Osteoporosis is a metabolic bone disease in which there is a decrease in the amount of bone present necessary to maintain the structural integrity of the skeleton. The rate of bone formation is often normal, whereas the rate of resorption is increased. Principal areas of demineralization are spine and pelvis, and compression fractures of the vertebrae are very common. Osteoporosis is often seen in postmenopausal women and can go undetected until a fracture occurs. Osteosarcoma is a spindle cell neoplasm that produces osteoid (unmineralized bone) or bone. About 60% of all osteosarcomas occur in children and adolescents in the second decade of life; males are affected twice as often as females. A patient usually presents with pain and swelling of the affected area, which is most often the distal femur, proximal tibia, and proximal humerus. Paget's disease is due to excessive bone resorption with replacement by soft, poorly mineralized osteoid in a disorganized fashion. It most often affects the skull, pelvis, femur, and vertebrae.

It generally presents in the fifth or sixth decades of life, and malignant transformation into osteosarcoma is seen in 1% of such cases. Stress fractures occur with overuse and generally present with chronic localized pain over the fracture site that becomes manifest with use. This patient's symptoms are unlikely due to a stress fracture, given the laboratory profile.

48. C. This patient has osteoarthritis due to morbid obesity, where extrusion of particles into synovial fluid results in destruction of articular cartilage, causing osteophytes to fracture and float in the joint space. Anti-IgG antibodies are found in rheumatoid arthritis, where phagocytosis of immune complex occurs. Antistreptolysin O titers, anti-DNase, and antihyaluronidase are elevated in post-streptococcal-related polyarthritis. Gram-negative rods, oxidase-positive, refer to *Pseudomonas aeruginosa*, which is commonly found in drug addicts with osteomyelitis. Lyme disease arthritis, which often affects knees and large joints, is polyarticular and migratory. Arthritis is a late sign of *Borrelia burgdorferi* infection. The picture shown reveals the presence of Heberden's nodes.

49. D. Osteoarthritis is the most common form of joint disease. The onset is insidious and usually presents with morning joint stiffness, seldom lasting longer than 15 min. Also, the pain is made worse with use and crepitus may be felt within the joint. Radiographs show narrowing of the joint space, sharpened articular margins, osteophyte formation, lipping of marginal bone, and thickened, dense subchondral bone. There is no evidence to suspect ankle sprain, since this patient also has knee pain. Crepitus would not be found with simple ankle strains. Ankylosing spondylitis is a chronic inflammatory disease of the spine's sacroiliac joints. It can result in stiff spine, uveitis, and aortic regurgitation. Reiter syndrome is associated with urethritis, conjunctivitis and arthritis. Osteoarthritis is associated with mechanical wear and tear of the joints, leading to destruction of articular cartilage, subchondral bone formation, and osteophytes.

50. D. Reiter's syndrome or reactive arthritis develops within days or weeks of either a dysenteric infection or a sexually transmitted disease. It is a clinical tetrad of urethritis, conjunctivitis, mucocutaneous lesions, and aseptic arthritis. It occurs most commonly in young men and is associated with HLA-B27. Osteoarthritis is the most common form of joint disease. The onset is insidious and usually presents with morning joint stiffness, seldom lasting longer than 15 min. Also, the pain is made worse with use and crepitus may be felt within the joint. Ankylosing spondylitis is a chronic inflammatory disease of the spine's sacroiliac joints. It can result in stiff spine, uveitis, and aortic regurgitation. Reiter's syndrome is associated with urethritis, conjunctivitis, and arthritis. Osteoarthritis is associated with mechanical wear and tear of the joints, leading to destruction of articular cartilage, subchondral bone formation, and osteophytes. Rheumatoid arthritis is an autoimmune disorder that affects the synovial joints (MCP and PIP), rheumatoid nodules, ulnar deviation, and subluxation.

51. B. Ewing's sarcoma is common in adolescents and typically involves the diaphyseal region of long bones and/or flat bones. Radiographs show a characteristic "onion peel" appearance with a soft tissue mass. The mass is composed of sheets of monotonous small round blue cells. The presence of p30/32, the product of the mic-2 gene, is a surface marker for Ewing's sarcoma. Chondrosarcoma is a tumor that most often affects flat bones and has a peak incidence in the fourth to sixth decades of life. This tumor can arise de novo, as a malignant transformation of an enchondroma, or as the cartilaginous cap of an osteochondroma.

52. B. People with severe osteoporosis often have depression due to their lack of independence and changing appearance. These patients can fracture verterbrae while coughing severely. Primary prevention of osteoporosis entails adequate calcium intake during youth; eating vegetables such as broccoli and kale, which are rich in calcium; and engaging in weight-bearing exercise such as walking, jogging, and aerobics. Alcohol and cheese should be avoided with the monoamine oxidase inhibitor class of antidepressants. Alcohol is known to accelerate osteoporotic changes. Estrogen replacement is secondary prevention. The use of stair rails is a good way to reduce injury after diagnosis. Swimming is not a weight-bearing exercise.

53. B. The best response is to assist the patient with pain management and teach her how to be more assertive about her needs and wants. The patient should avoid blaming family members for her illness. Making unrealistic demands and having the patient continue despite great pain would contribute to the patient's stress. Underlining the patient's negative thoughts about the permanence of her disease would be counterproductive.

54. A. Donning a scoliosis brace often requires assistance, and studies have shown that a mother's attitude to her child's illness greatly affects the child's acceptance of treatment. Counseling should be used if noncompliance continues or if the patient begins to withdraw from peers. Exercise is vital to the patient's sense of well-being and important for proper breathing and maintenance of muscle strength, but contact sports should be avoided to prevent injury to others. It is better to encourage discussion of a situation rather than to resort to reprimands if a patient is noncompliant. Switching to a higher-profile brace with a neck collar would make the patient more self-conscious.

55. D. Osteogenesis imperfecta, also known as brittle bone disease, is characterized by multiple fractures occurring with minimal trauma. This disease is caused by defective collagen synthesis, which results in generalized connective tissue abnormalities affecting the teeth, skin, eyes, and bones. The blueness of the sclerae is due to the translucence of thin connective tissue overlying the choroids. A history of multiple childhood fractures is a common clinical finding. Achondroplasia is an autosomal dominant cell-signaling defect of the fibroblast growth factor receptor 3. It results in dwarfism. Osteitis fibrosa cystica is a result of renally induced hypercalciuria. Achondroplasia is an autosomal dominant cell-signaling defect of the

fibroblast growth factor receptor 3. It results in dwarfism. Osteitis fibrosa cystica is a result of renally induced hypercalciuria.

56. B. Alcohol abuse leads to avascular necrosis via increased blood lipid levels that block vessels supplying the bone. Without proper treatment, collapse of the bone ensues. Patients display increased tolerance for alcohol. Blood smear shows megaloblastic anemia due to poor diet and lack of folic acid. A physician may not restrain a patient unless the patient can be committed under state law. Only police may restrain an intoxicated patient who attempts to drive.

57. C. Falls are the major cause of traumatic injury among the elderly. Activities that are not done on a daily basis put elderly patients at greatest risk for fractures, especially those who have sedentary lifestyles. Cycling is a low-impact sport that supports and stabilizes joints, hence puts an elderly person at lower risk for injury. Daily brisk walks increase bone density and reduce the risk of hip fracture. The third most likely cause of traumatic injury is being struck by a car. Being in a car during an accident is the second most common cause of traumatic injury among elderly individuals aged 65 to 75. Yoga and Tai Chi help to improve balance, flexibility, and breathing; they also help to reduce pain. Shoveling snow is done on an intermittent basis and thus can be associated with risk of injury.

58. D. Down's patients tend to have greater ligamentous laxity than the general population. Although injury is rare, the atlantoaxial joint is at greatest risk, and mild symptoms occur prior to complete dislocation. Bronchoconstriction is a concern for asthmatics. Exercise enhances cardiac function and decreases obesity risk. Cerebral palsy or spina bifida patients, not Down's patients, are at increased risk for falls. Shortness of breath can be a problem for cystic fibrosis patients who exercise.

59. I. Excessive twisting of the forearm causes lateral epicondylitis (tennis elbow); pain occurs over the lateral elbow where extensor muscles attach. The extensor carpi radialis brevis is torn at its origin on the lateral epicondyle. Extension of the wrist is compromised. In the chair-raise test, the patient puts his or her hands on the top of the back of the chair in front of the patient and lifts the chair. Patients with tennis elbow will have difficulty with this test. Treatment consists of rest, wearing a brace, and NSAID use, which provides relief for the majority of patients.

60. D. Osteoporosis involves a decrease in bone mass and is characterized radiographically by diffuse radiolucency of bone. It is associated with physical inactivity and aging. It can be caused by impaired synthesis or increased resorption of bony matrix protein. Fractures, especially compression fractures, which can cause kyphosis and shortened stature, are a hallmark of this disease. Patients typically have normal levels of calcium, phosphorus, alkaline phosphatase, parathyroid hormone, and potassium. Osteomalacia is vitamin D deficiency in adults. Bone and CT scan findings would not indicate pyogenic osteomyelitis. Scurvy is a deficiency of vitamin C. This vitamin is necessary for hydroxylation of proline and lysine in collagen synthesis.

61. A. Low thyroid levels contribute to a variety of symptoms seen in anorexia nervosa, such as bradycardia and hypothermia. Hypoalbuminemia and hypercholesterolemia are caused by protein deficiency. Patients who purge tend to develop hypokalemia, making them susceptible to cardiac arrhythmias. Gonadotropin levels are decreased, causing amenorrhea and decreased bone density. Starvation causes hypovolemia, leading to hypotension. IGF-1 stimulates DNA and collagen synthesis and decreases collagen degradation. Anorexic women are severely deficient in IGF-1, which increases with weight loss, improves with weight gain, and is correlated with bone loss.

62. G. Muscle mass and fat stores are equally lost in cachexia. In starvation, which can result in loss of bone density, muscle mass is proportionately preserved. The main cytokine involved in a cancer patient's cachexia is tumor necrosis factor alpha (TNF-α), which is produced by macrophages and inhibits lipoprotein lipase. TNF-α and -β are cachectins. Other cytokines, such as IL-1 and gamma interferon, act synergistically with TNF to indirectly promote cachexia. IL-1 stimulates other cells and induces fever. IL-2 stimulates cytotoxic T cells and activates NK cells. IL-3 stimulates hematopoiesis. IL-4 promotes B-cell growth. IL-5 is active in response to helminths via activation of eosinophils. Gamma interferon stimulates macrophages.

63. D. Type IV hypertriglyceridimia occurs secondary to alcoholism. In chronic alcoholics, the liver has a preference for ethanol over lipids as fuel, fat accumulates, and lipids are secreted in greater quantities. This hyperlipidemic state leads to fat emboli and obstruction of circulation to the femoral head, causing acute vascular necrosis (AVN). The femoral head bears great mechanical stress and is very vulnerable to AVN. Failure of full revascularization creates dead trabecular bone, which may include the subchondral plate, ultimately resulting in collapse of the femoral head. In type I, lipoprotein lipase is deficient and patients exhibit recurrent abdominal pain, rebound tenderness, and xanthomas. In type II, findings include xanthomas on the Achilles' tendon, corneal arcus, and recurrent polyarthritis. Patients with type III have claudication, elbow xanthomas, and hyperuricemia. Abdominal pain and peripheral neuropathy are seen in type V.

64. C. Energy for muscle contraction comes from ATP. ATP binds to the cross bridges between myosin heads and actin filaments. The release of energy powers the swiveling of the myosin head. Muscles store little ATP and so must recycle the ADP into ATP rapidly. Calcium ions are required for each cycle of myosin-actin interaction. Calcium is released into the sarcomere when a muscle is stimulated to contract. This calcium uncovers the actin binding sites. When the muscle no longer needs to contract, the calcium ions are pumped from the sarcomere and back into storage.

65. D. Being overweight exacerbates osteoarthritis once deterioration begins. There may be a relationship between obesity in women and osteoarthritis of the knees. The most effective way to reduce obesity is by awareness of food marketing practices, transportation patterns, and lack of physical activity and their influences on work, school, religious institutions, and health care facilities, especially in urban settings. Aggressive treatment of diabetes type II is for patients who are already obese; however, it is the obesity that is causing the knee pain. Follow-up of obese children is most effective when the program is family-oriented. Providing access to physical activity is one way to help reduce obesity but only addresses one facet of the problem. Reduction of alcohol consumption would reduce the occurrence of gout, but this is not primary prevention, nor is it relevant to the current complaint.

66. A. Ankylosing spondylitis is a rheumatic disease that causes arthritis of the spine and sacroiliac joints and usually affects adolescents and young adult males. It can cause inflammation of the eyes, lungs, and heart valves. It varies from intermittent episodes of back pain to a severe chronic disease that attacks the spine, peripheral joints, and other body organs, resulting in severe joint and back stiffness, loss of mobility, and deformity as life goes on. The cause is not known, but all of the spondyloarthropathies share a common genetic marker, called HLA-B27, that is used to make the diagnosis.

67. C. There are two initiating factors of diabetic ulcers: arterial occlusive disorders and diabetic neuropathy. These can lead to amputation of the lower extremity. In washing their feet, patients should test the water temperature first. Making it a point to wear well-fitting shoes prevents the breakdown of skin and protects it from shear forces. New shoes should be broken in slowly in order to prevent blisters. Checking oxygen saturation is a noninvasive vascular test to assess risk; use the toes, not the fingers. Using a mirror is a good way for diabetics to check their feet every day. Nails should be cut straight across to prevent ingrown toenails.

68. E. Causes of osteonecrosis include fractures, steroid use, vasculitis, and embolism. There is a correlation with osteonecrosis and meniscal surgery, but the cause of this is unknown. A subchondral infarct occurs most frequently with osteonecrosis, also known as avascular necrosis, and a wedge-shaped necrotic area is seen on x-ray. Replacement of necrotic tissue is delayed and may result in collapse. Joint replacement is often required to treat avascular necrosis. A patient with osteomyelitis would present with fever and acute onset. Hyperparathyroidism creates a "railroad track" appearance along the length of the trabeculae. A hematoma from ruptured blood vessels occurs after a fracture and the release of cytokines (PDGF, TGF, and interleukins) stimulates production of osteoclasts and osteoblasts. An osteoid osteoma with gritty tan hemorrhagic tissue is painful at night owing to the release of prostaglandins. Aspirin would relieve the pain from an osteoid osteoma.

69. D. This patient has Dupuytren's contracture, also known as palmar fibromatosis, which is seen more commonly in older men of European ancestry. It is rare in patients below age 30 and less frequent in women (M7:F1). This patient most likely has had the disorder for some time and waited to seek help until it severely hampered his lifestyle. Raynaud's disease (primary) is characterized by spasms of the vasculature. Raynaud's phenomenon (secondary), typically due to an autoimmune disease, is more common in women and may be seen in patients from colder climates. A trigger finger will click if there is enough force to move the tendon over the swollen sheath; the finger may extend or flex but will remain in position, and there may be pain at the base of the finger, unlike Dupuytren's, which is painful in later stages. A positive Tinel's sign reveals carpal tunnel syndrome, where flexion, abduction, and opposition of the thumb are all lost, as well as sensation over the thumb, index finger, and middle finger. In rheumatoid arthritis, there is symmetrical involvement, which may be accompanied by soft tissue swelling, vasculitis, pericarditis, or interstitial fibrosis of the lungs.

70. A. Dupuytren's contracture, a superficial fibromatosis, is a result of fibroblast deposition and collagen proliferation. Peyronie's disease is the penile equivalent. Glycosaminoglycan and collagen deposition occurs on the palmar fascia, where nodules proliferate, regress, and cause contracture of the fingers. IL-6 and TNF-α are acute-phase proteins involved respectively in opsonization and inhibition of lipoprotein lipase, causing cachexia. In Dupuytren's there is increased expression of PDGF, fibroblast growth factor, and TGF-β. Dupuytren's is more common in Caucasian males of northern European descent; Takayasu's arteritis is more common in Asian women. Nodular fasciitis is associated with immature spindle or stellate fibroblasts and develops rapidly, within a few weeks. This reactive pseudosarcoma does not recur, unlike Dupuytren's, which has a 50% recurrence rate.

71. A. Patients with Paget's disease are at high risk for developing osteosarcoma. Osteoblasts follow osteoclast resorption and create a disorganized mosaic of woven and lamellar bone. This leads to cellular pleomorphism and can ultimately lead to osteosarcoma. Laboratory tests may reveal elevated alkaline phosphatase without liver dysfunction, while calcium, phosphorus, and PTH levels are normal. Joints are typically spared. The tibia often looks bowed. Hearing loss in Paget's is due to temporal bone involvement. Bone thickening may cause narrowing of the spinal cord. Osteopetrosis is caused by osteoclast failure, while abnormal osteoclasts causing extensive bone resorption characterize Paget's. Osteomalacia is due to undermineralization of bone. Multiple myeloma appears as punched-out lesions on an x-ray. Blue droplets containing immunoglobulin, called Mott cells, may be seen in the cytoplasm of marrow cells. While IL-1 and IL-6 are osteoclast-activating factors, the cause of Paget's is unknown and the presence of these cytokines is only hypothesized. Osteoporosis is caused by prolonged negative calcium balance.

72. F. The outgrowths seen on x-ray are spurs, also known as osteophytes, and are caused by damage to the joint surface in osteoarthritis. Obesity is one cause, and Heberden's nodes on the DIPs and Bouchard's on the PIPs may be present. Abnormal curvature of the spine, kyphosis, and a Colles' fracture are seen in osteoporosis. A patient with gout, formerly called podagra, typically presents with an acutely hot and tender joint of the great toe; inflammation peaks quickly but may persist for days or weeks; the accompanying back pain is caused by nephrolithiasis. Fibroblast-like synovial cells degrade cartilage; they are seen in both rheumatoid arthritis and osteoarthritis but are more aggressive in rheumatoid arthritis. Many rheumatoid arthritis patients also express rheumatoid factor (anti-IgG Ab); muscle pain is a result of rheumatoid arthritis vasculitis; PIPs and MCPs, wrists, knees, elbows, and ankles are symmetrically affected; nodules are often found on pressure points. Renal disease in multiple myeloma is most often caused by Ig light chains; lytic lesions are seen on x-ray. Hypercalcemia may exacerbate obstruction of the nephrons and cause secondary osteoporosis. Prostate cancer is typically spread hematogenously to the axial skeleton and is detected on bone scan.

73. A. Renal osteodystrophy damages bones and joints in multiple ways. Retention of phosphate leads to low serum calcium levels and decreases 1-alpha hydroxylase. High aluminum content, sometimes found in the water used to prepare dialysis solutions, blocks deposition and results in osteomalacia. Beta$_2$ microglobulin, which is a component of amyloid fibrils and is normally catabolized in the proximal tubules, forms amyloid in patients on hemodialysis. Invasion causes destructive arthropathies as well as pathologic fractures. Chief cell hyperplasia is primary hyperparathyroidism, while renal osteodystrophy is secondary hyperparathyroidism. Patients with pseudohypoparathyroidism, called Albright's hereditary osteodystrophy, have round facies, short stature, and short metacarpal and metatarsal bones. For cell signaling, parathyroid hormone uses a stimulatory G protein, which increases intracellular cAMP. IL-2, which activates T cells, IL-5, which stimulates eosinophils, and gamma interferon, which stimulates macrophages, are involved in infectious processes, not bone resorption. IL-1, TNF-β, and TGF-β are cytokines involved in bone remodeling and may be implicated in osseous metastases of myeloma, lymphoma, and breast cancer. Patients with squamous cell carcinoma, typically male smokers, may have tissue that secretes PTH-related peptide and induces hypercalcemia. Biopsy may reveal the production of keratin.

74. C. This patient has Marfan's disease, which is the result of a defective fibrillin gene. Patients may also present with a pneumothorax, pectus excavatum, abnormally long arm span for height, arachnodactyly, or joint hypermobility. Progesterone and estrogen therapy may reduce the ultimate height of Marfan's patients. Testosterone injections to replace androgen deficiency are used for the treatment of Klinefelter's, which is caused by nondisjunction during parental gametogenesis and may result in gynecomastia, testicular dysgenesis, and mitral valve prolapse. Increased joint dislocations commonly occur in Ehlers-Danlos; patients have hyperextensible skin and joints. Duchenne muscular dystrophy, an x-linked recessive disease with defective dystrophin, results in fatty replacement of muscle, which presents as pseudohypertrophy of the calf muscles. Patients with Lesch-Nyhan syndrome, caused by deficient hypoxanthine-guanine phosphoribosyltransferase (HGPRT), are mentally retarded and display compulsive behaviors that may result in self-amputation of fingers, lips, or tongue.

75. A. Type I collagen is responsible for the formation of bone, tendons, skin, dentin, fascia, corneas, and late wound repair. Type II is found in cartilage, the vitreous body, and the nucleus pulposus. Skin, blood vessels, uterus, fetal tissue, and granulation tissue are made up of type III collagen. Type IV collagen makes up the basement membrane.

Chapter 9   Renal/Urinary System

Questions

1. A 27-year-old man with sensorineural hearing loss, cataracts, and a family history of nephritis presents for evaluation of hematuria. Examination of the heart, lungs and abdomen is within normal limits. Renal biopsy is performed. Irregular thickening of the glomerular basement membrane and splitting of the lamina densa is found. What is the most likely diagnosis?

   A. Alport's syndrome
   B. Goodpasture's disease
   C. Poststreptococcal glomerulonephritis
   D. Rapidly progressive glomerulonephritis
   E. Transplant rejection syndrome

2. A homeless 48-year-old man, a frequent visitor to the local emergency department because of alcohol abuse, presents again with similar issues. Today he complains of left-sided chest pain and decreased urinary output. His breath smells of alcohol. He also states that he was recently in a gas station while intoxicated. Laboratory studies reveal a serum creatinine of 2.8 mg/dL and serum blood urea nitrogen of 30 mg/dL. What is the most likely diagnosis?

   A. Bacterial cystitis
   B. Dehydration
   C. Ethylene glycol ingestion
   D. Fanconi's syndrome
   E. Pyelonephritis

3. A 40-year-old African American woman with a history of sarcoidosis presents to the emergency department complaining of left flank pain, nausea, and vomiting. On physical examination, cardiac and pulmonary findings are normal. She has left CVA tenderness. Urinalysis reveals microhematuria and crystals. A computed tomography (CT) scan reveals a left-upper-pole renal stone measuring 5 mm. What is the most likely explanation for these findings?

   A. Ammonium magnesium phosphate stones
   B. Calcium stones
   C. Cystine stones
   D. Ephedrine stones
   E. Uric acid stones

4. After a 3-hr football practice on a hot, sunny day, a player goes home and replaces more than the lost volume in sweat by drinking distilled bottled water. What will his volume and concentration status be?

	ECF Volume	ICF Volume	ECF Osmolarity
A.	Increased	No change	No change
B.	Decreased	No change	No change
C.	Increased	Decreased	Increased
D.	Decreased	Decreased	Increased
E.	Increased	Increased	Decreased
F.	Decreased	Increased	Decreased

5. A 3-year-old male child presents for evaluation of a palpable flank mass. The mass was found by the patient's mother while bathing the child. Physical examination reveals a 3-year-old who is severely behind in achieving his developmental milestones, suggesting mental retardation. Ophthalmologic examination reveals aniridia. CT scan reveals a left renal mass and a right-sided obstruction of the ureteropelvic junction. Which deletion of a tumor suppressor gene has been associated with this condition?

   A. BRCA-1
   B. BRCA-2
   C. p53
   D. WT-1
   E. WT-2

6. A 47-year-old man complains of gross hematuria for 6 months. He has worked in a factory on a mothball production line for 25 years and has a 40-pack-year smoking history. Physical examination of the heart, lungs, and abdomen is within normal limits. Urinalysis reveals hematuria, and urine cytology is positive for malignant cells. An intravenous pyelogram reveals a filling defect in the bladder. What is the most likely diagnosis?

   A. Pyelonephritis
   B. Renal stones
   C. Squamous cell carcinoma
   D. Transitional cell carcinoma
   E. Urinary tract infection

7. A 35-year-old man presents to his primary care physician for a follow-up evaluation. He has a history of diabetes mellitus and complains of generalized body swelling. Physical examination reveals edema of the lower extremities from ankles to knees. Urinalysis reveals elevated glucose. Serum glucose is 250 mg/dL. Blood urea nitrogen (BUN) and creatinine are within normal limits. Renal biopsy is performed (Figure 9-1). What is the most likely diagnosis?

   A. Acute renal failure
   B. Diabetic nephropathy
   C. Focal segmental glomerulosclerosis
   D. Goodpasture's syndrome
   E. Rapidly progressive glomerulonephritis

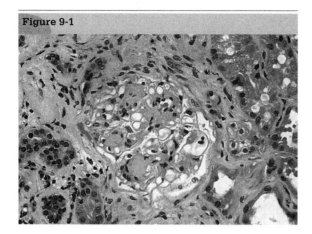

Figure 9-1

8. A 62-year-old truck driver complains of left flank and abdominal pain. She has a prior medical history of hypertension and diabetes mellitus. Physical examination of the heart, lungs, and abdomen is unremarkable. A CT scan of the abdomen reveals downward displacement of the left kidney and kinking of the left ureter with compression. What is the most likely diagnosis?

   A. Hiatal hernia
   B. Horseshoe kidney
   C. Nephroptosis
   D. Pelvic kidney
   E. Renal tumor

9. A 54-year-old patient complains of bright red blood (hematochezia) from his rectum but denies any prior history of blood loss or surgical issues. A colonoscopy is positive for multiple internal hemorrhoids. The patient asks why he has not had any discomfort or pain. You reply that a specific landmark separates the nerve innervations between the internal and external anus. Proximal to this line, there is no pain sensation. What is the name of that demarcating line?

   A. Crural line
   B. Dentate line
   C. Hilton's white line
   D. Sciatic line
   E. Toldt's line

10. The medical school anatomy group is dissecting the cadaver of an 82-year-old man who died in a motor vehicle accident. They come across a large nerve composed of tibial and peroneal parts. It is located between the ischial tuberosity and greater trochanter of the femur. What nerve is this?

   A. Hypogastric nerve
   B. Ilioinguinal nerve
   C. Pudendal nerve
   D. Sciatic nerve
   E. Superior gluteal nerve

11. A 28-year-old man, driving under the influence of alcohol and not wearing a set belt, is involved in a head-on collision with another vehicle. He is transported to the local emergency department, where he is given intravenous fluids and 2 U of packed red blood cells because of an initial hematocrit of 19%. Some 5 hr later, his hematocrit is at 33%. An infusion of isotonic sodium chloride with water is administered. His hematocrit is again taken 6 hr later and is 24%. Plasma protein levels are also decreased. What is the cause of the sudden decrease in hematocrit and plasma protein concentration?

   A. Autoimmune destruction by spleen
   B. Hemodilution
   C. Increased renal red blood cell excretion
   D. Shrinkage and lysis of red blood cells due to change in osmolarity
   E. Uremic pericarditis

12. A 3-year-old boy is brought to the emergency department with an acute onset, 1 hr earlier, of right testicular pain. His mother says he had been at on the playground when he first experienced this sharp pain in his right testicle. Examination reveals a horizontally riding erythematous right testicle. The left testicle is without injury and has a strong cremasteric reflex. What is the most appropriate initial step in the management of this condition?

   A. Antibiotics
   B. Doppler flow study
   C. Nonsteroidal anti-inflammatory agents
   D. Orchiectomy
   E. Watchful waiting

13. As a summer research project, a medical student is establishing a rabbit model to determine renal tubular dynamics. In regard to NaCl filtration and regulation, where is the site of glomerulotubular balance in the kidney?

   A. Collecting duct
   B. Distal convoluted tubule
   C. Proximal convoluted tubule
   D. Thick ascending limb (of Henle)
   E. Thin descending limb (of Henle)

14. A 32-year-old G2P1 in her twentieth week of pregnancy complains of voiding every 15 min, with a burning sensation. She denies seeing any blood in her urine and reports that she has had these symptoms for a week. Physical examination reveals no CVA tenderness. Urinalysis and culture are performed. Which of the following is the most likely cause of her complaints?

   A. *Escherichia coli* infection
   B. *Bacteroides fragilis*
   C. *Chlamydia pneumoniae*
   D. Nephrolithiasis
   E. Uremia

15. An 80-year-old retired worker presents to his local primary care physician complaining of having noted blood in his urine for 3 months. Physical exam reveals a well-appearing man who does not look his stated age. Other than a grade II/VI systolic ejection murmur (SEM), his exam is unremarkable. Past medical history is significant for non-Hodgkin's lymphoma. Which of the following is most likely responsible for his hematuria?

A. Complicated urinary tract infection

B. Cyclophosphamide use

C. Renal calculi

D. Renal cell carcinoma

E. Tuberculosis

16. A 22-year-old construction worker presents to his primary care physician because of gross hematuria with clots. His blood pressure is 160/98 mm Hg and heart rate is 82 bpm. Physical examination of the heart reveals no evidence of rubs, murmurs, or gallops. Pulmonary auscultation reveals no evidence of wheezes, rhonchi, or rales. There are decreased breath sounds at the bases bilaterally. Ultrasound is shown in Figure 9-2. What is the most likely explanation for this man's hypertension?

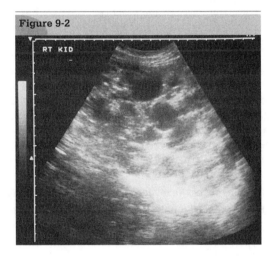

Figure 9-2

A. A defect in the PKD1 gene located on chromosome 16

B. Atherosclerotic plaques that partially occlude the lumens of both femoral arteries

C. Mutations in genes constituting the NC1 domain of type IV collagen

D. Necrosis and hyperplastic arteriolitis of afferent glomerular vessels

E. Defects in peripheral LDL receptors

17. A 40-year-old woman presents to her primary care physician complaining of irregular menstrual cycles. Physical examination reveals a blood pressure of 150/90 mm Hg. She has trunchal obesity, abdominal striae, and a round, moon-faced appearance. Serum glucose is 190 mg/dL. What is the most likely diagnosis?

A. Addison's disease

B. Cushing's disease

C. Cushing's syndrome

D. 17-Alpha-hydroxylase deficiency

E. 21-Beta-hydroxylase deficiency

F. Conn's syndrome

18. A 55-year-old man complains of malaise, fatigue, and flank pain. He presents to his primary care physician for further evaluation. He has a 35-pack-year smoking history. Physical examination reveals a palpable left flank mass. Laboratory studies obtained are shown below:

Electrolytes, serum

Sodium, serum	143 mEq/L
Chloride, serum	100 mEq/L
Potassium, serum	3.7 mEq/L
Bicarbonate, serum	24 mEq/L
Magnesium, serum	2.0 mEq/L
Creatinine, serum	1.0 mg/dL

Leukocyte count and differential

Leukocyte count	9,000/mm^3
Segmented neutrophils	75%
Bands	7%
Eosinophils	3%
Basophils	1%
Lymphocytes	27%
Monocytes	4%

Blood, plasma, serum

Alanine aminotransferase (ALT)	10 U/L
Amylase, serum	50 U/L
Aspartate aminotransferase (AST)	10 U/L
Calcium, serum	9 mg/dL
Glucose, serum	100 mg/dL
Hematocrit	55%
Urea nitrogen, serum (BUN)	10 mg/dL

Urinalysis

Urine pH	6.0
Red cells	25/HPF
White cells	2/HPF
Nitrates	Negative
Bacteria	Negative

Biopsy of mass histology shows polygonal cells with clearing of the cytoplasm. What is the most likely diagnosis?

A. Renal adenoma

B. Renal cell carcinoma

C. Teratoma

D. Transitional cell carcinoma

E. Wilms' tumor

19. A 29-year-old woman is pregnant for the first time. Her last menstrual period was some 10 or 20 weeks ago (she is a poor historian). She has a past medical history of seasonal allergies and recurrent urinary tract infections. Her mother has diabetes mellitus. Physical examination of the heart, lungs, and abdomen is unremarkable. Screening fetal ultrasound is performed and reveals both kidneys present and a distended bladder within the pelvic cavity. The most likely gestational age of this fetus is

A. 4 weeks

B. 8 weeks

C. 12 weeks

D. 15 weeks

E. 18 weeks

F. 20 weeks

20. Embryonic structures of the genitourinary system arise from the mesoderm and endoderm. From the chart below, select the appropriate embryonic structure and its correct male and female analog.

Embryonic Structure	Male	Female
A. Genital cords	Prostate	Gland of Skene
B. Genital cords	Cowper's glands	Gland of Skene
C. Genital glands	Testis	Clitoris
D. Müller's tubercle	Veromontanum	Veromontanum
E. Urogenital sinus	Bladder	Urethra

21. A 49-year-old man with a history of congestive heart failure, diabetes mellitus, and hypertension is hospitalized on the medical service because of an exacerbation of his lower extremity edema. Physical examination of the neck reveals jugular venous distension bilaterally. Cardiac and pulmonary examinations reveal bilateral rales. Lower extremities have 2+ pitting edema up to the knees. The patient is placed on intravenous furosemide in an attempt to reduce peripheral and central edema. Physiologically, which segment is most likely to have the smallest effect on reducing the amount of edema in the lower extremities after treatment with furosemide?

A. Collecting duct
B. Distal convoluted tubule
C. Loop of Henle (ascending limb)
D. Loop of Henle (descending limb)
E. Proximal convoluted tubule

22. A 38-year-old man undergoes an elective right inguinal hernia repair. He has no prior medical or surgical history. The surgical procedure is uneventful other than ligation of a neural structure overlying the spermatic cord. Postoperatively, the patient complains of decreased sensation over the lateral scrotum. Ligation of what structure is the most likely explanation of these findings?

A. Anterior femoral cutaneous nerve
B. Genitofemoral nerve
C. Ilioinguinal nerve
D. Posterior femoral cutaneous nerve
E. Pudendal nerve

23. A 67-year-old man sustains a gunshot wound to the left lower quadrant. Intravenous pyelography and CT scanning are performed and reveal a midureteral transection. Urologic consultation is obtained and the ureter is primarily reanastamosed with absorbable sutures. Blood supply to this segment will be maintained by which of the following vessels?

A. Anterior rectal artery
B. Anterior vesical artery
C. Lateral sacral artery
D. Lateral umbilical artery
E. Superior vesical artery

24. A 65-year-old man with a history of gross hematuria undergoes a CT scan. Findings include a 5- by 5-cm left-lower-pole

renal mass that enhances when the noncontrast images are compared with the contrast images. There is no evidence of thrombus in the renal veins or vena cava. There is no evidence of lymphadenopathy or pulmonary involvement. Left radical nephrectomy is performed. The specimen reveals the above-mentioned mass to be contained within Gerota's fascia, with areas of hemorrhage and necrosis. Tumor cells are likely to originate from which of the following structures?

A. Collecting duct
B. Distal convoluted tubule
C. Glomerulus
D. Loop of Henle
E. Proximal convoluted tubule

25. A 56-year-old telecommunications executive with no prior medical history complains of sharp, burning epigastric pain following a dinner with large shareholders who questioned the company's accounting practices. The man has experienced these symptoms throughout most workdays and much of his adult life but has felt that he controls them well with over-the-counter antacids. Although a full physical examination with lab work at a clinic for senior management revealed a positive urease test, the executive has not accepted pharmacologic treatment. Instead, he insists that a glass of nonfat milk and a piece of fruit keep him healthy. On the telephone with the company physician, the man does not report any fever, chills, or night sweats. Which of the following is the most likely complication of the man's treatment for his condition?

A. Destruction of the myenteric plexus of the esophagus
B. Elaboration of dilute urine with chronic inflammation of the kidneys
C. Hyperplasia of gastric glands secondary to ectopic production of gastrin
D. Metaplastic transformation of esophageal columnar epithelium
E. Pseudomembranous colitis with subsequent erosion of the colonic submucosa
F. Renal artery stenosis resulting from excess serum calcium

26. A 23-year-old woman presents to the clinic complaining that she has failed to develop pubic and axillary hair. She also complains of chronic headaches. Her blood pressure is 160/95 mm Hg. Laboratory studies reveal serum blood glucose of 60 mg/dL and serum potassium of 2.3 mEq/L. What is the most likely diagnosis?

A. Conn's syndrome
B. Developmental delay
C. 11-Hydroxylase deficiency
D. 17-Alpha-hydroxylase deficiency
E. 21-Beta-hydroxylase deficiency

27. Two police officers find a 27-year-old man found lying in an alleyway and bring him to the emergency department. Physical examination reveals cool, pale skin, rumpled clothing, a fetid odor, and matted hair. While checking his pulse, which is weak and rapid, the nurse notices what appear to be puncture marks at the tips of the man's fingers. Appropriate intravenous infusions stabilize the man over the next few hours. Which of the following are most likely to be found on further investigation over the next several days?

A. Contrecoup injury of the frontal cortex

B. Diffuse necrosis of the cortices of both kidneys

C. Eosinophilic proteinaceous renal casts resembling thyroid follicles on urinalysis

D. Foot ulcers

E. Ruptured berry aneurysm on cerebral imaging studies

28. A 56-year-old man presents to the emergency department with an acute onset of severe, colicky left flank pain that radiates down toward his groin. He is unable to remain comfortable and shifts his position frequently to relieve the pain. Physical examination reveals mild left CVA tenderness. There is no evidence of guarding or rebound tenderness. A CT scan of the abdomen is obtained (Figure 9-3). Should this patient have nephrolithiasis, which type of stone is most commonly found?

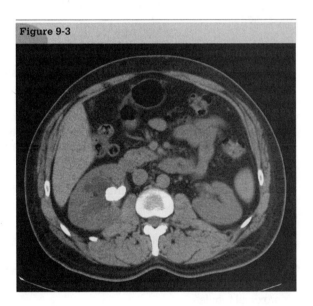

Figure 9-3

A. Calcium oxalate

B. Cholesterol

C. Cystine

D. Struvite

E. Uric acid

29. A 60-year-old retired railroad worker, having fallen down the front steps of his apartment building, is brought to the emergency department. On a skull x-ray, numerous areas of radiolucency are found. History reveals that the man has experienced periods of confusion, weakness, and lethargy that may have contributed to his fall, as well as recurrent bacterial infections in recent years. Subsequent lab work

reveals elevated levels of a monoclonal IgG in his blood and significant hypercalcemia. Which of the following additional findings is likely to be noted on further evaluation of this man's condition?

A. Cross-hatched fibrillary pattern on electron microscopy of glomeruli

B. Decreased serum levels of IL-6

C. Deposition of Bence Jones proteinaceous plaques on carotid arteries

D. Numerous cells containing Auer rods on peripheral blood smear

30. A pharmaceutical company is testing a series of compounds for potential use as topical analgesics. Laboratory data from a series of trials using paid subjects who are carefully monitored by an internal review board are shown below. Skin temperature is measured by continuous-feed thermocouple monitoring. Skin pH and sweat osmolarity are assessed by applying a neutrally moistened test strip to the surface of the skin after application of the compounds. Net (–) charge of basement membrane is measured by fine-needle aspiration of basement membrane after application.

Compound	Skin pH	Net (–) Charge BM	Skin Temp	Sweat Osmolarity
A	↑	↔	↓	↔
B	↓	↑	↑	↓
C	↑↑↑	↓	↓	↔
D	↓	↔	↑↑↑	↑↑↑
E	↓	↔	↓	↔
F	↔	↓↓↓	↔	↔
G	↓↓↓	↑	↓	↓
H	↑	↔	↓↓	↔

Subjects using Compounds A, B and E complain that the compounds sting excessively; they are therefore removed from the study. Subjects using compound H are similarly taken out of the study group after experiencing "nerve tingling." Assuming that a tolerable oral formulation may be devised and that its mechanism of action is identical to its topical effects, what potential side effect might be expected in patients who are prescribed compound F over a long time?

A. Ataxia

B. Clear cell renal carcinoma

C. Gross hematuria

D. Hemoptysis

E. Hydronephrosis

F. Proteinuria

G. T cell dyscrasias

H. Urethritis

I. Vomiting

J. Wire-loop effacement of glomeruli

31. A 58 year-old woman with well-controlled type II diabetes mellitus is enrolled into a clinical trial for an experimental drug (drug X) that increases sodium reabsorption and potassium secretion in the late distal tubule of the kidney yet does not impede normal hormonal feedback mechanisms for either electrolytes or glucose. Serum plasma and urine levels of this drug are carefully monitored and a titration curve is generated using experimental data over a period of several weeks. Which of the following statements best describes the behavior of this substance at plasma concentration below transport maximum in regard to renal metabolism?

A. Clearance of the substance relative to other substances may be described as inulin > drug X > K+ > urea > glucose > Na+.

B. Clearance of the substance relative to other substances may be described as Na+ > K+ > inulin > drug X > urea > glucose.

C. Clearance of the substance relative to other substances may be described as drug X > K+ > inulin > urea > Na+ > glucose.

D. Secretion of the substance will be inhibited by the relative hypokalemia induced by the drug.

E. Secretion of the substance will be enhanced by the woman's hyperglycemia.

32. A research engineer at a biomedical design firm has built a prototype of a device to filter biological fluids and maintain consistent levels of key metabolic substances. An experimental plasma analog (oncotic pressure 32 mm Hg) is channeled via metered valve (which prevents backflow) through a coiled 13-μm porous plastic tube at a pressure of 48 mm Hg and into a 200-μm-diameter nonporous pressurized chamber (40 mm Hg) composed of high-tensile-strength latex microfilaments. Inside is a second experimental aqueous solution of mouse anti–hRBC antibodies (oncotic pressure 21 mm Hg), which she has adapted for this study from another division of the company. Outflow from the coiled tube is collected in a sealed clear plastic graduated cylinder. In previous studies, the researcher has determined that both flow rate through the tube and size effects of constituent particles may be ignored. Furthermore, the antibodies do not fragment into constituent chains during experimental pressurization of the capsule, nor do they react with any of the other experimental fluids during any of the trial runs. What experimental results might be expected after a 2-hr trial of movement of fluid through this system?

A. Measured outflow in the graduated cylinder will lag inflow from the metered valve.

B. Measured outflow in the graduated cylinder will exceed inflow from the metered valve.

C. Pressure inside the chamber will increase by 8 mm Hg.

D. Pressure inside the coiled tube will decrease by 9 mm Hg.

E. Pressure inside the graduated cylinder will be 88 mm Hg.

F. Pressure inside the graduate cylinder will be 101 mm Hg.

33. A 26-year-old woman is brought to the emergency department complaining of blood in her urine. She informs the staff that she was playing her sport when her symptoms began. As part of a series of imaging studies to assess damage to internal organs, erect plain film intravenous urography reveals a kinked ureter with an approximately 2-cm inferior displacement of the kidney. Which of the following is the most likely causative agent?

A. Archery

B. Motocross

C. Sky diving

D. Soccer

E. Wrestling

34. A 26-year-old man is brought to the emergency department following a sports injury. As part of a series of imaging studies to assess damage to his spine, a plain film of the lumbar region is taken, revealing what appears to be a gas-filled segment of cylindrical tissue in the left renal fossa with a normal-appearing kidney and ureter on the right side. No additional masses are noted on this series. Which of the following pathological processes was most likely to result in this condition?

A. Chronic bacterial prostatitis

B. Chronic pyelonephritis

C. Failure of fusion of the paramesonephric ducts medially

D. Failure of induction of the metanephric vesicles

E. Persistence of the allantois

35. A 43-year-old man is scheduled to undergo significant reconstruction of his dentition following a motorcycle accident. Careful history by the dentist reveals that the man has been treated successfully for gout for the past few years and that he suffered from rheumatic fever as a child. What primary consideration must be given to this patient prior to undergoing his dental procedures?

A. Allopurinol must be stopped to prevent toxic nephropathy in the presence of nitrous oxide.

B. Penicillin V can be used for prophylaxis but its dosage must be increased because of increased secretion by the proximal tubule.

C. Penicillin V can be used for prophylaxis but its dosage must be decreased because of decreased urinary excretion.

D. *Staphylococcus aureus* osteomyelitis may be associated with termination of allopurinol therapy.

36. A 43-year-old man is brought into the emergency department after being involved in a motor vehicle accident where he lost control of his car and crashed head-on into a tree, sustaining an open skull fracture along with many lacerations. Careful history reveals that the man no longer has any urge to void and that a continuous dribble of urine may be observed from his penis. What part of the man's central nervous system is likely to have been affected by his injury?

A. Anterior pituitary

B. Inferior mesenteric plexus

C. Lateral spinothalamic tract

D. Posterior pituitary

E. Preganglionic fibers of the adrenal medulla

F. Superior mesenteric plexus

37. A 40-year-old man presents to the emergency department with chest pain, diaphoresis, headache, and anxiety. Physical examination reveals intermittent tachycardia, palpitations, diaphoresis, hypertension, and tremors. An initial cardiac workup with ECG, CK, CK-MB, and troponin enzymes is normal. CT scan of the abdomen is performed (Figure 9-4). In a 24-hr urine collection, vanillylmandelic acid is found to be elevated. Which of the following syndromes is most likely associated with this suprarenal mass?

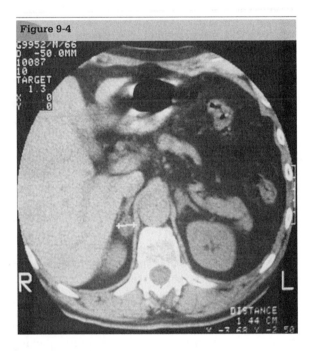

Figure 9-4

A. Carcinoid syndrome

B. Conn's syndrome

C. Sipple's syndrome

D. Sheehan's syndrome

E. Wermer's syndrome

F. Waterhouse-Friderichsen syndrome

38. A 39-year-old man is brought to a psychiatric unit by his wife, who explains that her husband, who is an air-traffic controller, has been drinking about 20 glasses of water a day over the past week. What is the most likely hormone to be found elevated on serum laboratory evaluation?

A. Aldosterone

B. Angiotensin II

C. Antidiuretic hormone

D. Atrial natriuretic peptide (ANP)

E. Cholecalciferol

F. Erythropoietin

39. A 16-year-old youth presents to the outpatient clinic for a routine high school sports physical. Examination of the heart, lungs and abdomen is unremarkable. Genitourinary examination reveals that the penis is uncircumcised and the foreskin cannot be retracted behind the glans. What is the most likely diagnosis?

A. Balanitis

B. Hypospadias

C. Epispadias

D. Paraphimosis

E. Peyronie's disease

F. Phimosis

G. Priapism

40. A 57-year-old man who has had a right inguinal hernia for 1 year elects to have it repaired. A third-year medical student is observing the case with the general surgeon. To begin the procedure, an oblique incision is made along the inguinal ligament. As the surgeon dissects through each layer with his scalpel, he begins to question the student on the anatomy of the region. In an attempt to remember the anatomy he studied 2 years earlier, he manages to recall the layers of the abdominal wall. Which of the following layers of the abdominal wall is the cremasteric muscle an extension of?

A. Antrerior superficial fascia

B. External oblique muscle

C. Internal oblique muscle

D. Transverse abdominal muscle

E. Transversalis fascia

41. A mother brings her 3-week-old infant son to the pediatric clinic reporting a new scrotal bulge that she found while changing a diaper yesterday. The infant is afebrile. Physical examination reveals a palpable mass in the scrotum while in the standing position, resolution of the mass in the supine position, and no transillumination of the scrotal sac. What is the most likely diagnosis?

A. Cryptorchidism

B. Direct inguinal hernia

C. Hydrocele

D. Indirect inguinal hernia

E. Varicocele

42. A 38-year-old man with HIV disease (secondary to intravenous drug abuse) and hepatitis complains of progressive fatigue and weight loss. He also has gross hematuria. Physical examination of the heart, lungs, and abdomen is within normal limits. Renal biopsy is performed (Figure 9-5). What is the most likely diagnosis?

A. Fanconi's syndrome

B. Focal segmental glomerulosclerosis

C. Hartnup disease

D. Membranous glomerulonephritis

E. Wegener's granulomatosis

Figure 9-5

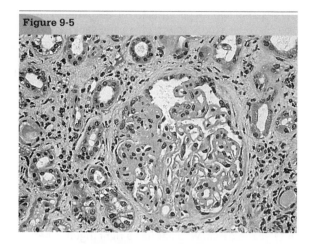

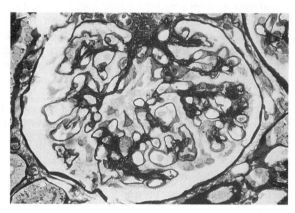

43. A 22-year-old woman visits her primary care physician with a 3-month history of nausea, vomiting, breast tenderness, and amenorrhea. Physical examination of the heart, lungs, and abdomen is unremarkable. Good bowel sounds are audible in all four quadrants. Peritoneal signs are absent. There is a firm suprapubic mass on abdominal palpation but no tenderness of the costovertebral angle. Urine beta-hCG testing is positive. Which of the following conditions is this woman at increased risk for over the next 6 to 8 months?

A. Bowman's space

B. Collapse of basement membrane with deposition of hyaline material in juxtamedullary glomeruli

C. Crescentic proliferation of parietal cells and accumulation of inflammatory cells

D. Duplication of glomerular capillary wall basement membrane

E. Hematuria and dysuria, with flank pain

F. Hypoalbuminemia

44. The permanent or definitive kidney arises from which of the following embryologic organs?

A. Mesonephros

B. Metanephros

C. Paramesonephric ducts

D. Pronephros

E. Telenephros

45. A 66-year-old man with a history of recurrent bladder cancer presents to his primary care physician for follow-up. He had multifocal transitional cell carcinoma resected transurethrally 3 months earlier. Which of the following environmental factors or chemicals is a known risk factor for transitional cell carcinoma of the bladder?

A. Aflatoxin B1

B. Beta-naphthylamine

C. Diethylstilbestrol (DES)

D. Chimney soot

E. Nitrosamines

F. Radon gas

G. Thorotrast

H. Vinyl chloride

46. A 57-year-old man presents to his primary care physician complaining of erectile dysfunction, which he has had for 3 years. He has no difficulty in obtaining an erection but loses it quickly after vaginal penetration. Physical examination of the heart, lungs, abdomen, and genitalia is within normal limits. The patient is given a prescription for sildenafil citrate (Viagra). What is the mechanism of action of this medication?

A. Beta$_2$ receptor agonist causing calcium/phosphatidyl-inositol system–mediated smooth muscle relaxation and increased blood flow in the corpora cavernosa

B. Beta$_2$ receptor agonist causing calcium/phosphatidyl-inositol system–mediated smooth muscle relaxation and increased blood flow in the corpora spongiosum

C. Phosphodiesterase-5 inhibitor that causes prolonged action of cAMP-mediated smooth muscle relaxation and increased blood flow in the corpora cavernosa

D. Phosphodiesterase-5 inhibitor that causes prolonged action of cAMP-mediated smooth muscle relaxation and increased blood flow in the corpora spongiosum

E. Phosphodiesterase-5 inhibitor that causes prolonged action of cGMP-mediated smooth muscle relaxation and increased blood flow in the corpora cavernosa

F. Phosphodiesterase-5 inhibitor that causes prolonged action of cGMP-mediated smooth muscle relaxation and increased blood flow in the corpora spongiosum

47. A 35-year-old man with a 3-day history of diarrhea comes to the emergency department. On physical exam, the only pertinent findings are dry mucous membranes and some abdominal tenderness. Bowel sounds are present in all four quadrants. The testes are descended bilaterally and are without masses. Complete blood count and serum electrolytes are within normal limits. In consideration of his presentation, which of the following will most likely cause a decrease in distal renal potassium secretion?

A. Acidosis

B. Alkalosis

C. Hyperaldosteronism

D. Loop diuretics

E. Luminal anions

F. Thiazide diuretics

48. A previously asymptomatic 45-year-old man presents to his primary care physician with a new onset of bilateral colicky flank pain and hematuria. Physical examination reveals hypertension and large palpable kidneys bilaterally. CT scan of the abdomen reveals multiple bilateral cysts throughout the renal parenchyma as well as renal enlargement. Which of the following is a possible complication that this patient may encounter during his lifetime?

A. Berry aneurysms
B. Charcot-Bouchard aneurysms
C. Epidural hematoma
D. Lacunar infarcts
E. Subdural hematoma

49. A 53-year-old man presents to the emergency department with a hernia of the lower abdominal wall. Anatomically it is classified as a direct inguinal hernia. Which of the following statements is true?

A. The hernia passes through the abdominal wall in "Hesselbach's triangle," which is bounded by the ilio-hypogastric nerve, rectus abdominis, and inferior epigastric vessels.
B. The hernia passes directly through the abdominal wall lateral to the inferior epigastric artery.
C. The hernia passes directly through both the internal and external rings of the abdominal wall.
D. Direct hernias more commonly occur in infants, owing to the failure of the processus vaginalis to close.
E. This condition can lead to damage of the ilioinguinal nerve.

50. A 62-year-old man is admitted to the hospital for diverticulitis after several days of nausea, diarrhea, and abdominal pain. Physical examination reveals an elevated blood pressure, orthostatic hypertension, tachycardia, a delayed capillary refill, and poor skin turgor. Serum BUN and creatinine are both elevated. On the basis of the following chart, determine the volume and concentration status of the patient.

	ECF Volume	ICF Volume	ECF Osmolarity
A.	Increased	No change	No change
B.	Decreased	No change	No change
C.	Increased	Decreased	Increased
D.	Decreased	Decreased	Increased
E.	Increased	Increased	Decreased
F.	Decreased	Increased	Decreased

51. A 57-year-old woman with a long history of hypertension presents to her primary care physician complaining of overgrowth of her gums. She is currently being treated with multiple antihypertensive medications. She also has a history of insulin-dependent diabetes mellitus. Her blood pressure today is 150/90 mm Hg. Physical examination of the heart, lungs, and abdomen is unremarkable. She does have

a liver span of 10 cm in the midclavicular line. What is the most likely explanation of these findings?

A. Amlodipine
B. Bepridil
C. Colchicine
D. Nifedipine
E. Trandolapril

52. A 63-year-old man has a chronic cough associated with chronic obstructive pulmonary disease. He also has hypertension with home blood pressures that ranges from 140 to 180 mm Hg systolic and 80 to 110 mm Hg diastolic. Physical examination reveals mild tachycardia without rubs, murmurs, or gallops. Which of the following would be the best antihypertensive agent for this patient?

A. Candesartan
B. Enalapril
C. Lisinopril
D. Moexipril
E. Trandolapril

53. A 50-year-old uncircumcised man presents to his primary care physician with a solitary, thickened, gray-white ulcerated and crusted plaque involving the skin of the penis shaft and the scrotum. His testes are descended bilaterally and are without masses. The prostate is 30 g in size; it is nontender and without masses. The remainder of his physical examination is within normal limits. What is the most likely diagnosis?

A. Bowen's disease
B. Bowenoid papulosis
C. Condyloma acuminatum
D. Erthroplasia of Queyrat
E. Fibrous dysplasia
F. Lentigo maligna
G. Paget's disease

54. A 35-year-old Caucasian man with a hepatitis B virus infection presents to the clinic with increased frequency of urination along with swollen lower legs. Exam reveals 2+ pitting edema of the lower extremities bilaterally. Cardiac examination shows no evidence of rubs, murmurs, or gallops. Pulmonary auscultation reveals no evidence of wheeze, rhonchi, or rales. Abdominal examination reveals mild hepatomegaly. Urinalysis revealed a protein level of 100 and a specific gravity of 1.060. The urine microscopy slide is shown in Figure 9-6. What is the most likely explanation of these findings?

A. Fanconi's syndrome
B. Focal segmental glomerulosclerosis
C. Hartnup's disease
D. Membranous glomerulonephritis
E. Wegener's granulomatosis

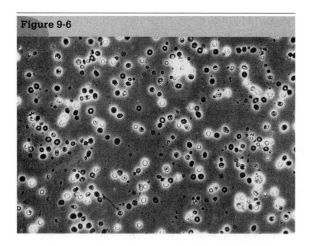

Figure 9-6

55. A 52-year-old man presents to the emergency department with an acute onset of pain, redness, and swelling of his first metatarsophalangeal joint. The remainder of the physical examination is within normal limits. Joint aspiration fluid reveals needle-shaped crystals with negative birefringence. Which of the following medications may the patient have taken prior to this incident?

A. Acetazolamide

B. Amiloride

C. Colchine

D. Furosemide

E. Probenecid

56. A 5-year-old child has new colicky abdominal pain with palpable purplish spots on his legs and buttocks bilaterally. According to his mother, he had an upper respiratory infection 2 weeks earlier. Physical examination of the heart, lungs, and abdomen is unremarkable. Bowel sounds are active in all four quadrants. Extremity examination reveals bilateral +1 ankle edema and arthralgia of the ankles and knees. Urinalysis shows microscopic hematuria and mild proteinuria. Histological examination of the patient's kidney would most likely show which of the following?

A. Crescent formation in Bowman's space

B. Dense deposits within the glomerular basement membrane

C. Fusion of foot podocytes

D. Mesangial deposits of IgA

E. Smooth and linear pattern of IgG in the glomerular basement membrane

F. Subepithelial humps

57. A 55-year-old woman with a history of mental retardation and seizure disorder presents for evaluation of a routine ultrasound that reveals bilateral echogenic renal masses. Renal biopsy is subsequently performed. Which of the following sets of biopsy characteristics would be linked to the increased incidence of renal cell carcinoma?

A. Closed cysts that are not contained within the collecting system

B. Large renal cyst

C. Multiple cysts, scarring, glomerular/tubular atrophy

D. Renal stones in dilated ducts, impaired tubular function, and small medullary cysts

E. Simple solitary renal cyst

58. A 3-year-old mentally retarded boy is brought to the pediatrics clinic because his mother feels something on his left side. Physical examination of the left eye reveals aniridia and a palpable smooth abdominal mass on the left side. Ultrasound reveals a solid mass arising from the left kidney. Chest x-ray is unremarkable. What chromosomal abnormality would you expect to find on chromosomal analysis?

A. APC gene mutations on chromosome 5

B. NF-1 gene mutations on chromosome 17

C. Rib gene mutations on chromosome 13

D. VHL gene mutations on chromosome 3

E. WT-1 gene mutations on chromosome 11

59. A neonate is evaluated immediately after birth. Physical examination of his heart reveals tachycardia and tachypnea. Abdominal examination shows that the bladder is exposed and everted on the lower abdominal wall. Which of the following additional anomalies would also be most likely be found in this patient?

A. Autosomal recessive polycystic kidney disease

B. Epispadias

C. Hypospadias

D. Narrowed pubic symphysis

E. Imperforate anus

F. Urachal cyst

60. A 65-year-old African-American man is referred for a urological consult for nocturia, urinary urgency, weakness of the urinary stream, an enlarged prostate, and serum prostate-specific antigen (PSA) of 27 ng/mL. Physical examination of the heart, lungs, and abdomen is within normal limits. Genitourinary examination reveals that the prostate contains a discrete, hard, nodular mass. Prostate size is 50 g. An ultrasound directed biopsy confirms prostatic carcinoma. Which zone of the prostatic parenchyma is most likely the site of the carcinoma?

A. Central

B. Peripheral

C. Periurethral

D. Transitional

E. Transcapsular

61. A 6-year-old boy is brought to his primary care physician because he has difficulty seeing the blackboard at school. He also has communication problems. Funduscopic examination reveals bilateral cataracts and lens discoloration. Cardiac, pulmonary, and abdominal examinations are within normal limits. The testes are descended bilaterally and are without masses. Urinalysis reveals microhematuria. An audiogram reveals bilateral sensorineural hearing loss. Which of the following would be seen on a renal biopsy?

A. Diffuse thinning of the glomerular basement membrane to < 225 nm

B. Foot process effacement

C. Kimmelstiel-Wilson lesions

D. Irregular thickening and splitting of the glomerular basement membrane

E. Wire-loop appearance

62. A surgeon who is performing an open nephrolithotomy for a staghorn calculus in a 37-year-old morbidly obese man makes an incision into a lower pole calyx. A preoperative x-ray of the kidneys, ureters, and bladder (KUB) is shown in Figure 9-7. If a probe were placed through the nephrotomy in the calyx, the most distal structure the probe would encounter is which of the following?

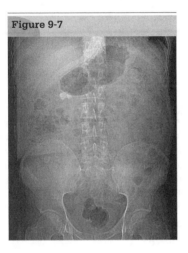

Figure 9-7

A. Column of Bertin

B. Cortex

C. Renal pelvis

D. Pyramid

E. Ureteropelvic junction

63. A 25-year-old man presents to the emergency department with hemoptysis and dyspnea. He has a past medical history of seasonal allergies and recurrent sinus infections. His past surgical history is notable for the repair of bilateral inguinal hernias. Physical examination of the heart, lungs and abdomen is within normal limits. Immunofluorescence reveals linear anti-GBM deposits. Which is the most likely diagnosis?

A. Alport's syndrome

B. Goodpasture's disease

C. Fanconi's syndrome

D. IgA Nephropathy

E. Wegener's granulomatosis

64. A 3-year-old boy presents with proteinuria > 3.5 g/day, generalized edema, hypoalbuminemia < 3 g/dL, and hyperlipidemia. Physical examination confirms generalized edema. Cardiac and pulmonary auscultation is within normal limits. Treatment with steroids leads to a complete recovery. What is the most likely diagnosis?

A. Alport's syndrome

B. Goodpasture's disease

C. Fanconi's syndrome

D. Hartnup's disease

E. IgA nephropathy

F. Minimal change disease

G. Wegener's granulomatosis

65. A 71-year-old man with diabetes mellitus presents to the emergency department with an acute onset of vomiting. Physical examination reveals a frail man who looks his stated age. His mucous membranes are dry and vital signs reveal a decreased blood pressure. The first test ordered by the physician is an arterial blood gas. Which of the following is the most likely diagnosis?

A. Metabolic acidosis

B. Metabolic alkalosis

C. Respiratory acidosis

D. Respiratory alkalosis

E. Respiratory arrest

66. A 50-year-old man presents to the emergency department with fever, weight loss, hematuria, bilateral pneumonitis, sinusitis, and hemoptysis. Nasopharyngeal examination reveals bilateral erythema and edema of the maxillary sinuses. Pulmonary auscultation reveals scattered bilateral rales. Which of the following is the most likely nephropathy?

A. Alport's syndrome

B. Goodpasture's disease

C. Hartnup disease

D. IgA nephropathy

E. Wegener's granulomatosis

67. A 28-year-old patient comes into the clinic with a recent onset of severe headaches and fatigue. His blood pressure is 160/100 mm Hg. Laboratory studies reveal a serum potassium of 2.6 mEq/L and decreased renin levels. Blood gas reveals metabolic alkalosis. CT scan reveals a nodular left adrenal gland. The kidneys are normal bilaterally with no evidence of stones, masses, or hydronephrosis. What is the most likely diagnosis?

A. Addison's disease

B. Conn's syndrome

C. Spironolactone overdose

D. Renal artery stenosis

E. Renal cell carcinoma

68. A 31-year-old man presents to the emergency department hyperventilating, and an arterial blood gas measurement is ordered. Exam is unremarkable besides the increased respiratory rate. When questioned about what caused his increased breathing rate, he responds by saying his roommate had given him some pills for a headache. Which of the following is the most likely causative agent for his symptoms?

A. Acetaminophen

B. Acetaminophen with codeine

C. Aspirin

D. Metoprolol

E. Morphine

69. A 45-year-old woman is scheduled for a left radical nephrectomy secondary to a diagnosis of left renal cell carcinoma. CT scan confirms the presence of a 7-cm left renal mass without evidence of vena caval involvement. There is no evidence of lymphadenopathy. What is the abdominal muscle on which the ureter descends?

    A. Gracilis

    B. Ligamentum flavum

    C. Psoas

    D. Quadratus lumborum

    E. Sartorius

70. A 36-year-old woman presents to her primary care physician with a complaint of feeling swollen and bloated. Physical examination of the heart, lungs, and abdomen is unremarkable. She does have some mild abdominal distension. Bowel sounds are present in all four quadrants. Peritoneal signs are absent. Her urinalysis reveals 5 g of protein, and blood tests show a serum protein of 1 g/100 mL and a total cholesterol of 270. Which of the following is likely to be the cause of her problem?

    A. Horseshoe kidney

    B. Nephrotic syndrome

    C. Potter's syndrome

    D. Renal dysplasia

    E. Renal ectopia

71. An 18-year-old woman is brought to the emergency department. She is thought to have a right renal vein thrombosis. In ascertaining a medical history, she reports being diagnosed with systemic lupus erythematosus and recalls being given steroids for her medical problem, which provided only minimal relief. She admits to having "some kidney problem" but is unable to recall the name of her disease. What is the most likely explanation of these findings?

    A. Alport's syndrome

    B. Focal glomerulosclerosis

    C. Membranous glomerulonephritis

    D. Minimal change disease

    E. Nephritis

72. A 17-year-old youth presents to his primary care physician for a follow-up examination of his chronic hypertension. He has had a 1-year history of gross hematuria that was evaluated only with ultrasound. Findings on ultrasound revealed bilaterally enlarged cystic kidneys of about the same size. His brother, sister, and mother have similar complaints and ultrasound findings. All have palpable kidneys on abdominal examination. All have serum creatinines in the range of 2.5 to 4.1 mg/dL. This patient later underwent a nephrectomy. Gross pathology is shown in Figure 9-8. Which of the following is a major concern for this patient and his other family members?

    A. Berry aneurysm

    B. Diplopia

    C. Diabetes mellitus

    D. Peripheral neuropathy

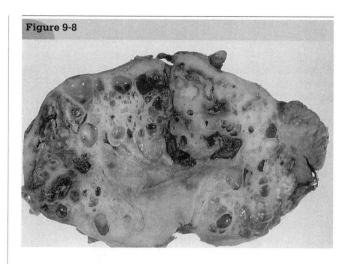
Figure 9-8

    E. Renal cell carcinoma

    F. Ventricular septal defect

73. A 23-year-old man presents to the emergency department 2 weeks after a tonsillitis infection, which resolved in its own. He complains of decreased urination, facial flushing and redness, and dark-colored urine. On light microscopy, the epithelial surface of the glomerular basement membrane shows protein deposits. Which of the following is most likely to have caused this situation?

    A. *Escherichia coli*

    B. *Entamoeba histolytica*

    C. Streptococcal impetigo

    D. Varicella

    E. Viral syndrome

74. A 17-year-old youth presents to his primary care physician with complaints of hematuria, facial flushing, headaches, and dizziness. Physical examination reveals bilateral palpable kidneys. While CT and labs are being ordered to confirm the suspected diagnosis, the primary differential diagnosis would include which of the following?

    A. Adult polycystic kidney disease

    B. Medullary cystic disease

    C. Medullary sponge kidney

    D. Simple renal cyst

    E. Tuberculosis

75. A 56-year-old man presents to his primary care physician complaining of fever, flank pain, and hematuria. He mentions being told of a chromosome 3 deletion but does not recall anything more. Laboratory studies reveal prominent polycythemia and pathology reports polygonal clear cells. What is the most likely diagnosis?

    A. McArdle's disease

    B. Peutz-Jeghers syndrome

    C. Turcot's syndrome

    D. Von Hippel-Lindau disease

    E. Von Willebrand's disease

Answer Key

1. A	**20.** A	**39.** F	**58.** E
2. C	**21.** C	**40.** C	**59.** B
3. B	**22.** C	**41.** D	**60.** B
4. E	**23.** E	**42.** B	**61.** D
5. D	**24.** E	**43.** E	**62.** E
6. D	**25.** B	**44.** B	**63.** B
7. B	**26.** D	**45.** B	**64.** F
8. C	**27.** B	**46.** E	**65.** B
9. B	**28.** A	**47.** A	**66.** E
10. D	**29.** A	**48.** A	**67.** B
11. B	**30.** F	**49.** E	**68.** C
12. B	**31.** C	**50.** B	**69.** C
13. C	**32.** B	**51.** D	**70.** B
14. A	**33.** B	**52.** A	**71.** C
15. B	**34.** D	**53.** A	**72.** A
16. A	**35.** C	**54.** D	**73.** C
17. B	**36.** C	**55.** D	**74.** A
18. B	**37.** C	**56.** D	**75.** D
19. F	**38.** D	**57.** C	

Answers and Explanations

1. A. Alport's syndrome is associated with nerve deafness, and ocular issues such as lens dislocation, and cataracts. Symptomatic nephritic disease with progression to end-stage renal disease by the early thirties is common. Alpha-5 chain of collagen IV is the mutation responsible for this syndrome. Goodpasture's disease, also known as anti–glomerular basement membrane disease, is caused by glomerular and alveolar basement membrane antibodies. Poststreptococcal glomerulonephritis is the classical presentation of nephritic syndrome. Most often, this complication follows infection with group A beta-hemolytic streptococci. Rapidly progressive glomerulonephritis is a nephritic syndrome that quickly leads to renal failure. Crescents in Bowman's capsule are a major histological finding. Transplant rejection syndrome usually occurs within the first 3 months of renal transplantation and is characterized by infiltrate of the interstitium and basement membrane.

2. C. This patient is exhibiting signs of acute tubular necrosis, which can be caused by a crush injury or direct injury to proximal renal tubules (high levels of mercuric chloride, gentamicin, or ethylene glycol). It is most frequently precipitated by renal ischemia secondary to hypotension and shock. This condition is reversible with dialysis, depending on the etiology. In the case of ethylene glycol, administration of ethyl alcohol will detoxify the kidneys and restore normal function. There is no evidence to suggest bacterial cystitis (no irritative voiding symptoms and no urinalysis provided that would suggest infection). Dehydration is unlikely in this patient with a ratio of BUN to creatine of 10 to 1. This patient has no evidence of Fanconi's syndrome by history (use of tetracycline antibiotics). Pyelonephritis is unlikely given that no urinalysis findings were provided and this patient does not have irritative voiding symptoms or flank pain.

3. B. Calcium stones are the most common stones found and are associated with hypercalciuria, hyperparathyroidism, malignancy, and the above three mentioned etiologies. Ammonium stones are radiolucent and usually formed secondary to infection (with *Proteus* or *Staphylococcus*). Uric acid stones are associated with hyperuricemia in 50% of the patients. Cystine stones are highly correlated with cystinuria or aminoaciduria. Ephedrine stones should be suspected in patients with a history of ephedrine abuse.

4. E. This is known as hyposmotic volume expansion. The football player has a net loss of NaCl without a net loss of water. The distilled water entering the extracellular space would increase its volume and decrease its osmolarity. As a result, water will flow from the extracellular fluid (ECF) to the intracellular fluid (ICF), thus increasing the ICF volume.

5. D. WT-1 is associated with the WAGR complex (Wilms' tumor, aniridia, genitourinary malformation, and mental retardation). WT-2 deletion is associated with Beckwith-Wiedemann syndrome. *BRCA-1*, *BRCA-2*, and *p53* are all associated with an increased incidence of breast cancer.

6. D. The classic presentation of transitional cell carcinoma (TCC) is that of a smoker with gross hematuria and no other symptomatic problems. Exposure to beta-naphthylamine or aniline dyes and chronic treatment with cyclophosphamide are also strongly connected contributory factors in this malignancy. Squamous cell carcinoma is usually associated with chronic inflammatory processes and *Schistosoma haematobium* infection. Pyelonephritis is associated with fever, increased white blood cell count, and infection. Renal stones would commonly present with lateral flank pain, possible family history of stones, and excruciating pain.

7. B. Diabetic nephropathy often shows signs of classic nephrotic syndrome. High urine glucose/poorly controlled sugars can suggest potential morbidities associated with diabetes. Renal biopsy may reveal an increase in the mesangial matrix, with resultant histologic changes such as diffuse glomerulosclerosis and nodular glomerulosclerosis (Kimmelstiel-Wilson nodules). Acute renal failure would not be accurate because this patient's BUN and creatinine levels are normal. Focal segmental glomerulosclerosis is seen in HIV patients and intravenous drug users. On light microscopy you see segmental sclerosis and hyalinization of the glomeruli. Goodpasture's syndrome is characterized by hemoptysis and glomerulonephritis (GN) with the classic IF finding of linear fluorescence and anti-GBM antibodies. Rapidly progressive GN is associated with renal failure, and you would see crescent-shaped GBM on LM. The slide from the renal biopsy shows the characteristic Kimmelstiel-Wilson nodules (rounded aggregations of hyaline) within the glomerulus, causing obstruction.

8. C. Nephroptosis is commonly found in truck drivers, motorcyclists, and horseback riders. This condition is caused by a loss of supporting fat around the kidney and causes the downward displacement. The ureteral kink/compression is caused by an aberrant inferior polar artery. Hiatal hernia is protrusion of the stomach through an esophageal hiatus and has nothing to do with this scenario. Horseshoe kidney is the fusion of the two lower kidney poles into one huge kidney and may also involve ureteral impingement. Pelvic kidney is caused by the failure of ascent of the kidneys, with one or both remaining in the pelvis. Renal tumor would not have the above appearance on imaging study and may not be associated with hydronephrosis.

9. B. The dentate or pectinate line is the demarcating line between the visceral and somatic nerve innervation. There is no somatic innervation above the dentate line and therefore no pain. Hilton's white line separates the internal and external anal sphincters and has no bearing on pain reception. The crural and sciatic lines are both nonexistent anatomy and have no physical location. Toldt's line is in the retroperitoneum.

10. D. The sciatic nerve, the largest nerve in the human body, is composed of both tibial and peroneal contributions. The superior gluteal nerve travels through the greater sciatic foramen and innervates the gluteal muscles. The pudendal nerve travels through the greater sciatic foramen and enters the perineum. The hypogastric nerve branches to the sigmoid colon and descending colon. The ilioinguinal nerve courses superiorly and anteriorly in the inguinal canal. It provides sensation to the lateral scrotum.

11. B. The "apparent" decrease of red blood cells is due to the addition of fluid into the extracellular fluid, which makes the concentration (hemoglobin) appear to be decreasing, when it is a dilutional change, not an empiric one. There would be no shrinkage and lysis of red blood cells due to the addition of the isotonic saline. Normal osmolarity will be maintained and there will be no shift, shrinkage, or lysis. There would be no justifiable cause for autoimmune destruction of the red blood cells based on the case presentation. There is no evidence to suggest either uremia or uremic pericarditis in this patient.

12. B. The diagnosis in this patient is testicular torsion. Typically you see a horizontally riding testicle. First step is to order a Doppler scan of the testicle to look at the blood flow. This is a surgical emergency calling for detorsioning of the testicle. Antibiotics are not useful because this is not an infectious process. Nonsteroidal anti-inflammatory drugs (NSAIDs) can be used for pain, but this is not first-line treatment. Orchiectomy is not the procedure of choice. Watchful waiting will cause the patient to lose the testicle, so it is not the treatment of choice either.

13. C. The proximal convoluted tubule is responsible for 67% of the reabsorption of filtered sodium, potassium, and water. There is an equal amount of sodium and water reabsorption, making this process isosmotic. The distal convoluted tubule is responsible for 5% of the sodium reuptake, the thin ascending limb for less than 1%, the thick ascending limb for 25%, and the collecting duct for approximately 3%.

14. A. This presentation is of a common urinary tract infection (UTI). *Escherichia coli* is the most common cause of urinary tract infections. Women are especially susceptible to this due to the short length of the female urethra in relation to that of the male. Pregnant women, owing to the physical presence of the fetus, are at an increased risk. Nephrolithiasis, also known as kidney stones, could present with similar complaints, but based on the patient's gender and age and no listed history of stones, UTI would be the most probable diagnosis.

15. B. Cyclophosphamide is one treatment for non-Hodgkin's lymphoma, and one of its side effects is hemorrhagic cys-

titis, leading to transitional cell carcinoma. Complicated UTI and renal calculi can present with hematuria, but the history does not support these diagnoses. One would expect to find flank pain on exam. Renal cell cancer does present with hematuria but is also associated with fever and a palpable flank mass.

16. A. A mutation of the *PKD1* gene is associated with about 85% of cases of adult polycystic kidney disease. This disease typically presents between the second and third decades with hypertension and gross hematuria. Progression to renal failure usually ensues. Atherosclerotic plaques are a likely consequence of this man's diet but they are unlikely to contribute significantly to his specific urinary symptoms. Antibodies to the NC1 domain of type IV collagen are implicated in Goodpasture's syndrome. Mutations of the genes coding for these proteins, however, are not involved in any of the polycystic kidney diseases. Fibrinoid necrosis is a consequence, not a cause of malignant hypertension. Furthermore, this patient's hypertension would not be considered malignant. Defects in peripheral LDL receptors are found in familial hypercholesterolemias, particularly type II. As such, they are unlikely to cause gross hematuria. The ultrasound shown reveals multiple bilateral renal cysts with kidneys measuring 16 cm in the longest dimension.

17. B. Cushing's disease presents with the classic symptoms of truncal obesity (along with buffalo hump and moon facies), hyperglycemia (secondary to increased cortisol production), and high protein catabolism leading to muscle wasting. All these features are attributed to an excess production of ACTH from the anterior lobe of the pituitary gland. Addison's disease is related to decreased function of the adrenal gland. Patients can be slow, sluggish, and have hypotension. Cushing's syndrome is attributed to an increase in ACTH production not related to pituitary disease. Such patients can have, for example, an oat cell carcinoma of the lung that produces ectopic ACTH. Deficiencies in 17-alpha and 21-beta hydrolase can result in ambiguous genitalia in the newborn. Conn's syndrome is associated with adrenal adenoma; it can produce signs related to hyperaldosteronism, such as hypertension, hypernatremia, and hypokalemia. Such tumors are often small (< 2 cm).

18. B. Renal cell carcinoma presents with the characteristics described in this case. It is the most common renal malignancy and is usually found in men between the ages of 50 and 70, with a higher incidence in smokers, and is associated with Von Hippel-Lindau disease. The occurrence of Wilms' tumor peaks at age 2 to 4 years, not in the mid-50s. Transitional cell carcinoma is most commonly found in smokers, but it is located in the bladder, not the kidneys. Teratoma is a neoplasm derived from all three germ layers, and is found in the ovaries/testes, not in the flank area. Renal adenoma is a pathological diagnosis. Most patients are asymptomatic.

19. F. This fetus is at approximately 20 weeks' gestation. The fetal kidney can reliably be detected at 15 weeks. Glomeruli and tubules develop from the metanephric blastema, while the ureter, renal pelvis, and collecting ducts arise from the mesonephric duct. The bladder starts to descend at the eighteenth week. By the twentieth week, the bladder is well separated from the umbilicus and the urachus becomes part of the medial umbilical ligament.

20. A. The embryonic structure of the genital cords gives rise to the prostate in the male and the gland of Skene in the female. Müller's tubercle gives rise to the veromontanum in the male and the hymen in the female. The urogenital sinus give rise to the bladder in both males and females. The genital glands gives rise to the testis in males and the ovary in females. Finally, the genital cords also gives rise to Cowper's glands in males and Bartholin's glands in females.

21. C. The ascending limb of the loop of Henle is impermeable to water. In this segment only sodium is reabsorbed, leading to a decrease in the osmolality of fluid as it exits the loop. In the proximal convoluted tubule, water and sodium reabsorption occur. Water reabsorption in the collecting duct is augmented by vasopressin. In the proximal convoluted tubule, sodium and chloride are resorbed along with water. The collecting duct is permeable to water under the influence of antidiuretic hormone.

22. C. This patient, who underwent an inguinal hernia repair, likely has damage to the ilioinguinal nerve. This structure runs atop the spermatic cord and can easily be injured in surgery of this kind. This nerve provides innervation to the anterior scrotum. Additional innervation to the scrotum is provided by the genital branch of the genitofemoral nerve, the posterior scrotal branch of the perineal branch of the pudendal nerve, and the perineal branch of the posterior femoral cutaneous nerve.

23. E. The ureter is a muscular tube that extends from the kidney to the urinary bladder. This structure is retroperitoneal. It receives its blood supply from the aorta and the renal, gonadal, common and internal iliac, umbilical, superior and inferior vesical, and middle rectal arteries.

24. E. Tumor stem cells can be considered to be developmentally based on the tissue cell in which they arose. Therefore kidney tumor stem cells are derived from proximal tubular cells. Bladder carcinomas arise from the basal cells, while testicular cancers arise from the germinal epithelium. Autosomal recessive polycystic kidney disease arises from the cells of the collecting duct. Inflammatory processes of the kidney often arise from the glomerulus.

25. B. Self-medication of peptic ulcers with milk and antacids is a significant cause of hypercalcemia and subsequent nephrocalcinosis. Calcified cellular debris helps occlude tubules and results in fibrosis and atrophy of nephrons. The earliest clinical sign of this condition is dilute urine. Excess serum calcium does not contribute to the formation of atheromatous plaques. In contrast, this patient's use of skim milk is likely to reduce his serum lipids and help to prevent such damage to his arteries. Destruction of the

myenteric plexus of the esophagus may result from infection of *Trypanosoma cruzi* but is unlikely to be affected by peptic ulcer. Similarly, Barrett's esophagus is more likely to result from long-standing gastroesophageal reflux disease (GERD). Although gastrin production may be elevated in cases of peptic ulcer caused by *H. pylori*, as suggested by the positive urease test, no clinical line of evidence points to ectopic production of the peptide in this patient. Hyperplasia of the gastric glands may result in Zollinger-Ellison syndrome. Pseudomembranous colitis is a complication of antibiotic treatment.

26. D. This patient is exhibiting the signs of 17-alpha-hydroxylase deficiency. Decreased levels of androgen cause the loss of axillary/pubic hair and hypoglycemia secondary to the decreased production of glucocorticoids. Increased aldosterone is responsible for the hypokalemia, as well as the current hypertension and related headache. With 11-hydroxylase deficiency you see decreased cortisol and aldosterone with increased sex hormones. Such patients present with masculinization and hypertension (due to 11-deoxycorticosterone). A deficiency of 21-hydroxylase presents with decreased cortisol and mineralocorticoids and increased sex hormones. Such patients look masculinized and are hypotensive. They have an increased renin level with volume depletion. Conn's syndrome is associated with elevated aldosterone level. Findings include hypertension, hypokalemia, and hypernatremia.

27. B. This patient has survived septic shock secondary to intravenous drug use, which creates profound venous pooling of the blood and hypovolemia in the absence of extravasation. Generalized ischemic infarction of the renal cortices is of paramount concern in such cases. A contrecoup injury of the cerebral cortex might be evident if the man had fallen suddenly, as might occur in an alcoholic patient. The case history suggests neither alcohol use nor a sudden fall. "Thyroidization" of the kidneys may result from chronic pyelonephritis. No evidence of such disease is apparent in this patient. Although many homeless people have severe problems managing their blood sugar, no evidence in this patient is suggestive of diabetes and subsequent ketoacidosis. Ruptured berry aneurysm is commonly seen as a complication of adult polycystic kidney disease and is unlikely in this case. Foot ulcers are uncommon in this situation.

28. A. Nephrolithiasis is most commonly caused (roughly 80% of the time) by calcium oxalate stones. Causes include idiopathic hypercalciuria, hyperparathyroidism, and alkaline urine. Cholesterol stones are the most common type of stone in cholelithiasis. Cystine stones, roughly 1%, are due to a defect in amino acid transport defects. Struvite stones, roughly 10%, are associated with urease-producing organisms such as *Proteus*. Uric acid stones, roughly < 10%, are associated with gout and states of high purine turnover.

29. A. Primary amyloidosis associated with immune cell dyscrasias is the most common form of amyloidosis (in the United States, up to 3,000 new cases are diagnosed each year). Renal amyloidosis is a serious and common association with multiple myeloma. Typical findings on renal biopsy are classic apple-green birefringence on staining with Congo red and a characteristic fibrillary pattern within the mesangium and subendothelium. Narrowing of capillaries by deposition of amyloid is apparent on lower magnification. Elevated levels of interleukin-6 (IL-6) are associated with multiple myeloma. Bence Jones proteins are, by definition, immunoglobin light-chain fragments found in the urine. Although these proteins are routinely found in the urine of patients with multiple myeloma, they are not normal components of arterial plaques. Auer rods are diagnostic of acute myelogenous leukemia.

30. F. The glomerular basement membrane contains excess negative charge as a means of preventing filtration of negatively charged plasma proteins via repulsive electrostatic forces. Any substance that reduces net negative charge of basement membrane, such as compound F, will allow filtration of proteins and thus result in proteinuria. Given that compound F seems to affect *only* the net charge on basement membrane, no other assumptions about its effects can be made with the information given. This style of question, in which seemingly overwhelming answer choices are present, is usually easy to answer if the single basic science question can be correctly gleaned.

31. C. The key to this question lies in understanding the fate of paraaminohippuric acid (PAH) as it passes through the kidney: filtration plus secretion from peritubular capillaries back into tubular fluid. The titration curve for the experimental drug is identical to that of PAH and thus, at submaximal concentrations, the drug may be assumed to have nearly identical clearance as PAH (i.e., higher than that of most other substances and a useful estimate of renal plasma flow [RPF]). The drug's action on sodium reabsorption in the distal tubule will not affect the clearance of the drug as long as normal serum electrolyte values are maintained, which can be surmised by the fact that normal feedback mechanisms are unimpeded by the drug. In essence, this drug seems to be an aldosterone analog and its actions will simply be compensated for by decreased secretion of the hormone by the adrenal cortex. Last, it is noted that the woman's glucose is well maintained; thus hyperglycemia and/or glucosuria will play no role in the drug's excretion.

32. B. Even in an artificial setting such as this, Starling forces determining glomerular filtration apply. Unlike a biological glomerulus, however, net flow *into* this manufactured capillary is favored by the following calculation: $(P_{GC} - P_{BS}) - (\pi_{GC} - \pi_{BS})$; substitution yields $(48 - 40) - (32 - 21) = -1$. Thus, fluid will flow from the pressurized chamber, or "Bowman's space," into the "capillary." The resulting outflow into the graduated cylinder then exceeds inflow via the metered valve. By carefully doing the math, one will quickly find that none of the other answers can be correct.

33. B. Nephroptosis, or downward displacement of the kidney with kinking of the ureter when the patient is upright, is attributable to deficiency or damage of supporting perirenal fat and surrounding fascia. Typically, this condition is found in persons whose occupations or pastimes call for excessive vertical jarring in a seated position over extended periods of time, such as equestrian team riders, motorcyclists, and commercial drivers. Sky diving, in which the person is free-falling much of the time, is unlikely to cause this condition. Soccer and wrestling, though fraught with their own orthopedic dangers, do not typically cause kidney displacement. Archery, in which the patient is standing most of the time, is even less likely to be damaging to the kidneys.

34. D. Induction of the metanephric vesicles results from failure of ureteric buds to develop and leads to either bilateral or unilateral renal agenesis. Cases are usually found incidentally and may involve the presence of the colon in the space normally occupied by the kidney. Unilateral renal agenesis is believed to be relatively common, but since most cases are asymptomatic, the true incidence is unknown. Chronic pyelonephritis and prostatitis may both result in hydronephrosis and scarring of the kidney, but these are not sufficient pathological processes to completely destroy the kidney. Persistence of the allantois leads to the formation of a urachal cyst, identified by urine outflow from the umbilicus. Fusion of the paramesonephric ducts leads to development of the uterus and vagina, and although they obviously have not fused in this male, this failure is unlikely to create any pathology.

35. C. With the patient's history of rheumatic heart disease, valvular defects must be considered and penicillin may be used as prophylaxis against bacteremia and subsequent recurrence of endocarditis. Probenecid, which inhibits the secretion of organic acids from the plasma to the renal tubules, was developed for use as an adjuvant to penicillin therapy. In this case, the man is already likely taking the drug as part of his gout treatment because it also inhibits reabsorption of uric acid. Allopurinol works by inhibiting xanthine oxidase and subsequent production of uric acid but has no significant nephrotoxicity. *Staphylococcus aureus* osteomyelitis may be initiated by seemingly innocuous bacterial insults such as dental work or even defecation, but it has no known association with termination of allopurinol therapy.

36. C. The lateral spinothalamic tract contains ascending fibers for bladder sensation that are brought to the spinal cord by the pudendal, pelvic, and hypogastric nerves. Lesions of this tract at any level above the sacral segments risk damage to these fibers and can result in the loss of the urge to void and overflow incontinence. Loss of upper motor input from the paracentral lobule via the corticospinal tract results in normal sensation but loss of control over voiding. The anterior pituitary and superior mesenteric plexus have no direct or indirect control over micturition. The inferior mesenteric plexus carries sympathetic fibers to the detrusor muscles, but damage to these fibers has no effect on the sensation of voiding or control of micturition. Preganglionic fibers of the adrenal medulla control secretion of catecholamines into the bloodstream, but loss of these fibers would have no effect on sensation of voiding or control of micturition.

37. C. The patient has a pheochromocytoma, a tumor derived from chromaffin cells that is characterized by excessive secretion of catecholamines, leading to hypertension, headache, diaphoresis, palpitations, and tremors. Diagnosis is by the finding of elevated urinary catecholamines (vanillylmandelic acid) in a 24-hr urine collection. Pheochromocytomas are associated with Sipple's syndrome, also called multiple endocrine neoplasia (MEN) IIA, or a triad of pheochromocytoma, medullary thyroid cancer, and hyperparathyroidism. Carcinoid syndrome occurs with about 5 to 10% of serotonin-secreting carcinoid tumors, which cause flushing, diarrhea, and right-sided valvular heart disease. Conn's syndrome is primary hyperaldosteronism, which presents with hypertension, hypokalemia, elevated aldosterone, and decreased renin. Sheehan's syndrome is ischemic necrosis of the pituitary secondary to hypotension from postpartum hemorrhage resulting in panhypopituitarism. Wermer's syndrome, also called MEN I, most commonly presents as tumors of the pituitary gland, parathyroids, and pancreas. Waterhouse-Friderichsen syndrome is acute adrenal insufficiency due to bilateral hemorrhagic infarction of the adrenal glands associated with a *Neisseria* infection.

38. D. Psychogenic polydipsia can result in a situation in which the water diuresis capability of the kidneys is overwhelmed and hypervolemia with dilution of electrolytes ensues. The increased volume increases stretch of the atria, with subsequent release of atrial natriuretic peptide (ANP), which exacerbates the dilutional hyponatremia yet ultimately helps reduce the hypervolemic state. Without dairy products and other sources of calcium and/or vitamin D in the diet, PTH will most certainly be elevated, particularly in children with significant bone growth demands. Hyopcalcemia may manifest itself as depression.

39. F. Phimosis is an acquired or congenital condition in which the foreskin cannot be pulled back behind the glans penis. In acquired phimosis, there likely is a history of poor hygiene, chronic balanoposthitis, or forceful retraction of a congenital phimosis. Balanitis is inflammation of the glans of the penis. Hypospadias is an anomaly in which the urethral meatus opens on the ventral surface of the penis. Epispadias is an anomaly in which the urethral meatus opens on the dorsal surface of the penis. Paraphimosis is an emergency condition in which the foreskin, once pulled back behind the glans penis, cannot be brought down to its original position. Peyronie's disease is a subcutaneous fibrosis of the dorsum of the penis. Priapism is an intractable, often painful erection. It can be due to intracavernosal injection therapy, sickle cell anemia, or hematologic malignancy.

40. C. The internal oblique fascia gives rise to the middle spermatic fascia, the conjoint tendon, and the cremasteric muscle of the spermatic cord. The superficial fascia consists of Camper's fascia, which is subcutaneous only, and Scarpa's fascia, which is continuous with the dartos fascia of the scrotum. The external oblique fascia gives rise to the external spermatic cord fascia. The transverse abdominal muscle fibers join with those of the internal oblique fascia to form the conjoint tendon. The transversalis fascia is continuous with the internal spermatic cord fascia.

41. D. An indirect inguinal hernia is the most common type of inguinal hernia in both males and females. It is due to a congenital patent processus vaginalis. Indirect inguinal hernias penetrate the abdominal cavity laterally to the inferior epigastric vessels, entering the internal inguinal ring and then the superficial external inguinal ring. Cryptorchidism is a developmental failure of the testes to descend into the scrotum. Direct inguinal hernias are acquired defects in the floor of Hesselbach's triangle, which usually occur more commonly in the adult population and are less common than indirect inguinal hernias. Hydrocele is a collection of fluid distending the tunica vaginalis and can be distinguished from a hernia when transillumination of the scrotum displays fluid in the tunica vaginalis. Varicocele is a dilation of the pampiniform plexus, usually due to torsion. It is often painful and feels like a "bag of worms" on palpation.

42. B. Focal segmental glomerulosclerosis is characterized by the sclerosis of some but not all glomeruli; in the affected glomeruli, only a portion of the capillary tuft is involved. The slide shown (Figure 9-5) reveals that the affected capillary loops have been replaced by collagen. This is also demonstrated by silver staining, which appears black. It is known to occur in the setting of HIV infection and intravenous drug use. Membranous glomerulonephritis is the most common adult nephropathy; 85% of the cases are idiopathic and the remaining ones can be caused by medications (penicillamine), infections (HBV, HCV, syphilis, malaria), or systemic diseases. Fanconi's syndrome is a manifestation of generalized dysfunction of the proximal renal tubules. It is characterized by impaired reabsorption of glucose, amino acids, and bicarbonate manifest as glycosuria, hyperphosphaturia and hypophosphatemia, aminoaciduria, and systemic acidosis. Hartnup disease is impaired renal tubular reabsorption of tryptophan, leading to pellagra-like manifestations. Wegener's granulomatosis is a necrotizing vasculitis with granulomas involving the nose, sinuses, lungs, and kidneys. It is classified as type III rapidly progressive glomerulonephritis (RPGN), also called pauci-immune nephritis, and defined by the lack of anti-GBM antibodies or immune complexes by immunofluorescence or electron microscopy. Most patients have classical antineutrophil cytoplasmic antibody (C-ANCA) in their serum.

43. E. In pregnant women, the enlarging fetus frequently compresses the ureters at the pelvic brim, leading to obstructed urine outflow and subsequent development of hydronephrosis. Simultaneously, however, increased progesterone *decreases* bladder tone, resulting in an increased residual bladder volume. Collectively, these factors predispose pregnant women to an increased risk of pyelonephritis. "Crescentic" proliferation of parietal cells and accumulation of monocytes in Bowman's space are found in RPGN. This disorder is characterized by extremely rapid loss of renal function and is not associated with pregnancy. Collapse of basement membranes with hyaline deposition in juxtamedullary glomeruli is characteristic of focal segmental glomerulosclerosis, which has known associations with HIV, heroin addiction, obesity, and sickle cell disease. "Tram tracking" (duplication) of capillary walls is the buzzword for membranoproliferative glomerulonephritis.

44. B. The metanephros or permanent kidney appears in the fifth week from both the ureteric bud and the metaneprhic mass. The ureteric bud is a diverticulum of the mesonephric duct that gives rise to the collecting system. The metanephric mass is derived from intermediate mesoderm of the lumbar and sacral regions and gives rise to the excretory units. The pronephros is a rudimentary and nonfunctional system that develops at the beginning of the fourth week and regresses by the end of the fourth week. The mesonephros is derived from intermediate mesoderm at the end of the fourth week, functions temporarily, and degenerates by the end of the eighth week. The paramesonephric ducts arise from the urogenital ridge epithelium and form the uterine canal.

45. B. Beta-naphthylamine is a known risk factor for transitional cell carcinoma of the bladder. The other options are risk factors for different types of cancers: aflatoxin B1, hepatocellular carcinoma; diethylstilbestrol (DES), clear-cell adenocarcinoma of the vagina occurring in daughters of patients who received DES; chimney soot, scrotal cancer; nitrosamines, gastric adenocarcinoma; radon gas, lung carcinoma; Thorotrast, hepatic hemangiosarcoma; vinyl chloride, hepatic hemangiosarcoma.

46. E. Sexual stimulation results in smooth muscle relaxation of the corpus cavernosum, increasing blood flow. The mediator of this response is nitric oxide. Nitric oxide activates guanylyl cyclase, which forms cGMP from GTP. cGMP produces smooth muscle relaxation. The duration of action is controlled by phosphodiesterase. Sildenafil is a phosphodiesterase-5 inhibitor that causes prolonged action of cGMP-mediated smooth muscle relaxation and therefore increases blood flow in the corpora cavernosa.

47. A. Acidosis, which decreases potassium secretion because hydrogen and potassium are effectively exchanged across the renal distal tubule's principal cell basolateral membrane. In acidosis, the blood contains excess hydrogen ions; this causes the potassium to leave the cell across the basolateral membrane in exchange for hydrogen ions, thus decreasing the intracellular concentration of potassium and the driving force for potassium secretion. Alkalosis increases potassium secretion because hydrogen and potassium are effectively exchanged across the renal distal tubule's principal cell basolateral membrane. In alkalosis the blood contains too few hydrogen ions, so these ions leave the principal cell across the basolateral membrane in exchange for potassium. As a result, the intracellular potassium concentration and driving force for potassium secretion are increased. Hyperaldosteronism increases potassium secretion because aldosterone increases sodium entry into the cells across the luminal membrane and increased pumping of sodium out of the cells by the sodium-potassium pump. Stimulation of this pump simultaneously increases potassium uptake in the principal cells, increasing the intracellular potassium concentration and the driving force for potassium secretion. Aldosterone also increases the number of luminal membrane potassium channels. Loop diuretics increase the flow rate through the distal tubule, causing dilution of the luminal potassium concentration and increasing the driving force for potassium secretion. Thiazide diuretics increase the flow rate through the distal tubule, causing dilution of the luminal potassium concentration and increasing the driving force for potassium secretion. Excess luminal anions cause an increase in potassium secretion by increasing the negativity of the lumen, which favors potassium secretion.

48. A. Intracranial berry aneurysms arise in the circle of Willis, and subarachnoid hemorrhages from these aneurysms account for death in about 4 to 10% of the patients with autosomal dominant polycystic kidney disease. Other extrarenal manifestations include liver cysts, mitral valve prolapse, and colonic diverticula. Charcot-Bouchard aneurysms are small arterial aneurysms, most frequently caused by hypertension; hypertension is often complicated by dilations at small arterial bifurcations. Epidural hematomas are intracranial hemorrhages commonly due to lateral skull trauma, resulting in a tear of the middle meningeal artery. Lacunar infarcts are caused by obstruction of small vessels and clinically manifest as focal motor or sensory deficits. Pure motor lacunar strokes often affect the internal capsule, and pure sensory lacunar strokes most often affect the thalamus. Subdural hematomas are intracranial hemorrhages that typically occur after head trauma, with resultant rupture of the bridging veins from the cortex to the dural sinuses.

49. E. The ilioinguinal nerve courses along the exterior fascia of the spermatic cord through the inguinal canal and can be damaged with herniation into the inguinal canal. The distribution of the ilioinguinal nerve innervates the scrotal skin, medial aspect of the thigh, and internal oblique and transverse abdominal muscles. Direct hernias usually occur in older men due to weakened abdominal wall muscles; they pass through Hesselbach's triangle (bounded by the inguinal ligament, inferior epigastric artery, and lateral border of the rectus abdominis). Direct hernias pass directly through the abdominal wall medial to the inferior epigastric artery and go through the superficial external ring only. Indirect hernias occur in infants due to the failure of the processus vaginalis to close. Indirect hernias pass through the abdominal wall lateral to the inferior epigastric arteries and through both the deep internal and external rings.

50. B. The patient is experiencing dehydration from several days of diarrhea, which involves a loss of isotonic fluid, also called isosmotic volume contraction. There will be a loss of ECF volume but no change in the effective ECF osmolarity. Because the ECF osmolarity is unchanged, there will be no change in the ICF volume.

51. D. This patient is likely taking nifedipine. This agent is a calcium channel blocker and can cause facial flushing, peripheral edema, gingival hyperplasia, and reflex tachycardia. It is useful in the treatment of vasospastic angina and hypertension. Amlodipine does not cause gingival hyperplasia. Bepridil is a calcium channel blocker associated with adverse effects such as agranulocytosis and arrhythmias. Colchicine is useful in the treatment of gout and does not cause gingival hyperplasia. Trandolapril is an angiotensin-converting enzyme inhibitor. Classic side effects include angioedema, agranulocytosis, cough, and hyperkalemia.

52. A. Candesartan is an angiotensin-receptor blocker. These agents have some advantages over angiotensin-converting enzyme (ACE) inhibitors because they are less likely to be associated with non–renin-angiotensin effects such as cough and angioedema. Therefore this agent is a good choice for a patient with a chronic cough. Enalapril is an ACE inhibitor used to treat hypertension. It is associated with risk of cough. Lisinopril is an ACE inhibitor with side effects that include cough. Moexipril is a long-acting ACE inhibitor that is also associated with side effects that include cough. Trandolapril is a very long-acting ACE inhibitor that is associated with risk of cough.

53. A. Bowen's disease is a penile carcinoma in situ and usually occurs in the fifth decade. It predominately affects uncircumcised men and is prone to involve the skin of the penile shaft and scrotum. Grossly, it usually presents as a single, solitary, thickened, gray-white opaque plaque with shallow ulcerations and crusting involving the penile shaft and scrotum. Bowen's disease evolves into invasive carcinoma < 10% of the time and is associated with an increased risk of visceral malignancy. Condyloma acuminatum are genital warts. Large conglomerations of warts are known as the Buschke-Lowenstein disease. Erythroplasia of Queyrat is penile carcinoma in situ of the glans penis.

54. D. Membranous glomerulonephritis is the most common adult nephropathy; 85% of the cases are idiopathic and the remainder can be caused by medications (penicillamine), infections (hepatitis B or C, syphilis, malaria), or systemic diseases. Fanconi's syndrome is a manifestation of generalized dysfunction of the proximal renal tubules. It is characterized by impaired reabsorption of glucose, amino acids, and bicarbonate manifesting as glycosuria, hyperphosphaturia, and hypophosphatemia, aminoaciduria, and systemic acidosis. Focal segmental glomerulosclerosis is characterized by the sclerosis of some but not all

glomeruli; in the affected glomeruli, only a portion of the capillary tuft is involved. It is known to occur in the setting of HIV infection and intravenous drug use. Hartnup disease is impaired renal tubular reabsorption of tryptophan, leading to pellagra-like manifestations. Wegener's granulomatosis is a necrotizing vasculitis with granulomas involving the nose, sinuses, lungs, and kidneys. It is classified as type III rapidly progressive glomerulonephritis (RPGN). RPGN is also called pauci-immune glomerulonephritis, defined by the lack of anti-GBM antibodies or immune complexes by immunofluorescence or electron microscopy. Most patients have classical antineutrophil cytoplasmic antibody (C-ANCA) in their serum. The slide shown (Figure 9-6) reveals dysmorphic red blood cells associated with glomerular bleeding.

55. D. Furosemide is a sulfonamide loop diuretic that inhibits sodium, potassium, and chloride cotransport in the thick ascending loop of Henle. In addition, it increases uric acid reabsorption in the proximal tubule, leading to hyperuricemia and acute attacks of gout. Acetazolamide is a carbonic anhydrase inhibitor; amiloride is a potassium-sparing diuretic; colchicine, which inhibits chemotaxis, is a treatment for acute gout; and probenecid, which increases renal urate excretion, is a prophylactic treatment for gout.

56. D. Mesangial deposits of IgA. The patient has Henoch-Schönlein purpura, which is a systemic childhood disorder often following an upper respiratory infection by 1 to 3 weeks. Clinically, patients present with palpable purpura on the legs and buttocks, arthralgia, gastrointestinal bleeding, abdominal pain, and IgA nephropathy. This last is characterized by mesangial deposition of IgA seen with immunofluorescence. Crescent formation in Bowman's space is a histological feature seen on light microscopy of rapidly progressive glomerulonephritis. Dense deposits within the glomerular basement membrane, also seen on electron microscopy, is a histological characteristic of membranoproliferative glomerulonephritis type II. Fusion of foot podocytes is an electron microscopic histological characteristic of minimal change disease. A smooth, linear pattern of IgG in the glomerular basement membrane is a histological pattern seen on immunofluorescence that is characteristic of Goodpasture's syndrome. The histological pattern of subepithelial humps is seen on electron microscopy in poststreptococcal glomerulonephritis.

57. C. Multiple cysts, scarring, and glomerular/tubular atrophy are characteristic of acquired cystic disease, which is associated with a higher incidence of renal cell carcinoma. Renal stones in dilated ducts, impaired tubular function, and small medullary cysts are associated with medullary sponge kidney and not related to renal cell carcinoma. Simple solitary renal cyst is an asymptomatic condition that is commonly found in adults. Closed cysts not contained within the collecting system are hallmarks of infantile polycystic kidney disease and prove fatal shortly after birth.

58. E. WT-1 gene mutations on chromosome 11. This child has WAGR syndrome (Wilms' tumor, aniridia, genital anomalies, and mental retardation), which is linked to WT-1 or WT-2 tumor-suppressor gene mutations on chromosome 11. Wilms' tumor is the most common renal tumor in children and is usually found between ages 2 and 7. An APC gene mutation on chromosome 5 is linked with adenomatous polyps and colon cancer; an NF-1 gene mutation on chromosome 17 is linked with neurofibromas; an Rb gene mutation on chromosome 3 is linked with retinoblastoma and osteosarcoma; and a VHL gene mutation on chromosome 3 is linked with von Hippel-Lindau disease.

59. B. This patient may have epispadias. Exstrophy of the bladder is a congenital ventral body wall defect in which the bladder wall mucosa is exposed. Epispadias and a widened pubic symphysis are constant features associated with bladder exstrophy. Surgical repair for bladder exstrophy consists of primary bladder closure, epispadias repair, and bladder neck reconstruction. The remaining choices are not associated with bladder exstrophy. Hypospadias is a urethral opening on the ventral surface of the penis. A urachal cyst is an embryological remnant of the allantois that has secretory activity resulting in a localized umbilical dilatation. An imperforate anus or lack of anal opening is a defect due to a lack of recanalization of the lower portion of the anal canal. Autosomal recessive polycystic kidney disease presents in infancy with progressive and often fatal renal failure.

60. B. The peripheral zone corresponds to the main prostatic gland and constitutes about 70% of the glandular tissue. This zone is most susceptible to inflammation and is the site of most prostatic carcinomas. The peripheral zone is palpable during the digital rectal examination. The central zone comprises about 25% of the glandular tissue and is not subject to inflammation and carcinoma. The periurethral zone may undergo pathologic growth in late stages of benign prostatic hypertrophy (BPH). The transitional zone frequently undergoes hyperplasia, which can cause obstruction of the prostatic urethra and lead to symptoms of BPH.

61. D. Alport's syndrome is a hereditary glomerulonephritis diagnosed in boys between the ages of 5 and 20. History reveals asymptomatic hematuria associated with nerve deafness, cataracts, and lens dislocations. Electron microscopy shows irregular GBM thickening and splitting. Thin membrane disease clinically manifests as familial asymptomatic hematuria and histologically as diffuse thinning of the GBM to < 225 nm compared to the normal 300- to 400-nm thickness. Minimal change disease histologically shows effacement of foot processes on electron microscopy. Kimmelstiel-Wilson lesions are nodular accumulations of mesangial matrix material seen in diabetic nephropathy. A wire-loop appearance is a light microscopic finding in lupus nephropathy resulting from immune complex deposition and gross thickening of the glomerular basement membrane.

62. E. The kidney is grossly divided into the cortex, medulla, calyces, and renal pelvis. If a probe is passed into the calyx, it will traverse the renal pelvis and then continue to the ureteropelvic junction (UPJ). From the UPJ, the ureter begins its descent into the pelvis to enter into the bladder at the ureterovesical junction (UVJ). The column of Bertin, renal cortex, and renal pyramids would be proximal to the probe in the calyx.

63. B. Goodpasture's disease, commonly seen in males between the ages of 20 and 40, is a glomerulonephritis with pulmonary hemorrhage and hemoptysis. Pulmonary involvement usually precedes renal involvement, which often results in rapidly progressive renal failure. Histology characteristically shows linear anti-GBM deposits on immunofluorescence staining. Alport's syndrome is a hereditary glomerulonephritis that affects males between the ages of 5 and 20. History reveals asymptomatic hematuria associated with nerve deafness, cataracts, and lens dislocations. Fanconi's syndrome is a manifestation of generalized dysfunction of the proximal renal tubules. It is characterized by impaired reabsorption of glucose, amino acids, and bicarbonate manifesting as glycosuria, hyperphosphaturia and hypophosphatemia, aminoaciduria, and systemic acidosis. IgA nephropathy clinically presents as benign recurrent hematuria in children, often following an upper respiratory infection. Wegener's granulomatosis is a necrotizing vasculitis with granulomas involving the nose, sinuses, lungs, and kidneys.

64. F. Minimal change disease is the most common cause of nephrotic syndrome in children; the peak age of diagnosis is 2 to 6 years. Light microscopy appears normal; however, electron microscopy shows fusion of epithelial foot processes. Treatment is with steroids, and patients usually recover fully. Alport's syndrome is a hereditary glomerulonephritis seen in males between the ages of 5 and 20. History reveals asymptomatic hematuria associated with nerve deafness, cataracts, and lens dislocations. Goodpasture's syndrome, seen in males between the ages of 20 and 40, is a glomerulonephritis with pulmonary hemorrhage and hemoptysis. Pulmonary involvement usually precedes renal involvement, which often results in rapidly progressive renal failure. Fanconi's syndrome is a manifestation of generalized dysfunction of the proximal renal tubules. It is characterized by impaired reabsorption of glucose, amino acids, and bicarbonate, manifesting as glycosuria, hyperphosphaturia, hypophosphatemia, aminoaciduria, and systemic acidosis. Hartnup disease is impaired renal tubular reabsorption of tryptophan, leading to pellagra-like manifestations. IgA nephropathy clinically presents as benign recurrent hematuria in children, often following an upper respiratory infection. Wegener's granulomatosis is a necrotizing vasculitis with granulomas involving the nose, sinuses, lungs, and kidneys.

65. B. A metabolic alkalosis is a process that causes a primary increase in bicarbonate; it is generated by either the loss of hydrogen ion or the gain of bicarbonate. Acute vomiting causes loss of gastric HCl, and this results directly in an increase in plasma bicarbonate concentration. The respiratory compensation for a metabolic alkalosis is decreased ventilation, which produces a secondary increase in $Paco_2$.

This mechanism produces up to a 0.7-mm Hg rise in $Paco_2$ for each 1.0-mEq/L increase in HCO_3. Respiratory acidosis is caused by hypoventilation, and one would see a decreased pH due to the increased CO_2 level. Respiratory alkalosis is caused by hyperventilation and leads to an increased pH and decreased CO_2 level.

66. E. Wegener's granulomatosis is a necrotizing vasculitis with granulomas involving the nose, sinuses, lungs, and kidneys. It is classified as type III rapidly progressive glomerulonephritis (RPGN). RPGN is also called pauci-immune glomerulonephritis, defined by the lack of anti-GBM antibodies or immune complexes by immunofluorescence or electron microscopy. Most patients have classical antineutrophil cytoplasmic antibody (C-ANCA) in the serum. Alport's syndrome is a hereditary glomerulonephritis diagnosed in males between the ages of 5 and 20. History reveals asymptomatic hematuria associated with nerve deafness, cataracts, and lens dislocations. Goodpasture's syndrome, seen in males aged 20 to 40, is a glomerulonephritis with pulmonary hemorrhage and hemoptysis. Pulmonary involvement usually precedes renal involvement, which often results in rapidly progressive renal failure. Hartnup disease is impaired renal tubular reabsorption of tryptophan, leading to pellagra-like manifestations. IgA nephropathy presents clinically as benign recurrent hematuria in children, often following an upper respiratory infection.

67. B. This patient likely has a primary aldosterone-secreting tumor, also known as Conn's syndrome. This patient is experiencing headaches and hypertension secondary to increased aldosterone, which increases Na+ reabsorption and increases the volume of blood volume and extracellular fluid. The increased Na+ reabsorption increases the secretion of K+ and H+, thus exacerbating the hypokalemia and metabolic alkalosis. Spironolactone, a K+-sparing diuretic, will be associated with an increased K+ level and gynecomastia. Renal cell carcinoma and renal artery stenosis are associated with hypertension, but this history makes these diagnoses unlikely.

68. C. Aspirin ingestion is associated with an increased respiratory rate (hyperventilation), which causes an elevation in the pH due to the decreased CO_2 concentration. Acute hyperventilation with hypocapnia causes a small early reduction in serum bicarbonate due to cellular uptake of bicarbonate. After a period of 2 to 6 hr, respiratory alkalosis is renally compensated by a decrease in bicarbonate reabsorption. The expected change in serum bicarbonate concentration $[HCO_3^-]$ can be estimated as follows: In acute hyperventilation, the $[HCO_3^-]$ falls 2 mEq/L for each decrease of 10 mm Hg in the $Paco_2$. (Limit of compensation: $[HCO_3^-] = 12 - 20$ mEq/L.) In chronic hyperventilation, the $[HCO_3^-]$ falls 5 mEq/L for each decrease of 10 mm Hg in the $Paco_2$. (Limit of compensation: $[HCO_3^-] = 12 - 20$ mEq/L.) Metoprolol causes a decrease in the pulse rate due to the blockage of the beta-receptor. You would then expect to see a decrease in the respiratory rate. Morphine, an opioid agonist, is associated with hypoventilation, therefore leading to a respiratory acidosis. Tylenol has no association with the respiratory rate.

69. C. The ureter, which is a muscular tube connecting the kidney and urinary bladder, traverses down the psoas muscle and crosses the common iliac artery at the bifurcation. The ligamentum flavum is located along the spinal column and has no bearing on the urinary system. The quadratus lumborum is located in the lower back but does not extend nearly the length of the kidney-ureter distance. The sartorius is located in area of the lateral to medial thigh and is not in any proximity to the genitourinary system.

70. B. Nephrotic syndrome is characterized by an increase in permeability of the basement membrane, which allows the loss of proteins (especially albumin) via urinary excretion. Generalized edema occurs from the decrease in plasma colloid pressure and resultant increase in fluid retention. Horseshoe kidney is more likely to cause urinary tract obstruction, secondary to physical impingement on the ureters. Potter's syndrome is a form of renal agenesis and associated with oligohydramnios. Renal ectopia, which is better known as a "pelvic kidney," would not necessarily cause the listed symptoms.

71. C. Membranous glomerulonephritis is a major cause of nephrotic syndrome, especially in the group comprising teenagers to young adults. Thickened capillary walls and basement membrane as well as a "spike and dome" appearance with stain are pathognomonic for this disease. There is also a 10% association with systemic lupus erythematosus as well as concomitant associations with hepatitis B, syphilis, and malarial infection. Focal glomerulosclerosis is clinically equivalent to minimal change disease but usually occurs in older patients. Minimal change disease is the classic presentation of nephrotic syndrome, with lipid-laden cortices and fusion of epithelial foot processes.

72. A. Berry aneurysm is commonly associated with adult polycystic kidney disease (ADPKD). It is important to check for this aneurysm when a diagnosis of APKD is made. The disease commonly appears from the midteens to the early thirties, although the condition appears at birth. Diplopia, ventricular septal defect, and peripheral neuropathy have no connection with the symptoms listed in the question. Diabetes mellitus and renal cell carcinoma can be considered due to the progression of kidney failure, but there were no indications suggesting these diagnoses. The gross specimen shows an enlarged kidney with multiple cysts of different sizes. Some of these cysts are hemorrhagic.

73. C. This is most likely descriptive of poststreptococcal glomerulonephritis, which is commonly found concurrent with or just after an infection with group A β-hemolytic streptococci. Most children and adults recover completely; labs will show decreased C3 and increased ASO levels. Light microscopy shows a "lumpy bumpy" pattern. *Escherichia coli* tends to be more of a urinary tract-based clinical infection, with increased frequency, dysuria, and a burning sensation. *Entamoeba histolytica* is a gastrointestinally based disorder, causing digestive problems and dysentery; it has no relation to the presented genitourinary issues. Varicella, classically known as chickenpox, has no correlation with the presented conditions.

74. A. Autosomal dominant polycystic kidney disease (APKD) usually appears between the midteens and late twenties and is the most common inherited kidney disorder. It occurs bilaterally, with notable enlargement of both kidneys. Simple renal cysts tend to be asymptomatic; therefore the clinical presentation would be more indicative of a different issue. Medullary cystic disease usually occurs in older children, not young adults. Medullary sponge kidney presents with small kidney cysts but not renal failure.

75. D. Von Hippel-Lindau disease is strongly associated with a deletion on chromosome 3 and with renal cell carcinoma. Based on his clinical and pathological presentation, both conditions exist in this patient. McArdle's disease is characterized by a deficiency in muscle phosphorylase, with glycogen accumulation in skeletal muscle as well as muscle weakness cramping after exercise. Peutz-Jeghers disease is clinically noted by darkening of the lips, hands, and genitalia along with benign hamartomatous polyps and not associated with any changes in chromosomal 3. Turcot's syndrome is characterized by multiple adenomatous polyps and tumors affecting the central nervous system. It has no known correlation with chromosome 3.

Chapter 10 Reproductive System

Questions

1. A 25-year-old G1P1001 with no major health problems presents to her primary care physician requesting information on oral contraceptives. Physical examination of the heart, lungs, and abdomen is within normal limits. A pill that has a large estrogen component is suggested. How does this pill most effectively help to avoid pregnancy in this woman?

   A. Blocking of endometrial proliferation, thereby impeding implantation

   B. By causing the cervical mucus to be more viscous, slowing sperm transport

   C. By decreasing menstrual blood flow

   D. Decreasing LH production

   E. Prevention of FSH production

2. A 56-year-old woman presents to her primary care physician with a recent onset of hot flashes and irregular menses for several months. She is a nonsmoker. Her body mass index (BMI) is 32. She states that she has become quite irritable recently in the presence of her husband of 32 years. She has not had any recent visual changes and no change in basal body temperature (BBT). You advise her to discontinue her hormone replacement therapy regimen and return in 8 to 12 days for a blood draw. Laboratory studies obtained reveal that her FSH level is 48 mIU/mL and her LH level is 32 mIU/mL. What is the most likely explanation of these findings?

   A. Chromophobic pituitary adenoma

   B. Decreased production of inhibin by atrophic ovaries

   C. Lack of direct feedback inhibition on the pituitary from decreased progesterone levels

   D. Menopausally mediated increase of pituitary releasing hormones from the hypothalamus

   E. Stimulation of FSH production by increased levels of estrone derived from adipocytes

3. A 26-year-old G0P0 presents to her primary care physician complaining of a bilateral nipple discharge that she describes as milky and sticky. She has been having this problem for 4 weeks, and it seems to be getting worse. She states that her menses have been of normal timing, duration, and quality, with her last menstrual period having occurred 6 days earlier. Urine beta-HCG is negative, and lab studies reveal a serum prolactin of 45 ng/mL and TSH 7 IU/mL. What is the most likely explanation for her nipple discharge?

   A. In situ ductal carcinoma

   B. Mammary duct ectasia

   C. Metochlopramide being taken for gastric stasis

   D. Secondary hypothyroidism

   E. Solitary pituitary adenoma

4. A 78-year-old woman presents to her family physician complaining of dysuria. She has no prior medical or surgical history. Physical examination is performed. The physician asks the patient to perform the Valsalva maneuver. Upon doing this, the cervix descends to protrude into the vagina. What is the most likely cause?

   A. Age-related laxity of the broad and round ovarian ligaments

   B. Endometrial hyperplasia

   C. Fecal impaction of the sigmoid colon

   D. Nulliparity

   E. Tear in the urogenital diaphragm

5. A 35-year-old G2P1001 in her forty-second week of gestation undergoes a cesarean section for a fetus weighing approximately 4500 g. Her prenatal care was up to date and unremarkable other than for some mild proteinuria during weeks 16 to 22 of her pregnancy. What defect is she at highest risk for developing during her next pregnancy?

   A. Abruptio placentae

   B. Brenner tumor

   C. Chorioamnionitis

   D. Disseminated intravascular coagulation

   E. Hydatidiform mole

   F. Mature teratoma (dermoid cyst)

   G. Placenta accreta

   H. Preeclampsia

6. An 82-year-old man receives a prostate examination by his primary care physician; it appears abnormal. On further clinical workup, it is found that he has an increased total PSA with a decreased fraction of free PSA. In which zone of the prostate is the lesion most likely located?

   A. Central zone

   B. Inferior zone

   C. Peripheral zone

   D. Periurethral zone

   E. Transitional zone

7. A 3-year-old boy is diagnosed with a malignant germ cell tumor, which is later determined to be the most common testicular tumor of infancy and early childhood. Which of the following hormones will be elevated in this tumor?

   A. Alpha-fetoprotein (AFP)

   B. Follicle-stimulating hormone (FSH)

   C. Human chorionic gonadotropin (hCG)

   D. Luteinizing hormone (LH)

   E. Thyroid-stimulating hormone (TSH)

8. A 70-year-old woman presents to her family physician complaining of a constant bloody vaginal discharge, which she has had for 3 months. Physical examination reveals a mass on the posterior wall of the vaginal fornix. A biopsy of the mass is obtained, and the pathology report suggests potentially metastatic squamous cell carcinoma of the vagina. Considering the location of the lesion, to which lymph nodes are the malignant cells most likely to metastasize first?

A. Deep inguinal

B. External iliac

C. Internal iliac

D. Superficial inguinal

E. Superficial internal pudendal

9. A 17-year-old girl presents to her family physician requesting a prescription for an oral contraceptive. Pelvic examination reveals vaginal inflammation. Biopsy is performed and reveals areas of columnar epithelium within the normal vaginal stratified squamous epithelium. What is the most likely etiologic agent(s) of this condition?

A. Contraceptive use by the mother during the pregnancy

B. Multiparity

C. Multiple sexual partners

D. Nulliparity

E. Use of superabsorbent tampons

10. A 31-year-old woman with a 3-year history of infertility has been determined to have persistent anovulatory cycles. You wish to treat this by giving her an estrogen receptor antagonist, thereby reducing suppression of the hypothalamic-pituitary axis. Which of the following medications could most specifically accomplish this?

A. Clomiphene

B. Danazol

C. Norgestrel

D. Raloxifene

E. Tamoxifen

11. A medical student is observing while the attending performs a pelvic examination on a nulligravida 16-year-old who has asked for oral contraceptives. In the process, a 0.6-cm firm white plaque is found on the left labia majora (see Figure 10-1). The lesion is biopsied and the pathology report reveals koilocytosis. What is the likely explanation for this finding?

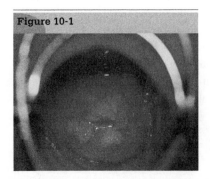

Figure 10-1

A. Condyloma acuminatum

B. Condyloma latum

C. Lichen sclerosus

D. Vaginal candidiasis

E. Vaginal adenosis

12. Which of the following poses the greatest risk of malignancy in an otherwise healthy 30-year-old woman?

A. Adenomyosis

B. Immature teratoma

C. Infection with HPV type II

D. Leiomyoma

E. Mature teratoma

13. A 23-year-old man presents to his primary care physician having been diagnosed with bilateral orchitis. Physical examination of the scrotum reveals erythema and edema. Both testicles are indurated. Urinalysis is normal. What is the most likely etiology of this condition?

A. Epstein-Barr virus

B. Herpes simplex II

C. Herpes zoster

D. Mumps virus

E. Varicella virus

14. A 39-year-old woman undergoes bilateral mastectomy after a diagnosis of infiltrating ductal carcinoma. Her mother, aunt, and three other relatives have had similar procedures performed, also in attempts to treat infiltrating ductal carcinoma in one or both breasts. Which of the following is the most likely etiology of the cancer in this woman?

A. A decrease in the expression of the c-erb allele

B. A mutant p53 allele

C. A mutant Rb allele

D. Expansion of a CCG trinucleotide repeat

E. Loss of a specific enzyme in the excision repair system

15. A 28-year-old woman presents to her primary care physician complaining of abdominal bloating coincident with her menses. Her physician notes a nodular texture of the uterus on bimanual examination, and ultrasound shows several asymmetric masses within and radiating from the uterine corpus on the left. Serum pregnancy test results are negative. What is the most likely explanation for this finding?

A. Adenomyosis

B. Endometrial hyperplasia

C. Endometriosis

D. Leiomyoma

E. Molar pregnancy

16. A 13-year-old girl presents to her family physician for her first pelvic examination. Physical examination reveals an overgrowth of the anterior vaginal fornix such that it obstructs the cervical os. Which of the following anatomical structures is responsible for the development of this portion of the vagina?

A. Paramesonephric ducts

B. Sinovaginal bulbs

C. Ureterovesical pouch

D. Urogenital sinus

E. Urogenital triangle

17. A 34-year-old G3P3003 presents to the pediatrician with her 3-year-old child. The mother is concerned that her son's testicles have yet to descend. Physical examination reveals bilateral undescended testicles, an empty scrotum, and a severely underdeveloped penis. An ultrasound of the abdomen reveals bilateral ovaries and the absence of testicles. What is the most likely cause of this condition?

A. Inadequate production of androgenic hormones by the adrenal gland

B. Inhibition of the enzymes needed for 21-hydroxylation

C. A lack of receptors for dihydrotestosterone on peripheral tissues

D. A karyotype of XO

E. Point mutations in the SRY gene

18. A 26-year-old G1P0 presents during her twenty-first week of pregnancy for a routine visit. She expresses extreme concern however, that her child may have a congenital anomaly, specifically Down's syndrome, despite the fact that she is at relatively low risk for this. She requests amniocentesis to assess the possibility. The physician explains that there are other techniques by which this may be ascertained, such as AFP levels, which can be measured much less invasively. He then adds that amniocentesis at this age presents much greater risk than benefit and that the chance of fetal compromise is large. The mother, however, insists that amniocentesis must be done as soon as possible and without further discussion. What should the physician do next?

A. Proceed with plans for the woman to undergo amniocentesis.

B. Refer the patient to a psychiatrist to further evaluate her desire to have this procedure performed.

C. Refuse to perform amniocentesis, and instead once again offer AFP screening.

D. Wait until a more favorable gestational age is reached and then perform amniocentesis.

E. Refer the patient to a tertiary care center.

19. A 36-year-old woman presents to her primary care physician with a complaint of persistent abdominal pain. She has had no change in her menses and no vaginal discharge; however, she has noticed a recent increase in her waist size. Abdominal examination reveals a solid mass just left of midline that is nontender to palpation. Abdominal x-ray is ordered; the film is shown below (Figure 10-2). What is the most likely diagnosis?

A. Adenocarcinoma

B. Choriocarcinoma

C. Granulosa cell tumor

D. Mature teratoma

E. Sertoli-Leydig cell tumor

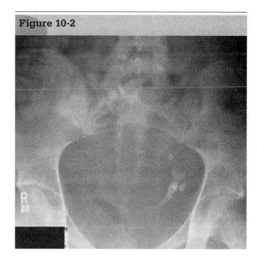

Figure 10-2

20. A 32-year-old man with a right testicular mass undergoes radical inguinal orchiectomy. Pathology reveals a seminomatous germ cell tumor. Which of the following statements is true of a seminoma?

A. It is a premalignant lesion.

B. It is analogous to teratoma, a tumor of the ovary.

C. It is the most common germ cell tumor, accounting for over 90%.

D. It is often associated with increased levels of follicle-stimulating hormone (FSH) or luteinizing hormone (LH).

E. It is very radiosensitive.

21. A 24-year-old woman who is approaching her fortieth week of gestation has not seen a physician since the start of her pregnancy. When she begins labor, a local midwife is able to make it to her home in time to deliver the baby. A successful delivery is achieved at week 40 with no major complications. Some 36 hr later, the neonate develops a conjunctivitis with a purulent discharge. What is the most likely causative organism?

A. *Chlamydia trachomatis* subtypes A-C

B. *Chlamydia trachomatis* subtypes D-K

C. *Haemophilus influenzae*

D. *Neisseria gonorrhoeae*

E. *Pseudomonas aeruginosa*

22. A 72-year-old nulliparous woman develops scant vaginal bleeding in the absence of any other symptoms. She presents to her primary care physician for further evaluation. Pelvic and bimanual exams are unremarkable. Urinalysis reveals trace blood; however, the Pap test shows a finding of adenocarcinoma. Which of the following is most closely associated with this finding?

A. Adenomyosis

B. Chronic use of oral contraceptives

C. Endometriosis

D. Endometrial hyperplasia

E. Leiomyoma

23. A 27-year-old man presents to your office with a recent diagnosis of choriocarcinoma. In looking to confirm the diagnosis of this tumor, you would expect to find which of the following lab results?

A. Decreased alpha-fetoprotein

B. Decreased hCG

C. Elevated alpha-fetoprotein

D. Elevated hCG

E. Leukocytosis

24. You are counseling a 27-year-old woman on her decision to become pregnant. You strongly encourage her to stop smoking and modify her diet. In order to reduce the risk that her child will be born with anencephaly or related conditions, which of the following dietary supplements must she consume during her pregnancy?

A. Biotin

B. Folate

C. Niacin

D. Riboflavin

E. Thiamine

25. A 35-year-old G3P2103 undergoes surgery for tubal ligation. Having located the ovaries, uterus, and adnexa, the surgeon wishes to locate the ovarian vessels. In which of the following structures should the surgeon look?

A. Round ligament of the uterus

B. Suspensory ligament of the ovaries

C. The broad ligament

D. The medial umbilical ligaments

E. Transverse cervical (cardinal) ligament

26. A 27-year-old sexually active man presents to the family medicine clinic complaining of multiple reddish brown papules on his penis. His testicles are descended bilaterally. Digital rectal examination reveals no evidence of hemorrhoids. What is the most likely diagnosis?

A. Balanoposthitis

B. Bowen's disease

C. Bowenoid papulosis

D. Erythroplasia of Queyrat

E. Paraphimosis

27. A 29-year-old nulliparous woman presents to her physician complaining of noncyclic vaginal bleeding and mild but persistent abdominal cramping. She has no other complaints and her past medical history is significant only for allergic rhinitis. She is not currently taking any medications. The physician is concerned about the possibility of a uterine mass, so a rectal exam is performed. What structure will most likely be compressed by palpation during this exam?

A. Ischiorectal fossa

B. Pouch of Douglas

C. Supralevator space

D. Urinary bladder

E. Vesicouterine pouch

28. A complete hysterectomy is performed on a 38-year-old G4P2113 after abdominal ultrasound reveals a unilateral ovarian mass obstructing the pelvic contents. An ultrasound is obtained (see Figure 10-3). The pathology report identifies the resected tumor as an ovarian fibroma. Prior to this procedure, paradoxical ascites had been identified in the absence of altered liver function tests or alcohol abuse. Which of the following physical exam findings is most likely to have been present in this person prior to the hysterectomy?

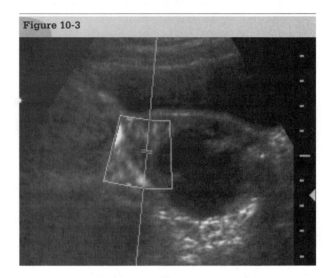

Figure 10-3

A. Decreased breath sounds

B. Elevated diastolic blood pressure

C. Inguinal lymphadenopathy

D. Macroscopic hematuria

E. Splenomegaly

29. Judging by her last menstrual period, a 25-year-old primigravida is in her tenth week of pregnancy. She also complains that she has had minor vaginal bleeding for a couple of weeks. Physical examination reveals her fundal height to be above the level of the umbilicus. Which of the following hormones would be markedly elevated in this condition?

A. 5-Hydroxyindolacetic acid

B. Alpha fetoprotein

C. Androgens

D. Beta-hCG

E. Estrogen

30. A 30-year-old nulliparous obese woman presents to the emergency department complaining of severe abdominal pain that began 18 hr ago. She complained of a similar pain approximately 4 weeks earlier. She states that she usually has monthly cramping with regular menses, but never of this severity. Physical examination reveals severe abdominal pain in both lower quadrants. Pelvic examination reveals uterosacral nodularity. The decision is made to perform an exploratory laparotomy after imaging studies prove inconclusive. What is the most likely diagnosis?

A. Endometriosis

B. Hematosalpinx

C. Pseudomyxoma peritonei

D. Stein-Leventhal syndrome

E. Struma ovarii

31. A 28-year-old woman presents to her family physician because of her inability to become pregnant. She does not complain of any specific problem, but express concern about her weight, as she has a strong family history of diabetes. Her partner has already been seen and has been shown to be fertile. She cannot remember when she had her last menstrual period but was not concerned, since her menses had never been heavy. Physical examination shows her BMI to be 34; she has prominent abdominal striae and hirsutism. Which of the following hormones would you expect to be elevated in this woman?

A. Estrogen

B. Follicle-stimulating hormone

C. Inhibin

D. Luteinizing hormone

E. T4

32. A 49-year-old sexually active G3P2103 presents to her primary care physician with multiple somatic complaints, including hot flashes, irregular menses, chronic diarrhea, and anxiety. All of these seem to have had their onset approximately 6 months earlier and no initiating factors can be identified. Abdominal examination reveals an abdominal mass that is painful to deep palpation. Ultrasound reveals a unilateral partially cystic ovarian mass. Which of the following laboratory studies will most likely be decreased in this case?

A. Alpha-fetoprotein

B. β-hCG

C. Follicle-stimulating hormone

D. Luteinizing hormone

E. Thyroid-stimulating hormone

33. A 55-year-old obese man with uncontrolled diabetes and a long history of unsatisfactory erections presents to his primary care physician to discuss possible treatment options. He reports having semierections but never getting fully erect. He wants to be examined and would like to be assured that there is no organic problem. Knowing his history, you explain that sexually he has a potential of developing:

A. Congestive heart failure

B. Paraphimosis

C. Peyronie's disease

D. Priapism

E. Retinopathy

34. During your third-year family medicine rotation, you interview a patient complaining of vaginal discharge and a burning sensation on urination. After obtaining a swab of the discharge and giving it to your preceptor for examination, he calls you over to the microscope, pointing out individual bacteria covering vaginal epithelial cells (see Figure 10-4). Which of the following organisms is mostly likely to be causative of this condition?

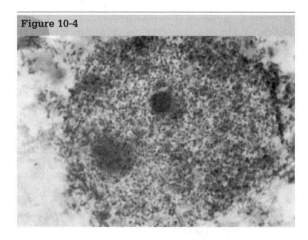

Figure 10-4

A. *Calymmatobacterium granulomatis*

B. *Candida albicans*

C. *Chlamydia trachomatis*

D. *Gardnerella vaginalis*

E. *Haemophilus ducreyi*

F. *Neisseria gonorrhoeae*

35. A 24-year-old G1P0 presents to her physician for a routine visit during her twentieth week of pregnancy. She complains of puffiness in her face and swelling around her wrists and hands, such that she has recently been unable to remove her wedding ring. Her blood pressure is recorded as 215/180 mm Hg in the right arm. Urinalysis reveals 2+ protein. Her total bilirubin is shown to be 3.2 mg/dL, LDH is 846 U/L, and AST is 103 U/L. Which of the following findings would you also expect to be most severely altered?

A. Alkaline phosphatase

B. Bleeding time

C. Creatine phosphokinase

D. GGT

E. Lipase

36. A 17-year-old sexually active man presents to the public health clinic complaining of dysuria, which he has experienced for 10 days. He admits to having had two unprotected sexual encounters in the previous month. A discharge is found on his underwear and cultures of the purulent discharge are taken from his urethra, demonstrating no bacteria. Which of the following organisms most likely explains these findings?

A. Anaerobic bacteria

B. *Candida albicans*

C. *Chlamydia*

D. *Neisseria gonorrhoeae*

E. *Treponema pallidum*

37. A 9-year-old child presents to her pediatrician for evaluation of her recent onset of menarche. She is not taking any medications and is not sexually active. Physical exam reveals Tanner stage 5 breasts, moderate amounts of pubic and axillary hair, and an increase in stature of 5 in. since her last visit 18 months earlier. Abdominal CT shows a left ovarian mass. Biopsy is undertaken. Which of the following characteristics would most likely be seen in this tissue?

   A. Call-Exner bodies
   B. Koilocytes
   C. Multinucleated giant cells
   D. Reinke crystals
   E. Signet-ring cells

38. A 39-year-old woman presents to her family physician complaining of a rash that has recently developed on the areola of her left breast. She states that the lesion has become itchy and has been accompanied by a watery red discharge for the last couple of days. Physical examination reveals that the lesion appears eczematous and the left nipple feels more solid and warm than the right. What is the most likely diagnosis?

   A. Intraductal papilloma
   B. Invasive ductal carcinoma
   C. Medullary carcinoma
   D. Nipple adenoma
   E. *Phyllodes* tumor

39. A healthy nulliparous 24-year-old woman undergoes regular 28-day menstrual cycles. Assuming no fertilization takes place, which of the following hormonal patterns would you expect to see on day 18 as compared to day 5 of the cycle? The number 0 represents no significant change.

	β-hCG	Estrogen	FSH	GnRH	LH	Progesterone
A.	↑	↑	↓	0	↓	↑
B.	0	↓	0	↓	0	↓
C.	0	↑	↓	↓	↓	↑
D.	↑	↓	↑	↑	↑	↓
E.	0	↑	0	↓	0	↑

40. A 12-year-old girl undergoes menarche and consequently up to 50 primordial follicles begin maturation. She is not sexually active and her reproductive development is appropriate for her age. She is not taking any medications and does not have a significant past medical history. Which of the following characteristics would you expect to be a feature of a unilaminar primary follicle in this girl?

   A. Dependent on follicle-stimulating hormone
   B. Liquor folliculi
   C. Theca interna
   D. Theca externa
   E. Zona pellucida

41. A 19-year-old man presents to the emergency department complaining of swelling and pain in the distal tip of his penis. He is uncircumcised, and upon further conversation, admits that he is unable to retract the foreskin past the tip of the glans and is in pain. What is the most likely diagnosis?

   A. Chlamydial infection
   B. Herpes simplex II
   C. Paraphimosis
   D. Phimosis
   E. Sickle cell crisis

42. A 42-year-old woman with a known history of endometrial carcinoma refuses medical and surgical therapy. This particular neoplasm can spread directly to the labia majora through lymphatics that follow the:

   A. Ovarian ligament
   B. Pubocervical ligaments
   C. Round ligament of the uterus
   D. Suspensory ligament of the ovary
   E. Uterosacral ligaments

43. A 19-year-old primigravida is giving birth to her first child. The baby is large for gestational age and the woman has a small introitus. Median episiotomy is performed to aid with vaginal delivery. Sequelae from this procedure might include impairment of which of the following muscles?

   A. Bulbospongiosus and ischiocavernosus
   B. Bulbospongiosus and superficial transverse perineal
   C. Ischiocavernosus and sphincter urethrae
   D. Obturator internus and deep transverse perineal
   E. Superficial anal and urethral sphincters

44. A 25-year-old woman is 12 weeks pregnant by dates. She denies prior medical or surgical history. Abdominal examination reveals normoactive bowel sounds with a nonpalpable fundal height. Urine beta-hCG testing is positive. Which of the following nutrients requires the *highest* percentage increase in supplementation during pregnancy?

   A. Calcium
   B. Niacin
   C. Vitamin A
   D. Vitamin D
   E. Vitamin E

45. A 57-year-old woman with endometrial carcinoma undergoes a radical hysterectomy and pelvic exenteration. Her ultrasound is shown in Figure 10-5. The lesion is found to have spread to the labia majora. This is plausible by which of the following lymphatic pathways?

   A. Cardinal ligament
   B. Pubic arcuate ligament
   C. Round ligament of the uterus
   D. Suspensory ligament of the ovary
   E. Suspensory ligament of the uterus

46. A 31-year-old woman seeks guidance to achieve pregnancy. She and her husband, who is age 28, have been having unprotected sexual intercourse for a year. However, their timing is erratic because of their work schedules. At which of the following times is the endometrial lining thickest and

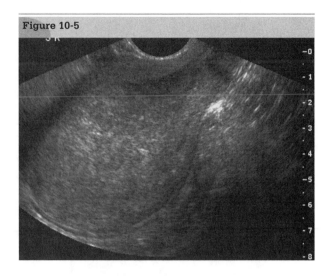

Figure 10-5

most conducive to implantation during the normal menstrual cycle?

A. Day 1

B. Day 4

C. Day 7

D. Day 12

E. Day 16

47. A 36-year-old GoPo complains of dysmenorrhea, dyspareunia, tenesmus, and pelvic pain and pressure. These symptoms seem to occur whenever she is ovulating. She and her husband have tried to have children but with no success. A laparoscopy is performed revealing chocolate cysts. What would be the most common location of these cysts?

A. Abdominal cholecystectomy scar

B. Fallopian tubes

C. Ovaries

D. Rectovaginal septum

E. Uterosacral ligament

48. A 17-year-old sexually active young woman presents to the emergency department with symptoms of diffuse lower abdominal pain, fever, and purulent vaginal discharge. Physical exam reveals cervical motion tenderness and adnexal tenderness. Bloodwork reveals leukocytosis. What bacteria will most likely be found on culture of the vaginal discharge?

A. *Neisseria meningitidis* and *Chlamydia trachomatis*

B. *Neisseria gonorrhoeae* and *Chlamydia trachomatis*

C. *Neisseria gonorrhoeae* and *Chlamydia psittaci*

D. *Escherichia coli* and *Chlamydia trachomatis*

E. *Escherichia coli* and *Neisseria meningitidis*

49. A 79-year-old nulliparous woman presents to her family physician with postmenopausal bleeding. After a thorough clinical workup, her physician determines that she has the most common gynecologic malignancy. Which of the following factors is most likely to predispose her to this malignancy?

A. Diabetes

B. Endometrial hyperplasia

C. Hypertension

D. Obesity

E. Parity status

50. A 19-year-old woman presents to her primary care physician regarding information about contraception. She has a past medical history of seasonal allergies. Physical examination of the heart, lungs, and abdomen is within normal limits. Pelvic examination reveals no evidence of cervical motion or adnexal tenderness. Which of the following contraceptive methods has the highest failure rate per 100 woman-years?

A. Intramuscular contraceptive implant

B. Intrauterine device-loop D

C. Oral contraceptive

D. Spermicide

E. Vasectomy of male partner

51. You are reviewing a histological report of a lesion found on the penis. The report describes a branching, villous, papillary connective tissue stroma that is covered by a thickened hyperplastic epithelium with superficial hyperkeratosis and acanthosis. Koilocytosis is also noted. Which of the following organisms most likely results in the histological description presented?

A. Anaerobic bacteria

B. *Candida albicans*

C. *Gardnerella*

D. Human papillomavirus

E. Pyogenic bacteria

52. An otherwise healthy 81-year-old man presents to his primary care physician complaining of dysuria, frequency, difficulty starting and stopping his stream of urine, hematuria, and severe acute-onset lumbosacral pain. After clinical examination and workup as well as needle biopsy of the prostate, he is diagnosed with Gleason 4 + 4 = 8 prostate cancer. Bone scan is positive for osteoblastic lesions. Which of the following treatments is most appropriate for this man's condition?

A. Clinical observation

B. Pharmacologic orchiectomy

C. Radiotherapy of the prostate

D. Surgical manipulation of the prostate

E. 5-alpha-reductase inhibitor

53. A 22-year-old sexually active woman presents to her primary care physician with vaginal itching and a profuse watery vaginal discharge. She gives a history of multiple unprotected sexual encounters over recent months. There has been an increased amount of watery vaginal discharge since she began menstruating 3 days earlier. The underlying cervical mucosa has a fiery red appearance. Which of the following organisms most likely results in the clinical description presented?

A. *Candida albicans*

B. *Condyloma acuminatum*

C. *Gardnerella vaginalis*

D. *Neisseria gonorrhoeae*

E. *Trichomonas vaginalis*

54. A 26-year-old sexually active woman presents to her primary care physician with small, painful vesicles and erythematous shallow ulcers involving her vulva and clitoris. She gives a history of multiple unprotected sexual encounters over recent months. Cytologic smears from the lesions show multinucleated giant cells containing small inclusions. Which of the following organisms is most likely responsible for her symptoms?

A. *Candida albicans*

B. *Chlamydia trachomatis*

C. *Gardnerella vaginalis*

D. Herpes simplex virus type 2 (HSV-2)

E. *Neisseria gonorrhoeae*

55. A 40-year-old woman with a history of endometriosis and polycystic ovaries presents to her primary care physician complaining of difficulty hearing. She denies any trauma to the ear. She did have a viral infection the previous week, which subsided. Her past medical history is insignificant. Physical examination reveals that the Weber test lateralizes to the deaf ear and Rinne test shows AC > BC in both ears. Otoscopy reveals no gross lesions in either ear. What is the most likely cause of her hearing loss?

A. Conductive defect

B. Cerumen impaction

C. Medication

D. Sensorineural defect

E. Viral infection

56. A 27-year-old sexually active woman is following up with her primary care physician to receive the results of her Pap smear. The report demonstrates dysplastic cervical epithelial cells with frequent koilocytosis. Which of the following viral proteins is responsible for inactivating the corresponding gene products of *p53* and *Rb*?

A. E4 and E5

B. E5 and E6

C. E6 and E7

D. E7 and E8

E. E8 and E9

57. A 10-year-old girl presents with nonpruritic papules on her hands. The lesions are approximately 3 mm in diameter with a central umbilication. Some of the lesions have already started to regress. Examination of the abdomen and pelvis reveals similar lesions. She also has a lesion lateral to her left labium. What is the most likely diagnosis?

A. Atopic dermatitis

B. Condylomata lata

C. Human papillomavirus infection

D. Molluscum contagiosum

E. Tinea versicolor

58. A 19-year-old man presents to the public health clinic with a painless, elevated, superficially ulcerated papule that has been present on his glans penis for 3 days (see Figure 10-6). On further questioning, the physician elicits a history of two unprotected sexual encounters in the previous month. Which of the following is true of this lesion?

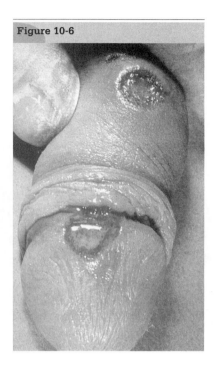

Figure 10-6

A. It is caused by *Neisseria gonorrhoeae*.

B. It usually involves the testis before the epididymis.

C. It is the most common cause of acute purulent urethritis.

D. No bacteria will be demonstrated in a culture of the purulent urethral discharge.

E. The lesion will most likely heal within 1 week.

59. A female patient is diagnosed with bilateral malignant ovarian tumors. Based on the general frequencies of the following malignant ovarian tumors, which one does she most likely have?

A. Carcinomatous mucocele of the appendix

B. Endometrioid tumor

C. Mucinous cystadenocarcinoma

D. Pseudomyxoma peritoneii

E. Serous cystadenocarcinoma

60. A 27-year-old pregnant woman presents to her primary care physician in the first trimester of pregnancy with vaginal bleeding and a rapid increase in the size of her uterus, which appears too large for the supposed stage of her pregnancy. It is later found that she has enlarged, edematous placental villi in a loose stroma. Which of the following characteristics is most commonly associated with this condition?

A. It is of maternal derivation.

B. It is thought to be due to the fertilization of the ovum by two or more spermatozoa.

C. It often results in the formation of a small embryo.

D. It progresses to choriocarcinoma in approximately 10% of cases.

E. It usually presents with a 46,XX karyotype.

61. A 37-year-old G4P4 presents to her primary care physician complaining of abdominal fullness. She has no prior medical history. Physical examination reveals a palpable uterine fundus. Urine beta hCG is positive. Serum beta hCG is markedly elevated. Ultrasound reveals a complex uterine mass. Chest x-ray reveals a lung mass. Which of the following statements is correct about this condition?

A. It is characterized by early hematogenous spread to the breast.

B. It is more frequent than ovarian choriocarcinoma.

C. It is most often preceded by a normal-term pregnancy.

D. It is most often preceded by the abortion of an ectopic pregnancy.

E. It is usually responsive to radiotherapy.

62. A woman presents with the triad of an ovarian tumor, abdominal ascites, and a large amount of fluid present in her lungs. Physical examination reveals decreased breath sounds at both bases. Cardiac examination reveals no evidence of rubs, murmurs, or gallops. Abdominal examination reveals a palpable left-lower-quadrant mass. Which of the following pathologies most likely resulted in this scenario?

A. Fibroma

B. Granulosa cell tumor

C. Krukenberg tumor

D. Sertoli-Leydig cell tumor

E. Thecoma

63. The parents of a newborn infant present to the office of their primary care physician seeming quite upset and confused. They were told that their son was born with a congenital defect called epispadias. In this situation, the opening of the urethral meatus is:

A. Dorsal

B. Fused

C. Narrow

D. Ventral

E. Widened

64. A 32-year-old African American man presents to the emergency department complaining of a painful erection that has now lasted for 8 hr. He denies any past history of this condition and has not taken any erectogenic medications. He admits to feeling run down, dehydrated, and really tired lately. He denies any drug use. Which of the following tests should be ordered in this patient?

A. Complete blood count

B. Chest x-ray

C. Hemoglobin electrophoresis

D. Neurological exam

E. Urinalysis

65. A 16-year-old teenager presents to his primary care physician; he has a long history of balanitis. He is uncircumcised and has significant erythema of the glans penis. His testes are descended bilaterally. What is the most likely etiology of this condition?

A. Blunt penile trauma

B. Diabetes

C. Poor eating habits

D. Poor hygiene

E. Unprotected sex

66. A 41-year-old woman with a history of vague abdominal pain, nausea, and vomiting presents to her primary care physician for evaluation. Ultrasound suggests the presence of a cervical mass. Which of the following statements about the mass is correct?

A. Its peak occurrence is in the elderly.

B. It is most often an adenocarcinoma.

C. It most frequently arises from preexisting vaginal intraepithelial neoplasia (VIN) at the squamocolumnar junction.

D. It has demonstrated only a moderate decrease in mortality since the introduction of the Pap smear.

E. Dysplastic cells commonly demonstrate koilocytosis.

67. A 61-year-old man presents to his primary care physician for evaluation of voiding dysfunction. He complains of a decreased urinary stream, urinary frequency, and urinary urgency. Physical examination of the prostate reveals no evidence of nodules. His most recent PSA is 2.1 ng/mL. What is the most likely etiology of his symptoms?

A. Androblastoma

B. Benign prostatic hyperplasia

C. Hydronephrosis

D. Prostatic cancer

E. Sexually transmitted diseases

68. A 37-year-old man visits his physician because he falls asleep several times a day while at work. He complains of daytime tiredness but claims that he gets 7 to 8 hr of sleep at night. His wife complains of the patient's snoring at night. He is 5 ft 10 in. tall and weighs 215 lb. He does not smoke and is not taking any medications. What is the most likely explanation for these findings?

A. Cataplexy

B. Depression

C. Narcolepsy

D. Obstructive sleep apnea syndrome

E. Tuberculosis

69. A 22-year-old woman presents to the emergency department with fever, vomiting, diarrhea, and decreased urine output. Her history is positive for the use of highly absorbent tampons 4 days earlier. Physical examination reveals a generalized rash that has begun to desquamate over her lower extremities. Which of the following organisms is the most likely cause of her symptoms?

A. An endotoxin produced by *Escherichia coli*

B. An endotoxin produced by *Staphylococcus aureus*

C. An endotoxin produced by *Staphylococcus epidermidis*

D. An exotoxin produced by *Staphylococcus aureus*

E. An exotoxin produced by *Staphylococcus epidermidis*

70. An otherwise healthy 26-year-old sexually active woman presents to her obstetrician/gynecologist with coalescing lesions that form large genital and inguinal ulcerations. Her genitals appear grossly distorted and she has inguinal lymphedema. Multiple organisms filling large histiocytes are found on histopathologic examination. Which of the following organisms is most likely responsible for her symptoms?

    A. *Calymmatobacterium granulomatosus*

    B. *Chlamydia trachomatis* L1, L2, or L3

    C. *Haemophilus ducreyi*

    D. Herpes simplex virus type 2

    E. *Neisseria gonorrhoeae*

71. A 46-year-old woman complains of vague pelvic pain. She presents to her primary care physician for evaluation. Physical examination reveals bilateral left-lower quadrant tenderness to deep palpation. Ultrasound reveals a pelvic mass. Serum alpha-fetoprotein levels are elevated. Which of the following etiologies most likely fits this clinical description?

    A. Dysgerminoma

    B. Endodermal sinus (yolk sac) tumor

    C. Immature teratoma

    D. Mature teratoma (dermoid cyst)

    E. Monodermal teratoma

72. A 42-year-old sexually active woman presents to her family physician with a sharply circumscribed, ulcerated nodule on her left labium major. On histologic examination of the nodule, it consists of a single layer of nonciliated columnar cells with a layer of flattened myoepithelial cells lying directly beneath the epithelium. Which of the following diagnoses is most likely in this patient?

    A. Bartholin's cyst

    B. Condyloma acuminatum

    C. Papillary hidradenoma

    D. Squamous hyperplasia

    E. Vestibular adenitis

73. A 72-year-old man presents to his primary care physician complaining of frequency, nocturia, difficulty starting and stopping urination, overflow dribbling, and dysuria. After clinical examination and workup, the urologist informs him that he has the most common urological condition found in men his age. For which of the following is he likely to be at increased risk due to the condition described?

    A. Azotemia (prerenal)

    B. Cancer of the prostate

    C. Diverticulum formation of the bladder

    D. Renal abscess

    E. Trabeculation of the kidney

74. A 32-year-old sexually active woman presents to the family medicine clinic with a white, patch-like mucosal lesion on her vulva, vulvovaginal pruritus, and a thick white vaginal discharge. Culture of the vaginal discharge demonstrates an organism that is commonly associated with diabetes mellitus, pregnancy, broad-spectrum antibiotic therapy, oral contraceptive use, and immunosuppression. Which of the following organisms is most likely responsible for this woman's clinical symptoms?

    A. *Candida albicans*

    B. *Chlamydia trachomatis*

    C. *Gardnerella vaginalis*

    D. *Neisseria gonorrhoeae*

    E. *Trichomonas vaginalis*

75. A 22-year-old sexually active woman has been diagnosed with a cystic-surface epithelial tumor of the ovary. She undergoes uncomplicated surgical removal. Which of the following statements about this lesion is correct?

    A. It is a rare benign tumor.

    B. It is a germ cell tumor.

    C. Its incidence is greatly increased in daughters of women who received thalidomide therapy during pregnancy.

    D. It often leads to vaginal adenosis, a condition characterized by mucosal columnar epithelium-lined crypts in areas normally lined by stratified squamous epithelium.

    E. It may be either solid or cystic.

Answer Key

1. E	20. E	39. E	58. B
2. B	21. D	40. E	59. E
3. C	22. D	41. D	60. E
4. A	23. D	42. C	61. B
5. G	24. B	43. B	62. A
6. C	25. B	44. A	63. A
7. A	26. C	45. C	64. C
8. D	27. B	46. E	65. D
9. A	28. A	47. C	66. E
10. A	29. D	48. B	67. B
11. A	30. A	49. E	68. D
12. B	31. D	50. D	69. D
13. D	32. E	51. D	70. A
14. B	33. C	52. B	71. B
15. D	34. D	53. E	72. C
16. A	35. B	54. D	73. C
17. B	36. C	55. A	74. A
18. A	37. A	56. C	75. E
19. D	38. B	57. D	

Answers and Explanations

1. E. Estrogen's primary function in the prevention of pregnancy is to inhibit FSH production, thereby inhibiting the development of the dominant follicle. Blockage of endometrial proliferation, increasing viscosity of the cervical mucus, and a decrease in LH production are all caused by progestin, another prominent hormone often employed in contraception. A decrease in menstrual blood flow is a noncontraceptive benefit seen in both estrogen- and progestin-containing oral contraceptive pills.

2. B. The period of perimenopause is marked by several "climacteric symptoms," including vasomotor symptoms ("hot flashes"), increasing menstrual irregularity, sleep disturbances, decreased libido, vaginal dryness, and periods of emotional irritability. One of the key mechanisms behind this is the progressive decrease in ovarian mass, leading to the underproduction of ovarian hormones, including inhibin. The decreased inhibin levels result in decreased inhibition of FSH release from the pituitary.

3. C. The lab results in this case are the deciding factor as to the etiology of the discharge. In assessing suspected galactorrhea, the prolactin and TSH levels should always be obtained. If prolactin levels are elevated, the next step should be to look for medications that could be interfering with the normal dopaminergic suppression of prolactin secretion. In this case, that medication is metoclopramide. The TSH level is within the normal range, ruling out secondary hypothyroidism and making a pituitary adenoma unlikely. The absence of irregular menses also suggests that the etiology is not an adenoma. Mammary duct ectasia, while often bilateral, most often presents with a serosanginous nipple discharge and normal prolactin levels. In situ ductal carcinoma is most often unilateral; it also presents with a serosanginous nipple discharge and normal prolactin levels.

4. A. A common result of normal aging is the increased laxity of the broad round ovarian and cardinal ligaments, usually combined with loss of tone in myofascial structures such as the urogenital diaphragm. This results in uterine prolapse into the vagina, most commonly presenting as dysuria. A tear in the diaphragm can also cause uterine prolapse but is less common and is usually accompanied by symptoms of incontinence. Fecal impaction, nulliparity, and endometrial hyperplasia are not associated with uterine prolapse.

5. G. Placenta accreta is the attachment of the placenta directly to the myometrium due to a defective decidual layer. It is predisposed by uterine scarring and inflammation, most commonly a result of scars from a previous cesarean sec-

tion. The major complication of this is impaired placental separation on delivery, possibly resulting in a massive hemorrhage. Placenta previa is also commonly seen in such scarring and often coexists with placenta accreta. Preeclampsia is the triad of hypertension, proteinuria, and edema. Hydatidiform mole is a pathological ovum resulting in cystic swelling of chorionic villi and proliferation of chorionic epithelium. Abruptio placentae is premature separation of the placenta. This condition can be associated with fetal death and disseminated intravascular coagulopathy. Teratomas constitute 90% of germ cell tumors of the ovary.

6. C. Adenocarcinoma of the prostate is extremely common in the older age group. It arises most often in the peripheral zone of the prostate and is usually diagnosed by rectal examination. In the early stages of the disease, it is associated with an increase in serum prostate-specific antigen (PSA). An increased total PSA with a decreased fraction of free PSA suggests malignancy, while an increase in total PSA with a proportionate increase in the fraction of free PSA suggests benign prostatic hypertrophy (BPH).

7. A. This child has an endodermal sinus (yolk sac) tumor. This is a malignant germ cell tumor that has its peak incidence in infancy and early childhood; it is the most common testicular tumor in this age group. It is analogous to endodermal sinus tumor of the ovary and causes an increase in serum alpha-fetoprotein, which is also associated with hepatocellular carcinoma.

8. D. Lymph from the lower 25% of the vagina (below the hymen) drains downward to the perineum, where it is received by the superficial inguinal lymph nodes. The upper three-quarters of the vagina, on the other hand, drains upward to the internal iliac nodes. Since the fornix lies adjacent to the cervix, it is classified as lying within the upper three-quarters of the vagina.

9. A. Vaginal adenosis is a benign condition characterized by areas of columnar epithelium within the normal stratified squamous epithelium of the vagina. It is also proposed to be a precursor to clear cell carcinoma of the vagina. Both are heavily associated with maternal use of diethylstilbestrol (DES), an estrogen-based contraceptive, during pregnancy. DES has since been removed from the market for this reason. The risk of developing vaginal adenosis is not known to correlate with the number of pregnancies or sexual partners. The use of superabsorbent tampons is notoriously related to the development of toxic shock syndrome but has no relation to the development of vaginal adenosis.

10. A. Antiestrogens interfere with the direct binding of estrogen with its receptor, some actually modulating the receptor on a molecular level such that it becomes less constitutively active. Both clomiphene and tamoxifen have such activity, but of the two, only clomiphene has been approved for the treatment of anovulation. Tamoxifen is specifically used for the treatment of estrogen-dependent breast tumors. Both drugs have the adverse effects of causing ovarian enlargement, hot flashes, nausea, and vomiting. Danazol is a combined antiestrogen and antitestosterone used to treat endometriosis and fibrocystic breast disease.

11. A. The term *koilocytosis* describes the cellular appearance of the typical genital wart, or condyloma acuminatum caused by human papillomavirus (HPV). The presence of only koilocytosis, however, says nothing about the potential malignancy of the lesion; therefore the specimen must be analyzed further to determine the particular strain of HPV causing this lesion. This condition must not be confused with condyloma latum, the lesion of secondary syphilis. Lichen sclerosus is a vulvar dystrophy often presenting as a white patch-like lesion, but it does not exhibit koilocytosis. Vaginal candidiasis, caused by *Candida albicans,* presents as a curdy white vaginal discharge but without adherent plaques or koilocytosis. Last, vaginal adenosis represents a benign condition marked by columnar epithelium–lined crypts in areas that normally exhibit stratified squamous epithelium.

12. B. Immature teratoma is usually a malignant tumor in females, as opposed to mature teratoma, which is usually benign. This is, however, reversed for males, in whom mature teratomas are more likely to be malignant. Human papillomavirus (HPV) type II is a benign strain of HPV. Leimyomas, or fibroids, are extremely common benign tumors of the uterus. They may very rarely transform into leiomyosarcomas. Adenomyosis is a benign extension of endometrial glands and stroma into the myometrium, most often causing uterine enlargement.

13. D. Mumps virus is the most likely causative agent for his orchitis. When this condition occurs bilaterally, there is a significantly increased risk of sterility, which would be a relevant cause for concern in a young man. Varicella, also known as chickenpox, and herpes zoster in adults can cause painful blisters and pruritus but is not known to cause orchitis. Epstein-Barr virus causes mononucleosis and swelling of the glands but is not the most likely cause of bilateral orchitis.

14. B. The presence of bilateral cancerous lesions, especially in such a young woman, is highly suggestive of a germline mutation. Of those listed, a derangement of the p53 allele is most highly correlated with the development of breast cancer. Genes implicated in the development of breast cancer include *BRCA-1, BRCA-2,* and *p53.* The c-erb allele is a growth factor receptor gene and is upregulated in some breast cancers. Increased trinucleotide repeats, Rb, and the excision repair system have yet to be implicated in the pathogenesis of breast cancers.

15. D. Leiomyomas, otherwise known as fibroids, are the most common benign tumors of the uterus. They are also commonly estrogen-responsive, causing them to enlarge in a cyclic pattern. When they are severe, they may cause mass effects in the abdomen, such as bloating. Adenomyosis also commonly causes uterine enlargement, but this is usually bilateral and nonnodular. The same is true for endometrial hyperplasia, which also rarely reaches the size of leiomyomas or adenomyosis. Endometriosis can result in chocolate cysts, but these rarely reach the size needed to cause mass effects. A molar pregnancy could also result in an asymmetric abdominal mass, but in this case the pregnancy test would have been positive.

16. A. The vagina has a dual origin; the upper portion (including the fornix) is derived from the paramesonephric ducts, whereas the lower portion comes from the sinovaginal bulbs, also known as the vaginal plate. The paramesonephric ducts then vacuolize to form the vaginal fornix and uterus. The sinovaginal bulbs also vacuolize, forming the distal vagina and vulva. The ureterovesical pouch is responsible for forming multiple elements, including the urinary bladder.

17. B. This question is a little tricky since the mother has the misconception that her child is male. The presence of ovaries in the absence of testicles, however, is definitive of the female gender. The child is therefore referred to as a female pseudohermaphrodite. The most common cause of this is the adrenogenital syndrome. It results from the body's inability to hydroxylate 17-hydroxyprogesterone adequately, leading to decreased or absent levels of 11-deoxycortisol. There is consequent congenital adrenal hyperplasia, decreased levels of cortisol, increased levels of ACTH, and increased production of androgens. Therefore these females are 46XX and have ovaries, but their external genitalia are masculinized. The lack of receptors for dihydrotestosterone is seen in androgen insensitivity syndrome. The XO karyotype is defined as Turner's syndrome and the gender is female, although the ovaries are fibrous streaks. Point mutations in the SRY gene and adrenal hypofunction are both variable according to the severity of the lesion; however, neither represent the most common cause of female pseudo-hermaphroditism.

18. A. Assuming that the patient understands the risks and benefits of the procedure (i.e., gives informed consent) and that other, less harmful procedures are available, the woman's choice is ultimately decisive. Thus, despite the potential risks to the fetus, amniocentesis should be performed.

19. D. This radiograph shows several calcified structures that represent fully developed teeth within a teratoma. Mature teratomas specifically represent the most common benign ovarian tumor or approximately 20% of ovarian tumors and 90% of germ cell tumors. This condition most often arises as a result of reduplication of paternal chromosomes, resulting in a 46XX genotype of purely maternal origin. None of the other tumors listed presents with distinct calcifications as seen in this radiograph.

20. E. It is very radiosensitive. A seminoma is a malignant lesion that is analogous to a dysgerminoma, a tumor of the ovary. It has a peak incidence in the mid-30s and is the most common germ cell tumor, accounting for 40% of such tumors. It is sometimes associated with increased serum human chorionic gonadotropin (hCG). Fortunately, because it is very radiosensitive, it can often be cured, even with lymph node metastases.

21. D. The scenario presented is typical of that seen with gonococcal ophthalmia. It usually appears within the first 5 days of life and is most common in the neonates of women who have not had standard medical care during birth or medical prophylaxis. The big difference between gonococcal ophthalmitis and trachoma is the amount of purulent discharge (which is much greater with the gonococcal infection) and the urgency of the condition. Trachoma and inclusion conjunctivitis, arising from infection by *C. trachomatis* subtypes A to C and D to K, respectively, produce a more chronic conjunctivitis that can cause blindness over time. However, gonococcal ophthalmia occurs soon after birth and is rapidly destructive; the blindness can occur in just days. Both organisms are acquired from the maternal birth canal during parturition.

22. D. Any bleeding in a postmenopausal woman should be assumed to be adenocarcinoma due to endometrial hyperplasia until proven otherwise. Endometrial hyperplasia itself results from excessive estrogen stimulation over time; sources of this stimulation include obesity, nulliparity, anovulatory cycles, and estrogen supplementation. Predisposition toward adenocarcinoma is not seen in any of the other choices.

23. D. Elevated hGC is a diagnostically significant marker of choriocarcinoma and is characterized by syncytiotrophoblasts and cytotrophoblasts. Elevated alpha-fetoprotein would be indicative of an endodermal sinus or yolk sac tumor. Leukocytosis is not a specific marker for any type of testicular tumor.

24. B. Folic acid represents the most common vitamin deficiency in the United States, and supplementation during gestation has been shown to drastically decrease the chances that the fetus will develop a neural tube defect. Folate is most commonly found in green leafy vegetables. Biotin deficiency is rare and is accompanied by several skin and gastrointestinal manifestations as well as mental status changes. Niacin deficiency is known to cause pellagra, which is characterized by dermatitis, diarrhea, and dementia. Deficiency of riboflavin is also very rare but manifests as cheilosis, glossitis, corneal vascularization, and seborrheic dermatoses. Lastly, thiamine deficiency has several manifestations, which include dry beriberi, wet beriberi, and Wernicke-Korsakoff syndrome.

25. B. The suspensory ligament of the ovaries houses the ovarian vessels. The transverse cervical ligament contains the uterine vessels. The broad ligament also carries uterine vessels as well as the uterine tubules and the round ligaments of the uterus and ovaries. The round ligament of the uterus itself contains no important anatomical structures. The medial umbilical ligaments carry the umbilical arteries.

26. C. Bowenoid papulosis is classified as a carcinoma in situ, along with erythroplasia of Queyrat and Bowen's disease.

Bowenoid papulosis occurs in sexually active adults and can be differentiated from erythroplasia of Queyrat and Bowen's disease by the younger age of patients in whom it presents. It is classified by multiple reddish brown papules on the penis, as opposed to Bowen's disease and erythroplasia of Queyrat, which usually become manifest as a single erythematous plaque. The plaque of Bowen's disease is found on the shaft of the penis or scrotum, whereas the plaque of erythroplasia of Queyrat most often involves the prepuce or glans penis. Paraphimosis results from forcibly retracting the prepuce over the glans penis and leads to marked swelling of the glans, which can cause extreme pain and urinary retention through urethral constriction. Balanoposthitis may result from infection of the glans and prepuce by a variety of organisms, such as *Candida albicans*, *Gardnerella*, and anaerobic bacteria.

27. B. Palpation within the rectum anteriorly against the uterus impinges upon the rectouterine pouch, also known as the pouch of Douglas. The ischiorectal fossa lies lateral and inferior to this, whereas the supralevator space lies lateral and superior. The urinary bladder is located at the anterior aspect of the uterus; the vesicouterine pouch lies between the two.

28. A. Meig's syndrome is the triad of ovarian fibroma, ascites, and pleural effusion. Hence, the most likely physical finding would be decreased breath sounds due to pleural effusion. Ascites results from direct irritation of the peritoneum by the solid tumor, whereas the pleural effusion is thought to be due to transport of the ascitic fluid by transdiaphragmatic lymphatic channels (although the size of the effusion is independent of the degree of ascites). Both the ascites and pleural effusion normally resolve on removal of the tumor. None of the other physical findings listed would be specific for Meig's syndrome.

29. D. This individual likely has hydatidiform mole. A molar pregnancy is often accompanied by vaginal bleeding, a larger uterus than normal for gestational age, and markedly elevated beta-hCG levels. It characteristically becomes symptomatic in the early months of pregnancy. AFP is found to be elevated in many yolk sac tumors. Estrogen levels are elevated in granulose-theca cell tumors, and androgen levels are elevated in Leydig cell tumors. 5-HIAA is a marker for carcinoid tumors.

30. A. The most common presenting complaint with endometriosis is cyclic abdominal pain, usually of increasing severity if the condition has developed recently. The image presented exhibits the characteristic chocolate cysts seen in this condition. Endometriosis is thought to arise from the reflux and proliferation of endometrial tissue onto the ovaries and into the peritoneum. Since the tissue is still functional, it is still responsive to estrogens and enlarges during menstruation, hence the cyclic pain. Hematosalpinx is a complication seen mostly in pelvic inflammatory disease. Pseudomyxoma peritonei is a result of the rupture or metastasis of a mucinous cystadenocarcinoma. Stein-Leventhal syndrome presents with amenorrhea and no cysts. Last, struma ovarii is a form of monodermal teratoma consisting solely of thyroid tissue.

31. D. The question stem presents all four of the key characteristics for polycystic ovarian syndrome: amenorrhea, infertility, obesity, and hirsutism. This condition may be caused by an excess of LH and/or androgens. It is also associated with peripheral insulin resistance and is an important risk factor for diabetes. All other hormone levels are within reference range or depressed in the case of polycystic ovarian syndrome.

32. E. This scenario describes the findings seen in struma ovarii, a rare type of monodermal teratoma consisting almost entirely of thyroid tissue. In approximately 15% of these, the ectopic thyroid tissue may become hyperactive, creating a hyperthyroid state. Struma ovarii may also coexist with serous or mucinous cystadenocarcinoma. Some of the symptoms seem climacteric; however, if this were the case, LH and especially FSH would be elevated due to loss of feedback inhibition by the decreased levels of estrogen. Also, the ovarian mass is not characteristic of menopause. AFP levels are increased in germ cell tumors, whereas beta-hCG levels are increased in ovarian choriocarcinoma and trophobastic disease.

33. C. Men with a history of partial erectile dysfunction who continue to have intercourse with a semierect penis are at increased risk for Peyronie's disease, which is a dorsal subcutaneous fibrosis of the penis. Congestive heart failure and retinopathy are both potential issues but not related in a sexual sense. Paraphimosis is limited to uncircumcised males, and there is no indication of foreskin issues. Priapism is described as a painful, nonsubsiding erection that lasts over 6 hours.

34. D. Clue cells are seen in cases of bacterial vaginosis; they represent individual bacteria, most commonly *Gardnerella vaginalis,* covering vaginal epithelial cells on Pap smear preparations. This bacterium is most commonly spread by sexual contact and accounts for many cases formerly classified as nonspecific vaginitis. *Chlamydia* (an intracellular parasite) is a cause of nongonococcal urethritis. Treatment for chlamydial infections is erythromycin or tetracycline. *Neisseria gonorrhoeae* is a Gram-negative organism that can cause urethritis and arthritis.

35. B. The information presented describes the HELLP syndrome, seen in some severe cases of preeclampsia. HELLP is an acronym for hemolysis, elevated liver enzymes, and low platelets. This syndrome complicates approximately 10% of cases of pregnancy-induced hypertension (PIH) and is primarily a microangiopathic process. Typical findings include prolonged bleeding time, increased levels of AST and ALT, and, when hemolysis is severe enough, increased levels of total bilirubin. Alkaline phosphatase and GGT levels are also nonspecific markers for liver pathology but are not often seen to be altered until severe systemic disease has occurred. CPK levels are not directly affected by the HELLP syndrome. Lipase is a marker of pancreatic destruction and hence is not directly affected by this syndrome.

36. C. A chlamydial infection is the most common cause of nongonococcal urethritis. It is a sexually transmitted disease that should be suspected when bacteria are not demonstrated in a purulent urethral discharge. Chlamydial infections can often lead to epididymitis. *Neisseria gonorrhoeae* most often presents as an acute purulent urethritis. Cultures of the purulent urethral discharge demonstrate intracellular Gram-negative diplococci. *Neisseria gonorrhoeae* may extend to the prostate, seminal vesicles, and epididymis but only rarely involves the testes.

37. A. Granulosa cell tumor is an estrogen-secreting neoplasm commonly implicated in precocious puberty in adolescents. Histologically, the tumor consists of cuboidal granulosa cells within anastomotic cords and Call-Exner bodies. These structures represent small follicles filled with an eosinophilic fluid. Granulosa cell tumors in adults are commonly sequelae of endometrial hyperplasia or carcinoma. Koilocytes are seen with viral infections such as HPV. Multinucleated giant cells are seen with chronic inflammatory conditions. Reinke crystals are seen with yolk sac tumors. Signet-ring cells are seen with adenocarcinoma.

38. B. An eczematoid lesion of the nipple or areola is characteristic of Paget's disease of the breast, which almost always signifies an underlying invasive ductal carcinoma of the breast. It is thought that the intraductal carcinoma undergoes retrograde extension into the overlying epidermis through mammary ductal epithelium. The large cells of the eczematous lesion have a typical histologic feature of being surrounded by a clear, halo-like area. None of the other options is related to Paget's disease of the breast. Intraductal papilloma is a benign lesion of the lactiferous ducts, which also produces a serosanguinous discharge. Medullary carcinoma is a highly malignant breast cancer containing little stroma and a fleshy histologic appearance. Nipple adenoma is a benign tumor of the nipple that produces a serosanguinous discharge and is often mistaken for malignancy. Phyllodes tumor is a large tumor of variable malignancy, often causing an ulceration of the overlying skin.

39. E. During the luteal phase, which occurs on days 15 to 28 of a regular 28-day cycle, the corpus luteum develops, producing estrogen and progesterone. Despite negative feedback of estrogen on the anterior pituitary early in the luteal phase, LH and FSH levels are still increased owing to the surge at ovulation, hence they are essentially unchanged compared to the follicular phase. Beta-hCG levels are not changed unless fertilization occurs.

40. E. Unilaminar primary follicles develop directly from primary follicles, and since they themselves possess a zona pellucida, so do unilaminar primary follicles. They are made up of a single layer of cuboid epithelial cells, contain no theca or liquor folliculi, and are responsive to local hormonal factors. Multilaminar primary follicles represent the next stage in development and consist of many layers of granulosa cells with both a theca interna and externa. Secondary follicles possess this plus an accumulation of liquor folliculi and are FSH-dependent. Graafian follicles represent the final stage of follicular development, are

FSH-dependent until they become dominant, and have an antrum filled with liquor folliculi.

41. D. Phimosis, or the inability to retract foreskin from the glans of the penis, is the most appropriate diagnosis for the young man in this scenario. This occurs only in uncircumcised males, owing to the presence of the foreskin. Paraphimosis is the inability to return the foreskin over the glans of the penis and causes pain. Both conditions can result from inflammation or trauma to the penis. In infants, it can also be a congenital issue. Herpes simplex II and chlamydial infection are both sexually transmitted diseases, neither of which present with the clinical issues described. Sickle cell crisis can present with priapism, not phimosis.

42. C. Carcinoma of the uterus can spread directly to the labia majora through the lymphatics that follow the round ligament of the uterus. The round ligament of the uterus extends from the uterus and merges with the subcutaneous tissue of the labia majora. The ovarian ligament is a fibromuscular cord that extends from the ovary to the uterus. The pubocervical ligaments are firm bands of connective tissue that extend from the pubis to the cervix. The suspensory ligament of the ovary is a band of peritoneum that transmits the ovarian vessels, nerves, and lymphatics. The uterosacral ligaments connect the uterus to the sacrum.

43. B. The perineal body is the central tendon of the perineum. It is a fibromuscular structure at the center of the perineum. It provides attachment for the bulbospongiosus, superficial and deep transverse perineal, and sphincter ani muscles.

44. A. Calcium must be supplemented during pregnancy to meet fetal needs and preserve maternal calcium stores. Milk is the recommended substance to promote calcium stores because it is inexpensive and provides 1 g of calcium and 33 g of protein per quart. The pregnant patient requires an additional 400 mg of calcium above the 800 mg required by nonpregnant individuals. Daily, 14 mg of niacin is required by the nonpregnant patient, while 16 mg is required in the pregnant state. Daily, 800 mg of vitamin A is required in the nonpregnant state while 1 g is required in the pregnant state. Daily, 200 mg of vitamin A is required in the nonpregnant state while 400 mg is required in the pregnant state. Daily, 8 mg of vitamin E is required in the nonpregnant state while 10 mg is required in the pregnant state.

45. C. The round ligament of the uterus runs laterally from the uterus through the deep inguinal ring, inguinal canal, and superficial inguinal ring. It becomes lost in the subcutaneous tissues of the labia majora. Therefore carcinoma of the uterus can spread directly to the labia majora by following the round ligament. Pathologically, this can imply a poor overall prognosis.

46. E. During the proliferative phase of the menstrual cycle, the stratum functionale proliferates and achieves maximum vascularity (thickness) at approximately day 16 of the menstrual cycle. The endometrial lining remains at this thickness until menstruation, which occurs on or about day 28 of the cycle in a normal female.

47. C. This patient has typical symptoms of endometriosis. Endometriosis is the finding of endometrial glands outside of the uterus. The most common site for endometriosis is the ovaries. The chocolate cysts result when the ovaries become distorted and filled with brown blood debris. Endometriosis can be found almost anywhere in the body, including old laparotomy scars, uterosacral ligaments, the rectovaginal septum, and the fallopian tubes. It has even been found in the nasal mucosa and lungs, but its most common location is in the ovaries. Endometriosis can cause pelvic pain, dysmenorrhea, dyspareunia, tenesmus, and infertility.

48. B. This patient is showing typical signs of pelvic inflammatory disease. The two most common bacteria found in PID are *Neisseria gonorrhoeae* and *Chlamydia trachomatis*. Typical treatment of PID involves dual coverage with ceftriaxone and doxycycline. *Neisseria meningitidis* and *Chlamydia psittaci* are not bacteria found in PID. Although rare, *Escherichia coli* can cause PID.

49. E. This woman most likely has an endometrial carcinoma, the most common gynecologic malignancy, which continues to increase in incidence. It more commonly affects nulliparous women and has its peak occurrence in older women. Endometrial carcinomas are most often manifest by postmenopausal bleeding, which frequently leads to early diagnosis. They are often preceded by high-grade endometrial hyperplasia and are predisposed to prolonged estrogen stimulation, as occurs with exogenous estrogen therapy or estrogen-producing tumors. Additional factors that predispose women to endometrial carcinomas include obesity, diabetes, and hypertension. The common factor may be obesity, because estrone is often synthesized in peripheral adipose tissue.

50. D. Spermicide use alone (without condom) has a failure rate of 11.9% per 100 woman-years. Regarding the distractor choices, all have a lower failure rate per 100 woman-years. Vasectomy has a failure rate of 0.02% per 100 woman-years, while oral contraceptives and intrauterine devices have failure rates of 1.5% or less.

51. D. Koilocytosis, or clear vacuolization of involved cells, is characteristic of human papillomavirus (HPV). The histological report describes a condyloma acuminatum, most frequently caused by HPV type 6 and less frequently by HPV type 11. Condyloma acuminatum is a benign tumor that may occur on any moist mucocutaneous surface of the external genitals of either sex. It is thought to be related to the common wart (verruca vulgaris), which may be caused by a variety of HPV types. Anaerobic bacteria cause a foul-smelling vaginal discharge. These infections of the female reproductive tract are rare. *Gardnerella vaginalis* would be identified by the presence of clue cells on microscopy. Pyogenic bacteria are the least likely culprit in this case.

52. B. This man suffers from a high-grade prostatic carcinoma, as indicated by the Gleason score of 8. Osteoblastic metastases to the lumbosacral spine should be suspected due to the severe acute-onset lumbosacral pain. Prostatic carcinoma is the most common form of cancer in men and the second leading cause of cancer death. Surgical manipulation and radiotherapy are more suited for the treatment of patients with localized prostatic carcinoma. Pharmacotherapy with a 5-alpha-reductase inhibitor and clinical observation is often useful in benign prostatic hyperplasia. Endocrine therapy is the treatment of choice for advanced, metastatic carcinoma. Because prostatic cancer cells depend on androgens for sustenance, endocrine therapy attempts to deprive the tumor cells of testosterone. This can be achieved by orchiectomy or administration of estrogen or luteinizing hormone–releasing hormone. The primary effect appears to be suppression of the secretion of luteinizing hormone by the pituitary, which leads to reduced testicular production of testosterone. Long-term administration of luteinizing hormone–releasing hormone agonists eventually suppresses the release of luteinizing hormone, essentially achieving a pharmacologic orchiectomy.

53. E. *Trichomonas vaginalis* is a sexually transmitted anaerobic, flagellated protozoan parasite. It is frequently associated with a loss of acid-producing normal flora of the vagina and leads to vaginal itching and the characteristic profuse watery vaginal discharge. This condition is exacerbated by menstruation and pregnancy and may cause urinary frequency and dysuria. Infants infected with *Trichomonas vaginalis* during birth spontaneously clear the parasite in a few weeks. *Trichomonas vaginalis* is best seen on fresh preparations diluted with warm saline and appears as flagellated, turnip-shaped trichomonads. Condyloma acuminatum is a benign tumor that may occur on any moist mucocutaneous surface of the external genitals of either sex. It is thought to be related to the common wart (verruca vulgaris), which may be caused by a variety of HPV types. *Trichomonas vaginalis* would be identified on microscopy.

54. D. Herpes simplex virus infection is common and may involve the cervix, vagina, vulva, clitoris, urethra, and perianal skin. The frequency of genital herpes has increased dramatically over the past two decades, and HSV-2 is now one of the major sexually transmitted diseases among teenagers and young women. Among affected individuals, clinical symptoms are seen in about one-third. The lesions begin 3 to 7 days after sexual contact and appear as painful erythematous papules in the vulva that progress to vesicles and then coalescent ulcers. The initial infection may produce systemic symptoms, such as fever, malaise, and tender inguinal lymph nodes. The vesicles and ulcers contain numerous virus particles, which appear as multinucleated giant cells with viral inclusions on cytologic smears. The lesions heal spontaneously in 1 to 3 weeks, but latent infection of regional nerve ganglia may persist. About two-thirds of women suffer recurrences, which are less painful. *Gardnerella* is a pleomorphic Gram-negative rod that causes vaginosis (green vaginal discharge) with a fishy smell. *Neisseria gonorrhoeae* is a Gram-negative coc-

cus that is sexually transmitted. It can cause vaginitis as well as arthritis. Chlamydial infections are associated with the presence of budding yeast on KOH preparation of secretions.

55. A. This is classic for a conductive hearing loss. The Weber test will lateralize to the affected ear. With sensorineural loss, Weber will lateralize to the good ear, while with the affected ear BC > AC with respect to the Rinne test. There is no evidence to suggest other possible causes for this patient's conductive hearing loss. This condition is not due to cerumen impaction, since the otoscopy is normal. There is no reason to suspect medication-induced hearing loss given her lack of medications.

56. C. The dysplastic cervical epithelial cells demonstrating koilocytosis indicate that this woman is infected with the human papillomavirus (HPV), most likely HPV type 16, 18, 31, or 33. After infection, HPV sequences are often integrated into dysplastic and malignant cervical epithelial cells. HPV viral proteins E6 and E7 bind and inactivate the gene products of *p53* and *Rb*, respectively.

57. D. This vignette is descriptive of molluscum contagiosum caused by the poxvirus. The characteristic finding with this is central umbilication with each lesion. It is similar to infection with HPV but is self-limiting. It will eventually regress on its own. Common warts caused by HPV are firm, hyperkaratotic papules with no umbilication. They are typically seen on the hands. Condylomata lata is the whitish wart-like lesion of secondary syphilis. Tinea versicolor infection is a fungal infection characterized by hypopigmented areas usually present on the trunk. It is usually an asymptomatic infection. Atopic dermatitis is a pruritic inflammation with preference for the face, neck, and flexor areas. It is usually associated with a personal or family history of asthma, allergic rhinitis, or hay fever.

58. B. It usually involves the testis before the epididymis. The lesion described is a chancre, which is the primary stage of syphilis. A chancre is a painless, elevated, superficially ulcerated and firm papule. Chancres are usually located on the glans penis or prepuce and most likely heal in 2 to 6 weeks. If left untreated, they will be followed by secondary and tertiary lues. Syphilis is caused by the spirochete *Treponema pallidum*, which can be easily demonstrated on dark-field microscopy.

59. E. A serous cystadenocarcinoma is a malignant cystic tumor lined with cells resembling the epithelium of the fallopian tube. It is frequently bilateral and accounts for approximately 50% of ovarian carcinomas. A mucinous cystadenocarcinoma is a malignant tumor characterized by multilocular cysts lined by mucus-secreting columnar epithelium and filled with mucinous material. It may often rupture or metastasize, leading to pseudomyxoma peritonei, with multiple peritoneal tumor implants all producing large quantities of intraperitoneal mucinous material. Pseudomyxoma peritonei can also be caused by a mucinous cystadenoma, carcinomatous mucocele of the appendix, and other mucinous tumors.

60. E. A hydatidiform mole characteristically occurs in the early months of pregnancy. It is clinically characterized by vaginal bleeding and a rapid increase in uterine size, in which the uterus is often too large for the supposed stage of pregnancy. A hydatidiform mole results in choriocarcinoma in only 2 to 3% of cases. It occurs in two varieties, a complete and an incomplete hydatidiform mole. A complete hydatidiform mole presents with a 46 XX karyotype and no embryo is present. It is exclusively paternal in derivation, a condition often referred to as androgenesis. A partial hydatidiform mole presents with triploidy and rarely tetraploidy and no embryo is present. It is thought to be due to the fertilization of the ovum by two or more spermatozoa and usually results in 69 chromosomes derived from two paternal and one maternal haploid set.

61. B. This patient has gestational choriocarcinoma. A gestational choriocarcinoma is characterized by an increased serum concentration of hCG, which is an important diagnostic sign. It is an aggressive malignant neoplasm that is characterized by early hematogenous spread to the lungs. It is more frequent than ovarian carcinoma and is usually responsive to chemotherapy. Gestational choriocarcinoma is preceded by a hydatidiform mole in 50% of cases and is less commonly preceded by a normal-term pregnancy in 20 to 30% of cases or an abortion of an ectopic pregnancy in 20% of cases.

62. A. A fibroma is a solid tumor that consists of bundles of spindle-shaped fibroblasts. It may be associated with Meig's syndrome, a triad of ovarian fibroma, ascites, and hydrothorax. A granulosa cell tumor secretes estrogen and often causes precocious puberty. In adults it is often associated with endometrial hyperplasia or endometrial carcinoma. It is characterized by Call-Exner bodies, which are small follicles filled with an eosinophilic secretion. A Krukenberg tumor occurs when the ovaries are replaced bilaterally by mucin-secreting signet-ring cells, which often originate in the stomach. A Sertoli-Leydig cell tumor secretes androgens and is associated with masculinization. A thecoma demonstrates round, lipid-containing cells as well as fibroblasts and occasionally secretes estrogen.

63. A. Epispadias is a congenital defect of the opening of the urethral meatus, where the opening is located in the dorsum of the glands rather than at the midline. It can be corrected by simple outpatient surgery, with minimal complications. A fused meatal opening would be a cause for concern and necessitate further investigation, due to the questionability of the existence of a urethra. Narrowing or stenosis of the urethral meatus is easily treatable via dilatation of the meatus. Ventral opening of the meatus is known as hypospadias, and like epispadias can easily be treated with simple outpatient surgery.

64. C. Hemoglobin electrophoresis would be the most direct way to diagnose a suspected sickle cell anemia. Sickle cell anemia can cause priapism due to sludging of blood in the corporal arterioles. This can lead to a prolonged penile erection unrelated to sexual desire. A complete blood count can show an anemic state but would not define or be able to designate a diagnosis. A chest x-ray would be of little or no use in this situation as the issue is hematologic in origin. A neurological exam would have no bearing on diagnosis of a priapic state, nor would a standard urinalysis.

65. D. Poor hygiene is the most common cause of balanitis. An accumulation of sweat, debris, and residue under the foreskin can cause irritation and produce inflammation of the glans, resulting in balanitis. Blunt penile trauma can cause phimosis but not balanitis. Eating habits will have no bearing on inflammation of the glans. Unprotected sex can cause irritation and inflammation, but it is not the main cause of this condition.

66. E. Invasive carcinomas most frequently occur in middle-aged groups and are most often squamous cell carcinomas; adenocarcinomas account for only 5% of cases. Invasive carcinomas most frequently arise from preexisting cervical intraepithelial neoplasia (CIN) at the squamocolumnar junction and have exhibited a striking decrease in mortality since the introduction of the Pap smear. They are associated with early sexual activity, multiple sexual partners, low socioeconomic status, and cigarette smoking. HPV types 16, 18, 31, and 33 are commonly found integrated into the genomes of dysplastic or malignant cervical epithelial cells, which explains the presence of koilocytosis.

67. B. Benign prostatic hyperplasia is the most frequent cause of urinary tract obstruction. In men, noncancerous prostatic enlargement is the most common cause of urinary obstruction. Androblastoma is a Sertoli cell tumor with endocrine manifestations and is benign. Hydronephrosis may be secondary to obstruction and can worsen over time owing to the failure to release urine steadily. Prostatic cancer is common but usually occurs in the periphery of the prostate, not the inner mucosal area. This entity is less likely in the presence of a normal PSA. Sexually transmitted diseases can cause irritation and inflammation as well as urinary obstruction, but this is quite rare in comparison with the other choices.

68. D. Obstructive sleep apnea syndrome (OSAS) presents with excessive daytime sleepiness and disruptive snoring. It is caused by an obstruction in the nose, mouth, or airway from a structural problem, such as an enlarged tongue or tonsils. When a person is in a supine position, fatty tissue in the neck can press down on the airway, narrowing it and causing OSAS. Risk factors include obesity and smoking. Cataplexy is a sudden collapse while awake due to emotional stimulation. It is a component of narcolepsy, a disease characterized by extreme daytime sleepiness and a sudden state of sleep. It is associated with hypnagogic and hypnapompic hallucinations. Depression must be associated with five of the seven criteria defining it for 2 weeks. Tuberculosis is a disease associated with fever, night sweats, and hemoptysis.

69. D. This young woman presents with a history and clinical symptoms associated with toxic shock syndrome, which was initially associated with the use of highly absorbent tampons. It is caused by an exotoxin produced by *Staphylococcus aureus*, which grows in the tampon. It is characterized by fever, vomiting, and diarrhea and is sometimes followed by kidney failure and shock. A generalized rash followed by desquamation is also commonly associated with toxic shock syndrome.

70. A. *Calymmatobacterium granulomatosus* is a Gram-negative rod that is probably sexually transmitted. It appears initially as a papule, which becomes superficially ulcerated. It progresses as adjacent lesions coalesce to form large genital or inguinal ulcerations, sometimes with lymphatic obstruction or genital distortion. *C. granulomatosus* is characterized by Donovan bodies, which are multiple organisms filling large histiocytes. Chancroid (*Haemophilus ducreyi*) is associated with small painful ulcers of the genitalia. Gonococcal infections are associated with the presence of Gram-negative diplococci on Gram's stain. *Chlamydia trachomatis* causes nongonococcal urethritis. Treatment involves tetracycline or erythromycin. Herpes simplex virus would be associated with the characteristic lesion of grouped vesicles on an erythematous base.

71. B. Endodermal sinus (yolk sac) tumors are tumors of germ cell origin that resemble extraembryonic yolk sac structures and produce alpha-fetoprotein. They are homologous to endodermal sinus tumors of the testis. Teratoma often is associated with a mixed echogenic picture on ultrasound. Teratomas constitute 90% of germ cell tumors of the ovary. They involve all three germ cell layers. Mature teratomas (dermoid cysts) are benign. Immature teratoma is an aggressive malignant tumor. Monodermal teratoma (struma ovarii) is typically composed only of thyroid tissue. Dysgerminomas are tumors of germ cell origin. Such tumors make up one-fourth of ovarian tumors and account for most ovarian tumors occurring in women below 20 years of age.

72. C. A papillary hidradenoma is identical in appearance to an intraductal papilloma of the breast. A papillary hidradenoma presents as a sharply circumscribed nodule, usually found on the labia majora or interlabial folds. It may be clinically confused with carcinoma owing to its tendency to ulcerate. On histologic examination, a papillary hidradenoma consists of tubular ducts lined by a single or double layer of nonciliated columnar cells, with a flattened layer of myoepithelial cells lying beneath the epithelium that are characteristic of sweat glands or sweat gland tumors. Vulvar intraepithelial neoplasia is diagnosed by vulvar biopsy. Vestibular adenitis is an inflammatory condition.

73. C. This man suffers from benign prostatic hyperplasia. This condition is present in 90% of men at 70 years of age, but clinical symptoms are present in only half of the men with the histologic changes of benign prostatic hyperplasia. The condition is related to the action of androgens, especially dihydrotestosterone (DHT), a metabolite of testosterone that is the ultimate mediator of prostate growth. DHT is synthesized in the prostate by the enzyme 5-alpha-reductase type 2. Therapy with 5-alpha-reductase inhibitor markedly reduces the amount of DHT present in the prostate and decreases prostatic volume and urinary obstruction in some patients. Benign prostatic hyperplasia may lead to secondary changes of the bladder, such as hypertrophy, trabeculation, and diverticulum formation. Hydronephrosis or acute urinary retention, with secondary urinary tract infection and even azotemia (postrenal) and uremia may develop. However, it should be noted that most current studies deny any association between benign prostatic hyperplasia and the formation of cancer of the prostate.

74. A. Candidiasis, or moniliasis, is the most common form of vaginitis and is caused by *Candida albicans*, a normal component of the vaginal flora. It is classically characterized by white, patch-like mucosal lesions, vulvovaginal pruritus, and a thick white vaginal discharge. Candidiasis is associated with diabetes mellitus, pregnancy, broad-spectrum antibiotic therapy, oral contraceptive use, and immunosuppression. *Chlamydia* causes arthritis, urethritis, and cervicitis. *Gardnerella vaginalis* is associated with the presence of clue cells on microscopy. *Neisseria gonorrhoeae* is associated with urethritis, cervicitis, prostatitis, epididymitis, and arthritis.

75. E. Clear cell adenocarcinoma is a rare malignant tumor. The 5-year survival rate is approximately 50% when it is confined to the ovaries; however, these tumors tend to be aggressive and to spread beyond the ovaries, resulting in a greatly decreased survival rate. Clear cell adenocarcinoma is a solid or cystic surface epithelial tumor of the ovary that is characterized by large epithelial cells with abundant clear cytoplasm. The incidence is greatly increased in daughters of women who received diethylstilbestrol (DES) therapy during pregnancy. Clear cell adenocarcinoma is often preceded by vaginal adenosis, a benign condition characterized by mucosal columnar epithelium-lined crypts in areas normally lined by stratified squamous epithelium.

Chapter 11 Respiratory System

Questions

1. A 38-year-old man who is watching a football game in the supine position aspirates a piece of popcorn. At which site of the lung will the aspirated particle most likely be lodged?

   A. Lingula of the left lower lobe

   B. Lower portion of the left lower lobe

   C. Lower portion of the right lower lobe

   D. Upper lobe of the left lung

   E. Upper lobe of the right lung

   F. Upper portion of the left lower lobe

   G. Upper portion of the right lower lobe

2. A 45-year-old sandblaster presents to his primary care physician for an annual physical required for work. A routine chest radiograph is obtained and fibrotic nodules are seen in the upper zones of the lungs. Calcified lymph nodes that produce an eggshell pattern are also seen. Despite these findings, the patient denies any coughing or shortness of breath. What is the most likely diagnosis?

   A. Anthracosis

   B. Asbestosis

   C. Berylliosis

   D. Byssinosis

   E. Silicosis

3. A 33-year-old man presents to his primary care physician with concerns about infertility. He and his wife have been trying to conceive for 2 years without success. He also complains about frequent viral infections and sinusitis. Physical examination reveals that the heart is auscultated on the right side of his chest. Where is the most likely defect in this patient?

   A. Actin

   B. Desmin

   C. Dynein

   D. Kinesin

   E. Vimentin

4. A mother brings her 10-month-old son in to the pediatrician because of his failure to thrive. The child has foul-smelling stools. He also has a chronic cough, which resulted in several previous visits to the emergency department. He is in the sixth percentile for height, weight, and head circumference. Which of the following tests would prove most helpful in diagnosis?

   A. Complete blood count

   B. HIV antibody test

   C. Lead level

   D. Stool culture

   E. Sweat test

5. A 29-year-old man presents to his physician for an annual checkup. He has a positive reaction to a PPD test. Chest x-ray reveals two calcified scars just above the interlobar fissure between the upper and lower lobes of the left lung. Hematoxylin-and-eosin (H&E) stain is shown in Figure 11-1. The pathologic organism implicated in the disease described is responsible for inducing:

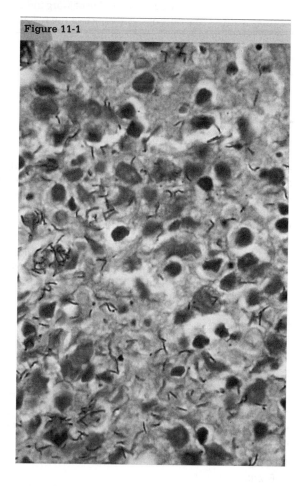

Figure 11-1

   A. Anaphylactic hypersensitivity

   B. Cell-mediated hypersensitivity

   C. Cytotoxic hypersensitivity

   D. Humoral immunity

   E. Immune-complex-mediated hypersensitivity

6. An 8-year-old girl is found to have a positive PPD test on a routine screening. She is otherwise healthy. Physical examination of the heart, lungs, and abdomen is unremarkable. She has a healed left-lower-quadrant scar from a prior inguinal hernia repair. Which of the following is the most likely to be found on her chest x-ray?

    A. Calcifications

    B. Cavitations

    C. Hilar adenopathy

    D. Lobar infiltrate

    E. No abnormal findings

7. Pneumoconioses are caused by inhalation of inorganic dust particles, such as coal dust or silica. Which of the following is common to all forms of pneumoconiosis?

    A. Caseating granulomas

    B. Formation of a lung abscess

    C. Increased susceptibility to tuberculosis

    D. Interstitial pulmonary fibrosis

    E. Noncaseating granulomas

    F. Plaques on the parietal pleura

8. A 58-year-old man with a history of chronic progressive dyspnea collapses in a shopping mall. He expires en route to the hospital. Autopsy is performed within 2 hr of death at the request of his family. A section of lung tissue is found to have undergone necrosis, and there is a loss of tissue architecture. The gross appearance of the tissue is cheese-like. On histological examination it has an amorphous eosinophilic appearance. Which of the following most likely resulted in the changes seen in the lung tissue?

    A. Adult respiratory distress syndrome

    B. Lung abscess

    C. *Mycobacterium tuberculosis*

    D. Pulmonary infarction

    E. Wegener's granulomatosis

9. The edematous fluid of a 40-year-old woman is examined and found to have increased protein, increased cells, and a specific gravity greater than 1.020. Which of the following is the most likely cause of her edema?

    A. Congestive heart failure

    B. Filaria

    C. Inflammation

    D. Nephrotic syndrome

    E. Portal hypertension

10. A 25-year-old man who is in the army presents to the emergency department complaining of a 3-week history of a dry hacking cough and episodic headache. Chest x-ray reveals diffuse infiltrates bilaterally. What is a unique feature of the causative agent in this patient?

    A. It is acid-fast.

    B. It contains cholesterol in the cell membrane.

    C. It is Gram-negative.

    D. It is Gram-positive.

    E. It will grow on chocolate agar.

11. A 2-month-old infant is brought to the emergency department with a 4-day history of cough, poor feeding, and a fever of 102°F (39°C). His respiratory rate is 30/min. Chest x-ray reveals patchy infiltrates bilaterally. Which of the following is the most likely explanation for these findings?

    A. Adenovirus

    B. Influenza A

    C. Respiratory syncytial virus

    D. *Staphylococcus aureus*

    E. *Streptococcus pneumoniae*

12. A 60-year-old patient develops a fever, chills, and a productive cough over the period of a week. Physical examination reveals dullness to percussion. A chest x-ray is obtained (Figure 11-2). What organism is most responsible for her pneumonia?

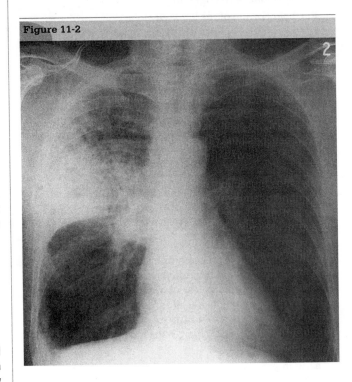

Figure 11-2

    A. *Bacteroides*

    B. *Haemophilus influenzae*

    C. *Mycoplasma pneumoniae*

    D. *Staphylococcus aureus*

    E. *Streptococcus pneumoniae*

13. A healthy woman who lives Colorado is found to have increased level of 2,3 diphosphoglycerate (2,3-DPG). What is the most likely effect on the hemoglobin-oxygen dissociation curve?

    A. No change to the dissociation curve

    B. Shifts the curve to the right, with hemoglobin having a decreased oxygen affinity

    C. Shifts the curve to the right, with hemoglobin having an increased oxygen affinity

    D. Shifts the curve to the left, with hemoglobin having a decreased oxygen affinity

E. Shifts the curve to the right, with hemoglobin having an increased oxygen affinity

14. A 28-year-old man with AIDS presents to his primary care physician with a productive cough, fever, and dyspnea. Physical examination reveals that he is febrile. Pulmonary auscultation demonstrates bilateral wheezes in the lower lung zones and dullness to percussion. Bronchoscopy is performed and lung tissue sampled and stained with a silver stain; it is found to grow an organism. What is the most likely diagnosis?

A. *Cryptococcus neoformans*

B. *Pneumocystis carinii*

C. *Pseudomonas aeruginosa*

D. *Staphylococcus aureus*

E. *Streptococcus pneumoniae*

15. A 33-week-old infant is born to a mother with gestational diabetes. The infant is hypoventilating and hypoxemic, apparently because of respiratory distress. Which of the following is an indication of lung immaturity?

A. Amniotic lecithin:sphingomyelin ratio < 2.0

B. Decreased amniotic fluid

C. Decreased alpha$_1$ antitrypsin in amniotic fluid

D. Elevated alpha-fetoprotein

E. Elevated maternal HbA$_{1c}$

16. A healthy 21-year-old student is preparing for a 5-km race. He has been training for 3 months, increasing his distance each week. What is the most likely effect on his body from the training regimen?

A. Mean arterial Po$_2$ increases

B. Mean arterial Po$_2$ decreases

C. Mean arterial Pco$_2$ increases

D. Pulmonary blood flow decreases

E. Venous Pco$_2$ increases

17. A lung biopsy is taken from a patient. In addition, a sputum culture taken from the same patient reveals Curschmann's spirals and Charcot-Leyden crystals. Which of the following cytokines are responsible for activating the cells responsible for this condition?

A. IL-2

B. IL-4

C. IL-5

D. TNF-α

E. IFN-γ

18. A 63-year-old retired shipyard worker presents to his physician complaining of dyspnea and a productive cough. A lung biopsy is performed and reveals a pleural plaque. What other histologic finding would likely be found?

A. Fibrotic nodules in the upper lung lobes

B. Hemosiderin-laden macrophages

C. Irregular linear densities in the lower lung lobes

D. Noncaseating granulomas

E. Oat cells

19. A 19-year-old man dies of rapidly progressive renal failure. On autopsy, his lungs are heavy, with areas of red-brown consolidation. There is also acute focal necrosis on the alveolar walls that is associated with intraalveolar hemorrhages. The alveoli also contain hemosiderin-laden macrophages. This disease is characterized by antibodies directed for which type of collagen?

A. I

B. II

C. III

D. IV

E. X

20. A 73-year-old man has been hospitalized for 6 days following a stroke. On the seventh day, he develops a fever and a productive cough. Physical examination reveals increased fremitus and crackles at the right lung base. Chest x-ray reveals patchy infiltrate in the right lower lobe. What is the most likely explanation for these findings?

A. Atypical *Mycobacterium*

B. *Haemophilus influenzae*

C. Influenza virus

D. *Moraxella catarrhalis*

E. *Pseudomonas aeruginosa*

21. A 65-year-old man presents to his primary care physician with chronic cough and difficulty breathing. He has worked as a stonecutter for 45 years. Pulmonary function tests reveal decreased lung volumes. No ferruginous bodies are seen on light microscopy. A chest x-ray is obtained (see Figure 11-3). Compared to the general population, this man has a significant risk of developing which of the following?

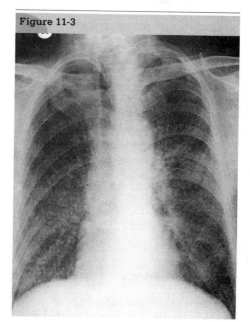

Figure 11-3

A. Asbestosis

B. Chronic bronchitis

C. Mesothelioma

D. Sinusitis

E. Tuberculosis

22. A 44-year-old woman presents to her primary care physician complaining of progressive dyspnea. She has never smoked and has no questionable occupational history. Physical examination of the chest reveals decreased fremitus, hyperresonance on percussion, and diminished breath sounds. Testing reveals that she is a homozygote for the PiZZ protein. This protein accounts for a deficiency in:

A. Eotaxin

B. Eosinophilic major basic protein

C. Alpha₁ antitrypsin

D. Neutrophil elastase

E. Prostaglandin D₂

23. A 53-year-old man is brought to the emergency department for evaluation of progressive dyspnea. Physical examination reveals decreased fremitus, hyperresonant percussion, and decreased breath sounds; furthermore, the trachea has shifted to the opposite side of the affected lung. What is the most likely diagnosis?

A. Atelectasis

B. Emphysema

C. Pleural effusion

D. Pneumonia

E. Pneumothorax

24. A 2-month-old infant is brought to the emergency department because he appears to be having difficulty breathing. The infant does not appear distressed and is not cyanotic. Cardiac auscultation reveals a harsh, continuous, machinery-like murmur. Which of the following is correct?

	Systemic Arterial Po₂	Pulmonary Arterial Po₂	Pulmonary Blood Flow	Pulmonary Arterial Pressure
A.	no change	↑	↑	↑
B.	no change	↓	↓	↓
C.	↑	↑	↑	↑
D.	↓	↓	↓	↓
E.	↓	↑	↑	↑

25. A 45-year-old alcoholic develops a cough and fever. CXR shows an air-fluid level in the superior segment of the right lower lobe. The most likely etiologic agent is which of the following?

A. Anaerobes

B. *Haemophilus influenzae*

C. *Legionella*

D. *Klebsiella*

E. *Streptococcus pneumoniae*

26. An infant born at the gestational age of 31 weeks has a lecithin/sphingomyelin (L/S) ratio of 1.7. The infant is having great difficulty breathing. Pulmonary auscultation reveals bilateral wheezes and rhonchi. Which of the following sequelae of this condition is possible?

A. Decrease in compliance

B. Decrease in intrapleural pressure

C. Increase in capillary filtration forces

D. Increase in lung recoil

E. Lower surface tension more in large than in smaller alveoli

27. A 68-year-old woman has been experiencing difficulty breathing for a week. She describes the sensation as if she could not generate her normal breathing rhythm. A CT scan reveals a pituitary mass lesion. Physical examination of the heart, lungs, and abdomen is unremarkable. What is the most likely part of the respiratory center that is affected?

A. Apneustic center

B. Dorsal respiratory group of the medulla

C. Cerebral cortex

D. Pneumotaxic center

E. Ventral respiratory group of the medulla

28. A 25-year-old marathon runner is completing his second marathon. He has no significant medical problems. He takes a nonsteroidal anti-inflammatory agent as needed for joint pain. His prior surgical history is arthroscopic surgery on both knees. At mile 13 of the race, he stops for an elective spirometry examination. What are likely findings on this examination for this patient?

A. Alveolar pressure equals atmospheric pressure

B. Alveolar pressure is higher than atmospheric pressure

C. Intrapleural pressure is negative

D. Intrapleural pressure is less negative than it is during expiration

E. Lung volume is less than the functional residual capacity (FRC)

29. A 7-year-old boy is brought to the emergency department with wheezing, dyspnea, and difficulty breathing, which wake him up in the middle of the night. He is afebrile. His respiratory rate is 35 bpm and his heart rate is 140/min. On auscultation, abnormal, high-pitched breath sounds are heard in all lung fields during inspiration and expiration. A chest x-ray is obtained (Figure 11-4). Which of the following findings is likely in this patient?

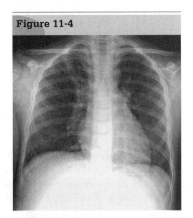

Figure 11-4

A. Acid fast organisms in sputum

B. Appearance of Curschmann's spirals in mucous plugs

C. Atypical activated T lymphocytes in the blood

D. Elevated serum cold agglutinins

E. Positive methenamine-silver stain of lung tissue

30. A 46-year-old man with a 35-pack-year smoking history has experienced shaking chills and shortness of breath for 2 days. His cough is productive of a yellowish sputum. He is on prednisone for psoriasis. Culture shows Gram-negative rods that are hard to see. What organism is most likely to be responsible for his symptoms?

A. *Legionella pneumophila*

B. *Listeria monocytogenes*

C. *Mycoplasma pneumoniae*

D. *Staphylococcus aureus*

E. *Streptococcus pneumoniae*

31. A 19-year-old woman attempts suicide by ingesting a large handful of barbiturates. Upon arrival in the hospital, her pulse is 105/min and her blood pressure is 95/60 mm Hg. Arterial blood gases are ordered. Which of the following values would be expected in this patient?

A. $P_{O_2} = 98$, $P_{CO_2} = 45$, pH $= 7.20$

B. $P_{O_2} = 45$, $P_{CO_2} = 45$, pH $= 7.45$

C. $P_{O_2} = 60$, $P_{CO_2} = 70$, pH $= 7.50$

D. $P_{O_2} = 65$, $P_{CO_2} = 30$, pH $= 7.45$

E. $P_{O_2} = 70$, $P_{CO_2} = 60$, pH $= 7.30$

32. A 40-year-old man presents to his primary care physician complaining of difficulty breathing and shortness of breath. Lung biopsy reveals pulmonary edema, hyaline membranes, and infiltration of the alveolar septa with mononuclear cells. There is also hyperplasia of type II pneumocytes. The lungs have a honeycomb appearance. Which of the following would most likely be seen upon further testing?

A. Decrease in lung volume

B. Increased airway resistance

C. Increased functional residual capacity (FRC)

D. Increased lung compliance

E. Increased tidal volume

33. A 56-year-old woman is admitted to the hospital because of a severe headache and irregular periods of apnea alternating with periods of noisy hyperventilation. Upon further testing, she is found to have viral meningitis. Which of the following respiration patterns is the woman experiencing?

A. Apneustic respirations

B. Biot respirations

C. Cheyne-Stokes respirations

D. Hyperpnea

E. Kussmaul respirations

34. A 58-year-old man with a 100-pack-year history of smoking presents to his primary care physician for evaluation of a chronic cough. Bronchoscopy and biopsy are undertaken. Which of the following metaplastic changes occurs in the respiratory tract of a chronic smoker?

A. Columnar epithelia to cuboidal epithelia

B. Columnar epithelia to squamous epithelia

C. Cuboidal epithelia to squamous epithelia

D. Squamous epithelia to columnar epithelia

E. Squamous epithelia to cuboidal epithelia

35. A 43-year-old man presents to the emergency department complaining of malaise, fever, and a productive cough. Chest auscultation and examination reveal decreased fremitus and dullness on percussion. Chest films show a consolidation immediately inferior to the horizontal fissure. What is the most likely site of localization of consolidation?

A. Inferior lobe of the right lung

B. Inferior lobe of the left lung

C. Middle lobe of the right lung

D. Superior lobe of the right lung

E. Superior lobe of the left lung

36. Two people both have a normal total ventilation of 7,500 mL/min. Person A, however, has a respiratory rate of 12 bpm while person B has a respiratory rate of 22 bpm. Which of the two has greater alveolar ventilation?

A. Person A

B. Person B

C. Both have equal alveolar ventilation

D. More information is needed

37. A neonate develops respiratory distress a few minutes after delivery and is taken to the neonatal intensive care unit (NICU) for observation. The following day the newborn becomes febrile and is short of breath. Examination of the sputum shows many neutrophils and Gram-negative rods growing pink colonies on MacConkey's agar. The organism most likely causing this neonate's symptoms belongs to which genus?

A. *Escherichia*

B. *Proteus*

C. *Salmonella*

D. *Shigella*

E. *Streptococcus*

38. A variety of factors can affect resistance in the airway. Which of the following would have the greatest impact on airway resistance?

A. Airway length

B. Airway pressure gradient

C. Airway radius

D. Airflow velocity

E. Viscosity of inspired gas

39. A 62-year-old woman presents to her primary care physician with a cough. She mentions occasionally coughing up blood. She states that she smoked 1 pack of cigarettes daily for 35 years but quit several years ago. Physical examination reveals bilateral wheezes. Laboratory values reveal hypercalcemia. Serum protein electrophoresis shows no abnormal spikes. A chest x-ray is obtained (Figure 11-5). What is the most likely diagnosis?

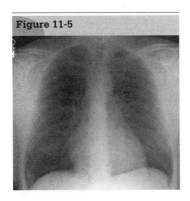
Figure 11-5

A. Goodpasture's disease

B. Multiple myeloma

C. Renal cell carcinoma

D. Small cell carcinoma of the lung

E. Squamous cell carcinoma of the lung

40. A 57-year-old obese woman presents to her primary care physician complaining of hemoptysis. She says that she has had a productive cough for several months, but only recently has she seen blood. She has had several episodes of coughing over the past few years. She has a 30-pack-year history of smoking. Which of the following patterns would be expected?

Total Lung Capacity	FEV$_1$	Forced Vital Capacity (FVC)	FEV$_1$/FVC	Residual Volume
A. ↓	↓	↓	↑	↓
B. ↓	↓	↓	normal	↓
C. ↑	↓	↓	↓	↑
D. ↑	↓	↓	normal	↑
E. ↑	↓	↓	↑	↑

41. A 12-year-old girl with cystic fibrosis presents to her pediatrician with a fever and a cough productive of blue-green-tinged sputum. Chest auscultation reveals crackles in the right middle lobe. Chest x-ray reveals a right-middle-lobe infiltrate. What is the most likely explanation for these findings?

A. *Klebsiella pneumoniae*

B. *Mycoplasma pneumoniae*

C. *Pneumocystis carinii*

D. *Pseudomonas aeruginosa*

E. *Streptococcus pneumoniae*

42. A 51-year-old man presents to his primary care physician with the following findings on examination of the right lung field: absent breath sounds, decreased resonance, decreased fremitus, and tracheal deviation to the affected side. What is the most likely diagnosis?

A. Bacterial pneumonia

B. Bronchial obstruction

C. Pneumothorax

D. Pleural effusion

E. Viral pneumonia

43. A 28-year-old woman presents to her primary care physician complaining of a cough, shortness of breath, intermittent hemoptysis, and sinusitis. Chest x-ray reveals large nodular densities. Serum studies reveal the presence of C-ANCA. What other finding might be present in this patient?

A. Arthritis

B. Changes in lips and oral mucosa

C. Hematuria

D. Hemorrhages

E. Nail-bed hemorrhages

F. Pericardial pain

44. A 5-year-old girl is brought to her pediatrician because of a high fever and a sore throat. Her mother states that she has had trouble swallowing and has been drooling a lot. You ask the child to lie down on the examining table and she refuses. Her mother then tells you that unless her daughter sits upright, she has difficulty breathing. What is the most likely explanation of these findings?

A. *Escherichia coli*

B. *Haemophilus influenzae*

C. *Mycoplasma pneumoniae*

D. *Rotavirus*

E. *Staphylococcus aureus*

F. *Streptococcus pneumoniae*

G. *Streptococcus pyogenes*

45. A 59-year-old man who is a heavy smoker presents to his primary care physician with chronic cough, acne, and increased urination. Physical examination reveals a protruding abdomen with purple striae, thin extremities, and a collection of fat between the shoulders. Lung biopsy reveals small round blue cells. What is the most likely diagnosis?

A. Adenocarcinoma

B. Bronchoalveolar carcinoma

C. Large cell carcinoma

D. Small cell carcinoma

E. Squamous cell carcinoma

46. A 75-year-old man presents to the emergency department with shortness of breath. Physical examination reveals tachycardia and decreased breath sounds throughout the lungs. He also has an increased anteroposterior diameter of the chest. Pulmonary function tests show a decreased infiltrate/exudate ratio. This man is found to have panacinar emphysema. If the cause of his condition is hereditary, which of the following organs might also be affected?

A. Brain

B. Heart

C. Kidney

D. Liver

E. Pancreas

F. Spleen

G. Thyroid

47. A 17-year-old African-American cheerleader falls during practice and is taken to the emergency department. Her history is unremarkable except for an episode a few months earlier when she had red bumps on her legs. A chest x-ray is obtained (Figure 11-6). Laboratory studies reveal hypercalcemia. Acid-fast stains are negative. Which of the following is also seen in patients with this condition?

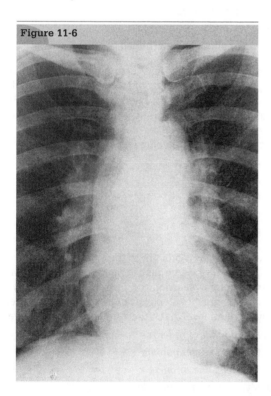

Figure 11-6

A. Anergy to tuberculin

B. Caseating granulomas

C. Decreased activity of serum angiotensin-converting enzyme

D. Hypocalciuria

E. Hypogammaglobulinemia

48. A lung specimen from a 68-year-old man living in New York City is examined at autopsy. Grossly the lungs have irregular black patches on them. Which of the following would most likely be found at biopsy?

A. Carbon-carrying macrophages

B. Fibrotic nodules filled with necrotic black fluid

C. Lung abscess

D. Prussian-blue–positive brown, rod-shaped bodies with clubbed ends

E. Silica nodules

49. An 82-year-old man presents to his primary care physician with dyspnea, wheezing, and cough. He sometimes feels as if he were gasping for air. His wife tells you that he has started sleeping with several pillows to avoid feeling short of breath when lying down. Chest x-ray reveals fluid around the lung space and an enlarged heart. Which of the following is a cause of his edema?

A. Decreased capillary permeability

B. Decreased hydrostatic pressure

C. Decreased oncotic pressure

D. Decreased sodium retention

E. Increased capillary permeability

F. Increased hydrostatic pressure

G. Increased oncotic pressure

50. A 17-year-old woman comes to your office complaining of difficulty breathing through her nose, so that she must breathe through her mouth. She sounds congested. She has a history of chronic rhinitis and sensitivity to aspirin. Physical examination reveals nasal polyps as the source of her breathing problem. Which of the following is this patient at an increased risk of developing?

A. Asthma

B. Bronchogenic carcinoma

C. Chronic bronchitis

D. Emphysema

E. Mesothelioma

51. A 35-year-old woman G2P0202 is currently 35 weeks pregnant. Her previous pregnancies were complicated by respiratory distress experienced by the baby at birth. She is curious about the development of the fetus and asks about the gestational age at which the lungs develop and function. What is the best answer to her question?

A. Week 5

B. Week 13

C. Week 20

D. Week 24

E. Week 35

52. Which of following cell types sits on the basal lamina of the alveolar epithelium and in the third trimester starts to secrete a substance that decreases surface tension on alveoli to prevent collapse?

A. Alveolar type I cells

B. Alveolar type II cells

C. Brush cells

D. Goblet cells

E. Macrophages

53. A 25-year-old man presents to the emergency department with wheezing and shortness of breath. Physical examination confirms bilateral scattered wheezes and increased fremitus bilaterally. Sputum cytology reveals Curschmann's spirals, eosinophils, and Charcot-Leyden crystals. Which of the following is a complication of this condition?

A. Lung abscess

B. Mesothelioma

C. Sinusitis

D. Squamous cell carcinoma

E. Status asthmaticus

F. Tuberculosis

54. A 35-year-old man who recently returned home from Europe presents to the emergency department with fever, weight loss, and hemoptysis. A sputum sample is obtained and found to be acid-fast. What would be the best medium to culture the organism on?

A. Charcoal yeast extract

B. Chocolate agar

C. Lowenstein-Jenson agar

D. Sabouraud's agar

E. Thayer-Martin media

55. A 69-year-old man with an 80-pack-year history presents to his primary care physician with chronic cough, dyspnea, chest pain, fatigue, and weight loss. A tumor is found in the hilar region of the lung and histologic examination reveals small round epithelial cells with little cytoplasm. In some of these tumor cells, neurosecretory granules are found. The doctor informs the patient that this type of cancer has a good initial response to chemotherapy. What is the most likely diagnosis?

A. Adenocarcinoma

B. Carcinoid tumor

C. Metastases

D. Small cell carcinoma

E. Squamous cell carcinoma

56. A 45-year-old man from Arizona was outside working on his farm when he suddenly became feverish (102°F, 38.85°C) with chills and difficulty breathing. Chest x-ray revealed bilateral infiltrates. Bronchoscopy revealed spherules in the tissue sample and dimorphic fungi grew as well. What organism is most likely responsible for this condition?

A. *Aspergillus*

B. *Blastomyces*

C. *Coccidioides*

D. *Histoplasma*

E. *Paracoccidioides*

57. A 22-year-old retired naval commander presents to his primary care physician with a 2-week history of scattered enlarged cervical lymph nodes. He denies any recent illnesses, and physical examination is unremarkable. Chest x-ray reveals bilateral hilar adenopathy. What is the most likely diagnosis?

A. Asbestosis

B. Berylliosis

C. Lymphoma

D. Pneumonia

E. Sarcoidosis

58. A 45-year-old man has been experiencing increased shortness of breath for 3 weeks, often after exertion. He has a 120-pack-year history. Chest x-ray shows a flattened diaphragm with increased expansion. What is the most likely finding on pulmonary function testing?

A. Ratio >1

B. Ratio <1

C. Ratio unchanged

D. $FEV_1 = FVC$

E. Ratio cannot be determined

59. A 45-year-old retired lawyer presents to the emergency department complaining of fever, chills, cough, and shortness of breath. Chest x-ray reveals bilateral patchy infiltrates. Coagulase-positive organisms are visible on culture and were shown to be resistant to the beta-lactams. What is the most appropriate treatment for this patient?

A. Ampicillin

B. Aztreonam

C. Ceftriaxone

D. Gentamicin

E. Methicillin

60. A 3-year-old boy is brought to the emergency department in respiratory distress; he has a temperature of 103°F (39.4°C). He has difficulty swallowing and, on exam, an inspiratory stridor is heard. X-ray shows epiglottic swelling. He has not received any vaccinations. What is the most likely causative agent?

A. *Haemophilus influenzae*

B. *Legionella pneumophila*

C. *Klebsiella pneumoniae*

D. *Mycoplasma pneumoniae*

E. *Streptococcus pyogenes*

61. A 35-year-old woman presents to her primary care physician with shortness of breath and chest pain. She is a smoker. Her medical history is unremarkable. She uses an oral contraceptive. Her travel history includes a very recent trip to Australia. Physical examination reveals respiratory distress and calf pain. She is afebrile. An arteriogram is obtained (Figure 11-7). What is the most likely diagnosis?

Figure 11-7

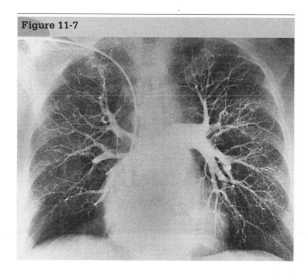

A. Dissecting aortic aneurysm

B. Fat embolus

C. Myocardial infarction

D. Pulmonary embolism

E. Syphilitic aneurysm

62. A 30-year-old woman presents to the clinic with a 3-day history of a dry, nonproductive cough that has been getting worse. She denies any episodes of fever or chills. She had been healthy up until these symptoms began. A tracheal aspirate is performed and Gram's stain fails to show any organism. Which of the following organisms is most likely the causative agent?

A. *Bacillus cereus*

B. *Chlamydia trachomatis*

C. *Clostridium difficile*

D. *Legionella pneumophila*

E. *Pseudomonas aeruginosa*

F. *Staphylococcus aureus*

G. *Streptococcus pneumoniae*

63. A 68-year-old woman living in a nursing home develops high fever, dyspnea, and a productive cough over 2 days. She is transferred to the community hospital after her mental status begins to deteriorate. Chest x-ray reveals a cavitary lesion in the right superior lobe. Which organism would be identified from her sputum?

A. *Legionella pneumophila*

B. *Mycoplasma pneumoniae*

C. *Pneumocystis carinii*

D. *Staphylococcus aureus*

E. *Streptococcus pneumoniae*

64. A 72-year-old man with a history of diabetes, hypertension, and COPD develops a productive cough for 3 days. Physical examination reveals labored breathing and auscultation of the chest reveals rales and rhonchi in the right middle lung field. Chest x-ray revealed a cavitary lesion in the right superior lobe. What is the empirical treatment for the causative organism?

A. Ciprofloxacin

B. Gentamicin

C. Nafcillin

D. Tetracycline

E. Vancomycin

65. A 45-year-old man is awakened one night by dyspnea and a cough productive of blood-tinged sputum. He has a history of alcoholism and diabetes. What is the most likely causative agent?

A. *Klebsiella pneumoniae*

B. *Legionella pneumophila*

C. *Mycoplasma pneumoniae*

D. *Pseudomonas aeruginosa*

E. *Streptococcus pneumoniae*

66. An immigrant from Chile comes to the United States to work. His routine chest x-ray reveals a lung mass as well as bilateral patchy infiltrates suggestive of pneumonia. Biopsy of the mass reveals fungal organisms—yeast forms with multiple buds in the shape of spokes on a wheel. What organism is most likely involved here?

A. *Blastomyces*

B. *Coccidiomyces*

C. *Cryptococcus*

D. *Histoplasma*

E. *Paracoccidiomyces*

67. A 65-year-old woman is found to have dyspnea, cough, and intermittent pleuritic chest pain. Gram's stain and culture of her sputum reveal *Streptococcus pneumoniae*, which is mildly resistant to penicillin. What is the most appropriate treatment?

A. Ceftriaxone

B. Cefuroxime

C. Erythromycin

D. Gentamicin

E. Vancomycin

68. A 35-year-old farmer from Wisconsin who watches birds and collects different exotic species in his spare time presents to the clinic with a 3-day history of a productive cough and fever. He is sexually active and has had numerous partners. Culture of the sputum reveals no organisms. What is the most likely organism implicated in this case?

A. *Chlamydia psittaci*

B. *Chlamydia trachomatis*

C. *Mycoplasma pneumoniae*

D. *Pseudomonas aeruginosa*

E. *Streptococcus pneumoniae*

69. A 59-year-old man with cystic fibrosis has a BUN/creatinine ratio of 30. He has a history of congestive heart failure and hypertension. He suddenly develops chills with a fever of 102°F (38.85°C) as well as a cough. Chest x-ray reveals bilateral patchy infiltrates in the lower lung fields. What drug should be avoided in this patient, given his history?

A. Cefuroxime

B. Erythromycin

C. Gentamicin

D. Penicillin

E. Piperacillin

70. A 4-year-old child aspirates a penny that becomes lodged in a peripheral airway. Which of the following changes in alveolar ventilation would occur in such an instance?

A. $\uparrow$ PaCO$_2$, $\downarrow$ PaO$_2$, $\uparrow$ VA/Q ratio

B. $\downarrow$ PaCO$_2$, $\uparrow$ PaO$_2$, $\downarrow$ VA/Q ratio

C. $\downarrow$ PaCO$_2$, $\uparrow$ PaO$_2$, $\uparrow$ VA/Q ratio

D. $\uparrow$ PaCO$_2$, $\downarrow$ PaO$_2$, $\downarrow$ VA/Q ratio

E. $\downarrow$ PaCO$_2$, $\downarrow$ PaO$_2$, $\downarrow$ VA/Q ratio

71. A 35-year-old man presents to his primary care physician with dyspnea and wheezing on expiration caused by episodic narrowing of the airways. He does not have any sneezing, nasal congestion, or cough. He states that he has not had this problem before and denies any family history. A chest x-ray is obtained (Figure 11-8). Which of the following is the most likely cause of his symptoms?

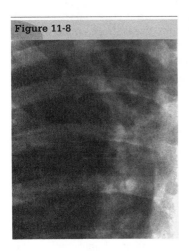

Figure 11-8

A. Adenovirus

B. Chronic bronchitis

C. Extrinsic asthma

D. Intrinsic asthma

E. Rhinovirus

72. A 45-year-old lawyer presents to his primary care physician with a fever, cough, nights sweats, and hemoptysis. He had been visiting his in-laws in Mississippi before his symptoms started. Culture and stain of his sputum revealed a positive Ziehl-Neelsen stain. What is the organism responsible for these findings?

A. *Klebsiella pneumoniae*

B. *Mycobacterium tuberculosis*

C. *Mycoplasma pneumoniae*

D. *Staphylococcus aureus*

E. *Streptococcus pneumoniae*

73. Regarding the patient presented in the above question, which of the following are extrapulmonary sites for infection?

A. Aorta

B. Gallbladder

C. Heart

D. Intervertebral disks

E. Spleen

74. A 50-year-old woman visits her primary care physician with the complaint of a cough productive of a yellowish substance and a fever, which she has had for 3 days. She denies having been around anyone who was sick. A Gram's stain and culture performed on her sputum shows a catalase-negative organism and demonstrates alpha hemolysis, resistant to optochin. Which of the following is the most likely causative organism?

A. *Peptostreptococcus*

B. *Streptococcus agalactiae*

C. *Streptococcus mutans*

D. *Streptococcus pneumoniae*

E. *Staphylococcus aureus*

75. A 30-year-old man comes to the otolaryngology clinic for evaluation of chronic lower respiratory tract infections. He has a medical history of seasonal allergies. His wife complains that he also has a snoring problem. Physical examination of the ears and throat are within normal limits. Nasal endoscopic examination reveals blue mucosa and multiple pseudopolyps. A biopsy of his respiratory epithelium is most likely to show abnormal:

A. Cilia

B. Cytoskeleton

C. Hemidesmosomes

D. Microvilli

E. Transport vesicles

Answer Key

1. G	20. E	39. E	58. B
2. E	21. E	40. C	59. E
3. C	22. C	41. D	60. A
4. E	23. E	42. B	61. D
5. B	24. A	43. C	62. B
6. E	25. A	44. B	63. D
7. D	26. E	45. D	64. E
8. C	27. E	46. D	65. A
9. C	28. C	47. A	66. E
10. B	29. B	48. A	67. C
11. C	30. A	49. F	68. A
12. E	31. E	50. A	69. C
13. B	32. A	51. D	70. D
14. B	33. B	52. B	71. D
15. A	34. B	53. E	72. B
16. E	35. C	54. C	73. D
17. C	36. A	55. D	74. C
18. C	37. A	56. C	75. A
19. D	38. C	57. B	

Answers and Explanations

1. G. Aspirated material usually enters the right lower lobar bronchus when an individual is in the supine position. It then lodges within the upper portion of the right lower lobe. If the person were sitting or standing, the aspirated material would most likely lodge in the lower portion of the right lower lobe. The right main bronchus is shorter and wider and turns at a shallower angle than the left main bronchus; therefore, unless the person were lying on his left side aspirated material would most likely end up lodged in the right lung.

2. E. All of the above findings are consistent with early silicosis. It is not until later in the course of silicosis that dyspnea, coughing, and other symptoms appear. Anthracosis is blackening of the lungs due to the inhalation of carbon particles. Asbestosis most commonly affects the lower lobes of the lung and is found in the shipbuilding, insulation, and roofing industries. Berylliosis and byssinosis are rare and are found in nuclear and aerospace workers and cotton workers, respectively.

3. C. The most likely diagnosis of this patient is Kartagener syndrome, characterized by bronchiectasis, sinusitis, and situs inversus. This stems from a defect in ciliary motility, most commonly absent or irregular dynein arms, which are responsible for ciliary movement. Males with this syndrome also tend to be infertile, due to ineffective spermatic motility. Actin is one of the contractile elements in skeletal muscular fibers. Desmin is a component of the intermediate filaments that copolymerize with vimentin to form constituents of connective tissue, cell walls, and filaments. Kinesin is another fibrous component found in axons, which aids in the transport of stimulus down the axon.

4. E. This patient has cystic fibrosis, the most common autosomal recessive disease in Caucasians. The primary defect is in the regulation of epithelial chloride transport by the CFTR protein encoded by the cystic fibrosis gene. This causes an increased chloride and sodium concentration in sweat, which explains the utility of the sweat test. Pancreatic abnormalities are involved in over 85% of CF patients, causing malabsorption of fat and fat-soluble vitamins. This leads to foul-smelling stools, abdominal distension, and poor weight gain. Pulmonary manifestations are seen in almost every case. The bronchioles are clogged with thick, viscous mucus, and *Pseudomonas aeruginosa* often colonizes the respiratory tract, causing pulmonary infections.

5. B. The patient had a scar due to a primary infection with *Mycobacterium tuberculosis*. Such an infection begins with inhalation of the mycobacterium and ends with a T-cell–mediated hypersensitivity response leading to a Ghon complex, which is a calcified scar in the lung. Anaphylactic hypersensitivity is a type 1 reaction characterized by IgE activation of mast cells with the release of histamine. Cytotoxic hypersensitivity is a type II reaction characterized by preformed antibodies against the body's antigens. An example of this is Graves' disease. Type III hypersensitivity (immune complex–mediated) causes the formation of immune complexes within the body. An example of this is serum sickness. Humoral immunity is due to B lymphocytes and is one mechanism of preventing infection from encapsulated organisms.

6. E. The positive PPD is a type of delayed hypersensitivity reaction. It indicates that this patient has been exposed to *Mycobacterium tuberculosis*. It represents relative immunity and hypersensitivity. *Mycobacterium tuberculosis* is spread by inhalation of droplets containing the organism. Most of these infections are asymptomatic and subclinical. Calcifications and cavitations are more commonly seen following reinfection in adults. Hilar adenopathy is seen in primary tuberculosis infections. Lobar infiltrates are typically seen with bacterial pneumonias.

7. D. The inhaled particles are ingested by macrophages, which release cytokines that drive fibrogenesis over the years. The hallmark of pneumoconiosis is diffuse fibrosis with a restrictive pattern of lung disease. Caseating granulomas are most commonly found in tuberculosis. Plaques on the parietal pleura are seen in asbestosis. Silicosis results in an increased susceptibility to tuberculosis. Lung abscesses occur following pulmonary infection. Noncaseating granulomas are characteristic of sarcoidosis.

8. C. The question describes caseous necrosis, which is most commonly seen as part of the granulomatous inflammation in *Mycobacterium tuberculosis*. In caseous necrosis, the tissue architecture is lost, but it is not liquefied. On histological section, it has an amorphous appearance with an increased affinity for acidophilic dyes. Lung abscesses result in liquefactive necrosis, which is characterized by digestion of the tissue. The tissue is soft and liquefied. This usually occurs following ischemic injury to the brain or suppurative infections. Pulmonary infarctions result in coagulation necrosis. In this type of necrosis, the architecture is preserved but there are nuclear changes. Increased cytoplasmic eosinophilia also occurs. Wegener's granulomatosis results in fibrinoid necrosis, which is characterized by a smudgy pink appearance in the vascular walls due to proteinaceous deposits. Adult respiratory distress syndrome (ARDS) results in the formation of intra-alveolar hyaline membrane composed of fibrin and cellular deposits.

9. C. Exudate is edema fluid that results from increased vascular permeability and inflammation. It has a high protein content, a specific gravity greater than 1.020, and large numbers of inflammatory cells. Transudate is edema fluid that results from an abnormality of Starling forces, as in congestive heart failure (CHF), portal hypertension, filarial, nephrotic syndrome, and liver disease. It does not contain any increased cells or increased protein. The specific gravity is less than 1.012. Edema from CHF and portal hypertension is due to increased hydrostatic pressure. Edema from nephrotic syndrome and liver disease is due to decreased oncotic pressure. Edema from filarial infestation, trauma, or surgery is due to lymphatic obstruction.

10. B. Mycoplasmal infection is common among the military and dorm residents. It does not show up on Gram's stain and is grown in Eaton's agar. It is unique in that it comprises the only bacterial membrane that contains cholesterol. Mycobacterial species, on the other hand, are acid-fast.

11. C. Respiratory syncytial virus is the most common cause of fever or pneumonia in infants less than 1 year of age. Reinfection can occur. Influenza A causes the systemic condition known as influenza, characterized by malaise, myalgias, fever, and headaches. Adenovirus is the most common cause of conjunctivitis. *Streptococcus pneumoniae* and *Staphylococcus aureus* cause pneumonia in older individuals.

12. E. *Streptococcus pneumoniae* is the most common cause of lobar pneumonia in the elderly. *Staphylococcus aureus* and *Haemophilus influenzae* cause a bronchopneumonia. *S. aureus* is seen in hospitalized patients. The incidence of *H. influenzae* pneumonia has decreased due to the advent of the *H. influenzae* type b (Hib) vaccine. *Mycoplasma pneumoniae* is responsible for walking pneumonia and causes a dry, hacking cough. CXR typically shows streaky infiltrates bilaterally. *Bacteroides* species cause aspiration pneumonia. CXR shows mediastinal enhancement.

13. B. 2,3 DPG shifts the curve to the right by binding to the beta chains of deoxyhemoglobin and decreasing the affinity of hemoglobin for O_2. This curve will have decreased, not increased, oxygen affinity.

14. B. *Pneumocystis carinii* is commonly seen to affect immunocompromised patients. Most infections are asymptomatic, and when sputum samples are stained with a silver stain, the yeast is seen. The other organisms do not stain with the silver stain but do cause pneumonia. *Cryptococcus neoformans* does affect immunosuppressed patients but causes meningitis.

15. A. An L:S ratio of less than 2.0 is diagnostic of infant respiratory distress syndrome (RDS). RDS is characterized by a deficiency of pulmonary surfactant. Surfactant reduces surface tension within the alveoli. If surfactant is deficient, the lungs collapse with each breath, requiring hard work by the infant to reinflate the lung. This accounts for the hypoventilation and hypoxemia. Because pulmonary secretions are discharged into the amniotic fluid, measurements of phospholipids provide a good estimate of the amount of surfactant found in the alveolar lining. Ele-

vated maternal alpha-fetoprotein levels can be associated with neural tube defects. Decreased amniotic fluid can lead to lung immaturity. Elevated maternal hemoglobin A1c is associated with maternal diabetes mellitus.

16. E. Mean values for both arterial P_{O_2} and P_{CO_2} do not change during exercise. Pulmonary blood flow increases because cardiac output increases during exercise. Venous P_{O_2} increases because excess CO_2 produced by the muscles is transported to the lungs by venous blood.

17. C. IL-5 is responsible for activating eosinophils, a major part of the acute- and late-phase reactions seen in atopic asthma. IL-4 activates the growth of mast cells. Both of these are involved in the hypersensitivity response seen in asthma. They as well as TNF-α are involved in the type I hypersensitivity reaction seen in asthma. IL-2 is secreted by helper T cells, which help to secrete cytotoxic and helper T cells. TNF-α is secreted by macrophages and is responsible for attracting and activating neutrophils. Interferon gamma (IFN-γ) is secreted by helper T cells and responsible for stimulation of macrophages.

18. C. The picture is that of a pleural plaque, the most common manifestation of asbestos exposure. These well-circumcised plaques are composed of dense collagen. Asbestosis usually affects the lower lung lobes; the upper lung lobes are affected in silicosis and coal worker's pneumoconiosis. Oat cells are characteristic of small cell carcinoma. Hemosiderin-laden macrophages are common in diffuse pulmonary hemorrhage syndromes.

19. D. This patient died of Goodpasture's syndrome, which is characterized by rapidly progressive glomerulonephritis and a necrotizing hemorrhagic interstitial pneumonitis. It mostly affects those in their teens and twenties, males more than females. It is caused by anti–basement membrane antibodies (type II hypersensitivity reaction). Basement membranes are composed of type IV collagen. Type I collagen is found in bone, tendon, skin, fascia, and dentin. Type II makes up cartilage. Type III is made of reticulin and is found in skin, blood vessels, and granulation tissue. Type X is found in the epiphyseal plate.

20. E. *Pseudomonas aeruginosa* is one of the most common organisms to cause hospital-acquired pneumonia. It causes a lobar infiltrate to be present on CXR and produces a blue-green pigment when cultured. Atypical *Mycobacterium* is associated with pneumonia in HIV-positive patients when the levels of CD 4 cells are decreased. *H. influenzae* can cause a pneumonia, but since the advent of Hib vaccine, the incidence has decreased. Influenza virus can cause pneumonia, but owing to its viral properties does not produce a lobar infiltrate. With influenza, bilateral streaky infiltrates are seen on CXR. *M. catarrhalis* is a common cause of otitis media.

21. E. This man has chronic silicosis, which is an occupational lung disease caused by exposure to free silica dust. It is seen in sandblasters, miners, stonecutters, and glassmakers. Silica is ingested by alveolar macrophages, which mount an inflammatory response. Nodules form and obstruct airways. The major complication of silicosis is tuberculosis. The risk is 10- to 30-fold higher than that of nonsilicotic populations. Mesothelioma and asbestosis are caused by exposure to asbestos. Asbestos exposure can be ruled out here because of this patient's occupational history and the absence of ferruginous bodies on light microscopy. Chronic bronchitis and sinusitis are not complications of silicosis. Chronic bronchitis is defined as productive cough occurring during at least 3 consecutive months over at least 2 consecutive years. A major cause is cigarette smoking. Sinusitis is inflammation of the sinuses.

22. C. A homozygote for the PiZZ protein has a severe deficiency of α-1-AT, which is responsible for inhibiting proteases, such as neutrophil elastase, which is capable of digesting lung tissue. Thus, with a deficiency of α-1-AT, neutrophil elastase and other proteases will not be inhibited. Individuals with the PiZZ protein are at increased risk for developing emphysema. Smokers have an even greater risk, so smoking cessation is advised. Eotaxin, major basic protein, and prostaglandin D_2 are both involved in the immune response seen in asthma.

23. E. Pneumothorax refers to air or gas in the pleural cavities. It can arise spontaneously or from trauma and is commonly associated with emphysema, asthma, and tuberculosis. Lung lobes affected by pleural effusions are dull on percussion. Emphysema and pneumonia cause no shift of the trachea. Lung lobes affected by pneumonia are also dull on percussion. Atelectasis causes the trachea to shift to the same side as the affected lung and produces a dull percussion.

24. A. This infant has a patent ductus arteriosus, which causes a left-to-right shunt. Blood from the aorta travels to the pulmonary trunk, exposing the normally low-pressure, low-resistance pulmonary circulation to increased pressure and/or volume. With this type of shunt, hypoxemia does not occur because there is increased pulmonary blood flow, pulmonary arterial pressure, and P_{O_2}.

25. A. The superior segment of the right lower lobe is the most likely segment to be involved in an aspiration pneumonia caused by anaerobic organisms. The remaining organisms do cause pneumonia but not the necrotizing type. Alcoholics are more susceptible to aspiration pneumonia.

26. E. Surfactant is produced by type II alveolar cells responsible for lowering surface tension in the alveoli. Therefore, it lowers lung recoil and increases compliance, which is associated with more effort to expand the lung. Premature infants with a low L:S ratio are more likely to develop respiratory distress owing to the lack of surfactant. A decrease in compliance is not associated with surfactant deficiency. This would cause less air to be present in the alveoli, which would also cause difficulty in respiration. A decrease in intrapleural pressure is associated with normal inhalation. An increase in capillary filtration forces would cause significant leakage of fluid from within the vessel, causing pulmonary edema.

27. E. The ventral respiratory group is responsible for expiration and is active during exercise. The apneustic center stimulates inspiration but is not responsible for the basic breathing rhythm. The pneumotaxic center inhibits inspiration. The cerebral cortex is responsible for voluntary control of breathing.

28. C. During the process of inspiration, intrapleural pressure becomes more negative than it is at rest or during expiration. Lung volume is greater than the functional residual capacity. Alveolar pressure is lower than atmospheric pressure. In obstructive lung diseases such as emphysema, there is a decrease in forced vital capacity and a decrease in peak expiratory flow rate. In cases of restrictive lung disease such as fibrosis, there is a decrease in forced vital capacity while the peak expiratory flow rate remains normal.

29. B. These symptoms are characteristic of asthma, which causes narrowing of airway passages. Attacks are often episodic and nocturnal. One of the most common microscopic findings is thick mucous plugs that occlude the airways. The mucous plugs contain shed epithelium, which give rise to Curschmann's spirals. Choice A is found in tuberculosis, choice D in mycoplasmal pneumonia, and choice E in *Pneumocystis carinii* pneumonia.

30. A. This is a typical presentation of pneumonia caused by *Legionella pneumophila*. Risk factors are smoking, steroids, and any immunocompromised state. The organism is hard to identify on Gram's stain. *Mycoplasma pneumoniae* causes an atypical pneumonia characterized by a dry, hacking cough. *Streptococcus pneumoniae* is a Gram-positive organism, as is *Staphylococcus aureus*. *Listeria monocytogenes* causes meningitis in newborns.

31. E. An overdose of barbiturates causes respiratory depression and thus a respiratory acidosis. This is characterized by a decreased P_{O_2}, an increased P_{CO_2}, and an acidotic pH. The normal P_{O_2} is approximately 80 to 110 mm Hg. The normal P_{CO_2} is 30 to 45 mm Hg. The normal pH is 7.35 to 7.45. The normal bicarbonate is 19 to 24 mEq/L. This value is sometimes provided in blood gas analysis, although it was not specifically asked for in this question.

32. A. The diagnosis is idiopathic pulmonary fibrosis, a restrictive lung disease. In restrictive lung diseases, lung volume decreases. Airway resistance does not change. Lung compliance is increased in obstructive diseases, such as emphysema, but decreases in restrictive diseases.

33. B. Biot respirations are caused by damage to the respiratory centers in the brainstem. This can occur in patients with brainstem strokes or vascular diseases that affect the brainstem. Kussmaul respiration is deep and rapid and is frequently seen in diabetic ketoacidosis. Cheyne-Stokes respiration is characterized by a gradual increase in the depth of respiration to a maximum, followed by a progressive decrease in the depth of respiration, resulting in apnea.

34. B. Pseudostratified ciliated columnar epithelium lines the entire respiratory tract excluding the vocal cords. Habitual cigarette smoking is considered a source of chronic irritation; thus the lining is replaced by stratified squamous epithelial cells, which are better suited for areas of "wear and tear." Persistent metaplasia can lead to cancer.

35. C. Only the right has a horizontal fissure. Immediately below this fissure is the middle lobe. The left lung does not have a horizontal fissure but rather an oblique fissure. Fissures divide the lungs into lobes.

36. A. Person B is performing rapid shallow breathing. Given that alveolar ventilation is equal to the difference between tidal volume and dead space then multiplied by the respiratory rate, person B will have a decreased tidal volume because there is a large component of dead-space ventilation. Thus, even though total ventilation may be normal, alveolar ventilation is depressed.

37. A. *Escherichia coli* is the most common cause for this neonate's pneumonia since it grows on MacConkey's agar and ferments lactose. This agar is used to identify lactose fermenters. *Salmonella* organisms are non–lactose fermenters that produce an inflammatory diarrhea. *Shigella* organisms are non–lactose-fermenting nonmotile organisms that produce dysentery. *Proteus* species are motile, non–lactose fermenters that are commonly associated with genitourinary symptoms. *Streptococcus* species are Gram-positive non–lactose fermenters.

38. C. There is an inverse fourth-power relationship between resistance and the radius of the airway. For example, if the airway radius decreases by a factor of 5, resistance will increase by a factor of 1,024 (4^5). This relationship is greater than that of any of the other answer choices.

39. E. The combination of cough, hemoptysis, wheezing, and smoking history suggests the diagnosis of lung cancer. Of the two lung cancers listed, squamous cell carcinoma is the one that may produce PTH-related peptide protein. PTHr leads to hypercalcemia. Small cell carcinomas commonly produce ADH or ACTH. In a patient with Goodpasture's, hemoptysis may present before the hematuria, but because of the other symptoms squamous cell carcinoma is the better choice. Renal cell carcinoma (RCC) may produce ectopic PTHrP and smokers do have an increased risk, but these patients present with hematuria, a palpable mass, flank pain, and a fever. The lack of an IgG or IgA spike on serum protein electrophoresis should rule out multiple myeloma.

40. C. The disease described is chronic bronchitis, which is productive coughing for 3 months or more for 2 consecutive years. Patients are often obese. Chronic bronchitis is an obstructive disease, therefore the key to answering this question is to know that the FEV_1/FVC ratio decreases with obstructive diseases, which leaves only choice C. Choices A and B are characteristic of restrictive lung diseases, where the ratio is normal or increased.

41. D. Cystic fibrosis patients are susceptible to infection by *Pseudomonas aeruginosa*. This organism usually forms a blue-green pigment. *Streptococcus pneumoniae* causes a lobar pneumonia in the elderly. *Mycoplasma pneumoniae* causes an atypical pneumonia that presents with a dry, hacking cough. *Pneumocystis carinii* affects immunocompromised patients (AIDS). *Klebsiella pneumoniae* is associated with alcoholism and diabetes.

42. B. In a bronchial obstruction, you would find absent breath sounds over the area, decreased resonance and fremitus, and tracheal deviation toward the side of the lesion. With a pneumothorax, the lung will collapse owing to air in the pleural space. It is characterized by hyperresonance, absent fremitus, and tracheal deviation away from the affected side. In a pleural effusion, you would find decreased breath sounds over the effusion, dullness to percussion, decreased fremitus, and no tracheal deviation. In viral pneumonia, there is no consolidation or volume loss. Findings such as decreased fremitus are not necessarily present. In bacterial pneumonia, since consolidation occurs, there will be increased fremitus, and bronchial breath sounds may be heard.

43. C. This patient has Wegener's granulomatosis, which is characterized by necrotizing granulomatous vasculitis of the vessels of the respiratory tract, kidney, and other organs. It presents with chronic sinusitis, hemoptysis, otitis media, cough, and dyspnea. Common findings are C-ANCA, a chest-ray with large nodular granules, hematuria, and red cell casts. Changes in the lips and oral mucosa may be seen in Kawasaki disease, which is an acute necrotizing vasculitis of small and medium-sized vessels. It is a disease of infants and children. Nail-bed hemorrhages are seen in bacterial endocarditis. Pericardial pain is seen in pericarditis.

44. B. Acute epiglottitis is most common in children between 2 and 6 years of age and is usually caused by the bacterium *Haemophilus influenzae*. It is a life-threatening disease that usually begins with a high fever and very sore throat. Other symptoms include drooling, stridor, hoarseness, cyanosis, difficulty breathing (the patient may have to sit upright and lean slightly forward to breathe adequately). *Streptococcus pneumoniae* is the leading cause of pneumonia in adults (40 to 65 years of age) and the elderly. *Staphylococcus aureus* causes acute bacterial endocarditis, food poisoning, and toxic shock syndrome. *Streptococcus pyogenes* causes rheumatic fever, scarlet fever, pharyngitis, and cellulitis. Rotavirus is a common cause of diarrhea. *Mycoplasma pneumoniae* is the leading cause of pneumonia in adults (18 to 40 years of age) and the second leading cause in children (6 weeks to 18 years of age). *Escherichia coli* most commonly causes urinary tract infections and diarrhea.

45. D. This man has Cushing's syndrome secondary to small cell carcinoma. Small cell carcinomas can produce ACTH or ACTH-like peptide. These neoplasms present with the described symptoms and biopsy findings. They are linked to smoking and found centrally in the lung. Squamous cell carcinoma can produce PTH-related peptide, not ACTH. Adenocarcinoma is a peripheral lung cancer that often arises in scars. Bronchoalveolar carcinoma is not linked to smoking. Large call carcinoma is an aggressive, undifferentiated carcinoma.

46. D. Panacinar emphysema can be associated with deficiency of alpha₁ antitrypsin, which is an alpha₁-protease inhibitor. This deficiency is due to a variant in the *pi* gene on chromosome 14. The variant results in an alteration in the protein that interferes with its hepatic secretion. This can ultimately lead to liver damage and possibly liver cirrhosis.

47. A. This patient has sarcoidosis, which is characterized by noncaseating granulomas often involving multiple organ systems. It is seen frequently in African Americans. It becomes clinically apparent during the teenage or young adult years. People with sarcoidosis often show reduced sensitivity and sometimes anergy to skin test antigens. Lab findings include hypercalcemia, hypercalciuria, hypergammaglobulinemia, and increased activity of serum angiotensin-converting enzyme.

48. A. Anthracosis is caused by the inhalation of carbon dust. It is characterized by carbon-carrying macrophages. These macrophages are the cause of the irregular black patches. Anthracosis is commonly found in people living in urban areas and usually causes no harm. Fibrotic nodules filled with necrotic black fluid are commonly found in patients with progressive massive fibrosis due to coal worker's pneumoconiosis. Silicotic nodules are seen in silicosis. Brown rod-shaped bodies with clubbed ends that stain for Prussian-blue are ferruginous bodies. These are characteristic of asbestosis. Lung abscesses are seen owing to pulmonary infection.

49. F. This man has pulmonary edema secondary to left-sided heart failure. The edema is due to increased hydrostatic pressure. Patients typically present with dyspnea, wheezing, orthopnea, cough, a feeling of drowning, and anxiety. Increased capillary permeability leads to edema, but this is usually secondary to inflammation. Decreased oncotic pressure leads to edema. The decreased oncotic pressure results from hypoalbuminemia from various causes, such as cirrhosis of the liver or nephrotic syndrome. Sodium retention from heart failure may cause edema, but it would be increased, not decreased.

50. A. Asthma is a pulmonary disease characterized by increased sensitivity of the airways to stimuli. It is divided into extrinsic asthma, which includes allergic asthma, and intrinsic asthma, which includes pharmacologic asthma. Pharmacologic asthma is often related to aspirin sensitivity. These patients have recurrent rhinitis and nasal polyps. Aspirin results in an excess production of leukotrienes. These cause bronchoconstriction, which initiates the asthmatic response. Bronchogenic carcinoma is related to cigarette smoking, asbestos, and radiation. Mesothelioma is due to asbestos exposure. The diagnosis requires a productive cough for at least 6 consecutive months for at least 2 consecutive years.

51. D. Lung development can be divided into four stages. In the glandular stage (weeks 5 to 17), respiration is not possible. At the second or canalicular stage (weeks 13 to 25), respiratory bronchioles and terminal sacs form. Fetuses born prior to week 20 rarely survive. At the third or terminal sac stage (weeks 24 to birth), type I and II alveolar cells are present and respiration is possible. Premature infants born between 25 and 28 weeks' gestation are capable of survival with intensive care. The last stage is the alveolar stage (birth to year 8). In this stage the bronchioles, terminal sacs, alveolar ducts, and alveoli proliferate. Week 35 is when type II alveolar cells start to secrete surfactant.

52. B. The substance described is surfactant. It is composed of mainly of phospholipids. Surfactant is typically made after 35 weeks of gestation by type II alveolar cells. Infants born prior to 35 weeks may not have produced enough surfactant, which leads to respiratory distress. Type I alveolar cells also sit on the basal lamina of the alveolar epithelium; however, they do not produce surfactant, but form part of the blood-air barrier. Goblet and brush cells are both found in the respiratory mucosa. Goblet cells produce mucus. Brush cells are columnar cells with microvilli. They have a general sensory function. Macrophages are the mononuclear phagocytes. In the alveoli of the lungs, they ingest small inhaled particles.

53. E. This man has extrinsic bronchial asthma. This is a type I hypersensitivity reaction caused by hyperplasia of bronchial submucosal glands and goblet cells, which causes an overproduction of mucus and plugs up the airways. The Charcot-Leyden crystals are breakdown products of eosinophilic granules. The Curschmann's spirals are whorls of sloughed surface epithelium in the mucin. Complications of asthma include chronic bronchitis, pulmonary emphysema, and status asthmaticus. Tuberculosis is caused by infection with *Mycobacterium tuberculosis*. Mesothelioma is caused by asbestos infection. Smoking increases the incidence of squamous cell carcinoma. Lung abscesses are due to pulmonary infection. Sinusitis is inflammation of the paranasal sinuses and is not caused by asthma.

54. C. This patient has tuberculosis. *Mycobacterium tuberculosis* is best cultured on Lowenstein-Jensen agar. Chocolate agar is used to grow *Haemophilus influenzae*. Fungi grow on Sabouraud's agar. Charcoal yeast extract helps to identify *Legionella* species, and *Neisseria gonorrhoeae* will grow on Thayer-Martin medium.

55. D. Small cell carcinomas have a strong relationship to cigarette smoking (> 98%). Most tumors are hilar or central and the type of epithelial cell described in the question is an oat cell, characteristic of small cell carcinoma. Small cell carcinomas are also responsive to chemotherapy initially, unlike non–small cell carcinomas. Squamous cell carcinoma is also very strongly associated with smoking but lacks the oat cell characteristic of small cell carcinoma. Squamous cell carcinoma is clearly linked to smoking and can be associated with the production of ectopic hormones, such as ACTH. Given the lack of other imaging studies, metastasis is unlikely in this case. Carcinoid tumor can cause carcinoid syndrome (flushing, sweating, wheezing, and diarrhea).

56. C. The patient has San Joaquin Valley Fever secondary to the fungus *Coccidiomyces*. This fungus lives in the southwestern region of the United States. It can cause pneumonia or disseminate into other tissue systems. The other organisms also cause systemic mycotic infections but are found in different areas of the country. *Aspergillus* is a cause of interstitial lung disease and can cause restrictive changes such as decreased lung volumes. *Blastomyces* and *Histoplasma* are also considered to be pneumoconioses and also cause interstitial lung diseases. They too can be associated with reduced lung expansion and decreased lung volumes. *Paracoccidiomyces* is a rare cause of interstitial lung disease, particularly in patients with HIV.

57. B. Berylliosis is a disease associated with hilar adenopathy on CXR in individuals who have been exposed to nuclear weapons, ceramics, or fluorescent lights. Since this patient is a retired naval commander, he probably had previous exposure to nuclear weapons. Sarcoidosis, a multisystemic disease of unknown cause, is more prevalent in the African-American population. The typical CXR finding is bilateral hilar lymphadenopathy; histologically, noncaseating granulomas are seen. Asbestosis causes a pulmonary fibrosis due to asbestos exposure, common in shipbuilders. With pneumonia, one more commonly finds cough and fever associated with the history. Lymphoma is a possibility, but is unlikely with this history. One would see systemic findings along with more areas of lymphadenopathy.

58. B. Typically the ratio is < 1 in an obstructive lung disease—for example, asthma. The patient has a hard time expiring air, so the FEV_1 decreases, which leaves more air in the lungs, thus increasing FVC. In restrictive lung disease, the ratio is either unchanged or increased slightly in severe cases. The patient cannot inspire air into the lungs because of the restriction, so therefore the FVC decreases, which causes an increase in the ratio. The FEV_1 is never equal to the FVC.

59. E. Methicillin is the drug of choice for resistant *Staphylococcus aureus*. This drug is penicillinase-resistant and usually does pretty well for this species. Ceftriaxone and ampicillin are in the beta-lactam category so would not be helpful in this situation. Gentamicin is used to treat infections with Gram-negative rods. Aztreonam is resistant to beta-lactamases but offers no coverage against Gram-positive organisms.

60. A. *Haemophilus influenzae* is the most common cause of epiglottitis in young children who have not been vaccinated against the *Haemophilus influenzae* type b capsule. Symptoms are similar to those described in the question. *Klebsiella pneumoniae* is another cause of pneumonia. *Legionella pneumophila* causes pneumonia in humans. *Mycoplasma pneumoniae* causes an atypical pneumonia in middle-aged adults. *Streptococcus pyogenes* is the most common cause of pharyngitis.

61. D. This patient has a pulmonary embolism (PE). Her symptoms, history of oral contraceptives, and prolonged bed rest all point to a PE. Most often these originate from venous thrombosis in the lower extremities. Although myocardial infarction should always be in the differential for chest disorders and dyspnea, her history points to a PE. A dissecting aortic aneurysm would present with severe tearing chest pain. These patients have a history of hypertension. Syphilitic aneurysms are a manifestation of tertiary syphilis. There is no reason to believe that this patient has syphilis. Fat emboli are associated with long bone fractures and liposuction.

62. B. Of the organisms listed, only *Chlamydia* is resistant to Gram-staining because of its intracellular nature. Others include *Rickettsia, Mycobacterium*, and *Mycoplasma*. *Streptococcus pneumoniae, S. aureus, Clostridium*, and *Bacillus* are all Gram-positive. The others are all gram-negative.

63. D. Of the organisms listed only *Staphylococcus aureus* would be responsible for causing a lung abscess. Elderly patients are usually infected with the influenza virus and acquire pneumonia after infection. *Mycoplasma pneumoniae* is an atypical pneumonia that does not cause abscess formation. *Streptococcus pneumoniae* causes pneumonia in elderly patients but does not cause lung abscesses. *Legionella pneumophila* pneumonia is associated with smokers and immunocompromised patients. *Pneumocystis carinii* causes pneumonia in immunocompromised patients, typically those with AIDS.

64. E. *Staphylococcus aureus* is the culprit here because of the likelihood of abscess formation. Empirically vancomycin should be started until sensitivities are established. Then nafcillin is a reasonable drug to use. Tetracycline has no coverage against Gram-positive organisms. Gentamicin is used for Gram-negative infections, as is ciprofloxacin.

65. A. This is a pneumonia caused by *Klebsiella pneumoniae*, which typically affects alcoholics and diabetics. Sputum looks like red currant jelly. *Streptococcus pneumoniae* does not give a characteristic appearance to the sputum. *Legionella pneumophila* affects smokers and the immunocompromised. *Mycoplasma pneumoniae* causes a pneumonia characterized by a dry, hacking cough. *Pseudomonas aeruginosa* can cause a pneumonia in diabetics but typically gives a blue-green tinge to the sputum.

66. E. This disease is caused by *Paracoccidioides*, which is found in rural Latin America. It is a dimorphic yeast with buds in a pattern resembling a captain's wheel. Coccidiomycosis should be suspected if a patient lives in the southwestern United States and has spherules with endospores. Blastomycosis is found in areas around the Mississippi river. Histoplasmosis demonstrates tiny yeast forms in macrophages and is found in the Ohio or Mississippi River Valleys. *Cryptococcus* is an encapsulated yeast that causes meningitis; it is associated with pigeons.

67. C. Erythromycin is the drug of choice for a mildly resistant strain of *Streptococcus pneumoniae*. If a highly resistant strain occurs, then ceftriaxone is used. Vancomycin is reserved for patients resistant to ceftriaxone. Gentamicin has no coverage against *S. pneumoniae*. Cefuroxime has little to no coverage for *S. pneumoniae*.

68. A. The clue to the answer here is the hobby of bird collecting and watching, significant for *Chlamydia psittaci* atypical pneumonia. This organism is intracellular and therefore lacks Gram-staining capabilities. *Chlamydia trachomatis* is responsible for causing urethritis. *Mycoplasma pneumoniae* also causes an atypical pneumonia but has a dry cough associated with it. *Streptococcus pneumoniae* does cause a productive cough but is not associated with birds. *Pseudomonas aeruginosa* also can cause a pneumonia but typically does so in cystic fibrosis patients.

69. C. This patient has prerenal failure with a BUN/Cr ratio of 30. Because of his condition, an aminoglycoside would be avoided since it poses a risk of renal toxicity and ototoxicity. A good choice for this patient would either be ceftazidime or piperacillin. Penicillin and erythromycin offer no coverage against *P. aeruginosa*.

70. D. Blocking the airway will decrease the ventilation/perfusion (V/Q) ratio. This leads to a decrease in P_AO_2 and an increase in P_ACO_2.

71. D. This patient has asthma, which is related to increased sensitivity of air passages to stimuli. Intrinsic asthma usually begins in adult life and is not associated with a history of allergy. It includes nonreaginic asthma and pharmacologic asthma. It may be complicated by chronic bronchitis. Extrinsic asthma is a type I hypersensitivity response that begins in childhood. Patients usually have a family history of allergy. Chronic bronchitis is characterized by a productive cough for greater than 3 consecutive months in 2 or more years. This patient does not have a cough. Rhinovirus and adenovirus are causes of the common cold. These patients typically present with coryza, sneezing, nasal congestion, and mild sore throat.

72. B. This is a typical presentation of tuberculosis infection. The patient's recent visit might suggest that he was in contact with someone who had tuberculosis. Positive Ziehl-Neelsen stain indicates acid-fast organisms. The other possibilities can cause a cough but do not cause hemoptysis. They are also not seen on acid-fast stain.

73. D. Pott's disease is an extrapulmonary manifestation of tuberculosis. It can affect the intervertebral disks and cause spinal problems. Other sites include the central nervous system, kidneys, gastrointestinal tract, and lymph nodes. The other sites listed are not possibilities for extrapulmonary involvement. Pott's disease does not affect the aorta. Syphilis can cause aortitis. The gallbladder is not typically involved with tuberculosis. The heart is not typically involved with tuberculosis. Myocarditis is typically viral in nature. The spleen is not a typical extrapulmonary site for infection with tuberculosis.

74. C. This is a very important classification system used to identify different types of organisms. *Staphylococcus aureus* is catalase-positive, so that omits it from the choices. *Streptococcus pneumoniae* does undergo partial hemolysis (alpha), but is sensitive to optochin. *Peptostreptococcus* does not undergo hemolysis. *Staphylococcus agalactiae* is beta-hemolytic organism (clear zones around colony), so it is out as well. That leaves *Streptococcus mutans*, which is alpha-hemolytic and resistant to optochin.

75. A. This patient suffers from immotile cilia syndrome, which results from a genetic defect causing an absence of beat or an abnormal ciliary beat. The cilia have several abnormalities, including axonemes that lack ciliary dynein arms. This syndrome is associated with recurrent lower respiratory tract infections, sterility in men, and decreased fertility in women.

Chapter 12   Skin and Related Connective Tissue

Questions

1. A 1-year-old boy is brought to the pediatrician for evaluation of diffuse erythematous lesions over the front and back of the trunk and over the scalp. Physical examination also reveals hepatosplenomegaly and lymphadenopathy. Biopsy shows that the cells are CD1a-positive and, on electron microscopy, Birbeck granules are seen. What is the most likely diagnosis?

   A. Basal cell carcinoma
   B. Histiocytosis X
   C. Malignant melanoma
   D. Seborrheic keratosis
   E. Squamous cell carcinoma

2. A 39-year-old man with a history of allergic rhinitis presents for evaluation of persistent erythema of the non-hair-bearing skin over his left iliac crest. He has no other medical or surgical history. Which of the following layers of the epidermis is present only in areas of hairless skin?

   A. Stratum basale
   B. Stratum corneum
   C. Stratum granulosum
   D. Stratum lucidum
   E. Stratum spinosum

3. What cell type, the most prominent cell type of the epidermis, is chiefly responsible for producing material that will make an extracellular water barrier?

   A. Adipocyte
   B. Keratinocyte
   C. Langerhans cell
   D. Melanocyte
   E. Merkel cell

4. These are large, ovoid structures found in the deeper dermis and hypodermis. They are deep pressure receptors for mechanical and vibratory sense. They appear microscopically as concentric layers of lamellae, much like an onion sliced in half. Which of the following is described?

   A. Eccrine sweat gland
   B. Hair follicle
   C. Meissner's corpuscle
   D. Pacinian corpuscles
   E. Ruffini endings

5. A 50-year-old man presents to his primary care physician with a pearly nodule on his face. This nodule is heaped up, with translucent borders and telangectasias. Microscopy of a punch biopsy reveals nests of basaloid cells with a palisading growth pattern. Based on this description and the image in Figure 12-1, what is the most likely diagnosis?

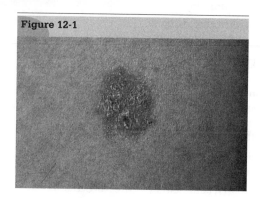

Figure 12-1

   A. Basal cell carcinoma
   B. Malignant melanoma
   C. Psoriasis
   D. Seborrheic keratosis
   E. Squamous cell carcinoma

6. A 20-year-old man presents complaining of fatigue and an alarming change in his skin. Examination of the skin reveals a diffuse bronze tint. Blood analysis shows a blood glucose level of 500 mg/dL; ALT and AST are also significantly elevated. What is the most likely pigment described?

   A. Bilirubin
   B. Iron
   C. Keratin
   D. Lipofuscin
   E. Melanin

7. A 38-year-old man presents to his primary care physician for evaluation of an ingrown left great toenail. Physical examination is undertaken. Cardiac, pulmonary, and abdominal examinations are within normal limits. The edge of the skin fold covering the root of the toenail, which is composed of keratin and thus does not desquamate, is called which of the following?

   A. Eponychium
   B. Hyponychium
   C. Lunula
   D. Matrix
   E. Nail bed

8. An 8-year-old boy presents to the pediatrician with a macu-lopapular rash covering his body; his mother reports that it began on his axillae, groin, and neck. The rash is accentu-ated in the skin folds. For 3 days, he has also had a mild fever, which is now increasing, as well as pharyngitis, head-ache, emesis, and chills. Physical examination reveals an erythematous appearance of the tongue. What is the most likely explanation for these findings?

    A. Human herpesvirus 6
    B. Morbillivirus
    C. Group A beta-hemolytic streptococcus
    D. Parvovirus B19
    E. *Staphylococcus aureus*

9. A 6-year-old boy presents to the emergency department with a skin eruption that began as a coalesced maculopapular rash on his face and then progressed down his body. As the rash proceeded downward, it developed into more pinpoint lesions; it then cleared after 3 days. Physical examination reveals posterior cervical and occipital adenopathy and spots on the soft palate. What is the most likely diagnosis?

    A. Herpesvirus 6
    B. Measles
    C. Group A beta-hemolytic streptococcus
    D. Parvovirus B19
    E. Rubella

10. A child has been diagnosed with chickenpox. His parents ask you about the possibility of transmission to other members of the family who live with them. In addition to the infected child, there is one sibling who has never had chickenpox or varicella vaccine, the two parents, who both had chickenpox as a child, and a grandmother who had shingles 2 years ear-lier. The grandmother is especially worried that she may get shingles again. What advice would you give the family?

    A. All of them are susceptible to catching chickenpox from the child.
    B. The sibling may catch chickenpox and the parents and grandparents may catch shingles, since they have already had chickenpox.
    C. The sibling may catch chickenpox, the parents will not catch anything, but the grandmother may redevelop shin-gles, since she has had them before.
    D. The sibling may catch chickenpox, but everyone else will be OK, since they have been exposed to varicella before.
    E. There is no threat of infection; chickenpox is not conta-gious.

11. A healthy 38-year-old man who is planning to run his first marathon does an exercise test on a treadmill. Which of the following nerve types provide for vasodilatation of blood vessels in the skin to dissipate excess body heat, which is important in temperature regulation?

    A. Cutaneous parasympathetic
    B. Cutaneous sympathetic
    C. Somatic afferent
    D. Somatic efferent
    E. Visceral parasympathetic

12. A 67-year-old woman presents to the clinic complaining of a fluctuant mass on her thumb, which she states began as a hard nodule. When she returns the next day, the lesion has begun to break down and ulcerate. She cannot remem-ber any specific injury but states that she likes to work in her rose garden, for which she has won many local awards. What is the most likely explanation for these findings?

    A. *Borrelia burgdorferi*
    B. *Candida albicans*
    C. *Plasmodium falciparum*
    D. *Sporothrix schenckii*
    E. *Tinea corporis*

13. A 47-year-old man with a history of skin cancer presents for a follow-up examination. A picture of his original lesion is shown in Figure 12-2. His treatment included wide excision with periodic surveillance examinations. Melanocytes, the cells responsible for producing pigmentation in the skin, arise from what cell origin?

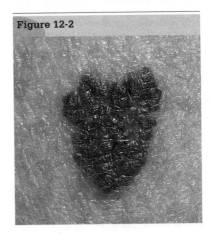

Figure 12-2

    A. Differentiation of epithelial cells
    B. Endoderm
    C. Mesenchyme
    D. Neural crest
    E. Surface ectoderm

14. A 17-year-old youth presents for evaluation of severe acne. He has had this condition for 4 years and has tried multiple treatments, including facial washes and over-the-counter creams and ointments, along with multiple courses of anti-biotics. He is asking for a more effective treatment. Which of the following is the most effective acne treatment?

    A. Gentamicin
    B. Isopropyl alcohol
    C. Isotretinoin
    D. Penicillin G
    E. Vancomycin

15. A 42-year-old woman presents to the emergency depart-ment with swelling, heat, and redness around a break in the skin of her thigh. Two hours later, the redness has spread rapidly to include her entire leg. The diagnosis of necrotizing fasciitis is tentatively made. What is the most likely bac-terium responsible for this infection?

A. *Chlamydia trachomatis*

B. *Enterococcus*

C. *Escherichia coli*

D. Group A beta-hemolytic streptococcus

E. Group B streptococcus

16. A 38-year-old woman with a history of diabetes mellitus and hyperlipidemia has an infected hair follicle that penetrates deep into the subcutaneous tissue and has produced multiple contiguous, painful lesions that communicate beneath the skin. What is the most likely diagnosis?

A. Abscess

B. Carbuncle

C. Cellulitis

D. Furuncle

E. Impetigo

17. A 28-year-old woman presents to the physician with discrete, scaly lesions on her face, scalp, pinnae, and neck. She has otherwise been normal with no past medical history of any diseases or surgeries, and she denies taking any medications. She tells you that she has no other complaints whatsoever but that she had recently tested positive for antinuclear antibody (ANA) by her family doctor. What is the most likely diagnosis?

A. Dermatomyositis

B. Discoid lupus erythematosus

C. Psoriasis

D. Scleroderma

E. Systemic lupus erythematosus

18. The sensory receptors are located in the papillary layer of thick skin; they are tapered cylinders oriented perpendicular to the skin surface and are responsive to low-frequency stimuli. Which of the following is described?

A. Eccrine sweat gland

B. Hair follicle

C. Meissner's corpuscle

D. Pacinian corpuscles

E. Ruffini endings

19. A 38-year-old woman presents to her primary care physician with symmetric thickening, tightening, and induration of the skin of the fingers. She has similar changes in her arms, face, and neck. Which of the following other disorders is most commonly associated with her disease?

A. Coarctation of the aorta

B. Enlargement of the third ventricle

C. Raynaud's phenomenon

D. Renal failure

E. Truncus arteriosus

20. Which of the lettered structures in Figure 12-3 is responsible for producing sebum, which coats the hair shaft and skin?

A. A

B. B

C. C

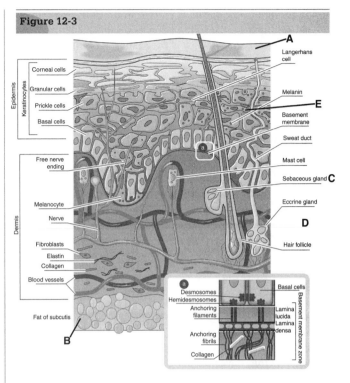

Figure 12-3

D. D

E. E

21. A 23-year-old woman presents to her primary care physician complaining of hives, which she noted after swimming in her family's pool. She says she also gets these hives when she has been inside too long with the air conditioner on as well as during the winter after being outside for long periods of time. She has no illnesses and no recent travel history; she takes oral contraceptives. She has no known drug allergies and has complaints only of allergies to pollen and dust. Physical examination of the skin, heart, lungs, and abdomen is within normal limits. What is the most likely diagnosis?

A. Angioedema

B. Cold-induced urticaria

C. Contact dermatitis

D. Eczema

E. Fixed drug reaction

22. A 40-year-old woman is brought to the emergency department after having been struck by a motor vehicle an hour earlier. She has no obvious external physical trauma but is having difficulty breathing, and there is diffuse swelling of her face, especially her lips. She requires intubation for maintenance of her airway and improves within a few hours. She is tentatively diagnosed with hereditary angioedema. Which enzyme level should be checked to confirm her diagnosis?

A. Creatine kinase

B. C1 esterase

C. Dystrophin

D. Fibrillin

E. Troponin I

23. An excited young father is present in the delivery room as his wife gives birth to their son. His wife is a 26-year-old G1P0 in her fortieth week of pregnancy. He is distressed to see that there is a white, cheese-like substance covering the baby; this, however, wipes off easily as the nurses clean him. The father approaches you nervously and asks what needs to be done. What should you tell him?

A. "Don't worry about it, it's no big deal."

B. "Stand back this is an emergency."

C. "Nothing is wrong with your baby, the white substance protects the baby's skin from the amniotic fluid in the uterus."

D. "Your baby may have a serious infection; we are going to have to take him to the ICU to observe him for a few hours."

E. "I have never seen anything like this before, we will have to consult with experts in the field to figure out what is wrong with your son."

24. A concerned parent brings her 2-month-old baby boy to the pediatrician because of two small spots under his armpit and one near his groin. She has noticed the spots since he was born but thought that they would disappear in time. She says they have not changed size or color. Physical examination reveals that the baby has small pigmented macules located in each axilla and on the right lower abdomen just above the inguinal ligament. These are not tender and have symmetric, regular borders. The physician's diagnosis is accessory nipples. What is the next most appropriate step in the evaluation of this patient?

A. Biopsy of one of the accessory nipples

B. Complete blood count

C. CT scan of the abdomen

D. Genetics referral for chromosome testing

E. Offer reassurance to the parent

25. A physician wishes to deliver a local anesthetic subcutaneously. Which of the following epidermal skin layers will the physician penetrate first?

A. Stratum basale

B. Stratum corneum

C. Stratum granulosum

D. Stratum lucidum

E. Stratum spinosum

26. A 65-year-old man presents to his dermatologist with a lesion on his nose. Examination reveals a raised shiny papular lesion with small blood vessels. What is the most likely diagnosis?

A. Basal cell carcinoma

B. Histiocytosis X

C. Malignant melanoma

D. Seborrheic keratosis

E. Squamous cell carcinoma

27. A deficiency of which of the following essential nutrients will directly impair oxidation of lysyl residues on collagen?

A. Copper

B. Folic acid

C. Iron

D. Vitamin C

E. Vitamin D

28. A 10-year-old boy is brought to the dermatology clinic by his mother, who is worried about the appearance of a new mole. His mother tells the dermatologist that he has had many malignant melanomas and basal cell carcinomas in the past and she is worried that this may be another one. Physical examination reveals an irregular macular lesion on the boy's neck. What is the most likely defect in this patient?

A. Addition of mannose-6-phosphate to newly synthesized proteins

B. Excision of pyrimidine dimers in DNA

C. Glycosylation of asparagine residues in newly synthesized proteins

D. Removal of deaminated cytosine bases in DNA

E. Repair of mismatched base pairs in newly replicated DNA

29. A 15-year-old boy, brought into clinic by his mother, complains of vision problems in both eyes. Physical examination shows that the patient is 6 ft tall and extremely thin. His joints can be extended considerably beyond a normal range. The sternum appears to be depressed inward and auscultation of the heart reveals a holosystolic murmur with a midsystolic click. This presentation is most likely consistent with defective synthesis of which of the following:

A. Elastin

B. Glycogen

C. Lysosomal enzymes

D. Type I collagen

E. Type II collagen

30. A 46-year-old man who has chewed tobacco for over 30 years develops a large raised brown lesion on his lower lip. He also has a nodule on his face (Figure 12-4). What is the most likely diagnosis?

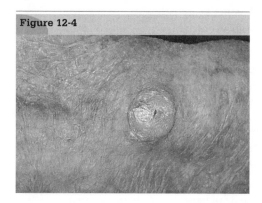

Figure 12-4

A. Basal cell carcinoma

B. Squamous cell carcinoma

C. Malignant melanoma

D. Merkel cell carcinoma

E. Histiocytosis X

31. A pathologist is attempting to study a punch biopsy of a skin lesion from a patient suspected of having a malignant melanoma. From which embryologic tissue is the skin layer is the pathologist's tissue sample derived?

    A. Ectoderm
    B. Endoderm
    C. Mesoderm
    D. Neural crest
    E. Notochord

32. A 9-year-old mentally retarded boy is brought to his pediatrician for a follow-up evaluation. Physical examination reveals a musty odor as well as light-colored skin and hair. This child's condition is due to the inability to manufacture which of the following amino acids?

    A. Alanine
    B. Arginine
    C. Phenylalanine
    D. Tryptophan
    E. Tyrosine

33. A 6-year-old child is brought into her primary care physician by her mother because of multiple skin lesions. Physical examination reveals eight discrete coffee-colored macular lesions over the thoracic and abdominal areas. A defect in which gene is most likely responsible for this disorder?

    A. *BRCA-1*
    B. *HFE*
    C. *NF-1*
    D. *Rb*
    E. *WT-1*

34. An 8-year-old boy fell on a rusty nail and complained of pain on his right leg. A few days later, he developed a fever and discoloration of skin in the area. He was admitted to the hospital, where progressive involvement of the lower leg, buttock, and abdomen was noted. Skin lesions consisted of gas-filled blebs with surrounding tissue necrosis. What is the most likely etiology of this condition?

    A. *Clostridium botulinum*
    B. *Clostridium difficile*
    C. *Clostridium perfringens*
    D. *Staphylococcus aureus*
    E. *Streptococcus pyogenes*

35. After being stung by a bee, a 15-year-old boy develops severe pruritus immediately around the area of the sting. Which of the following cell types is responsible for releasing the mediator that is most likely causing the pruritus?

    A. CD8+ T cells
    B. Eosinophils
    C. Macrophages
    D. Mast cells
    E. Plasma cells

36. A researcher wishing to study the synthesis of collagen is able to manufacture radioactively labeled oligosaccharides that can be used in the analysis. At which point in collagen synthesis would the researcher first begin to detect radioactivity on the collagen precursors?

    A. Golgi complex
    B. Lysosome
    C. Plasma membrane
    D. Rough endoplasmic reticulum
    E. Smooth endoplasmic reticulum

37. A 30-year-old woman visits her family physician complaining of weakness in her arms and thighs. She has had difficulty getting up after sitting in her chair and has noticed this for about 2 weeks now. She has also noticed the appearance of a rash on her face. Physical examination reveals a rash predominantly involving the upper eyelids, with a trace of periorbital edema. What is the most likely diagnosis?

    A. Dermatomyositis
    B. Myotonic dystrophy
    C. Polymyositis
    D. Scleroderma
    E. Systemic lupus erythematosus

38. A nurse injects lidocaine in order to anesthetize an area of skin so as to allow for painless insertion of an intravenous catheter. Which of the following nerve fibers in the skin will the lidocaine injection predominantly affect?

    A. A-alpha fibers
    B. A-beta fibers
    C. A-gamma fibers
    D. Beta fibers
    E. C fibers

39. A 59-year-old man presents to his primary care physician with severe itching, burning, and a sharp pain in his right flank. He says that he has also felt bumps along the right side of his back. Physical examination reveals several groups of vesicles that extend from the right midaxillary line to near the midline of the patient's back. What is the most likely diagnosis?

    A. Chickenpox
    B. Herpetic whitlow
    C. Molluscum contagiosum
    D. Scabies
    E. Shingles

40. Two days after going on a hike, a 12-year-old girl develops erythematous plaques and vesicles on her legs. Some plaques appear to be developing crusts. She also complains that the plaques are severely pruritic. Examination reveals a trace of periorbital edema. What is the most likely diagnosis?

    A. Atopic dermatitis
    B. Acute contact dermatitis
    C. Erysipelas
    D. Impetigo
    E. Lyme disease

41. A 48-year-old man presents to the emergency department complaining of extreme ocular irritation. He mentions that he has several blister-type lesions that continue to grow and "burst" on his back, trunk, and mouth. He states that when the lesions burst, a white milky fluid comes out of them. He says that the lesions become painful after they open up. He is currently on morphine for pain control. Immunofluorescence imaging is shown in Figure 12-5. Which of the following diseases does this patient most likely have?

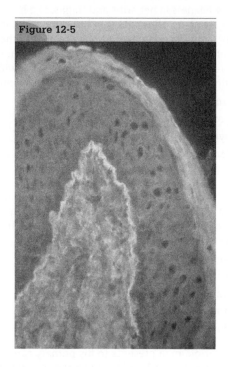

Figure 12-5

A. Bullous pemphigoid

B. Cicatricial pemphigoid

C. Eczematous dermatitis

D. Erythema multiforme

E. Vitiligo

42. A 29-year-old athlete complains of increased sweating during his workouts for his company's softball team. He has no pertinent medical or surgical history. Physical examination reveals a male patient in normally good health, but he appears to have a profuse buildup of sweat on his anterior and posterior trunk. The sweat glands found in almost all the skin of the body can be described as what type?

A. Apocrine

B. Eccrine

C. Endocrine

D. Holocrine

E. Paracrine

43. A 27-year-old man applies for a job as a hospital unit secretary. He has no prior medical or surgical history. As part of the employment process he is required to have a purified protein derivative (PPD) test. The basis for the skin reaction from a positive PPD is which of the following?

A. CD8+ T cells inducing apoptosis in skin cells exposed to antigen

B. Degranulation of mast cells leading to release of inflammatory mediators

C. Formation of antigen-antibody complexes in the epidermal layer of the skin

D. Interaction of CD4+ T cells and macrophages near the skin surface

E. Specific antibodies cross-reacting to "self" antigens present on skin cells

44. A defect in the formation of the embryological germ layer that gives rise to the epidermal layer of the skin would also affect which of the following?

A. Dura mater

B. Heart

C. Lens of eye

D. Pancreas

E. Spleen

45. If one were to do an immunofluorescence study of a patient with dermatitis herpetiformis, an antibody to which human immunoglobulin would be needed?

A. IgA

B. IgG1

C. IgG2

D. IgE

E. IgM

46. A patient is diagnosed at birth with phenylketonuria (PKU) and the mother is told that the patient will have symptoms of albinism. Which of the following is involved in the pathogenesis of this condition?

A. Bilirubin

B. Iron

C. Keratin

D. Lipofuscin

E. Melanin

47. Aging cells, when viewed under the microscope, have a visible "wear and tear" pigment. What is the name of this pigment?

A. Bilirubin

B. Iron

C. Keratin

D. Lipofuscin

E. Melanin

48. A 53-year-old man presents to his primary care physician for a routine exam. He states that he has spent his entire summer out fishing on a lake. Physical examination reveals a 5-mm mass above his nose. The lesion consists of pearly papules with visible telangiectatic vessels. Biopsy is performed. Which of the following histopathologic findings would most likely be seen under microscope?

A. Keratin pearls

B. Onionskin appearance

C. Palisading nuclei

D. Perivascular pseudorosette pattern of cells

E. Psammoma bodies

49. A 25-year-old man presents to his primary care physician complaining of a recurrent rash. He states that the rash consists of blisters that occur in groups on the extensor surfaces of his elbows, knees, and upper back (see Figure 12-6). Biopsy of the lesions shows deposits of IgA at the tips of dermal papillae, along with dermal microabscesses heavily filled with neutrophils and eosinophils. The patient is instructed to go on a gluten-free diet. What is the most likely diagnosis?

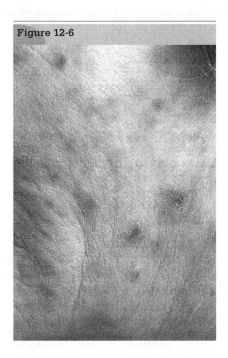

Figure 12-6

A. Bullous pemphigoid

B. Cicatricial pemphigoid

C. Dermatitis herpetiformis

D. Eczematous dermatitis

E. Erythema multiforme

50. A 48-year-old farmer comes to clinic asking about a suspicious lesion on his hand that has progressively grown in size over a 2-month period. He mentions that he has recently been working in the fields all day and that, because of his recent interest in glass making, he may have been exposed to amorphous arsenic. Physical examination reveals a lesion on the patient's hand consistent with actinic keratosis. What is this lesion most likely a precursor of?

A. Basal cell carcinoma

B. Chondrosarcoma

C. Melanoma

D. Seborrheic keratosis

E. Squamous cell carcinoma

51. An 8-year-old child presents to her primary care physician because of a newly developed rash. Her mother states that her daughter just recently recovered from a weeklong upper respiratory infection and continues to have abdominal pain. Physical examination reveals a temperature of 101.2°F (38.4°C). The patient has bright red urticaria-type lesions on the extensor surfaces of her arms and legs. What is the most likely diagnosis?

A. Churg-Strauss syndrome

B. Kaposi's sarcoma

C. Hypersensitivity vasculitis

D. Henoch-Schönlein purpura

E. Polyarteritis nodosa

52. A 35-year-old man presents to his primary care physician with a rash on the extensor surfaces of his extremities. He states that the rash does not itch. Physical examination reveals erythematous papules and plaques with characteristic silver scaling on his arms and legs. Which of the following histologic findings is likely to be seen on biopsy of these lesions?

A. IgA deposits at the tips of dermal papillae

B. IgG antibodies directed against epidermal basement membrane

C. IgG antibodies directed against epidermal intercellular cement substance

D. Munro abscesses within parakeratotic epidermis

E. Vacuolated cells in the granular cell layer of epidermis

53. A 33-year-old man with paresthesias of his fingertips presents for evaluation. What modified epidermal cells located in the stratum basale and most abundant in the fingertips are responsible for cutaneous sensation?

A. Adipocytes

B. Keratinocytes

C. Langerhans cells

D. Melanocytes

E. Merkel cells

54. A 33-year-old Caucasian man presents to his primary care physician for removal of recurrent suspicious lesions that appear to be basal cell carcinomas. The patient also has a history of recurrent actinic keratosis. His hair is white and his skin has a pink tone. His eyes appear very light. What enzyme has failed to make the proper intermediates, leading to this patient's symptoms?

A. Oxaloacetate decarboxylase

B. Phenylalanine hydroxylase

C. Tyrosinase

D. Tyrosine hydroxylase

E. Tyrosine kinase

55. A 10-year-old girl comes to the pediatrician with a rash on her cheeks, which has raised borders and is bright red. Her mother states that she was on her way to the park to play, since it was such a sunny day; then, when she looked at her daughter in the back seat, she noticed this rash. The child had a headache, fever, chills, and myalgias 2 to 3 days earlier but is not feeling sick today. What is the most likely explanation of these findings?

    A. Herpesvirus 6
    B. Morbillivirus
    C. Group A beta-hemolytic streptococcus
    D. Parvovirus B19
    E. *Staphylococcus saprophyticus*

56. A 14-year-old boy is brought to his primary care physician for a general checkup. The patient states that he bruises easily. Physical examination reveals hyperextensible joints in his hands, and his skin shows hyperelasticity. Funduscopic evaluation reveals bilateral angioid streaks. The patient's mother states that the father had similar findings. Which of the following extracellular matrix molecules is most likely affected in this condition?

    A. Fibronectin
    B. Laminin
    C. Types I and III collagen
    D. Type II collagen
    E. Type IV collagen

57. A 20-year-old woman present to her primary care physician complaining of recurrent cold sores around her lips. She states that she noticed a similar lesion once on her boyfriend's lower lip. She thinks she might have gotten her cold sores by kissing her boyfriend while he had the lesion. Which nerve axon is the disease most likely traversing as it continues to cause the recurrent cold sores in this patient?

    A. Cranial nerve V1
    B. Cranial nerve V2 and cranial nerve VII, mandibular branch
    C. Cranial nerves V2 and V3
    D. Cranial nerve V1 and cranial nerve VII, buccal branches
    E. Cranial nerve VII, buccal and mandibular branches

58. A 35-year-old woman presents to her primary care physician for evaluation of an increasingly itchy and hardened area of skin over the dorsa of her legs and feet. The patient states that she has found herself to be more irritable lately; she has also noted significant weight loss and insomnia. Physical examination reveals proptosis of the globe bilaterally. Her skin appears warm and moist, and she has a mild tremor in her fingers. The skin on the dorsa of her feet and legs appears red and plaque-like. Which of the following laboratory test results is consistent with the clinical picture?

    A. Decreased serum T4
    B. Decreased T3 resin uptake
    C. Increased thyroid-binding globulin
    D. Increased serum thyroid-stimulating hormone
    E. Positive antibodies against the thyroid-stimulating hormone receptor

59. A 27-year-old Caucasian man presents to the dermatology clinic with a significant rash consisting of macules, papules, and vesiculobullous lesions. A skin biopsy is performed. Histologically, the specimen is significant for a split between the epidermal and dermal layers. There is evidence of subepidermal edema, nuclear dust in the dermis, and perivascular lymphoplasmacytic infiltrate. What is the most likely diagnosis?

    A. Bullous pemphigoid
    B. Dermatitis herpetiformis
    C. Erythema multiforme
    D. Pemphigus vulgaris
    E. Varicella

60. A 50-year-old woman presents to the ambulatory care clinic for follow-up of her gastric malignancy. She has noticed significant weight loss and a loss of appetite. Her health continues to decline slowly, so it is decided that she should undergo a gastrectomy. Retrospectively, which of the following could have alerted the physicians to this patient's condition and helped identify her malignancy at an earlier stage?

    A. Hyperpigmented areas of skin involving the armpits and dorsa of the knees
    B. Presence of a dome-shaped nodule filled with soft gray-white material on the skin
    C. Pedunculated lesion with numerous capillaries and edematous stroma in the mouth
    D. Rough, scaling, poorly demarcated plaques on the face and upper trunk
    E. Sheets of lesions on the face resembling keratin "pearls"

61. A 1-month-old infant is brought to the emergency department for evaluation of a purple-red area of skin discoloration on one side of her face. The mother states that the child was born with this skin defect. Physical examination reveals increased intraocular pressure in the eye ipsilateral to the skin discoloration. Ophthalmology consultation is obtained and reveals significant retinal detachment and hemorrhaging of choroidal tissue. As the physician is leaving the room, the mother remembers that her child occasionally has convulsing seizures. An MRI of the brain and spinal cord is performed and reveals extensive hemangiomatous involvement of the meninges. What is the most likely diagnosis?

    A. Kaposi's sarcoma
    B. Osler-Weber-Rendu syndrome
    C. Sturge-Weber syndrome
    D. Temporal arteritis
    E. Von Hippel-Lindau disease

62. A 42-year-old woman presents to the ambulatory care clinic complaining of increasing ocular irritation. She states that her eyes always feel itchy and often as though there were sand in them. She also states that she has had difficulty chewing her food properly, making swallowing difficult. Physical examination reveals a lack of tear film over the corneas. Using fluorescein, the presence of corneal abrasions is noted. On palpation, her parotid glands feel enlarged bilaterally. What is the most likely diagnosis?

    A. Dermatomyositis
    B. Mixed connective tissue disease

C. Osteoarthritis

D. Polyarteritis nodosa

E. Polymyositis

F. Progressive systemic sclerosis

G. Sjögren's syndrome

H. Wegener's granulomatosis

63. A 23-year-old woman presents to her primary care physician for a yearly follow-up on her medical conditions. She states that she has been doing well except for her progressive difficulty with swallowing. She has occasional dyspnea and is short of breath. Physical examination reveals hard, immobile nodules in her elbows and knees and the skin on her digits seems quite thin, fragile, shiny, and somewhat flexed at the interphalangeal joints. She has tiny red dots over her trunk. You place a few cubes of ice in her hands and notice a resultant pallor and cyanosis. She does not appear to show much facial expression during the exam. ANA tests are positive and show anticentromere activity. What is the most likely diagnosis?

A. Mixed connective tissue disease

B. Osteoarthritis

C. Polyarteritis nodosa

D. Progressive systemic sclerosis

E. Wegener's granulomatosis

64. A 40-year-old man presents to the clinic complaining of bright red blood in his urine. He does not complain of any dysuria, urgency, frequency, or postvoid dribbling. He has some mild flank discomfort bilaterally. He mentions that he has noticed that he sometimes has a productive cough, in which he spits out a thick mucus-like material that has bright red streaks in it. He complains of trouble with epistaxis during sleep. The patient has no history of respiratory or urinary problems. He denies any recent travel outside the country. Physical examination reveals some dried blood around the inside border of his nares. An ultrasound of the kidneys shows no evidence of renal calculi. A renal biopsy is performed and shows infiltration by neutrophils and granulomas with giant cells in the small arteries. What is the most likely diagnosis?

A. Dermatomyositis

B. Mixed connective tissue disease

C. Osteoarthritis

D. Polyarteritis nodosa

E. Sjögren's syndrome

F. Systemic lupus erythematosus

G. Wegener's granulomatosis

65. A 45-year-old man comes to clinic with multiple complaints that have troubled him over recent weeks. He has had headache, fever, abdominal discomfort, chest pain, cough, dyspnea, and occasional hemoptysis. He was recently diagnosed with a urinary tract infection and was put on trimethoprim-sulfamethoxazole to treat the infection. He notices that his symptoms began shortly after his UTI was treated. What is the most likely diagnosis?

A. Mixed connective tissue disease

B. Osteoarthritis

C. Polyarteritis nodosa

D. Polymyositis

E. Wegener's granulomatosis

66. A 35-year-old woman comes to clinic complaining of pain in her joints and muscles. She has pain in her muscles when she presses on them. She also complains of some difficulty swallowing, describing it as "the food feels like it gets stuck in my chest." ANA titers are drawn and come back high for anti-nRNP ANAs. Analysis of the ANA shows an immunofluorescent speckled nuclear appearance. What is the most likely diagnosis?

A. Dermatomyositis

B. Mixed connective tissue disease

C. Osteoarthritis

D. Polyarteritis nodosa

E. Polymyositis

67. A 33-year-old woman presents to her primary care physician clinic complaining of fever and a feeling of malaise, which she has had for the 2 weeks. She also states that she has noticed a 15-lb weight loss over the previous month, as well as pain in her joints on and off for a month or two. She says that the "sun is bad" for her face because she develops a rash on her cheeks when she is out in the sun. Which of the following other finding can be associated with this condition?

A. Immune complexes at the dermal-epidermal junctions

B. Kidney microscopy antibody study showing linear pattern immunofluorescence

C. Positive titer for anti-IgG antibodies

D. Positive titer for antimitochondrial antibodies

E. Increased serum complement

68. During embryological development, the epidermal layer of the skin overlying the head and neck is derived from what embryologic layer?

A. Endoderm

B. Mesoderm

C. Neural crest

D. Neuroectoderm

E. Surface ectoderm

69. A 68-year-old man presents to his primary care physician with painful skin lesions on his chest that developed over recent days. He had similar episodes of these lesions several years ago. He states that some lesions are new and filled with pus, while others seem to be healing. Physical examination reveals that the lesions are only on the left side of his chest and stop at the level of the sternum horizontally. The lesions are isolated to the area around his nipple and seem to all be in a horizontal line. This disease has affected the dorsal root ganglia of which ganglion?

A. C4

B. C4 and C5

C. T2

D. T4

E. T10

70. A 35-year-old woman presents for evaluation of recent complaints of weakness when she combs her hair and when she has to walk upstairs to check on her 11-year-old son. She also says she has had to wear more makeup lately because her eyes have a funny-looking color above them. A CPK level and muscle biopsy are ordered. What condition should be of the highest in priority on the differential diagnosis?

A. Dermatomyositis

B. Discoid lupus erythematosus

C. Psoriasis

D. Scleroderma

E. Systemic lupus erythematosus

71. A 27-year-old man has suffered second- and third-degree burns during a fire in his home. He was rescued and immediately taken to the burn unit of the closest hospital. After his airway, breathing, and circulation are secured, he is started on intravenous fluids and electrolytes to reestablish homeostasis. During the first week, the patient remains stable and seems to be improving slightly. However, during week 2, he develops a high-grade fever and has a blood pressure of 90/50 mm Hg. What is the most likely cause of this patient's fever and hypotension?

A. Autoimmune reactions against the damaged tissue

B. Loss of adequate fluid volume with resultant severe dehydration

C. Sepsis secondary to fungal infection

D. Sepsis secondary to *Pseudomonas* infection

E. Sepsis secondary to staphylococcal infection

72. A 15-year-old boy presents to his primary care physician complaining of an itchy rash in both of his armpits. Physical examination reveals that the rash has well-defined borders and consists of spongiosis with vesicle formation. He is instructed to change the type of deodorant he uses and is sent home. What was this patient's most likely problem?

A. Bullous pemphigoid

B. Cicatricial pemphigoid

C. Dermatitis herpetiformis

D. Eczematous dermatitis

E. Erythema multiforme

73. A 33-year-old man presents to his primary care physician with multiple complaints. He states that his eye itches and burns, and he has had some change in his vision in recent weeks. He also states that he has some burning on urination. He states that most of the day he lies in bed because it hurts to move around. He has never had any kidney infection or stones. He has not been taking any medications. He states that he has never traveled outside the country and cannot recall being bitten by any animal or insect. Physical examination reveals that the patient has a red eye with a ciliary flush and purulent discharge. On urinalysis, his urine shows traces of blood. The joints in his fingers appear stiff, and he is hesitant to move them. Which of the following did this patient most likely suffer from prior to his recent symptoms?

A. Chlamydial infection

B. Gout

C. Juvenile rheumatoid arthritis

D. Malignancy

E. Sarcoidosis

74. A 45-year-old man presents to his primary care physician because of painful sores in his mouth. He states he had similar sores a few years back and later developed blisters on his back, chest, legs, and toes (Figure 12-7). A biopsy of one of the lesions is done and shows eosinophilic infiltrate surrounding the dermis. Serum tests are positive for IgG antibodies directed against the basement membrane of the epidermis. What is the most likely diagnosis?

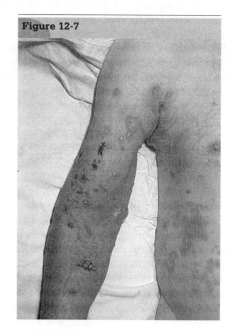

Figure 12-7

A. Bullous pemphigoid

B. Cicatricial pemphigoid

C. Dermatitis herpetiformis

D. Eczematous dermatitis

E. Erythema multiforme

75. A 25-year-old African American woman comes to clinic because she fears she has a cancer on her ear. She states that she had her ear pierced for the first time a week earlier, and after a few days noticed that her ear seemed to have developed a growth on it quite rapidly. She had never had her ear pierced before. What is the most likely diagnosis?

A. Basal cell carcinoma

B. Blue nevus

C. Epidermal inclusion cyst

D. Keloid

E. Malignant melanoma

Answer Key

1. B	20. B	39. E	58. E
2. D	21. B	40. B	59. C
3. B	22. B	41. B	60. A
4. D	23. C	42. B	61. C
5. C	24. E	43. D	62. G
6. B	25. B	44. C	63. D
7. A	26. A	45. A	64. G
8. C	27. A	46. B	65. C
9. E	28. B	47. D	66. B
10. D	29. B	48. C	67. A
11. B	30. B	49. C	68. E
12. D	31. C	50. E	69. D
13. D	32. E	51. D	70. A
14. C	33. C	52. D	71. D
15. D	34. C	53. E	72. D
16. B	35. D	54. C	73. A
17. B	36. D	55. D	74. A
18. C	37. A	56. C	75. D
19. C	38. E	57. C	

Answers and Explanations

1. B. Histiocytosis X (Langerhans cell histiocytosis) is caused by a proliferation of Langerhans cells, which are normally found in the epidermis. These cells are CD1a-positive and Birbeck granules are seen on electron microscopy. Histiocytosis X occurs most frequently in children less than 2 years of age but may occasionally be seen in adults. Untreated, the disease is rapidly fatal. With extensive chemotherapy, 50% of patients survive 5 years. Squamous cell carcinoma is most often seen among people who have high sun exposure and usually presents on sun-exposed areas such as the face, arms, and hands. Prognosis is good in that this condition rarely metastasizes and can be cured with complete excision. Seborrheic keratosis is a benign squamoproliferative neoplasm. Malignant melanoma is a common tumor with significant risk of metastasis. It is associated with sunlight exposure. Fair-skinned persons are at increased risk. Depth of tumor correlates with risk of metastases.

2. D. The stratum lucidum is found only in thick skin and contains eosinophils in which the keratinization process is matured. The nucleus and cytoplasmic organelles become disrupted and disappear as the cells gradually fill with keratin. The other layers of the skin—the stratum basale, stratum spinosum, stratum granulosum, and stratum corneum—are found in both thin and thick skin.

3. B. Keratinocytes produce keratin, which creates an extracellular water barrier. These cells are located in the basal layer and contain numerous free ribosomes, giving it a basophilic appearance on histologic section. Melanocytes produce melanin, a pigment. Langerhans cells present antigens to T cells. Merkel cells are epidermal cells that function in cutaneous sensation. Adipocytes are fat-storage cells.

4. D. Pacinian corpuscles are deep pressure receptors for mechanical and vibratory sense. They have a concentric shape and contain fluid in their lamellae which, when displaced, detects pressure on the skin surface. Hair follicles produce the keratinized cells that form hair. Meissner's corpuscles are touch receptors responsive to low-frequency stimuli. Ruffini endings respond to mechanical displacement of adjacent collagen fibers. Eccrine sweat glands produce sweat in all areas of the body except the lips and part of the external genitalia.

5. C. Basal cell carcinoma is the most common tumor in adults in the United States. It is most commonly seen in middle-aged to elderly individuals; risk factors are chronic sun exposure, fair complexion, immunosuppression, and xeroderma pigmentosum. It is most commonly seen on sun-exposed, hair-bearing areas. It grows slowly and rarely metastasizes but may be locally aggressive. Complete excision is usually curative. Squamous cell carcinoma most often is seen among people who have high sun exposure and usually presents on sun-exposed areas such as the face, arms, and hands. Prognosis is good in that this condition rarely metastasizes and can be cured with complete excision. Seborrheic keratosis is a benign squamoproliferative neoplasm. Malignant melanoma is a common tumor with significant risk of metastasis. It is associated with sunlight exposure. Fair-skinned persons are at increased risk. Depth of tumor correlates with risk of metastases.

6. B. This patient is exhibiting signs of hereditary hemochromatosis, an inherited defect in iron metabolism. In this disease, iron cannot be metabolized and rapidly accumulates in the body. Organs commonly affected by this disease include the skin (giving a bronze tint to the skin), the liver (hepatic cirrhosis occurs because of the iron accumulation), pancreas (the pancreas is essentially destroyed by accumulating iron and blood glucose control is impaired, giving rise to the term "bronze diabetes"), and the central nervous system. Bilirubin is a breakdown product of hemoglobin and is normally recycled and excreted. Lipofuscin, commonly called the "wear-and-tear pigment," is an intracellular pigment composed of polymers of lipids and phospholipids complexed with protein. It is a normal accumulation in cells. Bilirubin is a breakdown product of hemoglobin and is normally recycled and excreted. Cirrhosis of the liver impairs the ability of the liver to conjugate and eliminate bilirubin. Unconjugated bilirubin accumulates in the blood and gives a yellowish tint to the skin.

7. A. The eponychium, also known as the cuticle, is the edge of the skin fold covering the nail root. Because it is thin, it tends to break off or is trimmed and pushed back. The hyponychium secures the free edge of the nail plate at the fingertip. The lunula is the crescent-shaped white area at the root of the nail. The matrix is the germinative zone of the cells of the nail. The nail bed consists of epithelial cells, on which the nail plate rests.

8. C. This disease is scarlet fever, which was first described in 1627. Before the antibiotic era, the mortality rate was up to 10%. Today, with antibiotic administration, the prognosis is good, but the fatality rate remains at 1 to 15% if the disease is not treated. Morbillivirus causes measles. *Staphylococcus aureus* can cause a similar disease, called Filatov-Dukes' disease. Human herpesvirus 6 is thought to cause roseola. Parvovirus B19 causes fifth or "slapped cheeks" disease.

9. E. The disease being described here is rubella. Caused by the rubivirus, it proceeds as described and is usually gone in 3 days, giving it the name "3-day measles" and German measles. It is vaccinated against by the mumps-measles-rubella (MMR) vaccine, not for the danger it presents to children but for the threat it poses to a fetus if a pregnant woman contracts rubella. Some of the outcomes of this infection during pregnancy are congenital cataracts, microcephaly, and thrombocytopenia. Morbillivirus causes measles. Human herpesvirus 6 causes roseola. Parvovirus B19 causes fifth or "slapped cheeks" disease.

10. D. Chickenpox is caused by the varicella virus, a member of the herpesvirus family. Anyone who has never had chickenpox or who has not been vaccinated against it is susceptible to acquiring the disease. Once someone has contracted the varicella virus, the virus lies dormant in the dorsal root ganglions. Shingles is caused when the virus is reactivated and reemerges along the dermatomal distribution of the nerves from a particular dorsal root ganglion. Shingles cannot be caused by exposure to the chickenpox virus. However, since there are vesicles containing live virus, any nonimmunized children should avoid an adult with shingles, as there is a risk of contracting chickenpox from them.

11. B. Cutaneous sympathetic nerves innervate the vessels of the skin and provide for vasodilation, which allows excess body heat to be dissipated. Parasympathetic nerves play little role in temperature regulation. Somatic afferent nerves are sensory nerves. Somatic efferent nerves are motor nerves. Visceral parasympathetic nerves innervate the viscera and have little role in temperature regulation.

12. D. Sporotrichosis is a cutaneous fungal infection caused by *Sporothrix schenkii* and is most commonly associated with getting stuck by the thorn of a rose bush. The lesions start as a hard nodule that becomes fluctuant, then breaks down and ulcerates. There can be regional lymphatic spread, which results in the same progression of lesions. *Tinea corporis* is the cause of ringworm, a dermatophyte infection. *Borrelia burgdorferi* causes Lyme disease. *Plasmodium* species cause malaria. *Candida albicans* is a member of the normal flora; it can cause infections in the vagina and mouth as well as systemic infections.

13. D. During the first 3 months of development, the epidermis is invaded by cells arising from the neural crest; these are called melanocytes and synthesize melanin. The surface ectoderm gives rise to the epidermis. The endoderm does not give rise to skin structures. Epithelial cells do not differentiate to form melanocytes. The dermis develops from mesenchyme.

14. C. Isotretinoin (13-*cis*-retinoic acid) has brought about much improvement in the treatment of severe acne that is refractory to other forms of treatment. This medicine is derived from vitamin A. Severe birth defects are an important side effect. For this reason, women are required to be on birth control while taking isotretinoin. Penicillin G binds to penicillin-binding protein and blocks transpeptidase cross-linking of the cell wall. It is bactericidal for Gram-positive cocci and rods. Vancomycin inhibits cell wall mucopeptide formation by binding the D-ala-D-ala portion of cell-wall precursors. It is used for serious Gram-positive multi-drug-resistant organisms. Isopropyl alcohol is rubbing alcohol and may be applied topically to help reduce a fever.

15. D. The only bacterium of those listed that can cause necrotizing fasciitis is group A beta-hemolytic streptococcus. This is an important infection that must be recognized quickly, as it spreads along fascial planes and can rapidly cause widespread infection. This infection can also be caused by *Clostridium* and *Staphylococcus aureus*. *Chlamydia trachomatis* can cause arthritis, conjunctivitis, and urethritis. Enterococci cause enteric (GI tract) infections. Group B streptococcal infections cause pharyngitis.

16. B. A carbuncle is formed when there are multiple, contiguous painful lesions under the skin. An abscess is a collection of pus. A furuncle exists when an abscess extends deep into the subcutaneous tissue. Cellulitis is a deep infection of cells. Impetigo consists of pustules that crust over to become honey-colored, wet, and flaky.

17. B. Discoid lupus erythematosus is a disease involving the cutaneous findings of systemic lupus erythematosus (SLE) with none of the systemic findings. The lesions are characteristically as described and lab testing most commonly shows a positive antinuclear antibody. Scleroderma is a multisystemic disease characterized by abnormalities of small blood vessels, fibrosis of the skin and internal organs, immune system activation, and autoimmunity. SLE is a systemic disease that is not limited to the skin involvement presented in this case. Psoriasis is associated with scaly lesions but not with a positive ANA. Dermatomyositis is associated with proximal muscle weakness and heliotrope rash.

18. C. Meissner's corpuscles are touch receptors particularly responsive to low-frequency stimuli in the papillary layer of hairless skin, particularly that of the fingers and toes. They are present just below the epidermal basal layer. On stains, these corpuscles appear as a skein of loosely twisted wool. Hair follicles produce keratinized cells forming hair. Ruffini endings respond to mechanical displacement of adjacent collagen fibers. Pacinian corpuscles are deep pressure receptors for mechanical and vibratory sense. Eccrine sweat glands produce sweat in all areas of the body except the lips and part of the external genitalia.

19. C. Raynaud's phenomenon is the condition in which the fingers and toes undergo changes in color in response to temperature changes due to vasospasm. The disease in the question stem is scleroderma, which can be associated with Raynaud's phenomenon in a spectrum of related symptoms known as CREST syndrome, which stands for calcinosis, Raynaud's phenomenon, esophageal dysmotility, sclerodactyly or scleroderma, and telangectasias. The other question choices are not part of the CREST syndrome.

20. B. The sebaceous gland is responsible for producing sebum. A is the epidermis, C is the arrector pili muscle, D is the matrix of the hair follicle, and E is the hair itself.

21. B. Cold-induced urticaria is an allergic type of reaction mediated by IgE, which is stimulated by a cold environment such as the swimming pool, air conditioners, and wintertime cold temperatures. Treatment is currently aimed at avoidance of cold environments and the use of antihistamic agents. Eczema is characterized by raised, scaly plaques, not hives. Angioedema is closely related to urticaria but is characterized by deeper edema of the dermis and subcutaneous fat. There is no evidence of a specific substance that the patient is in contact with to suspect contact dermatitis. The patient's only medication is oral contraceptive pills, which do produce a waxing and waning hive-type reaction.

22. B. The enzyme deficiency in hereditary angioedema is C1 esterase. This condition can be brought on by stress and trauma. It is classically described as in the question stem, with edema of the face and lips. It can also cause laryngeal edema, sometimes requiring intubation for airway management. Creatine kinase and troponin 1 are enzymes in muscle; they are monitored for acute myocardial infarction. Fibrillin is deficient in Marfan's syndrome. Dystrophin is deficient in Duchenne muscular dystrophy.

23. C. The white substance on the baby is called the vernix caseosa, which is formed by secretions from sebaceous glands and degenerated epithelial cells and hairs. It protects the skin from the macerating effects of the amniotic fluid while the fetus is in the uterus. The other answers are inappropriate for this situation.

24. E. Polythelia is the medical name for supernumerary nipples. This is caused by the persistence of the mammary line, which usually regresses during fetal development. The nipples may appear anywhere along a line extending from the axillae though the nipples to the groin and upper thigh. The condition is benign and no further tests are needed. The parents should be reassured that nothing is wrong with their child.

25. B. Histologically, the epidermis has five layers, which are demarcated based upon microscopic morphology. The most superficial layer, the stratum corneum, is characterized by anucleate cells filled with keratin filaments. Beneath the stratum corneum is the stratum lucidum, which is seen well only in thick skin and is considered actually to be a subdivision of the stratum corneum. The stratum granulosum is beneath the stratum lucidum and comprises cells containing keratohyalin granules. The stratum spinosum beneath the stratum granulosum is composed of spiny-looking cells. Finally, the stratum basale, the deepest layer of the epidermis, is composed of a single layer of stem cells from which keratinocytes arise.

26. A. Basal cell carcinomas are the most common skin tumors. They tend to involve sun-exposed areas, most often on the head and neck. Grossly, they are characterized by a pearly papule with overlying telangiectatic vessels. The lower lip is actually the most common site on which a tobacco user might develop squamous cell carcinoma. Malignant melanomas are the most likely primary skin tumors to metastasize systemically. Histiocytosis X (Langerhans cell histiocytosis) is caused by a proliferation of the Langerhans cells normally found in the epidermis. These cells are CD1a-positive, and Birbeck granules are seen on electron microscopy. Seborrheic keratosis is a benign squamoproliferative neoplasm associated with sun exposure. Fair-skinned persons are at increased risk. Depth of tumor correlates with risk of metastasis.

27. A. The enzyme lysyl oxidase requires copper as a cofactor. Therefore a deficiency of copper will impair the ability of lysyl oxidase to function and ultimately will impair the ability of collagen to cross-link, decreasing its strength. A deficiency of folic acid is known to cause neural tube defects in developing fetuses as well as megaloblastic anemia in adults. Iron deficiency causes microcytic anemia and is the most common cause of anemia in the United States. A deficiency of vitamin C impairs the functioning of enzymes responsible for hydroxylating proline and lysine residues in procollagen. The condition that results is known as scurvy and is characterized by impaired wound healing, splinter hemorrhages, and bleeding gums. A deficiency of vitamin D impairs the absorption of dietary calcium. Disease states characterized by a vitamin D deficiency are rickets in children and osteomalacia in adults.

28. B. This patient most likely has xeroderma pigmentosum, due to an autosomal recessive trait in which pyrimidine dimers (especially between thymines) formed in ultraviolet light cannot be excised. This leads to a huge increase in potential cancer-causing mutations in sun-exposed individuals. Typically, such people will have many different skin cancers, including malignant melanomas and basal cell carcinomas. A defect in the addition of mannose-6-phosphate to newly synthesized proteins is characteristic of I-cell disease. Patients with I-cell disease present with coarse facial features, gingival hyperplasia, macroglossia, and die owing to cardiorespiratory failure in the first decade of life. A defect in the glycosylation of asparagine residues has not been associated with the development of skin carcinomas. A defect in the removal of deaminated cytosine bases in DNA and in the repairing of mismatched base pairs may produce skin carcinomas but is not consistent with the classic pathology underlying xeroderma pigmentosum.

29. B. The patient most likely has Marfan's syndrome, which is a multisystemic disorder due to a defect in the fibrillin gene. Patients with Marfan's syndrome have a variety of symptoms including bilateral lens dislocation, hyperextensible joints, mitral valve prolapse, arachnodactyly, tall thin build, and pectus excavatum. A defect in glycogen synthesis may present in any number of ways, such as hepatomegaly and cardiomegaly, depending on the enzyme deficiency. Examples of glycogen storage diseases include McArdle's disease and Pompe's disease. Lysosomal storage diseases may present with systemic manifestations such as CNS dysfunction, hepatic dysfunction, and so on, but these are inconsistent with the patient's symptoms. Examples include Tay-Sachs and Krabbe disease. Types I and II collagen defects will lead to different types of Ehlers-Danlos syndrome, which can be characterized by a variety of symptoms, such as joint hyperextensibility. However, the other symptoms of this patient are classic for Marfan's syndrome.

30. B. This patient most likely has a squamous cell carcinoma. People who chew tobacco for a long time are at an increased risk of developing squamous cell carcinomas near or in the oral cavity. The lower lip is actually the site at which a tobacco user is most likely to develop squamous cell carcinoma. Basal cell carcinomas are the most common skin tumors. They tend to involve sun-exposed areas, most often on the head and neck. Grossly, they are characterized by pearly papules with overlying telangiectatic vessels. Malignant melanomas are the most likely primary skin tumors to metastasize systemically. Histiocytosis X (Langerhans cell histiocytosis) is caused by a proliferation of the Langerhans cells normally found in the epidermis. These cells are CD1a-positive and Birbeck granules are seen on electron microscopy. This patient has no evidence to suggest a tumor involving the Merkel cells.

31. C. The dermis of the skin is derived from mesoderm, since it is mostly connective tissue. Ectodermal skin gives rise to tissue including the epidermis and associated appendages, including hair and nails. Endodermal structures include GI epithelium, pancreas, gallbladder, and liver. Neural crest cells develop into peripheral neural structures. The notochord, which defines the anteroposterior axis of the embryo, becomes the nucleus pulposus of the intervertebral disk.

32. E. Patients with phenylketonuria lack the enzyme phenylalanine hydroxylase. This enzyme is needed to generate tyrosine, which is a precursor for the skin pigment melanin. As a result of this functional lack of tyrosine, PKU patients, if they are not supplemented with tyrosine, may present with signs of albinism, including light-colored skin and hair. Alanine is not an essential amino acid, so no deficiency state will occur in adequate nutritional states. No classical pathology is associated with arginine deficiency. Phenylalanine actually accumulates in patients with PKU and leads to the overproduction of metabolic by-products, which cause the symptoms. Tryptophan deficiency may be seen in Hartnup disease, which is characterized by an inability to absorb tryptophan in the intestine. Patients present with the pellagra-like symptoms of dermatitis, dementia, and diarrhea.

33. C. This patient most likely suffers from neurofibromatosis type I, which is linked to a defect in the NF-1 gene. Patients with this autosomal dominant disorder will usually have multiple café au lait spots, which are classically described as coffee-colored multiple neurofibromas and pigmented nodules of the iris (Lisch nodules). Defects in the BRCA-1 gene are associated with an increased risk of breast and ovarian cancers in women. Defects in the HFE gene are linked to hereditary hemochromatosis, which is an inability to metabolize iron. Defects in the WT-1 gene are linked to the development of a renal tumor known more commonly as a Wilms' tumor. A defect in the Rb gene is linked to familial retinoblastoma, characterized by a predisposition to develop tumors of the retina.

34. C. This patient most likely has gas gangrene as a result of *Clostridium perfringens* infection. These particular organisms produce a lecithinase, which causes severe necrosis of the surrounding tissue. Gas from the bacterial metabolism builds up in the necrotic areas, producing the classic gas-filled blebs. *C. perfringens* can also cause a gastroenteritis if ingested. *Clostridium botulinum* causes botulism, a disease characterized by descending paralysis of skeletal muscles ultimately leading to respiratory failure. Botulism is associated with home-canned foods. *Clostridium difficile* can cause a mild gastroenteritis in healthy individuals and can also cause a disease known as pseudomembranous colitis in individuals undergoing antibiotic therapy. *Staphylococcus aureus* can cause a wide variety of skin problems including impetigo, scalded skin syndrome, and abscesses. *Streptococcus pyogenes*, although most known for causing streptococcal pharyngitis, can also cause skin disorders including impetigo and erysipelas (a classic facial cellulitis).

35. D. The patient is most likely suffering from a type I hypersensitivity reaction caused by release of histamine from mast cells. The hallmark of the type I hypersensitivity is severe pruritus occurring immediately upon exposure to a particular antigen. CD8+ T cells are involved in destroying cells infected with viruses or fungi. Eosinophils are known to play a role in parasitic infections as well as certain allergic reactions. Although they are increased in certain patients with type I hypersensitivity reactions, they do not release the histamine involved in the reaction. Macrophages are nonspecific phagocytic cells of the immune system that may participate in type IV hypersensitivity reactions. Plasma cells are antibody-producing B cells seen in a variety of situations, including infection.

36. D. The researcher would be able to detect radioactivity on the collagen precursors when the oligosaccharides become attached to them. This occurs in the rough endoplasmic reticulum (RER). Posttranslational modification, such as hydroxylation and glycosylation of proteins, occurs in the RER in general. Ribosomes associated with the RER are also where proteins bound for the cell membrane, lysosomes, and secreted proteins are synthesized. The Golgi complex is where the packaging of proteins for shipping to their appropriate location takes place. Proteins generally enter the Golgi complex after being synthesized in the RER. Radioactivity on the collagen precursors would be detected here, but not before the RER. Lysosomes are responsible for digesting material ingested by the cell as well as digesting intracellular organelles. Radioactivity would not be detected at the lysosome level. The plasma membrane is responsible for imparting structural stability to the cell as well as serving as a barrier. The smooth endoplasmic reticulum serves as a site of steroid synthesis and drug detoxification.

37. A. Dermatomyositis is autoimmune disease characterized by a distinctive skin rash that may accompany or precede the onset of muscle disease. The rash generally involves the upper eyelids and may be associated with periorbital edema. Muscle weakness develops; it generally affects the proximal muscles initially, making tasks such as rising from a chair extremely difficult. Myotonic dystrophy is a congenital weakness of various skeletal muscles, with other symptoms including cataracts, frontal balding, and cardiomyopathy. Polymyositis is an autoimmune disease that has the same clinical features of dermatomyositis; however, skin involvement does not occur. Scleroderma is an autoimmune disease characterized by progressive deposition of collagen throughout the body. Symptoms involve the skin, GI tract, musculoskeletal system, and kidneys. SLE is an autoimmune disease characterized by deposition of immune complexes throughout various organ systems, including the skin, kidneys, and lungs.

38. E. Local anesthetics predominantly affect C fibers, which are responsible for carrying slow pain sensations from the periphery to the CNS. A-alpha fibers are efferent motor neurons supplying skeletal muscle. A-beta fibers are predominantly responsible for carrying sensations of touch and pressure to the CNS. A-gamma fibers innervate the intrafusal fibers of muscle spindles. In being stimulated by these fibers, the sensitivity of the muscle spindle is continually modulated by the CNS. Beta fibers are preganglionic autonomic fibers and do not carry pain sensations.

39. E. This patient has classical signs and symptoms of herpes zoster, or shingles. Shingles is caused by the varicella zoster virus (VZV) and occurs commonly in the elderly as a result of a less effective immune system. After the primary infection of the VZV during childhood, known commonly as the chickenpox, the VZV remains latent in dorsal root ganglia and may recur many years later in the form of shingles. Vesicular lesions occur along a unilateral dermatomal distribution, usually not crossing the midline. Patients typically complain of itching, burning, and sharp pain due to neuritis. Chickenpox is the initial infection of the VZV during childhood and would not be likely in a 59-year-old man. Herpetic whitlow is caused by herpes simplex virus type I (HSV-I); it is characterized by vesicular lesions beneath the fingernails. Molluscum contagiosum, caused by the poxvirus, is characterized by flesh-colored papules with central umbilication usually on the hands. Scabies is caused by the mite *Sarcoptes scabiei* and is characterized by burrows on the interdigital skin, palms, and wrists. Patients complain of itching and burning in these areas.

40. B. This patient has an acute contact dermatitis (ACD) from poison ivy exposure. ACD is characterized by a type IV hypersensitivity reaction from an irritating antigen, in this case poison ivy resin. Symptoms typically occur 24 to 48 hr after exposure. Atopic dermatitis is an inherited inflammatory disorder of skin with a predilection for flexor surfaces, face, hands, and feet. Atopic dermatitis occurs in conjunction with a wide variety of disorders, including asthma and allergic rhinitis. Erysipelas is a facial cellulitis generally caused by *Streptococcus pyogenes*. The classic presentation is a sunburn-like rash comprising most of the face. Impetigo is a skin infection, usually with either *Streptococcus pyogenes* or *Staphylococcus aureus*, and is characterized by honey-colored, crusting lesions. Lyme disease is a multisystemic disease caused by the spirochete *Borrelia burgdorferi*, which is transmitted by deer ticks. The initial manifestation of Lyme disease is the characteristic bull's-eye rash known as erythema migrans. Cardiovascular, rheumatic, and parasympathetic nervous symptoms can develop if the disease is not treated.

41. B. Cicatricial pemphigoid is a subset of the mucous membrane pemphigoid family. It often has ocular manifestations as well as affecting the skin and other mucous membranes. It is caused by an autoimmune reaction to adhesion molecules in the hemidesmosome-epithelial membrane complex. The pustule-like lesions on the skin continue to grow and burst, causing a great deal of pain. Fibroblast activation secondary to inflammatory cytokines causes progressive fibrosis in the eye, leading to tear insufficiency and later to corneal damage. Vitiligo is a disease caused by an acquired loss of melanocytes in discrete areas of the skin, resulting in a lack of pigment. It is much easier to appreciate the depigmented skin in darker skinned individuals. Eczematous dermatitis can have multiple etiologies including infection, chemicals, and allergy contact. Bullous pemphigoid is caused by an autoimmune dysfunction where IgG antibodies attack the basement membranes of the epidermis, compromising the stability of the epidermis and resulting in bullae. Erythema multiforme is associated with drug hypersensitivity. Targetoid cells are seen histologically.

42. B. Eccrine glands constitute the vast majority of sweat glands in the body. They are found virtually everywhere and discharge directly onto the skin surface. They discharge a watery solution and are innervated by cholinergic sympathetic neurons. Apocrine sweat glands are found in the axillary, areolar, and anal regions of the body. They open into hair follicles and discharge a foul-smelling substance. These glands are innervated by adrenergic sympathetic neurons. Endocrine glands are ductless glands that secrete their products into the bloodstream. The products of these glands are generally called hormones. Holocrine glands actually secrete their product after they undergo apoptosis. As a result, both the secretory product and cellular debris are discharged into the glandular lumen. Paracrine glands secrete their products into nearby connective tissue, so that nearby cells are affected.

43. D. A positive PPD test indicates a past infection with the genus *Mycobacterium* and is characterized as a type IV hypersensitivity reaction. A type IV hypersensitivity is characterized by an interaction between T-helper type 1 cells, macrophages, and their associated cytokines. The type IV hypersensitivity reaction typically occurs 24 to 48 hr after the second contact with the antigen. CD8+ T cells inducing apoptosis in skin cells exposed to antigen is not characteristic of any hypersensitivity reaction. The degranulation of mast cells is characteristic of an immediate type I hypersensitivity reaction seen in such things as bee stings. Formation of antigen-antibody complexes in the skin would be a type III hypersensitivity reaction, characteristic of such things as the Arthus reaction and serum sickness. Specific antibodies cross-reacting to self-antigens present on skin cells would be characteristic of a type II hypersensitivity reaction. Type II hypersensitivity reactions are found in such disorders as Graves' disease and myasthenia gravis.

44. C. The epidermal layer of the skin comes from ectoderm, as does the lens of the eye. The dura mater comes from mesoderm. The heart is also derived from mesoderm. The pancreas derives from endoderm. The spleen derives from mesoderm.

45. A. Dermatitis herpetiformis is characterized by deposits of IgA along the rete ridges of the skin. Therefore, in order to utilize immunofluorescence to diagnose dermatitis herpetiformis, an antibody to IgA is needed. IgG1 and IgG2 may be found on immunofluorescence in the skin manifestations of systemic lupus erythematosus as well as other conditions. IgE and IgM are not known to be involved in any autoimmune skin disease.

46. B. Patients with PKU lack the enzyme phenylalanine hydroxylase, which leads to an inability to manufacture tyrosine. Tyrosine is an immediate precursor for the skin pigment melanin. A lack of melanin leads to symptoms of albinism in PKU patients. Lipofuscin, commonly called the "wear-and-tear pigment," is an intracellular pigment. Bilirubin is a breakdown product of hemoglobin and is normally recycled and excreted. Keratin is the protective layer overlying skin.

47. D. Lipofuscin, commonly called the "wear-and-tear pigment" is an intracellular pigment composed of polymers of lipids and phospholipids complexed with protein. It is a normal accumulation in cells. Bilirubin is a breakdown product of hemoglobin and is normally recycled and excreted. Keratin is the protective layer overlying skin. Iron accumulation results in hemosiderosis.

48. C. This patient most likely has a basal cell carcinoma, which is most common in sun-exposed areas of the skin. It is described as looking like "pearly papules," often with visible telangiectasias. Typical histopathologic findings include palisading nuclei. Keratin pearls are seen in squamous cell carcinoma. Onionskin appearance of bone is seen in Ewing's sarcoma, which is an anaplastic small cell malignant tumor; it appears most commonly in the diaphysis of long bones, pelvis, scapula, and ribs. A perivascular pseudorosette pattern of cells is associated with medulloblastomas, which are highly malignant cerebellar tumors that can compress the fourth ventricle, leading to hydrocephalus. Psammoma bodies, spindle cells concentrically arranged in a whorled pattern, are typical of meningioma, the second most common type of primary brain tumor.

49. C. This patient has typical findings of dermatitis herpetiformis. This disease mainly affects people in the age range of 20 through 40 years. It is characterized by recurrent blisters that tend to occur in groups on the extensor surfaces, upper back, and sacral areas. Deposits of IgA and microabscesses with neutrophils and eosinophils are characteristic on biopsy. Dermatitis herpetiformis is associated with gluten sensitivity and often resolves with a gluten-free diet. Eczematous dermatitis can have multiple etiologies including infection, chemicals, and allergy contact. Cicatricial pemphigoid is a subset of the mucous membrane pemphigoid family. It often has ocular manifestations as well as affecting the skin and other mucous membranes. It is caused by an autoimmune reaction to adhesion molecules in the hemidesmosome-epithelial membrane complex. Erythema multiforme is associated with drug hypersensitivity. Targetoid cells are seen histologically. Bullous pemphigoid is caused by an autoimmune dysfunction where IgG antibodies attack the basement membranes of the epidermis, compromising the stability of the epidermis and resulting in bullae.

50. E. Actinic keratosis is a known precursor of squamous cell carcinoma. Squamous cell carcinoma is a very common form of skin cancer whose risk factors include both excessive sun exposure and arsenic exposure. It commonly occurs on the hands and face. Squamous cell carcinoma is usually only locally invasive and does not often metastasize. Chondrosarcoma is a malignant cartilaginous tumor not associated in any way with sun or arsenic exposure or with actinic keratosis. Melanoma is a common skin cancer with high metastasizing potential. It is associated with sun exposure and is more common in light-skinned people. However, it is not related to actinic keratosis. Seborrheic keratosis is not related to actinic keratosis.

51. D. Henoch-Schönlein purpura is characterized by hemorrhagic urticaria on the extensor surfaces of the hands, legs, and buttocks. It is often accompanied by fever, gastrointestinal involvement, and renal symptoms (i.e., IgA nephropathy). It is closely linked with upper respiratory infections, most likely streptococcal in origin. Churg-Strauss syndrome is a necrotizing vasculitis that is prominent in the respiratory tract and is often associated with asthma. Kaposi's sarcoma is caused by the HSV8 virus and affects individuals with AIDS. Hypersensitivity vasculitis is characterized by acute inflammation of small blood vessels, showing as palpable purpura that is not isolated to the skin. It is not more likely to occur on the extensor surfaces of the hands, legs, and buttocks than at any other site or organ. Polyarteritis nodosa does not often appear in the skin.

52. D. This patient has the typical presentation of psoriasis, which is a chronic inflammatory process. Histologically, Munro abscesses, or minute neutrophilic abscesses, are seen within the parakeratotic stratum corneum. IgA deposits at the tips of dermal papillae are seen in dermatitis herpetiformis. IgG antibodies directed against epidermal basement membrane are seen in bullous pemphigoid. IgG antibodies directed against epidermal intercellular cement substances are seen in pemphigus vulgaris. Vacuolated cells in the granular cell layer of the epidermis are characteristic of verruca vulgaris, or the common wart.

53. E. Merkel cells are chiefly responsible for cutaneous sensation. They are most abundant in the areas where sensory perception is acute, as in the fingertips. These cells are closely associated with the expanded terminal bulb of an afferent myelinated nerve fiber. Melanocytes produce melanin, a pigment. Keratinocytes produce keratin, which forms a waterproof layer. Langerhans cells are antigen-presenting cells. Adipocytes are fat storage cells.

54. C. This patient suffers from oculocutaneous albinism in which there is a synthetic defect in melanin production. In tyrosinase-negative albinism there is a failure of tyrosinase to convert tyrosine to dihydroxyphenylalanine, which is required for proper melanin synthesis. The other enzymes listed do not have anything to do with melanin production and do not contribute to albinism.

55. D. Parvovirus B19 causes fifth disease or "slapped cheeks," as it is sometimes called. This disease is normally followed by a full recovery in a normal host but can cause aplastic anemia in patients with sickle cell anemia or other hemoglobinopathies. Parvovirus B19 is also the most common cause of nonimmune hydrops in newborns. Morbillivirus causes measles. *Staphylococcus saprophyticus* can cause urinary tract infections. Group A beta-hemolytic streptococcus causes scarlet fever. Human herpesvirus 6 causes the childhood exanthem known as roseola.

56. C. This patient has findings most consistent with Ehlers-Danlos syndrome type VI, a connective tissue disorder inherited as an autosomal recessive trait. Ehlers-Danlos comprises a spectrum of disorders in collagen synthesis. The defect in type VI Ehlers-Danlos affects the skin, bones, tendons, and vessels, sites where type I and III collagen is mostly found. Fibronectin is secreted by endothelial cells and fibroblasts and is not related to Ehlers-Danlos. Laminin is the most important protein in basement membranes and is not affected in Ehlers-Danlos. Type II collagen is found in cartilage and vitreous humor. Type IV collagen is found in basement membranes.

57. C. The recurrent cold sores are most likely caused by herpes simplex virus I, which usually affects the oral and inferior nasal regions. HSV establishes a latent state in the ganglia of cranial nerve V, most commonly the V2 and V3 branches; this becomes obvious, as these branches innervate the areas affected by the sores. The branch of CN V1 is less commonly affected by HSV1; however, in some circumstances it can be. CN VII is almost never affected by HSV1.

58. E. This patient shows signs and symptoms of hyperthyroidism, more specifically Graves' disease (i.e., proptosis is found in Graves' disease, not in all types of hyperthyroidism). Graves' disease is caused by antibodies directed toward the TSH receptors, providing unregulated stimulation of the thyroid gland. Serum T_4 levels are not usually very helpful in determining thyroid state. A decreased T_3 resin uptake and increased thyroid-binding globulin indicate low serum T_3, which would be a hypothyroid state. Increased serum TSH is usually seen in hypothyroid states because of the feedback between the hypothalamus-pituitary system and the thyroid gland.

59. C. Bullous pemphigoid, dermatitis herpetiformis, and erythema multiforme all show a split between the epidermis and dermis. However, suepidermal edema, a dermis with significant nuclear dust, and superficial perivascular lymphoplasmacytic infiltrate are more typical of erythema multiforme. In bullous pemphigoid, subepidermal bullae with eosinophilic infiltrate would be characteristic. Dermatitis herpetiformis shows dermal microabscesses with neutrophils, eosinophils, IgA, and fibrin at the tips of dermal papillae. Pemphigus vulgaris and varicella do not show the splitting between the epidermal and dermal layers of the skin. Prominent intraepidermal acantholysis and sparing of the basal layer is characteristic of pemphigus vulgaris. Varicella would show various stages of lesions ranging from active vesicles to crusting lesions.

60. A. Acanthosis nigricans, characterized by acanthosis and hyperpigmentation of skin involving the flexural regions, should often clue the physician to consider an underlying malignancy, most commonly in the stomach, lung, breast, and uterus. Dome-shaped nodules filled with soft gray-white material are characteristic of an epidermal inclusion cyst and have no relationship with underlying malignancies. Vascular pedunculated lesions with edematous stromas common to the skin and mucous membranes are characteristic of granuloma pyogenicum, which has no relationship to internal malignancies. Rough, scaling, poorly demarcated plaques are typical of actinic keratosis. Actinic keratosis can often lead to squamous cell carcinoma of the skin; however, this condition is not likely to be a marker for internal malignancies of the GI tract. Keratin "pearls" are seen with squamous cell carcinoma. Squamous cell carcinoma of the skin does not usually have the potential to metastasize to internal organs.

61. C. The lesion on the child's face is a port-wine stain, a type of capillary hemangioma that occurs on the face and neck. Port-wine stains are classic signs of Sturge-Weber syndrome. These patients have hemangiomatous involvement throughout their meninges, which can often lead to convulsions. Ocular findings including glaucoma and retinal detachment are also common. Infants with Sturge-Weber syndrome are often mentally retarded. Kaposi's sarcoma is a malignant vascular tumor that is more common in adults with AIDS. This type of Kaposi's sarcoma is associated with herpesvirus type VIII. Osler-Weber-Rendu syndrome, also known as hereditary hemorrhagic telangiectasia, is an inherited condition characterized by dilated and convoluted capillaries and venules of the skin and mucous membranes. Patients with Osler-Weber-Rendu syndrome are prone to develop internal hemorrhages (GI bleeds). Temporal arteritis is a systemic vasculitis often manifesting in the elderly. Common symptoms of temporal arteritis include headache, jaw claudication, and visual impairment. Von Hippel-Lindau disease is marked by cavernous hemangiomas, not capillary hemangiomas. It is characterized by multiple vascular tumors (hemangioblastomas) commonly located in the cerebellum and brainstem as well as by adenomas and cysts in the liver, kidneys, and pancreas.

62. G. This patient shows signs and symptoms of Sjögren's syndrome, which consists of the triad: xerostomia (dry mouth), keratoconjunctivitis sicca (dry eyes), and a connective tissue or autoimmune disease. Most often, this last is rheumatoid arthritis. The corneal abrasions are caused by lack of a protective tear film over the cornea due to lacrimal duct's involvement in Sjögren's syndrome. Tears are responsible for providing the anterior cornea with nutrition as well. The parotid glands, which are salivary glands, are likely obscured by cellular infiltration, causing difficulty in chewing and swallowing. Progressive systemic sclerosis, also known as scleroderma, is a connective tissue disease that occurs mostly in younger women. Wegener's granulomatosis is a disease of unknown etiology characterized by necrotizing granulomatous vasculitis mainly affecting the lungs and kidneys. It is most often associated with C-ANCAs, cytoplasmic antibodies with a cytoplasmic staining pattern. Polyarteritis nodosa is the one connective tissue disease that predominates in men. The rest predominate in women. Anti-nRNP titers are found in patients with mixed connective tissue disease (MCTD). MCTD is like other connective tissue diseases except that it usually spares the kidneys, whereas other connective tissue diseases do not.

63. D. Progressive systemic sclerosis (PSS), also known as scleroderma, is a connective tissue disease that occurs mostly in younger women. This patient exhibits the CREST syndrome variant, with the characteristic physical findings of calcinosis (nodules in the elbows and knees), Raynaud's phenomenon (cyanosis and pallor of the hand as it holds ice), esophageal dysfunction (difficulty swallowing), sclerodactyly, and telangiectasias. This patient's fixed facial expression is caused by hypertrophied collagen fibers in the subcutaneous tissue, which tighten the skin. Other common findings in PSS include pulmonary fibrosis and hypertension. Wegener's granulomatosis is a disease of unknown etiology characterized by necrotizing granulomatous vasculitis mainly affecting the lungs and kidneys. It is most often associated with C-ANCAs, cytoplasmic antibodies with a cytoplasmic staining pattern. Polyarteritis nodosa is the one connective tissue disease that predominates in men. The rest predominate in women. Anti-nRNP titers are found in patients with mixed connective tissue disease (MCTD). MCTD is like other connective tissue diseases except that it usually spares the kidneys, as other connective tissue diseases do not.

64. G. This patient likely has Wegener's granulomatosis, which is a disease of unknown etiology characterized by necrotizing granulomatous vasculitis mainly affecting the lungs and kidneys. It is most often associated with C-ANCAs, cytoplasmic antibodies with a cytoplasmic staining pattern. The hematuria and hemoptysis are caused by bleeding of the vasculature in the lungs and kidneys secondary to the inflammation. Lack of recent travel can help rule out any tropical microbial diseases like leischmaniasis. Wegener's granulomatosis is a disease of unknown etiology characterized by necrotizing granulomatous vasculitis mainly affecting the lungs and kidneys. It is most often associated with C-ANCAs, cytoplasmic antibodies with a cytoplasmic staining pattern. Polyarteritis nodosa is the

one connective tissue disease that predominates in men. The rest predominate in women. Anti-nRNP titers are found in patients with mixed connective tissue disease (MCTD). MCTD is like other connective tissue diseases except that it usually spares the kidneys, as other connective tissue diseases do not. Sjögren's syndrome consists of the triad: xerostomia (dry mouth), keratoconjunctivitis sicca (dry eyes), and a connective tissue or autoimmune disease. Most often, the associated connective tissue or autoimmune disease is rheumatoid arthritis.

65. C. Polyarteritis nodosa is the one connective tissue disease that predominates in men. The rest predominate in women. It is an immune complex vasculitis that causes fibrinoid necrosis of small and medium-sized arteries. The antigens often responsible for leading to the activation of immune complexes include the hepatitis B antigens and drugs such as sulfonamides and penicillins. Patients with polyarteritis nodosa may complain of multiple problems because the vasculature of virtually any organ can be affected. Wegener's granulomatosis is a disease of unknown etiology characterized by necrotizing granulomatous vasculitis mainly affecting the lungs and kidneys. It is most often associated with C-ANCAs, cytoplasmic antibodies with a cytoplasmic staining pattern. Anti-nRNP titers are found in patients with mixed connective tissue disease (MCTD). MCTD is like other connective tissue diseases except that it usually spares the kidneys, as other connective tissue diseases do not.

66. B. Anti-nRNP titers are found in patients with mixed connective tissue disease (MCTD). MCTD is like other connective tissue diseases except that it usually spares the kidneys, whereas other connective tissue diseases do not. It affects mainly women in their late 30s to early 40s. Common symptoms include arthralgias, myalgias, and myositis, esophageal hypomotility, and Raynaud's phenomenon. Polyarteritis nodosa is the one connective tissue disease that predominates in men. The rest predominate in women. Osteoarthritis is associated with degeneration of joints and can be associated with Heberden's nodes.

67. A. This patient likely has systemic lupus erythematosus (SLE), a connective tissue disease that mainly affects women of childbearing age. It is characterized by immune complex–mediated inflammatory lesions throughout the body, most importantly in the kidney. Skin biopsies of patients with SLE often show immune complexes at the dermal-epidermal junction. Kidney microscopy studies would show a "wire-loop" appearance. The linear pattern of immunofluorescence is seen in Goodpasture's syndrome. ANA titers are usually positive for anti–double stranded DNA antibodies and anti–Smith antigen antibodies. Anti-histone antibodies are seen in the drug-induced forms of lupus. Anti-IgG antibodies are found in rheumatoid arthritis. Antimitochondrial antibodies are seen in primary biliary cirrhosis. Serum complement levels are usually decreased in SLE.

68. E. Surface ectoderm is responsible mainly for the derivation of the adenohypophysis, the ocular lens, and the epithelial linings and epidermis of skin. Endoderm is responsible mainly for gut tube epithelium in organs throughout the GI tract as well as lungs, liver, thymus, thyroid, and parathyroid glands. Mesoderm is responsible for connective tissue, muscle, bone, cardiovascular structures, urogenital structures, lymphatics, spleen, adrenal cortex, and serosal linings. Neural crest is responsible for dorsal root ganglia, melanocytes, Schwann cells, pia mater, chromaffin cells of the adrenal medulla, and enterochromaffin cells. Neuroectoderm is responsible for the neurohypophysis, CNS neurons, oligodendrocytes, astrocytes, and the pineal gland.

69. D. The disease described most resembles shingles, which characteristically affects only one side of a dermatome. In this case, the dermatome affected is T4. The T4 dermatome is at the level of the nipple and extends horizontally across the chest at this level. The C4 dermatome is at the level of the anterior portion of the trapezius and the lower portion of the neck. The T2 dermatome extends horizontally across the chest at the level of the armpit. The T10 dermatome extends horizontally across the abdomen at the level of the umbilicus.

70. A. The disease being described is dermatomyositis, which presents with proximal muscle weakness and a heliotrope (lilac-colored) rash on the eyelids. The diagnosis can be sealed with a creatine phosphokinase level, electromyography, and a muscle biopsy. Scleroderma is a multisystem disease characterized by abnormalities of small blood vessels, fibrosis of the skin and internal organs, immune system activation, and autoimmunity. Systemic lupus erythematosus affects the skin, joints, kidneys, nervous system, and immune system. Discoid lupus erythematosus is limited to the skin involvement, which is usually found in SLE as well. Psoriasis is associated with scaly lesions, with arthritis developing later in some cases.

71. D. Infection with *Pseudomonas aeruginosa* is a major cause of sepsis in patients who suffer severe burns. Without the proper defense barrier provided by the skin (destroyed by the burns), *Pseudomonas* can easily gain access to internal organs. The sepsis is due to this patient's inability to fight off infection because of the defective chemotactic ability of his mononuclear leukocytes. Autoimmune reactions against the damaged tissue are not a likely occurrence in burn patients. Loss of adequate fluid volume and dehydration would not usually cause a fever. This patient was kept adequately hydrated with intravenous fluids and electrolytes. Fungal and staphylococcal infections are possibilities; however, in burn patients, the most common cause of infection is *P. aeruginosa*.

72. D. Eczematous dermatitis can have multiple etiologies including infection, chemicals, and allergy contact. This patient most likely had an allergic type of hypersensitivity reaction to the deodorant, hence the well-demarcated rash on both armpits. Spongiosis with vesicle formation is characteristic of the acute stage. In chronic acanthosis, hyperkeratosis and lichenification are commonly seen. There is also a subacute stage, which has characteristics of both the acute and chronic stages. Atopic eczematous dermatitis is most often caused by a type IV delayed

hypersensitivity reaction. Cicatricial pemphigoid is a subset of the mucous membrane pemphigoid family. It is often associated with ocular manifestations as well as affecting the skin and other mucous membranes. It is caused by an autoimmune reaction to adhesion molecules in the hemidesmosome–epithelial membrane complex. Erythema multiforme is associated with drug hypersensitivity. Targetoid cells are seen histologically. Bullous pemphigoid is caused by an autoimmune dysfunction whereby IgG antibodies attack the basement membranes of the epidermis, compromising the stability of the epidermis and resulting in bullae.

73. A. This patient is showing the classic triad of Reiter's syndrome, which includes uveitis/conjunctivitis, urethritis, and arthritis. Reiter's syndrome commonly follows a chlamydial or a gastrointestinal infection. It is linked to HLA-B27. The rest of the choices would not cause his symptoms. Gout is caused by the deposition of uric acid crystals in joints, such as the metatarsophalangeal joint of the big toe. Juvenile rheumatoid arthritis would not be associated with kidney or ocular manifestations. There is no indication here of metastatic malignancy. Sarcoidosis would usually present with respiratory manifestations, such as a cough. It can, however, cause uveitis.

74. A. This patient shows characteristics of bullous pemphigoid, which is characterized by supepidermal bullae. Bullous pemphigoid is caused by an autoimmune dysfunction where IgG antibodies attack the basement membranes of the epidermis, compromising the stability of the epidermis and resulting in bullae. A linear band of immunofluorescence can be seen along the basement membrane on electron microscopy. Cicatricial pemphigoid is a subset of the mucous membrane pemphigoid family. It often has ocular manifestations as well, as affecting the skin and other mucous membranes. It is caused by an autoimmune reaction to adhesion molecules in the hemidesmosome–epithelial membrane complex. Erythema multiforme is associated with drug hypersensitivity. Targetoid cells are seen histologically.

75. D. A keloid is an abnormal proliferation of connective tissue with a very abnormal arrangement of collagen. This abnormal proliferation, which contains a lot of collagen, looks very similar to tumor-like scar. Keloids are much more common in African-American individuals and usually follow some sort of trauma, in this case the ear piercing. The problem with keloids is that they tend to recur even after resection. The spitz nevus can be often confused with malignant melanoma. However the lack of color change or change in size would make melanoma a little less likely. Also, this patient is much younger than the average patient who presents with melanomatous lesions. Spitz nevus is also known as juvenile melanoma; however, because the lesion is benign, this name is falling out of use. However, one should always consider melanoma when a lesion of this kind is seen and make sure that proper testing is done to rule melanoma out. Molluscum contagiosum is a viral disease caused by the DNA poxvirus. It is contracted by direct contact. The lesions are characteristically pink, umbilicated, and dome-shaped.

Chapter 13 Pharmacology

Questions

1. A 49-year-old man who has been hospitalized for 3 weeks for spinal surgery and rehabilitation develops a fever of 103.1°F (39.5°C) and hypotension. Initial Gram's stain of blood cultures shows Gram-positive cocci in grape-like clusters. The cultures are sent for identification and sensitivities. While waiting for the results of the sensitivities, which antibiotic should be started?

   A. Amoxicillin
   B. Ceftriaxone
   C. Ciprofloxacin
   D. Vancomycin
   E. Penicillin

2. A 56-year-old woman who is currently being treated for atrial fibrillation tells her physician that she has been quite tired recently and that she has become extremely sensitive to the cold. She also notes a color change in her skin. Physical examination reveals that the patient's skin has a bluish tone. What sort of drug toxicity is the most likely explanation for this patient's symptoms?

   A. Amiodarone
   B. Digoxin
   C. Flecainide
   D. Lidocaine
   E. Procainamide

3. A 29-year-old man presents to his family physician complaining of a headache in the region of his forehead. After a thorough physical examination, the physician diagnoses the patient with acute sinusitis and is ready to prescribe amoxicillin. The patient alerts the physician to the fact that when he was a child, he received penicillin for pneumonia and, as a result, broke out in a severe itchy rash. Which antibiotic would be absolutely contraindicated in this patient?

   A. Chloramphenicol
   B. Ceftriaxone
   C. Doxycycline
   D. Erythromycin
   E. Vancomycin

4. A 54-year-old woman with diabetes mellitus presents to her primary care physician for a follow-up examination. Her current medications include glyburide. Ophthalmoscopic examination reveals bilateral retinal changes. Her vision is 20/200 without glasses. Her neck is supple and she has mild jugular venous distension bilaterally. Cardiac examination reveals no evidence of rubs or murmurs. Pulmonary and abdominal examinations are unremarkable. What is the mechanism of action of glyburide?

   A. Close calcium channels in alpha-cell membranes
   B. Close calcium channels in beta-cell membranes
   C. Close potassium channels in alpha-cell membranes
   D. Close potassium channels in beta-cell membranes
   E. Open calcium channels in alpha-cell membranes
   F. Open calcium channels in beta-cell membranes
   G. Open potassium channels in alpha-cell membranes
   H. Open potassium channels in beta-cell membranes

5. A 25-year-old patient presents to his primary care physician complaining of a rash on his trunk. The patient states that he went hiking with friends about 2 weeks earlier and that, a few days after the hike, he developed a fever and headache, which have not yet resolved. Shortly thereafter, he developed a rash on his palms and soles, which slowly migrated to his wrists, ankles, and now his trunk. Assuming that a tick bite caused this patient's symptoms, which of the following treatments should be considered?

   A. Amantadine
   B. Ceftriaxone
   C. Penicillin
   D. Rifampin
   E. Tetracycline
   F. Watchful waiting

6. A mother brings her 6-year-old son to the ambulatory care clinic because he has not been eating properly, with his diet consisting mainly of "junk food." She states that he seems to be clumsy at night because he bumps into things, but he is fine in the morning. She also states that his eyes appear increasingly irritated and dry. The child had blood in his urine once during the previous week. What is the most likely explanation for these symptoms?

   A. Hypovitaminosis A
   B. Hypervitaminosis D
   C. Vitamin A deficiency
   D. Vitamin C deficiency
   E. Vitamin K deficiency

7. A 42-year-old woman presents to her primary care physician with new complaints of fatigue and morning stiffness, which she has been experiencing every day for roughly 2 months. She states that it takes her a good hour to get going in the morning but that her symptoms improve with activity. Her pain is localized to her wrists, ankles, and knees bilaterally. She has noticed that these areas have often appeared swollen and felt warm. Her past medical history is significant for peptic ulcer disease and hypertension. Her current medications include a beta-blocker. Physical examination of the heart, lungs, and abdomen is within normal limits. Musculoskeletal exam is positive for warm, swollen wrist, ankle, and knee joints bilaterally. What is the most appropriate treatment for pain/inflammation in this patient?

A. Allopurinol
B. Aspirin
C. Celecoxib
D. Gold salts
E. Indomethacin

8. A 55-year-old man presents to the ambulatory care clinic complaining of severe pain and redness in his first metatarsophalangeal joint. The pain woke him up from a sound sleep the previous night. He has had several similar episodes in the past and had been taking allopurinol chronically to eliminate attacks; however, he ran out of pills about a month ago and has not been able to afford to get his prescription refilled. Physical examination shows that the skin overlying the joint is red and painful. He also has a discrete tophus on the pinna of his left ear. The physician prescribes colchicine to help alleviate the pain. What is the mechanism of action of this medication?

A. At therapeutic doses, it blocks proximal tubular resorption of uric acid.
B. It binds to tubulin, causing its depolymerization and thus disrupting cellular function and decreasing granulocytic migration to the affected area.
C. It is a COX-1 and COX-2 inhibitor and thereby reduces inflammation.
D. It is a purine analog that reduces the production of uric acid by competitively inhibiting the last two steps in uric acid biosynthesis.
E. It is an immunosuppressive agent that helps to suppress the immune system, thereby quelling the localized attack on the joint.

9. A 54-year-old woman presents to her primary care physician because she has developed a maculopapular pruritic dermatitis and loss of taste sensation after using a medication for the treatment regimen for her rheumatoid arthritis. What is the most likely explanation for these findings?

A. Aspirin
B. Chloroquine
C. Ibuprofen
D. Indomethacin
E. Methotrexate
F. Naproxen
G. Penicillamine

10. A 58-year-old man is hospitalized for treatment of a deep venous thrombosis in his left lower extremity. Diagnosis was made postoperatively after right hemicolectomy performed for a colon mass. He is currently being given an intravenous anticoagulant. Which of the following statements is most correct?

A. This agent has a half-life measured in hours.
B. This agent is a small ionic polymer.
C. This agent has limited effect on coagulation effects in vitro.
D. This agent is monitored via the extrinsic pathway.
E. This agent has a site of action in the liver.

11. A 14-year-old girl presents to the ambulatory care clinic after developing a rash on her face. The patient's mother states that the rash seemed to appear after the patient had been outdoors all day at a picnic in the park. A picture of the patient's skin is shown in Figure 13-1. The patient states she has been taking medication for a skin problem. Physical examination reveals, aside from the rash, a yellowish discoloration of her teeth. Which of the following drugs could be responsible for this patient's symptoms?

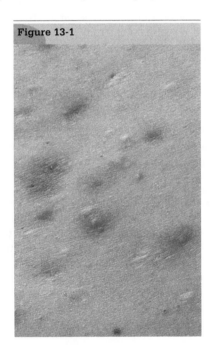

Figure 13-1

A. Benzoyl peroxide
B. Chloramphenicol
C. Erythromycin
D. Minocycline
E. Phenytoin

12. A 54-year-old woman presents to her primary care physician with signs and symptoms consistent with the early stages of rheumatoid arthritis. She was started on acetaminophen and methotrexate therapy, which provided adequate relief. However, after several years of this therapy, her symptoms began to worsen. Radiologic studies of her hands show progressive destruction in the joints of several fingers. Treatment with a

new second-line agent for rheumatoid arthritis is considered. The particular drug is available only in a parenteral formulation and its mechanism of action is antagonism of tumor necrosis factor. Which drug is being considered?

A. Cyclosporine

B. Etanercept

C. Indomethacin

D. Naproxen

E. Penicillamine

13. A 37-year-old man is brought to surgery after a motor vehicle accident because of a suspected perforation of the bowel. The anesthesiologist decides to utilize phenobarbital for induction of anesthesia. What is the mechanism of action of this drug?

A. Acts as a competitive antagonist at GABA receptors.

B. Facilitate GABA-A action by increasing the duration of Cl– channel opening.

C. Facilitate GABA-A action by increasing the frequency of Cl– channel opening.

D. Facilitate GABA-B action by decreasing the frequency of Cl– channel opening.

E. Inhibit the actions of glutamine diffusely throughout the CNS.

14. An infant born at 29 weeks' gestation is in respiratory distress. The lecithin-to-sphingomyelin ratio in the amniotic fluid is 1.2. Histological changes are noted. What treatment of the mother prior to the birth of the infant could have prevented this condition?

A. Aminocaproic acid

B. Aspirin

C. Corticosteroids

D. Flumazenil

E. Protamine

15. A 25-year-old woman with cystic fibrosis and infected with *Pseudomonas aeruginosa* was hospitalized with a pneumonia, treated with ceftazidime, and sent home. The next day she called complaining of persistent vomiting and nausea. What is the most likely reason for the nausea and vomiting?

A. Alcohol use

B. Gastroenteritis

C. Pregnancy

D. Sexually transmitted illness

E. Upper respiratory infection

16. A 64-year-old woman presents to her family physician for an annual checkup. She reports having fallen asleep sitting up for several recent nights, as well as shortness of breath in walking from the living room to the kitchen. Physical examination reveals an S_3 heart sound and bilateral pitting edema of the lower extremities. She is given a prescription for digoxin and put on a salt-restricted diet. She returns a week later with unchanged symptoms. What is the most appropriate treatment for this patient?

A. Captopril, propranolol

B. Diltiazem, furosemide

C. Furosemide

D. Furosemide, digitalis, captopril

E. Hydrochlorothiazide, digitalis, and spironolactone

F. Nitroglycerin, aspirin

17. A 42-year-old motorcyclist presents to the emergency department after crashing into an embankment. He claims that he laid his bike down to prevent a crash. Physical examination reveals multiple abrasions on both arms and legs. X-rays of the chest, abdomen, and pelvis reveal no evidence of fractures. What antibiotic should be prescribed to prevent infection from the abrasions?

A. Ampicillin

B. Ceftriaxone

C. Ciprofloxacin

D. Gentamicin

E. Trimethoprim

18. A 2-month-old infant is brought to the pediatrics clinic with a fever and profound neck stiffness. For several days she has had an upper respiratory infection, which was treated with acetaminophen. A spinal tap reveals an increased white blood count, decreased glucose, and increased protein. The fluid is cloudy in appearance. Which set of antibiotics would be most appropriate for the treatment of this patient?

A. Cefotaxime, vancomycin

B. Nafcillin, moxifloxacin

C. Ofloxacin, penicillin

D. Tobramycin, ceftriaxone

E. Trimethoprim/sulfamethoxazole

19. A 13-year-old basketball player has an asthma attack during a workout with the team. She had forgotten her inhaler, but several other players had their asthma medications with them. She therefore took a medication but still had persistent symptoms approximately 10 min later. Which of the following medications did she most likely take?

A. Albuterol

B. Epinephrine

C. Isproterenol

D. Salmeterol

E. Terbutaline

20. An 18-year-old Asian-American woman presents to her primary care physician for her first prenatal visit. It is estimated that she is 9 weeks pregnant. Her fluorescent treponemal antibody test is positive, although she has been completely asymptomatic. What medication and/or recommendation should be made to this patient?

A. Cefazolin

B. Discontinue the theophylline

C. Doxycycline

D. Ketoconazole

E. Levofloxacin

F. Penicillin G

G. Piperacillin

H. Streptomycin

I. Tetracycline

21. A 17-year-old girl went camping in Ohio for 2 weeks. Approximately a week later, she presents to her primary care physician complaining of a red macule on her right leg. The lesion has a central clear area. She also has a similar lesion on her lower back. She does not remember being bitten by a spider. What is the most appropriate treatment for this patient?

   A. Cephalexin

   B. Ceftriaxone

   C. Chloramphenicol

   D. Ciprofloxacin

   E. Doxycycline

   F. Gentamicin

   G. Penicillin G

22. A 54-year-old man presents to the emergency department complaining of excruciating pain in his left toe. Physical examination reveals a red toe that is very sensitive to touch. What is the most appropriate treatment for this patient?

   A. Aspirate fluid from the joint and send it for cultures.

   B. Give allopurinol and follow up in 1 week.

   C. Give the patient allopurinol and admit him to the hospital for 12 hr so the drug can take effect.

   D. Give sulfinpyrazole and admit the patient overnight.

23. A 65-year-old man presents to his primary care physician complaining of a cough and shortness of breath, which he has had for 2 days. He reports that he recently had root canal surgery. A sputum culture is taken and oragnisms are identified with silver stain. Gram's stain reveals Gram-negative rods. What is the most appropriate treatment of this condition?

   A. Ciprofloxacin

   B. Erythromycin

   C. Gentamicin

   D. Penicillin

   E. Sulfamethoxazole

24. A 78-year-old woman with lung cancer metastatic to bone presents to the emergency department with lethargy, dehydration, and mental confusion. A complete blood count reveals a hematocrit of 29%. Serum potassium is 3.5 mEq/L. Serum calcium is 14 mg/dL. Serum transaminases are mildly elevated. What is the most appropriate treatment for this patient?

   A. Alendronate

   B. Dialysis

   C. Ergocalciferol (vitamin D_2)

   D. Furosemide

   E. Rehydration with normal saline and then furosemide

25. A 53-year-old truck driver presents to his primary care physician for a routine examination. He reports that he has spent most of his summer driving across the country. Physical examination reveals a 7-mm lesion on the left dorsal aspect of his left arm (Figure 13-2). Further evaluation reveals pearly papules with visible telangiectatic vessels. The lesion is biopsied and found to contain palisading nuclei. What is the most appropriate treatment for this patient?

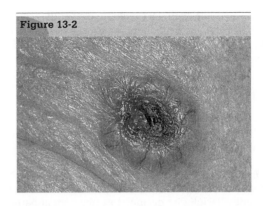

Figure 13-2

   A. 5-Fluorouracil

   B. 6-Mercaptopurine

   C. Bleomycin

   D. Busulfan

   E. Cyclophosphamide

   F. Watchful waiting

26. A 35-year-old woman arrives at the emergency department after a motor vehicle accident. She sustained bilateral femoral fractures, a small cerebral contusion with bleeding, and a collapsed left lung. After the insertion of a chest tube and appropriate treatment of the femoral fractures, she is instructed to maintain strict bed rest for the following 3 weeks. What is the best antithrombotic treatment for this patient?

   A. Compression pulse devices around both lower extremities

   B. Low-molecular-weight heparin

   C. Subcutaneous heparin injections and warfarin for 3 days and then only warfarin

   D. Subcutaneous heparin

   E. Warfarin

27. A 26-year-old HIV-positive patient has granuloma lesions in both lung fields and intracranial lesions on CT scan. On physical examination, he has decreased breath sounds at both lung bases and scattered rales. Cardiac examination reveals no evidence of rubs, murmurs, or gallops. What is the most appropriate treatment for this patient?

   A. Amoxicillin

   B. Amphotericin B

   C. Ampicillin

   D. Ceftriaxone

   E. Cefuroxime

   F. Ciprofloxacin

   G. Gentamicin

28. A 62-year-old man presents to his primary care physician complaining of severe headaches. Physical examination reveals several telangiectasias on his chest. The liver is palpable 7 cm below the ribs. Which test and/or intervention is most likely to cause an adverse effect/reaction in this patient?

   A. Advise the patient to drink more water and consider taking a vitamin supplement

   B. Order complete blood count and liver enzymes tests

C. Prescribe amitriptyline to control migraine headaches

D. Question the patient about ethanol use and suggest Alcoholics Anonymous if response is appropriate

29. A 46-year-old woman presents to her primary care physician complaining of a 1-week history of a painful thrombotic vein in her upper thigh. She has a history of diabetes mellitus. Physical examination of the heart, lungs, and abdomen is unremarkable. Examination of the right upper thigh shows that the vein is visible; the patient reports that it also occasionally itches. What is the treatment of choice for this patient?

A. Heparin and warfarin for 3 days followed by warfarin for 6 months

B. Low-molecular-weight heparin

C. Subcutaneous heparin and warfarin for 3 days then warfarin for 16 weeks

D. Warfarin for 1 year

E. Warfarin for 6 weeks

F. Warm compresses and ibuprofen

30. A 47-year-old man is scheduled for a kidney transplant in 2 days. He has a history of diabetes mellitus and hypertension. His diabetes has resulted in end-stage renal disease. He currently undergoes dialysis 3 days a week. What immunosuppressant drugs should be initiated postoperatively to prevent kidney rejection?

A. Azathioprine

B. Cyclosporine

C. Cyclosporine and azathioprine

D. Mycophenolate mofetil

E. Prednisone

F. Tacrolimus, OKT3, and azathioprine

31. A 56-year-old man with occasional anginal symptoms was given nitroglycerin by his cardiologist to take during an anginal attack; he was also advised, if his symptoms persisted, to proceed to the emergency department. What is the mechanism of action of nitroglycerin?

A. It is a beta-blocker.

B. It is a calcium channel blocker.

C. It decreases the heart rate at the AV node.

D. It has a positive inotropic effect.

E. It causes venodilation and relaxation of vascular smooth muscle.

32. A 15-year-old boy is brought to the emergency department after an attempted suicide. He took an entire bottle of acetaminophen and followed it with a pint of whiskey. What is the most appropriate treatment for this patient?

A. Deferoxamine

B. Ethanol

C. Methylene blue

D. *N*-acetylcysteine

E. Naloxone

F. Protamine

G. Vitamin K

33. A 78-year-old Caucasian man presents to the emergency department because he has had slurred speech and right arm weakness for about 30 min. A CT scan is performed and reveals no evidence of cerebral bleeding. The patient is then diagnosed with a transient ischemic attack (TIA) and is started on clopidogrel. The mechanism of action of this agent is which of the following?

A. It acts as a thrombolytic, dissolving fibrin clots.

B. It inhibits vitamin K–dependent clotting factors.

C. It irreversibly inhibits cyclooxygenase.

D. It prevents the formation of clots by inhibiting thrombin.

E. It prevents the formation of clots by irreversibly inhibiting the binding of adenosine diphosphate.

34. A 68-year-old woman has been hospitalized for 3 weeks with endocarditis of the mitral valve. During that time, she has been treated with intravenous antibiotics. Physical examination of the heart reveals no evidence of rubs, murmurs, or gallops. Pulmonary auscultation reveals no wheezes, rhonchi or rales. The abdomen is soft and nontender. Bowel sounds are audible in all four quadrants. Today she begins to experience bloody diarrhea. What is the most appropriate treatment?

A. Bismuth subsalicylate

B. Diphenoxylate

C. Infusion of sodium chloride

D. Lactulose

E. Loperamide

F. Metronidazole

35. A 16-year-old boy presents to the emergency department accompanied by two friends, who report that they were injecting heroin. A few minutes after his injection, the patient lost consciousness and was driven to the hospital by his friends. What is the most appropriate treatment for this patient?

A. Administer ipecac.

B. Administer naloxone.

C. Administer pralidoxime.

D. Arouse the patient with a painful stimulus and call the police to take him to jail for the night.

E. Start an intravenous line and monitor patient overnight.

36. A 63-year-old woman presents to her primary care physician complaining of cough and a skin rash. While taking her history, you discover that she is taking a medication for high blood pressure, but she could not name it, saying only that it was a little white pill. Which of the following antihypertensive drugs could cause the reported symptoms in drug toxicity?

A. Captopril

B. Clonidine

C. Hydralazine

D. Phentolamine

E. Prazosin

F. Sodium nitroprusside

37. A 14-year-old girl is brought to the emergency department with nausea and vomiting, muscle cramps, weakness, and confusion. Physical examination of the heart and lungs is within normal limits. Laboratory studies reveal a serum potassium of 9 mEq/L. Which of the following treatments would be unlikely to be of benefit to this patient?

A. Calcium

B. Dialysis

C. Insulin and glucose

D. Kayexalate

E. Thiazide diuretic

38. A 45-year-old man presents to his primary care physician with a rash on the left side of his face and just below the left eye and back as far as the hairline. He has no history of trauma to this area and has made use of no new cosmetic products. He reports having had a kidney transplant 3 years earlier. What is the most appropriate treatment for this patient?

A. Aspirin to decrease inflammation

B. Doxycycline

C. Intravenous acyclovir

D. No drugs at this time to reduce the risk of drug interactions with his current immunosuppressant drugs

E. Oral acyclovir

39. A 65-year-old Caucasian man presents to the emergency department with complaints of fever, chest pain (which is unrelieved by nitroglycerin), and fatigue. His past medical history is notable for a myocardial infarction, which occurred approximately 3 weeks earlier. The patient's current electrocardiogram shows diffuse ST-segment elevations and PR depressions. What is the most appropriate first-line treatment for this patient?

A. Acetaminophen

B. Corticosteroids

C. Enalapril

D. Furosemide

E. Ibuprofen

40. A 54-year-old African American man presents to his primary care physician with a new onset of hypertension; at a local health fair, his blood pressure was found to be 173/98 mm Hg. In the office today, his blood pressure is 164/95 mm Hg. He also has a history of diabetes mellitus. Which of the following would be the most appropriate medication for this patient?

A. Amlodipine

B. Clonidine

C. Hydrochlorothiazide

D. Lisinopril

E. Losartan

41. While mowing his lawn, a 55-year-old man developed severe substernal chest pain radiating to his neck and left arm. He is brought to the emergency department for evaluation. His electrocardiogram is shown in Figure 13-3. What is the most appropriate treatment for this patient?

A. Aspirin, captopril, digoxin, diltiazem

B. Aspirin, diltiazem, acetazolamide, nitroglycerin

C. Captopril, propranolol, aspirin, nitroglycerin

D. Digoxin, nitroglycerin, aspirin, spironolactone

E. Hydrochlorothiazide, aspirin, epinephrine, digoxin

42. An ambulance brings a 35-year-old Caucasian woman to the emergency department after she began seizing some 30 min earlier, as she is still doing. After treating her with benzodiazepines as per protocol, the physician speaks to the family, who give no history of seizure; in fact, they report that the patient's only medical history involved a bout of tuberculosis, for which she is still being treated. What is the most likely explanation for this patient's seizures?

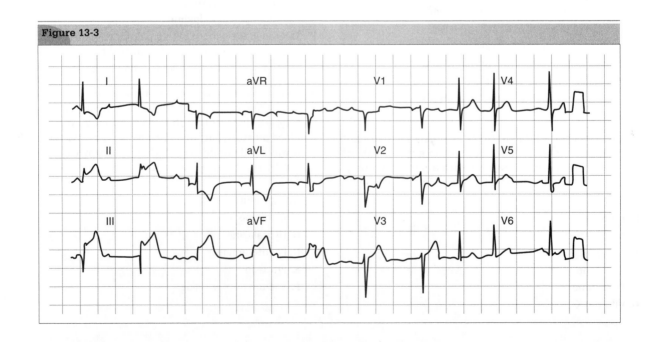

Figure 13-3

A. Ethambutol
B. Isoniazid
C. Pyrazinamide
D. Rifampin
E. Streptomycin

43. A 54-year-old African-American woman presents to her primary care physician with complaints of a facial rash, myalgias, fatigue, fever, and oral ulcers, which she has now had for 4 weeks. Her only significant medical history involves a ventricular arrhythmia, diagnosed some 8 weeks earlier, for which she is currently under treatment. ANA testing reveals positive antihistone antibody. What is the most likely explanation for these findings?

A. Disopyramide
B. Flecainide
C. Procainamide
D. Propafenone
E. Sotalol

44. A 12-year-old boy is brought to the pediatrician because of persistent fatigue and a tremor in his right hand that has progressed over the course of a year. Aside from the tremor, physical examination is unremarkable except for what appears to be a dark brown ring around both irises. Laboratory studies reveal a serum ceruloplasmin level of 12 mg/dL and an AST/ALT of 89 and 105, respectively. Which of the following medications is most appropriate for this patient?

A. Deferoxamine
B. Dimercaprol
C. EDTA
D. Methylene blue
E. Penicillamine

45. A 73-year-old woman presents to her primary care physician with hand soreness and color changes when her hands get cold. She says that her hands first turn white, then bluish, and finally red. Her current medications include ibuprofen for osteoarthritis, vitamin E once a week to help her skin heal, propranolol to control a supraventricular arrhythmia, ciprofloxacin for a recent urinary tract infection, and desloratidine for her seasonal allergies. Which of the following medications should be discontinued?

A. Ciprofloxacin
B. Desloratidine
C. Ibuprofen
D. Propranolol
E. Vitamin E

46. A 64-year-old man with a 5-year history of hypertension presents to his primary care physician for follow-up. His medications include a calcium channel blocker and an angiotensin-converting enzyme (ACE) inhibitor. Today his blood pressure is 160/105 mm Hg. You decide to add clonidine to his regimen. What is its mechanism of action?

A. It blocks central alpha$_2$ receptors.
B. It blocks peripheral alpha$_2$ receptors.
C. It potentiates central alpha$_2$ receptors.
D. It potentiates the effects of anticholinergics centrally.
E. It potentiates the effects of GABA centrally.

47. A 55-year-old man presents to his primary care physician with new-onset hypertension. He is given clonidine 0.2 mg to be taken twice a day; however, he mistakenly takes it four times a day. Which of the following will be the most likely result?

A. Bradycardia
B. Diarrhea
C. Erectile dysfunction
D. Excess salivation
E. Hypertension
F. Polyuria
G. Ventricular arrhythmia

48. A 47-year-old woman presents to the emergency department because she has had several episodes of epistaxis within the past several weeks as well as some generalized fatigue. Physical examination is significant for scattered petechiae in her mouth and bruises over her trunk and limbs that are at various stages of resolution. Laboratory studies reveal a platelet count of 3,000. The remainder of her hematologic evaluation is within normal limits. Microscopy of the peripheral smear shows very few platelets without clumping. What is the most appropriate treatment for this patient?

A. Bone marrow transplant
B. Corticosteroids
C. Heparin
D. Immunoglobulin infusion
E. Splenectomy

49. While undergoing an appendectomy for presumed appendicitis, a 23-year-old man begins to become tachycardic. This is soon followed by rigidity and cyanosis. His body temperature is 40°C (104°F). What is the most appropriate treatment for this patient?

A. Acetaminophen
B. Aspirin
C. Dantrolene
D. Diazepam
E. Lorazepam
F. Phenobarbital
G. Phenoxybenzamine
H. Phenytoin

50. A 67-year-old man presents to his primary care physician with increasing muscle weakness, diplopia, and ptosis. He also complains of easy fatigability. Physical examination of the heart, lungs, and abdomen is unremarkable. He appears to be breathing heavily and seems somewhat dyspneic. On administration of edrophonium, his strength and breathing improve. The mechanism of action of this drug is:

A. To activate acetylcholine receptors in the postsynaptic membrane

B. To activate antiacetylcholinesterase and decrease the acetylcholine in the synapse

C. To inhibit acetylcholine receptors in the presynaptic membrane

D. To inhibit acetylcholine receptors in the postsynaptic membrane

E. To inhibit antiacetylcholinesterase and increase the acetylcholine in the synapse

51. A 54-year-old African-American man presents to his primary care physician with complaints of a headache and a visual disturbance that he describes as blurriness at the edges of his visual field. He also complains of erectile dysfunction. His serum prolactin level is elevated. Which of the following medications is most appropriate to treat this patient?

A. Bromocriptine

B. Chlorpromazine

C. Haloperidol

D. Risperidone

E. Thioridazine

52. A 21-year-old man presents to his primary care physician complaining of severe cramps and diarrhea, which have troubled him for several weeks. He also reports that he has lost approximately 30 lb in the last month. Colonoscopy reveals inflammation of the right colon and terminal ileum. Biopsy reveals transmural inflammation with granuloma formation. A histologic slide is shown in Figure 13-4. What is the most appropriate treatment for this patient?

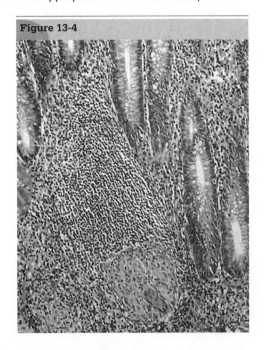

Figure 13-4

A. Ampicillin and aspirin

B. Aspirin and protamine sulfate

C. Ampicillin and sulfasalazine

D. Fluoroquinlone and pantoprazole

E. Pantoprazole and corticosteroids

F. Sulfasalazine and aspirin

G. Sulfasalazine and corticosteroids

53. A 39-year-old African American woman with a 10-year history of sarcoidosis develops polyuria and increased thirst. Laboratory studies reveal a urine specific gravity of 1.002 and a plasma osmolality of 308. What is the most appropriate treatment for this patient?

A. Demeclocycline

B. Desmopressin

C. Furosemide

D. Lithium

E. Methoxyflurane

54. A 9-year-old girl is brought to her pediatrician because of a rash, fever, and headache that developed about a week after she visited her grandmother in Maine. Physical examination reveals a blanchable macular rash on her wrists, ankles, palms, and soles. A Weil-Felix test is positive. What is the most appropriate treatment for this patient?

A. Ciprofloxacin

B. Doxycycline

C. Erythromycin

D. Imipenem

E. Penicillin G

F. Pyrimethamine

G. Trimethoprim-sulfamethoxazole

55. A 9-year-old boy with a history of Lesch-Nyhan syndrome presents to his primary care physician with the onset of acute lymphoblastic leukemia. He is given a prescription for 6-mercaptopurine (6-MP). Which of the following drugs would be contraindicated in this patient if he has a history of gout?

A. Allopurinol

B. Aspirin

C. Colchicine

D. Cytarabine

E. Methotrexate

56. A 64-year-old woman presents to her primary care physician with a new onset of hyperlipidemia. Her recent laboratory values are as follows: total cholesterol, 167; high-density lipoprotein (HDL) cholesterol, 32; low-density lipoprotein (LDL) cholesterol, 105; triglycerides, 204. After reading the results, you decide to treat her low HDL. Which of the following would be the best medication for this patient?

A. Atorvastatin

B. Cholestyramine

C. Gemfibrozil

D. Lovastatin

E. Niacin

57. A 57-year-old African American woman presents to her primary care physician for follow-up treatment of locally advanced breast cancer. Physical examination of the heart reveals transient tachycardia. She has no rubs or murmurs. Pulmonary auscultation reveals no rales, rhonchi, or wheezes bilaterally. The abdominal examination is noncontributory. Pelvic examination is deferred. She is begun on a treatment regimen that includes cyclophosphamide. Which of the following toxicities is of concern with this medication?

A. Hemorrhagic cystitis

B. Hepatotoxicity

C. Nephrotoxicity

D. Pulmonary fibrosis

E. Secondary leukemia

58. A 54-year-old Caucasian woman with a 35-year history of insulin-dependent diabetes mellitus presents for follow-up. She has recently received an orthotopic kidney transplant. Physical examination of the heart reveals an S_3 gallop. She also has a grade II systolic ejection murmur. Pulmonary auscultation reveals decreased breath sounds at both lung bases. She is on an immunosuppressive regimen with cyclosporine. What is the mechanism of action of this medication?

A. Binding to the FK-binding protein and thus inhibiting IL-2 secretion

B. Blocking of IL-2 receptors

C. Blocking of NF-kappa B protein formation

D. Inhibiting the transcription of IL-2

E. Interfering with the metabolism of nucleic acid

59. A 5-year-old boy presents to his family physician complaining of an earache. Otoscopy reveals bulging of the right tympanic membrane with an effusion. Which antibiotic is contraindicated in this child?

A. Ampicillin

B. Ciprofloxacin

C. Metronidazole

D. Penicillin

E. Vancomycin

60. A 52-year-old man with type I diabetes mellitus presents to his primary care physician for evaluation of his blood pressure. He has a history of chronic renal insufficiency and a baseline creatinine of 2.5 mg/dL. His current medications include metformin. Physical examination reveals no evidence of cardiac, pulmonary, or abdominal abnormalities. Genitourinary examination reveals an uncircumcised penis with descended testicles bilaterally. He has a right epididymal head cyst. What significant toxicity of metformin must the treating physician be aware of?

A. Cardiotoxicity

B. Edema

C. Hepatotoxicity

D. Hypoglycemia

E. Lactic acidosis

61. An 81-year-old man with metastatic prostate cancer presents to his primary care physician for follow-up. He complains of weight loss and bone pain. He has lost 10 lb in 3 months without dieting. His PSA is 25 ng/mL and his most recent bone scan reveals osteoblastic lesions in the sacrum and lumbar spine. He is begun on leuprolide. Digital rectal examination reveals induration of the prostate gland. Which of the following should also be administered to this patient?

A. Finasteride

B. Flucytosine

C. Flutamide

D. Ketoconazole

E. Leucovorin

62. The cardiac exam of a neonate at birth reveals a continuous, machine-like murmur. Further studies reveal that the newborn has transposition of the great vessels with a patent ductus arteriosus (PDA). In order to keep this patient's PDA open until surgical intervention is possible, which of the following should be administered?

A. Aspirin

B. Indomethacin

C. Misoprostol

D. Prostacyclin

E. Ticlopidine

63. A 63-year-old Caucasian woman with a history of deep venous thrombosis treated by warfarin develops recurrent gastroesophageal reflux. She decides to utilize the over-the-counter medication cimetidine. Four weeks later, she complains of several bruises, saying that she is unaware of their origin. Her international normalized ratio (INR) is 9.15. What is the most likely explanation for these findings?

A. Cimetidine binds to plasma proteins and displaces warfarin.

B. Cimetidine causes hepatotoxicity and decreases warfarin's metabolism.

C. Cimetidine causes nephrotoxicity and decreases warfarin's metabolism.

D. Cimetidine is an inducer of CYP450.

E. Cimetidine is an inhibitor of CYP450.

64. A 43-year-old alcoholic woman presents to the emergency department complaining of fatigue, dizziness, and rapid heartbeat. Rectal examination is positive for blood. Upper gastrointestinal endoscopy is performed (Figure 13-5) and octreotide administered. This agent is an analog of which of the following?

A. Cholecystokinin

B. Dopamine

C. Norepinephrine

D. Secretin

E. Somatostatin

F. Vasopressin

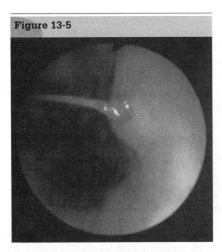

Figure 13-5

65. A 53-year-old man with a 3-year history of congestive heart failure (CHF) presents to the emergency department with an exacerbation of his condition. He is allergic to sulfa medications. His baseline laboratory values indicate a serum calcium of 14.5 mg/dL and a serum creatinine of 2.5 mg/dL. A CT scan of the head and neck reveals a parathyroid mass. Which of the following diuretics is most appropriate for this patient?

A. Acetazolamide

B. Captopril

C. Ethacrynic acid

D. Furosemide

E. Hydrochlorothiazide

F. Mannitol

G. Spironolactone

66. A 66-year-old man presents to the emergency department with a blood pressure of 234/111 mm Hg. He has a history of hypertension, diabetes mellitus, and recurrent priapism. His medications include a calcium channel blocker. He is on other medications but does not know their names. His cardiac, pulmonary, and abdominal examinations are within normal limits. Examination of the lower extremities reveals evidence of venous stasis bilaterally. Infusion of hydralazine is begun. What is this drug's mechanism of action?

A. To block alpha$_1$ receptors peripherally

B. To block alpha$_2$ receptors centrally

C. To increase cGMP and primarily vasodilate arteries

D. To increase cGMP and primarily vasodilate veins

E. To potentiate beta$_2$ receptors peripherally

67. A 29-year-old woman with a 7-year history of HIV presents to her primary care physician saying that she just found out she is pregnant. She has been treated with highly active antiretroviral therapy (HAART) therapy for 6 months, since her CD4 cell counts dropped below 200 mm^3. In light of this new information, there is concern about potential teratogenic effects. Which of the following medications is most concerning?

A. Delavirdine

B. Efavirenz

C. Nevirapine

D. Saquinavir

E. Zidovudine

68. A 31-year-old man with new-onset AIDS is begun on HAART. When he comes in 4 weeks later to have follow-up blood work done, he reports that he is doing well. His cardiac, pulmonary, and abdominal examinations are unremarkable. He has evidence of healing balanitis. He is uncircumcised. He has a left grade II varicocele. His mean corpuscular volume (MCV) is now 109, and his hemoglobin is 9.5 mg/dL and hematocrit 29%. Which of the following medications could be the cause of his new-onset anemia?

A. Amprenavir

B. Didanosine

C. Ritonavir

D. Stavudine

E. Zidovudine

69. A 14-year-old boy presents to his primary care physician with what appears to be mild to moderate acne spread diffusely over his face. His past medical history is notable for recurrent bouts of otitis media. His past surgical history notes a right inguinal hernia/hydrocele repair. Physical examination of the heart, lungs, and abdomen is unremarkable. He is begun on therapy with tetracycline. Which of the following potential side effects of this drug is most concerning?

A. Epistaxis

B. Fanconi's syndrome

C. Nephrotoxicity

D. Ototoxicity

E. Tooth discoloration

70. A confused 19-year-old woman is brought to the emergency department by her college roommate. The roommate reports that her friend was fine the previous night, but that she awoke this morning complaining of chills, myalgias, and neck stiffness. Physical examination reveals a heart rate of 110 bpm, blood pressure of 90/60 mm Hg, and a diffuse petechial rash. After empiric therapy is begun, a lumbar puncture is performed, revealing pairs of Gram-negative cocci that have a polysaccharide capsule and ferment maltose. Which of the following drugs would be considered as prophylaxis for this patient's contacts?

A. Ceftriaxone

B. Doxycycline

C. Ertapenem

D. Meropenem

E. Piperacillin

F. Polymyxin B

G. Rifampin

H. Vancomycin

71. A 34-year-old man presents to his primary care physician with a sinus infection and is treated with cefazolin for 21 days. At about day 15, he complains of multiple episodes of diarrhea and diffuse cramping. Toxin examination of his stool reveals *C. difficile* exotoxin. What is the most appropriate treatment for this patient?

A. Ampicillin

B. Aztreonam

C. Ciprofloxacin

D. Metronidazole

E. Vibramycin

72. A 79-year-old woman presents to your clinic complaining of the continuous shaking of her right hand as well as some difficulty moving her right arm; she has had these problems continuously for some 6 months. She ambulates in slow, shuffling fashion. Physical examination of the heart, lungs, and abdomen is within normal limits. She is begun on an oral drug that has also been used as an antiviral agent. What is this drug's mechanism of action in this disease?

A. It augments the effect of dopamine on the pars compacta.

B. It blocks central GABA receptors.

C. It blocks the effect of dopamine on the globus pallidus.

D. It causes the release of dopamine from intact nerve terminals.

E. It potentiates the effect of dopamine on the globus pallidus.

73. A medical student is involved in a summer research project designed to determine the effects of inotropic agents on the hemodynamics of a rat. The rat is given a dose of phentolamine, followed by a dose of epinephrine. What will the net effect on the rat's blood pressure be, and how is this explained?

A. There will be a depressor effect due to unopposed beta₁ stimulation.

B. There will be a depressor effect due to unopposed beta₂ stimulation.

C. There will be an increase in blood pressure due to unopposed alpha₁ stimulation.

D. There will be an increase in blood pressure due to unopposed alpha₂ stimulation.

E. There will be an increase in blood pressure due to unopposed beta₂ stimulation.

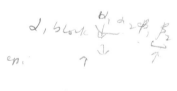

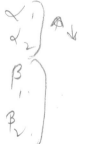

74. A 59-year-old man presents to his primary care physician for a new patient evaluation. He has a 5-year history of diabetes and hypertension. His previous physician currently has his diabetes under adequate control. The patient wants to establish care in your practice and restart treatment for his hypertension. He remembers that in the past he was given a prescription for an antihypertensive drug that caused him to have a severe coughing episode. What would be an appropriate pharmacological treatment for this patient?

A. Captopril

B. Diltiazem

C. Enalapril

D. Lisinopril

E. Losartan

75. A 48-year-old, somewhat disoriented woman is brought to the emergency department with nausea and vomiting. She is oriented only to person and time but not to place. The patient has a normal complete blood count and the electrolyte panel is within normal limits except for a potassium level of 5.9 mEq/L. Later that evening, the patient's husband arrives and states that his wife has had no recent change in her diet but that she did change her hypertension medication about a month ago. He is not aware of what drug she is now taking and did not bring her medication to the emergency department. What drug would be highly likely to be causing this patient's side effects?

A. Amiloride

B. Ethacrynic acid

C. Furosemide

D. Hydrochlorothiazide

E. Mannitol

Answer Key

1. D	20. F	39. E	58. D
2. A	21. E	40. D	59. B
3. B	22. A	41. C	60. E
4. D	23. B	42. B	61. C
5. E	24. E	43. C	62. C
6. C	25. A	44. E	63. E
7. C	26. A	45. D	64. E
8. B	27. B	46. C	65. C
9. G	28. C	47. C	66. C
10. A	29. F	48. B	67. B
11. D	30. C	49. C	68. E
12. B	31. E	50. E	69. B
13. B	32. D	51. A	70. G
14. C	33. E	52. G	71. D
15. A	34. F	53. B	72. D
16. E	35. B	54. B	73. B
17. A	36. A	55. A	74. E
18. A	37. E	56. E	75. A
19. D	38. C	57. A	

Answers and Explanations

1. D. From the Gram's stain, the most likely bacterium would be *Staphylococcus aureus*. In a hospital setting, the concern for methicillin-resistant *S. aureus* (MRSA) should be high. This is a skin flora carried by many and often acquired in the hospital setting owing to overuse of antibiotics. Of the antibiotics listed, the only one that would cover MRSA is vancomycin.

2. A. This patient is most likely suffering from amiodarone toxicity. Amiodarone is a class III antiarrhythmic used for the treatment of atrial fibrillation and ventricular arrhythmias. Toxicities include symptoms relating to thyroid dysfunction, such as cold sensitivity and fatigue, as well as a unique bluish tint to the skin, commonly called "smurf" skin. Digoxin is used as a positive inotropic agent for patients with congestive heart failure (CHF), although it can be used in certain arrhythmias. The toxicity profile includes GI upset, headache, blurred vision, and possible cardiac arrhythmias. Flecainide is a class IC antiarrhythmic; its toxicity profile includes increased risk of arrhythmias. Lidocaine is a class IB antiarrhythmic drug whose toxicities include CNS dysfunction at high doses. Procainamide is a class IA antiarrhythmic whose toxicity profile includes a lupus-like syndrome in patients who are slow-acetylators.

3. B. Studies have shown that 2 to 3% of patients who are allergic to any of the penicillins will have similar reactions to any of the cephalosporins. Ceftriaxone is a third-generation cephalosporin and would be contraindicated in this patient. Erythromycin, a macrolide antibiotic, would most likely be the drug of choice in this scenario. Although chloramphenicol, doxycycline, and vancomycin would not likely be prescribed for this patient's sinusitis, they would not be absolutely contraindicated, as these antibiotics do not generally cross-react with penicillins.

4. D. Sulfonylureas like glyburide and glipizide act by closing potassium channels in beta-cell membranes and thus depolarize the cell. This leads to an increased influx of calcium and triggers insulin release. These agents do not close or open calcium channels in either alpha- or beta-cell membranes. Sulfonylureas do not open potassium channels in either alpha- or beta-cell membranes.

5. E. This patient exhibits typical findings of Rocky Mountain spotted fever, which is caused by *Rickettsia rickettsii*. All rickettsial diseases are treated with tetracycline. A rash on the palms and soles is commonly seen in Rocky Mountain spotted fever, syphilis, and coxsackie A virus infection; however, only Rocky Mountain spotted fever is caused by a tick bite. Amantadine is helpful in preventing influenza A and rubella by blocking viral penetration and viral replication. Ceftriaxone is commonly used in meningitis and to treat gonococcal infections. Penicillin is used against Gram-positive cocci and rods, Gram-negative cocci, and spirochetes (such as *Treponema pallidum*, the cause of syphilis). Rifampin is used in prophylaxis against *Mycobacterium tuberculosis* and in the contacts of children infected by *Haemophilus influenzae* and *Meningococcus*.

6. C. Vitamin A, which is found in a variety of meats and vegetables, is essential to the maintenance of mucus-secreting epithelium and is a precursor to retinol, a component of visual pigment. People who are deficient in vitamin A suffer from night blindness and squamous cell metaplasia, which can cause dry eyes or even corneal softening. The squamous metaplasia can also manifest as renal calculi, which can cause hematuria. Hypervitaminosis A causes alopecia, liver damage, and changes in bone composition. Hypervitaminosis D becomes manifest as growth retardation and renal calculi but has no relationship to night blindness. Vitamin C deficiency causes scurvy, which leads to hemorrhages and bone changes. Vitamin K deficiency is seen in some newborns and causes hemorrhagic disease due to the defective production of clotting factors.

7. C. Nonsteroidal anti-inflammatory medications such as aspirin and indomethacin are generally used as first-line treatments for pain and inflammation in patients with rheumatoid arthritis. However, the patient presented here has a history of peptic ulcer disease, which means that she is at a greater risk of recurrent disease with chronic use of these agents. Thus, the best first-line agent would be the selective COX-2 inhibitor Celecoxib, which would be less likely to cause GI toxicity (i.e., bleeding and ulcers). Allopurinol is a purine analog used in the chronic treatment of gout. Gold salts are considered disease-modifying antirheumatic agents (DMARDs) and are used only to treat rheumatoid arthritis that does not respond to salicylates or other NSAID therapy.

8. B. Gout is a metabolic disorder characterized by high levels of uric acid in the blood. It most commonly affects men but can also affect postmenopausal women. Acute gouty attacks are treated with colchicine and nonsteroidal anti-inflammatory drugs (NSAIDs). Colchicine helps alleviate the pain of gout by binding to tubulin and causing its depolymerization. This binding disrupts key cellular functions, such as migration. Thus the movement of granulocytes into the affected area is prevented and pain is reduced. NSAIDs, which are inhibitors of COX 1 and 2, are also used to help decrease pain and inflammation. It is important to note that aspirin is contraindicated because it competes with uric acid for the organic acid secretion mechanism in the proximal tubule of the kidney. Probenecid and sulfinpyrazone are uricosuric agents commonly used in the treatment of gout. At therapeutic doses, they block proximal tubular resorption or uric acid. Allopurinol is a purine analog used in the chronic treatment of gout. It functions to reduce the production of uric acid by competitively inhibiting the last two steps of uric acid production, which are both catalyzed by xanthine oxidase. There are several immunosuppressive agents used to treat autoimmune conditions such as rheumatoid arthritis. Gout is not an autoimmune condition; an immunosuppressive agent would not be helpful in its acute treatment.

9. G. Penicillamine is an effective agent in acute, severe rheumatoid arthritis in those patients who can tolerate it. Penicillamine is not a first-line treatment for rheumatoid arthritis but is gaining acceptance in some centers as an alternative to gold, chloroquine, and the cytostatic agents. Side effects necessitate discontinuation of penicillamine in one-third of patients taking the drug. The most common side effects are a maculopapular pruritic dermatitis, gastrointestinal upset, a loss of taste sensation, thrombocytopenia, and leukopenia. Salicylates are the drugs of choice in the treatment of the milder forms of inflammatory disease. These include acute rheumatic fever, rheumatoid arthritis, osteoarthritis, and mild systemic lupus erythematous. Chloroquine is used in the treatment of infections with *Plasmodium* (malaria). Ibuprofen, indomethacin, and naproxen are NSAIDs.

10. A. Heparin has a half-life measured in minutes. It is a large anionic polymer that can inhibit coagulation in vitro; its site of action is in the blood. Heparin is monitored by the intrinsic pathway utilizing the partial thromboplastin time (PTT).

11. D. This patient has been treated for acne with minocycline, a common treatment for acne. Minocycline is a tetracycline drug that has been shown to cause discoloration in the teeth of children, abnormal bone development, and photosensitivity. All patients put on minocycline should be advised to avoid sun exposure as much as possible. Benzoyl peroxide is a topical ointment used to treat acne and can rarely cause a skin rash; however, discoloration of the teeth is not a known side effect. Chloramphenicol is often used to treat meningitis. The most common side effects of chloramphenicol include aplastic anemia and

"gray-baby syndrome." Erythromycin is an antibiotic medication; it is not used to treat acne. Common side effects of erythromycin include GI discomfort, acute cholestatic hepatitis, and eosinophilia. Phenytoin is an antiseizure medication. The more common side effects of phenytoin include gingival hyperplasia, ataxia, diplopia, and megaloblastic anemia.

12. B. Etanercept is a recombinant protein that binds to tumor necrosis factor and prevents its inflammatory effects. It is a second-line agent in the treatment of rheumatoid arthritis (RA). Cyclosporine is a peptide antibiotic that interferes with T-cell function by binding to immunophyllins. It is used for immunosuppression in patients who have received organ transplants. Indomethacin and naproxen are NSAIDs used to treat inflammation when salicylates are no longer effective or tolerated. Penicillamine is used in the treatment of RA, but it has no anti-inflammatory effect. Phenylbutazone is used in the acute treatment of RA; however its mechanism of action is not antagonism to TNF. Sulfasalazine is an anti-inflammatory medication that was once used to treat RA; now it is commonly used to treat inflammatory bowel disease.

13. B. By increasing the duration of Cl– channel opening, phenobarbital decreases neuronal firing and thus allows for induction of anesthesia or sedation. Benzodiazepines act at the same receptor but increase the frequency of Cl– channel. This agent does not act as a competitive antagonist at GABA receptors. Benzodiazepines do not inhibit the actions of glutamine diffusely throughout the CNS.

14. C. This infant is suffering from neonatal distress syndrome, which is due to a deficiency of surfactant in the lungs, leading to increased surface tension and ultimately respiratory collapse. Surfactant is typically made after 35 weeks of gestation by type II pneumocytes. The lecithin-to-sphingomyelin ratio is often < 1.5 in this syndrome. Treatment includes the administration of steroids to the mother before birth or artificial surfactant to the infant. Aspirin would not help in this situation. Flumazenil is a treatment for benzodiazepine overdose. Protamine is a treatment for heparin overdose. Aminocaproic acid is a treatment for an overdose of streptokinase or tissue plasminogen activator (t-PA).

15. A. Cephalosporins are associated with a disulfiram-like reaction. When alcohol is ingested by a patient taking this antibiotic, the patient will immediately experience vomiting and nausea. She should have been warned about this side effect. The other choices are possible but unlikely in the situation given. Gastroenteritis, pregnancy, sexually transmitted diseases, and upper respiratory infections will not precipitate disulfiram-like reactions.

16. E. Patients with CHF who require adjunctive therapy may be given a thiazide diuretic initially; the loop diuretics are generally saved for those who fail to respond to thiazide. Digitalis increases myocardial contractility but has a very narrow therapeutic window. Hypokalemia predisposes patients to digitalis intoxication; therefore the potassium-sparing diuretic spironolactone is added. Propranolol and diltiazem both decrease heart rate and may worsen the CHF. Nitroglycerin, aspirin, and captopril are more appropriately used in myocardial infarction.

17. A. Ampicillin covers Gram-positive bacteria, the most common flora found on the skin. Ciprofloxacin inhibits DNA gyrase type II. It works well against Gram-negative rods in the urinary and gastrointestinal tracts. Trimethoprim inhibits dihydrofolate reductase, is bacteriostatic, and is often used in combination with sulfonamides. Current use includes the urinary tract and respiratory tracts. Gentamicin is an aminoglycoside that inhibits the formation of initiation complex and causes misreading of mRNA.

18. A. Cefotaxime and vancomycin cover the most likely organisms in this scenario (*Pneumococcus, Meningococcus,* and *Haemophilus influenzae*). The other combinations provide less effective coverage. Nafcillin is an extended-spectrum penicillin agent. Other members of the extended-spectrum penicillin class include oxacillin, cloxacillin, and dicloxacillin. Trimethoprim/sulfamethoxazole is useful in the treatment of uncomplicated urinary tract infections.

19. D. Salmeterol is not a rapid-onset medication and takes a while to provide relief from asthma symptoms. It should be used to prevent symptoms from occurring, not to relieve current symptoms. Epinephrine should have a rapid onset in relief of these symptoms. Isproterenol is a nonspecific beta agonist that relaxes bronchial smooth muscle. Albuterol is a beta agonist that also relaxes bronchial smooth muscle and is useful during an acute exacerbation of asthma. Terbutaline is a beta$_2$ agonist that is useful in the treatment of asthma. This agent also has beta$_1$ effects.

20. F. Penicillin G is the drug of choice for treatment of syphilis. Doxycycline and tetracycline are alternative treatments. Tetracycline and doxycycline should not be used in pregnant women. The other drugs do not effectively treat syphilis. Cefazolin is useful in presurgical prophylaxis against wound infections. Doxycycline is an oral tetracycline antibiotic and can be used to treat urethritis and prostatitis. Ketoconazole is an antifungal agent and is also used to treat hormone-refractory prostate cancer.

21. E. Lyme disease in its initial stages is treatable with oral doxycycline. Doxycycline is the drug of choice unless the patient has a history of an allergy to it. The other antimicrobials are not considered first-line treatment for Lyme disease. Cephalexin is a cephalosporin antibiotic. Ceftriaxone is a third-generation cephalosporin. Chloramphenicol inhibits 50S peptidyltransferase. This agent is bacteriostatic. Ciprofloxacin is a quinolone that inhibits DNA gyrase. This agent is bactericidal. Doxycycline is bacteriostatic, binds to the 30S ribosomal subunit, and prevents attachment of the amino acyl-tRNA.

22. A. Infection must first be ruled out via aspiration and culture. The next treatment may be an anti-inflammatory agent to decrease the pain. Allopurinol or sulfinpyrazone can be prescribed after gout (uric acid in joints) is diagnosed; however, these drugs will take a few days to have

an effect. Allopurinol inhibits xanthine oxidase and prevents hypoxanthine and xanthine from being converted to uric acid. Uricosuric agents (e.g., sulfinpyrazone) increase the elimination of uric acid by inhibiting its proximal tubular reabsorption.

23. B. Erythromycin, part of the macrolide class of antibiotics, is commonly used to treat upper respiratory infections and pneumonias. It has excellent coverage against *Legionella* species. Penicillin is good for Gram-positive cocci and rods and Gram-negative cocci. Ciprofloxacin is good for Gram-negative rods of the genitourinary and gastrointestinal tract. Gentamicin has no coverage for *Legionella* species.

24. E. Rehydration is required before giving furosemide, so that the patient does not become hypotensive. Then pharmacologic treatment may be given. Furosemide will increase urinary excretion of calcium, thus lowering serum calcium. Furosemide is a loop diuretic. Dialysis is not necessary at this time. Alendronate and ergocalciferol will not help a patient's hypercalcemia.

25. A. This patient has signs of a basal cell carcinoma, which is most common in sun-exposed areas of the skin. It is described as looking like "pearly papules," often with visible telangiectasias. Typical histopathologic findings include palisading nuclei. Topical 5-fluorouracil has often been shown to be effective in treating basal cell carcinoma by inhibiting thymidylate synthase, which results in decreased dTMP and inhibits the S-phase of DNA replication, hence stopping growth. 6-Mercaptopurine is used in the treatment of leukemias and some lymphomas. Bleomycin is used in testicular cancer and lymphomas. Busulfan is used to treat chronic myelogenous leukemia (CML). Cyclophosphamide is used to treat non-Hodgkin's lymphoma as well as breast and ovarian cancer and as an immunosuppressant in transplant patients.

26. A. This patient has a possible cerebral bleed, and in this case anticoagulation with heparin or warfarin could increase the likelihood of bleeding in the brain. Therefore, the only correct treatment would be compression pulse devices to prevent deep venous thrombosis. Low-molecular-weight heparin has better bioavailability and a longer half-life than traditional subcutaneous heparin. However, it is quite expensive and not the best agent for this patient. Warfarin interferes with the normal synthesis of vitamin K–dependent clotting factors.

27. B. This patient most likely has a fungal infection with *Cryptococcus neoformans* or some fungal agent, which would be best treated with amphotericin B. Ampicillin achieves therapeutic concentration in cerebrospinal fluid, but only during inflammation. Amoxicillin does not reach therapeutic concentration in cerebrospinal fluid. Amoxicillin is a broad-spectrum penicillin that is penicillinase-sensitive. Ampicillin is similar to amoxicillin except that amoxicillin has greater bioavailability. Ceftriaxone is a third-generation cephalosporin that is used to treat serious Gram-negative infections. Ciprofloxacin is a quinolone antibiotic that inhibits DNA gyrase.

28. C. Amitriptyline should not be used in conjunction with ethanol. Since this patient has classic signs of alcoholism, this drug should not be prescribed until alcoholic liver damage is ruled out. Advising the patient to drink water and consider taking a vitamin supplement is appropriate. This patient should have a complete blood count and liver enzyme tests ordered; he should also be questioned about ethanol use, and Alcoholics Anonymous should be suggested.

29. F. This patient has thrombosis of a superficial vein; the treatment of choice is an anti-inflammatory drug and warm compresses. Anticoagulation is not needed for this type of thrombosis. Heparin and warfarin are used to treat deep venous thrombosis and for prophylaxis in hypercoagulable states. They are not used in ambulatory patients or to treat vessel injury.

30. C. The role of immunosuppressive therapy is to provide maintenance suppression in order to prevent rejection as well as to treat episodes of acute rejection. In this case all that is needed is maintenance therapy. Agents are used in combination because no single agent provides adequate therapy; also combination therapy allows lower doses of each drug to be used and thus helps to avoid side effects. The best agents for this patient are cyclosporine and azathioprine. Cyclosporine and corticosteroids are used in acute rejection; they are not appropriate for this patient. Tacrolimus (FK506) is similar to cyclosporine. It binds to FK-binding protein and inhibits secretion of IL-2 and other cytokines. It has a strong immunosuppressive effect in organ transplant recipients.

31. E. This patient has angina pectoris. Nitroglycerin is used in the management of angina pectoris and congestive heart failure. The medication works to dilate the vascular bed. Common side effects are headache, light-headedness, and hypotension. This agent is not a beta-blocker or a calcium channel blocker. Digoxin has a positive inotropic effect.

32. D. N-acetylcysteine inactivates the toxic metabolite and should be given to this patient. Protamine neutralizes heparin ionically. Naloxone displaces opioids from their receptors. Ethanol is the proper treatment of methanol ingestion. Methylene blue reduces methemoglobin to hemoglobin in arsenic poisoning. Vitamin K stimulates the synthesis of coagulation factor in overdoses of warfarin. Deferoxamine forms an inactive complex with metal in iron overload.

33. E. After a TIA it is imperative to minimize the risk of stroke; this is often done with either aspirin or clopidogrel. Normally, adenosine diphosphate, which is released by activated platelets, antagonizes the subsequent binding of platelets, thus helping to decrease the formation of clots. Aspirin irreversibly inhibits cyclooxygenase. Tissue plasminogen activator is a thrombolytic agent. Heparin acts to inhibit thrombin by activating anti-thrombin III. Warfarin inhibits vitamin K–dependent clotting factors.

34. F. This patient has been treated with many different antibiotics over 3 weeks to treat her endocarditis. She is most likely experiencing an overgrowth of *Clostridium difficile*. The appropriate treatment in this situation is metronida-zole, which is effective against *C. difficile*. Diphenoxylate, infusion of sodium chloride, and lactulose will all slow down peristalsis but will not treat the problem. Lactulose can increase the bulk of the stool and is used mostly for constipation. Intravenous infusion of sodium chloride may be needed to prevent dehydration, but it will not treat the patient's underlying problem.

35. B. Naloxone can cause complete or partial reversal of opioid depression. It is a competitive inhibitor of opioids. Ipecac is used after the ingestion of certain poisons in order to induce vomiting. This patient may have to be observed overnight, but naloxone should be administered first. Pralidoxime reverses nicotinic stimulation, which leads to skeletal muscle relaxation.

36. A. Captopril, an ACE inhibitor, has the common side effects of dry cough and skin rash. Prazosin is an alpha$_1$ antagonist; cough and skin rash are not common side effects. Hydralazine causes release of nitrous oxide from blood vessel endothelium, which promotes vasodilation. Phentolamine is a competitive blocker of alpha-receptors; dry cough and skin rash are not common side effects. Sodium nitroprusside increases intracellular production of cyclic guanosine monophosphate (cGMP); dry cough is not a common side effect. Clonidine is a central alpha$_2$ receptor agonist.

37. E. Thiazide diuretics are often used to treat hypercalcemia but not hyperkalemia. The other options are all possible treatments for hypercalcemia. Calcium is important, as it can stabilize myocardial membranes. Dialysis may be required for this patient if the serum potassium does not decrease with more conservative methods. Insulin will shift potassium into cells and is a useful treatment for this patient. Kayexalate binds potassium in the gut and is also a treatment of choice for this patient.

38. C. This patient is most likely experiencing herpes zoster infection due to the immunosuppressant he is currently taking. Intravenous acyclovir is recommended for immunocompromised individuals, whereas oral acyclovir is used for immunocompetent patients. This patient needs treatment for two reasons: he is immuosuppressed and the lesion involves the eye. Doxycycline and aspirin will not treat the infection.

39. E. Nonsteriodal anti-inflammatory drugs (NSAIDs), such as ibuprofen, are the first-line treatment in this patient with Dressler's syndrome (an autoimmune pericarditis that typically occurs between 2 and 4 weeks after a myocardial infarction). Of the remaining options, only corticosteroids would be used in this particular pathology and only after treatment with NSAIDs had failed.

40. D. In initiating antihypertensive medication in an African American patient, a calcium channel blocker is recommended, because clinical studies have shown that African Americans respond better to that class of medications. However, in Caucasians and diabetics, it should be noted that ACE inhibitors are currently the first-line treatment. This patient is an African American and a diabetic; therefore, an angiotensin-converting enzyme inhibitor such as lisinopril should be the first line treatment.

41. C. This patient is experiencing a myocardial infarction. This is best treated with an ACE inhibitor, beta-blocker, aspirin, and nitroglycerin. Diltiazem, a calcium channel blocker, is not as appropriate as a beta-blocker at this time. Digoxin is used to treat congestive heart failure. Spironolactone, a potassium-sparing diuretic, is not indicated in this patient. The ECG shown reveals evidence of an acute inferior myocardial infarction.

42. B. This patient is currently in status epilepticus due to isoniazid toxicity. This condition is also treated with pyridoxine. Some other toxicities of isoniazid are a peripheral neuropathy (which can be prevented with pyridoxine prophylaxis), drug-induced lupus, and hepatitis. Ethambutol is not associated with status epilepticus. The other three agents are not commonly associated with causing an epileptic condition. Pyrazinamide and rifampin are first-line antituberculosis agents. Rifampin is classically associated with a red-orange discoloration of body fluids such as urine, stool, sweat, and tears (thus discoloring contact lenses).

43. C. Procainamide is the most common offender in idiopathic drug-induced lupus. However, this lupus is differentiated from systemic lupus erythematosus by the presence of antihistone antibodies and complete resolution of the disease after withdrawal of the offending drug. Sotalol and disopyramide also treat ventricular arrhythmias, but they are not usually associated with lupus. Flecainide and propafenone are known to be proarrhythmic, but they are not associated with lupus. Some other drugs that may cause drug-induced lupus include hydralazine, isoniazid, quinidine, chlorpromazine, and penicillamine.

44. E. Wilson's disease is an autosomal recessive disorder marked by the accumulation of copper in tissues such as the brain, liver, and eye. Besides decreased ceruloplasmin, there is also an increase in the urinary excretion of copper. Penicillamine acts as a chelator and is currently listed as first-line treatment. Deferoxamine is used in iron toxicity, dimercaprol in mercury toxicity, and EDTA in lead toxicity. Methylene blue is not used in heavy metal toxicity.

45. D. This patient is most likely experiencing Raynaud's syndrome. The initial treatment consists of discontinuing any medications that reduce cardiac output or cause vasospasm (e.g., beta-blockers, ergotamines, oral contraceptives). The other listed drugs are not known to cause vasospasm or to decrease cardiac output. Ciprofloxacin is a quinolone antibiotic that inhibits DNA gyrase. Vitamin E has some mild anti-inflammatory effects. Ibuprofen is an NSAID.

46. C. Clonidine stimulates alpha$_2$ receptors centrally. This produces a negative feedback–like mechanism by causing the presynaptic neuron to release less norepinephrine, thus decreasing the blood pressure. Clonidine does not block central alpha$_2$ receptors; it stimulates these receptors. It has no mechanism to potentiate the effects of anticholinergics, nor does it potentiate GABA centrally.

47. C. The most common side effect of excess clonidine is impotence. Other side effects include dry mouth and sedation. Also, it should be noted that clonidine can be used as an antidiarrheal (in diabetics), since it increases the absorption of sodium chloride and decreases the secretion of bicarbonate in the gastrointestinal tract. Abrupt cessation of a clonidine regimen can result in a rebound hypertensive crisis.

48. B. This scenario describes a patient with immune thrombocytopenic purpura (ITP). Although intravenous immunoglobulin and splenectomy are utilized in ITP, high-dose corticosteroids are always tried first. Heparin is a potential cause of ITP, and transplantation has no role. Bone marrow transplantation is not appropriate for this patient. Immunoglobulin infusion is not indicated for this patient.

49. C. Dantrolene is the treatment of choice for malignant hyperthermia (an inherited myopathy thought to be due to a reduction in the uptake of calcium by the sarcoplasmic reticulum, thus interfering with normal muscle relaxation after contraction). Dantrolene acts to decrease muscle contraction by directly interfering with the release of calcium ions from the sarcoplasmic reticulum within skeletal muscle cells. Acetaminophen and aspirin are useful for the treatment of low-grade fevers but are not indicated in malignant hyperthermia. Diazepam and lorazepam can be useful in the setting of seizures. This is not the case with malignant hyperthermia.

50. E. Patients with myasthenia gravis harbor antibodies to the acetylcholine receptor. Edrophonium is an antiacetylcholinesterase inhibitor that helps to overcome the loss of receptors by increasing the amount of acetylcholine in the synapse, which can then react with the remaining receptors. This agent does not activate acetylcholine receptors in the postsynaptic membrane, nor does it decrease the acetylcholine in the synapse.

51. A. Bromocriptine is a dopamine agonist that would decrease elevated prolactin levels. The other drugs act as dopamine antagonists, which would worsen this man's condition. Chlorpromazine and haloperidol are antipsychotic agents, as is thioridazine, which is used in the management of schizophrenia. Each of these agents can raise serum prolactin levels; therefore such patients should be monitored appropriately.

52. G. This patient has Crohn's disease. The biopsy slide shows intense mucosal inflammatory cell infiltration and a giant cell granuloma. Sulfasalazine contains a sulfonamide moiety that is linked to the aspirin analog 5-aminosalicylate. When given orally, it passes into the distal ileum and colon and is cleaved by bacteria. As a result, the sulfonamide portion is absorbed and the 5-ASA is then available to the intestinal mucosa, where it inhibits the cyclooxygenase pathway. Corticosteroids would also be useful in helping to inhibit this patient's inflammatory condition. Aspirin is a good inhibitor of cyclooxygenase, but it, unlike sulfasalazine, is not targeted to the mucosa of the distal small intestine and colon. Antibiotics are not indicated in this instance but may be required if an abscess or signs of infection are found. Pantoprazole, a proton-pump inhibitor, is not indicated in this patient.

53. B. This woman has central diabetes insipidus, which, like sarcoidosis, can be caused by neurosyphilis, encephalitis, or posterior pituitary/hypothalamic damage. Desmopressin is an analog of antidiuretic hormone and thus acts to correct the deficiency. The other drugs are known to either cause (lithium, demeclocycline, methoxyflurane) or worsen (furosemide) diabetes insipidus.

54. B. This patient has Rocky Mountain spotted fever, which is caused by *Rickettsia rickettsii* and transmitted by the female *Dermacentor* tick. Doxycycline is a bacteriostatic antibiotic that binds to the 30S ribosomal subunit and prevents aminoacyl tRNA from reaching its acceptor site on the mRNA. Ciprofloxacin is a quinolone antibiotic; it is not a first-line agent for this condition. Erythromycin is a macrolide antibiotic. Imipenem is an extended-spectrum penicllin. Trimethoprim/sulfamethoxazole is useful in the treatment of respiratory and urinary tract infections.

55. A. Children with Lesch-Nyhan syndrome are often susceptible to attacks of gout owing to the overproduction of uric acid because of a deficiency of hypoxanthine guanine phosphoribosyl transferase (HGPRT) with increased urinary excretion of uric acid. For chronic treatment of gout, allopurinol (which blocks xanthine oxidase) is often prescribed, but it should be avoided in this patient because 6-MP is also metabolized by xanthine oxidase. The combination of the two can lead to increased bone marrow, gastrointestinal, and liver toxicity. Methotrexate is an S phase–specific antimetabolite. It is a folic acid analog that inhibits dihydrofolate reductase. Cytarabine inhibits DNA polymerase and is used in the management of acute myelogenous leukemia.

56. E. Of the choices given, niacin is known to have the greatest effect in increasing HDL cholesterol. Cholestyramine is a bile acid resin that decreases the LDL cholesterol. The statins are HMG-CoA reductase inhibitors and have their greatest effect in decreasing LDL cholesterol. Gemfibrozil is a lipoprotein lipase stimulator in endothelial cells and is most beneficial in treating hyperlipidemia.

57. A. Cyclophosphamide is classically associated with hemorrhagic cystitis acutely and may even lead to transitional cell carcinoma with chronic treatment. It is the acrolein metabolite of this agent that causes the toxicity. Cyclophosphamide acts as an alkylating agent in that it cross-links DNA at guanine N-7. This agent has minimal hepatotoxicity and nephrotoxicity. Bleomycin is associated with pulmonary fibrosis. Secondary leukemia is uncommon with cyclophosphamide. Cyclophosphamide is not associated with nephrotoxicity. That side effect is common with the aminoglycoside class of antibiotics.

58. D. Cyclosporine is used as an immunosuppressant after an organ transplant. It acts by binding to cyclophins (peptidyl proline *cis*-trans isomerase). This complex will inhibit calcineurin (which is required to activate the NFAT transcription factor) and subsequently inhibit the transcription and production of IL-2. This agent does not bind to the FK-binding protein and inhibit IL-2 secretion; rather, it acts on inhibition of transcription of IL-2. This agent does not block IL-2 receptors nor does it interfere with nucleic acid metabolism.

59. B. Ciprofloxacin, a fluoroquinolone, can interfere with the growth plate. All the other antibiotics are safe to use in children. Ampicillin is a reasonable choice to treat otitis media. Some antimicrobial resistance has been associated with this agent. Middle-ear aspiration and culture may be necessary to determine sensitivities. Metronidazole is useful for anaerobic infections.

60. E. Lactic acidosis can occur in diabetics who have either renal insufficiency or hepatic dysfunction when metformin (which acts to decrease hepatic gluconeogenesis and increase glucose removal from the bloodstream) is administered. Of the other toxicities, second-generation sulfonylureas often cause hypoglycemia. The glitazones are responsible for edema and hepatotoxicity. No particular oral hypoglycemic has an association with cardiotoxicity.

61. C. Flutamide is a nonsteroidal competitive antagonist at androgen receptors. It is given concomitantly with leuprolide because the initial effects of leuprolide include a transient burst of LH and FSH; however, this increase in LH and FSH decreases with time as the negative feedback mechanism is activated. Finasteride is a 5 alpha reductase inhibitor that has been shown to decrease prostate size and improve voiding symptoms in patients with benign prostatic hyperplasia. Ketoconazole blocks androgen synthesis at the level of the adrenal gland and may be useful for patients with prostate cancer who do not respond to traditional medications such as leuprolide and flutamide.

62. C. Misoprostol (PGE-1) keeps a PDA open by decreasing vascular tone. Its other actions include increasing uterine tone, decreasing bronchial tone, and preventing NSAID-induced peptic ulcers by increasing the production of the gastric mucosal barrier. Indomethacin is an NSAID utilized to close a PDA. Aspirin is not an appropriate agent to keep a PDA open. Ticlopidine will decrease platelet viscosity.

63. E. Warfarin is metabolized by the CYP450 system; when it is inhibited by cimetidine (a reversible blocker of H_2 receptors), more warfarin is made available in the circulation and anticoagulation is potentiated. Other P450 inhibitors include ketoconazole, grapefruit, erythromycin, isoniazid, and sulfonamides.

64. E. Octreotide is an analog of somatostatin and is used in the treatment of carcinoid, acromegaly, and bleeding esophageal varices. Figure 13-5 shows an actively bleeding varix. Vasopressin is sometimes also used in esophageal varices but is not the analog of octreotide. There is no reason to administer cholecystokinin to this patient. Dopamine should be considered in patients who have hypotension; it can also be used to increase renal blood flow. Norepinephrine is an inotrope that can increase blood pressure and cardiac output.

65. C. Ethacrinic acid is the best option for this patient. It acts similarly to a loop diuretic like furosemide (thus decreasing serum calcium), but it can also be used in those with a sulfa allergy, as it is a derivative of phenoxyacetic acid. Also, it should be noted that furosemide is known to cause an allergic reaction in sulfa-sensitive patients. Hydrochlorothiazide would not be used because it increases the serum calcium and can cause a sulfa allergy as well. Acetazolamide is a carbonic anhydrase inhibitor. It can cause self-limited bicarbonate diuresis. Captopril is an angiotensin-converting enzyme inhibitor that leads to a reduction of angiotensin II and prevents inactivation of bradykinin. Hydrochlorothiazide inhibits sodium chloride reabsorption from the distal tubule. Mannitol is an osmotic diuretic. Spironolactone is a potassium-sparing diuretic.

66. C. Hydralazine is an antihypertensive agent often used in hypertensive emergencies (systolic BP > 200). By increasing cGMP and dilating arteries, it acts to decrease the afterload that the left ventricle must pump against. Nitrates act to increase cGMP and also dilate veins. Hydralazine does not potentiate beta$_2$ receptors peripherally.

67. B. Efavirenz (Sustiva) is a nonnucleoside reverse transcriptase inhibitor that acts to prevent the transcription of viral RNA to DNA. Of the other choices given, zidovudine (a nucleoside analog) is used in pregnancy to prevent transmission of HIV to the fetus. Other side effects of efavirenz are rash, nightmares, and CYP450 inhibitor and inducer. Delviradine is a reverse transcriptase inhibitor used in the treatment of HIV. Saquinavir is a protease inhibitor that inhibits assembly of new virus by blocking protease enzymes. Zidovudine is a nucleoside reverse transcriptase inhibitor.

68. E. Zidovudine is a nucleoside reverse transcriptase inhibitor that classically causes megaloblastic anemia. It is often a component of HAART, which consists of three drugs: two nucleoside reverse transcriptase inhibitors plus either a nonnucleoside reverse transcriptase inhibitor or a protease inhibitor. Ritonavir is a protease inhibitor that interferes with the cytochrome P450 system of the liver. Didanosine and stavudine are nucleoside reverse transcriptase inhibitors.

69. B. Tetracycline is a bacteriostatic agent that binds to the bacterial 30S subunit and prevents the attachment of aminoacyl-tRNA. Fanconi's syndrome is an acquired disorder due to a proximal tubule defect that results in a decreased blood pH, bicarbonate, phosphate, glucose, and amino acids because of leakage in the kidney. Of the other toxicities, tetracycline also causes tooth discoloration, but this is usually seen only in those below 7 years of age. Another side effect seen in this age group is inhibition of bone growth.

70. G. Rifampin is used as treatment for prophylaxis in close contacts of those infected by *Neisseria meningitidis*. Rifampin, which is normally used in combination with other agents (such as isoniazid or ethambutol) to treat tuberculosis, acts by blocking mRNA synthesis. The penicillins are the drugs of choice to treat infections caused by streptococci, meningococci, penicillin-susceptible pneumococci, and for *T. pallidum*. Ertapenem and meropenem are carbapenems; they are used to treat a wide range of infections, including septicemia.

71. D. Pseudomembranous colitis develops in patients after their normal enteric flora is depleted by the use of broad-spectrum antibiotics such as the cephalosporins, penicillins, and classically clindamycin. Treatment includes metronidazole or oral vancomycin. Intravenous vancomycin cannot be used because not enough of the drug reaches the intestinal lumen, where the clostridia lie. Ampicillin can cause pseudomembranous colitis, as can vibramycin.

72. D. In Parkinson's disease, the dopaminergic neurons in the pars compacta of the substantia nigra are slowly lost. Amantadine, which is most notable for treatment of influenza A and rubella, is often used as initial treatment. This agent is well absorbed from the GI tract and 90% is excreted by the kidneys. This agent does not work on the pars compacta nor does it block GABA receptors. It does not potentiate the action of dopamine on the globus pallidus.

73. B. Phentolamine is a reversible nonselective alpha-blocker. It allows epinephrine (which binds to alpha$_1$, alpha$_2$, beta$_1$, and beta$_2$ receptors) to bind only to beta-receptors. The result is a depressor effect primarily because of the beta$_2$ stimulation. There is no depressor effect due to unopposed beta$_1$ stimulation. There will not be an increase in blood pressure due to unopposed alpha$_1$, alpha$_2$, or beta$_2$ stimulation.

74. E. Losartan is an angiotensin II–receptor blocker. It works by blocking the effects of angiotensin II. It is not an (ACE) inhibitor, so it does not cause cough. ACE inhibitors are known to cause cough, and since the patient remembers a coughing episode from the previous medication, he was most likely on an ACE inhibitor. Diltiazem is a calcium channel blocker used in some antihypertensive regimens, but it is not a first-line agent for the treatment of hypertension. Captopril and lisinopril are ACE inhibitors.

75. A. Amiloride is one of the diuretics in the potassium-sparing class. It is a competitive aldosterone antagonist in the cortical collecting tubule. It has the known side effect of causing hyperkalemia. Furosemide and ethacrynic acid both act by inhibiting the cotransport system in the ascending loop of Henle. They are not potassium-sparing diuretics and, with excessive use, actually cause potassium wasting. Hydrochlorothiazide is a thiazide diuretic that inhibits NaCl reabsorption in the early distal tubule. This diuretic also does not spare potassium. Mannitol is an osmotic diuretic that works in the proximal convoluted tubule to increase tubular fluid osmolarity, which increases urine flow.

Index

Note: Page numbers followed by f indicate figures.

Diagnostic Test   Answer Sheet

BLOCK 1

1. _____
2. _____
3. _____
4. _____
5. _____
6. _____
7. _____
8. _____
9. _____
10. _____
11. _____
12. _____
13. _____

14. _____
15. _____
16. _____
17. _____
18. _____
19. _____
20. _____
21. _____
22. _____
23. _____
24. _____
25. _____
26. _____

27. _____
28. _____
29. _____
30. _____
31. _____
32. _____
33. _____
34. _____
35. _____
36. _____
37. _____
38. _____
39. _____

40. _____
41. _____
42. _____
43. _____
44. _____
45. _____
46. _____
47. _____
48. _____
49. _____
50. _____

BLOCK 2

51. _____
52. _____
53. _____
54. _____
55. _____
56. _____
57. _____
58. _____
59. _____
60. _____
61. _____
62. _____
63. _____

64. _____
65. _____
66. _____
67. _____
68. _____
69. _____
70. _____
71. _____
72. _____
73. _____
74. _____
75. _____
76. _____

77. _____
78. _____
79. _____
80. _____
81. _____
82. _____
83. _____
84. _____
85. _____
86. _____
87. _____
88. _____
89. _____

90. _____
91. _____
92. _____
93. _____
94. _____
95. _____
96. _____
97. _____
98. _____
99. _____
100. _____

Diagnostic Test   Answer Sheet

BLOCK 3

101. _____

102. _____

103. _____

104. _____

105. _____

106. _____

107. _____

108. _____

109. _____

110. _____

111. _____

112. _____

113. _____

114. _____

115. _____

116. _____

117. _____

118. _____

119. _____

120. _____

121. _____

122. _____

123. _____

124. _____

125. _____

126. _____

127. _____

128. _____

129. _____

130. _____

131. _____

132. _____

133. _____

134. _____

135. _____

136. _____

137. _____

138. _____

139. _____

140. _____

141. _____

142. _____

143. _____

144. _____

145. _____

146. _____

147. _____

148. _____

149. _____

150. _____

BLOCK 4

151. _____

152. _____

153. _____

154. _____

155. _____

156. _____

157. _____

158. _____

159. _____

160. _____

161. _____

162. _____

163. _____

164. _____

165. _____

166. _____

167. _____

168. _____

169. _____

170. _____

171. _____

172. _____

173. _____

174. _____

175. _____

176. _____

177. _____

178. _____

179. _____

180. _____

181. _____

182. _____

183. _____

184. _____

185. _____

186. _____

187. _____

188. _____

189. _____

190. _____

191. _____

192. _____

193. _____

194. _____

195. _____

196. _____

197. _____

198. _____

199. _____

200. _____

Diagnostic Test   Answer Sheet

BLOCK 5

201. _____
202. _____
203. _____
204. _____
205. _____
206. _____
207. _____
208. _____
209. _____
210. _____
211. _____
212. _____
213. _____

214. _____
215. _____
216. _____
217. _____
218. _____
219. _____
220. _____
221. _____
222. _____
223. _____
224. _____
225. _____
226. _____

227. _____
228. _____
229. _____
230. _____
231. _____
232. _____
233. _____
234. _____
235. _____
236. _____
237. _____
238. _____
239. _____

240. _____
241. _____
242. _____
243. _____
244. _____
245. _____
246. _____
247. _____
248. _____
249. _____
250. _____

BLOCK 6

251. _____
252. _____
253. _____
254. _____
255. _____
256. _____
257. _____
258. _____
259. _____
260. _____
261. _____
262. _____
263. _____

264. _____
265. _____
266. _____
267. _____
268. _____
269. _____
270. _____
271. _____
272. _____
273. _____
274. _____
275. _____
276. _____

277. _____
278. _____
279. _____
280. _____
281. _____
282. _____
283. _____
284. _____
285. _____
286. _____
287. _____
288. _____
289. _____

290. _____
291. _____
292. _____
293. _____
294. _____
295. _____
296. _____
297. _____
298. _____
299. _____
300. _____

Diagnostic Test   Answer Sheet

BLOCK 7

201. _____   314. _____   327. _____   340. _____
302. _____   315. _____   328. _____   341. _____
303. _____   316. _____   329. _____   342. _____
304. _____   317. _____   330. _____   343. _____
305. _____   318. _____   331. _____   344. _____
306. _____   319. _____   332. _____   345. _____
307. _____   320. _____   333. _____   346. _____
308. _____   321. _____   334. _____   347. _____
309. _____   322. _____   335. _____   348. _____
310. _____   323. _____   336. _____   349. _____
311. _____   324. _____   337. _____   350. _____
312. _____   325. _____   338. _____
313. _____   326. _____   339. _____

Chapter 1   Answer Sheet

1. _____
2. _____
3. _____
4. _____
5. _____
6. _____
7. _____
8. _____
9. _____
10. _____
11. _____
12. _____
13. _____
14. _____
15. _____
16. _____
17. _____
18. _____
19. _____

20. _____
21. _____
22. _____
23. _____
24. _____
25. _____
26. _____
27. _____
28. _____
29. _____
30. _____
31. _____
32. _____
33. _____
34. _____
35. _____
36. _____
37. _____
38. _____

39. _____
40. _____
41. _____
42. _____
43. _____
44. _____
45. _____
46. _____
47. _____
48. _____
49. _____
50. _____
51. _____
52. _____
53. _____
54. _____
55. _____
56. _____
57. _____

58. _____
59. _____
60. _____
61. _____
62. _____
63. _____
64. _____
65. _____
66. _____
67. _____
68. _____
69. _____
70. _____
71. _____
72. _____
73. _____
74. _____
75. _____

Chapter 2   Answer Sheet

1. _____

2. _____

3. _____

4. _____

5. _____

6. _____

7. _____

8. _____

9. _____

10. _____

11. _____

12. _____

13. _____

14. _____

15. _____

16. _____

17. _____

18. _____

19. _____

20. _____

21. _____

22. _____

23. _____

24. _____

25. _____

26. _____

27. _____

28. _____

29. _____

30. _____

31. _____

32. _____

33. _____

34. _____

35. _____

36. _____

37. _____

38. _____

39. _____

40. _____

41. _____

42. _____

43. _____

44. _____

45. _____

46. _____

47. _____

48. _____

49. _____

50. _____

51. _____

52. _____

53. _____

54. _____

55. _____

56. _____

57. _____

58. _____

59. _____

60. _____

61. _____

62. _____

63. _____

64. _____

65. _____

66. _____

67. _____

68. _____

69. _____

70. _____

71. _____

72. _____

73. _____

74. _____

75. _____

Chapter 3   Answer Sheet

1. _____

2. _____

3. _____

4. _____

5. _____

6. _____

7. _____

8. _____

9. _____

10. _____

11. _____

12. _____

13. _____

14. _____

15. _____

16. _____

17. _____

18. _____

19. _____

20. _____

21. _____

22. _____

23. _____

24. _____

25. _____

26. _____

27. _____

28. _____

29. _____

30. _____

31. _____

32. _____

33. _____

34. _____

35. _____

36. _____

37. _____

38. _____

39. _____

40. _____

41. _____

42. _____

43. _____

44. _____

45. _____

46. _____

47. _____

48. _____

49. _____

50. _____

51. _____

52. _____

53. _____

54. _____

55. _____

56. _____

57. _____

58. _____

59. _____

60. _____

61. _____

62. _____

63. _____

64. _____

65. _____

66. _____

67. _____

68. _____

69. _____

70. _____

71. _____

72. _____

73. _____

74. _____

75. _____

Chapter 4   Answer Sheet

1. _____
2. _____
3. _____
4. _____
5. _____
6. _____
7. _____
8. _____
9. _____
10. _____
11. _____
12. _____
13. _____
14. _____
15. _____
16. _____
17. _____
18. _____
19. _____

20. _____
21. _____
22. _____
23. _____
24. _____
25. _____
26. _____
27. _____
28. _____
29. _____
30. _____
31. _____
32. _____
33. _____
34. _____
35. _____
36. _____
37. _____
38. _____

39. _____
40. _____
41. _____
42. _____
43. _____
44. _____
45. _____
46. _____
47. _____
48. _____
49. _____
50. _____
51. _____
52. _____
53. _____
54. _____
55. _____
56. _____
57. _____

58. _____
59. _____
60. _____
61. _____
62. _____
63. _____
64. _____
65. _____
66. _____
67. _____
68. _____
69. _____
70. _____
71. _____
72. _____
73. _____
74. _____
75. _____

Chapter 5   Answer Sheet

1. _____
2. _____
3. _____
4. _____
5. _____
6. _____
7. _____
8. _____
9. _____
10. _____
11. _____
12. _____
13. _____
14. _____
15. _____
16. _____
17. _____
18. _____
19. _____

20. _____
21. _____
22. _____
23. _____
24. _____
25. _____
26. _____
27. _____
28. _____
29. _____
30. _____
31. _____
32. _____
33. _____
34. _____
35. _____
36. _____
37. _____
38. _____

39. _____
40. _____
41. _____
42. _____
43. _____
44. _____
45. _____
46. _____
47. _____
48. _____
49. _____
50. _____
51. _____
52. _____
53. _____
54. _____
55. _____
56. _____
57. _____

58. _____
59. _____
60. _____
61. _____
62. _____
63. _____
64. _____
65. _____
66. _____
67. _____
68. _____
69. _____
70. _____
71. _____
72. _____
73. _____
74. _____
75. _____

1. _____

2. _____

3. _____

4. _____

5. _____

6. _____

7. _____

8. _____

9. _____

10. _____

11. _____

12. _____

13. _____

14. _____

15. _____

16. _____

17. _____

18. _____

19. _____

20. _____

21. _____

22. _____

23. _____

24. _____

25. _____

26. _____

27. _____

28. _____

29. _____

30. _____

31. _____

32. _____

33. _____

34. _____

35. _____

36. _____

37. _____

38. _____

39. _____

40. _____

41. _____

42. _____

43. _____

44. _____

45. _____

46. _____

47. _____

48. _____

49. _____

50. _____

51. _____

52. _____

53. _____

54. _____

55. _____

56. _____

57. _____

58. _____

59. _____

60. _____

61. _____

62. _____

63. _____

64. _____

65. _____

66. _____

67. _____

68. _____

69. _____

70. _____

71. _____

72. _____

73. _____

74. _____

75. _____

Chapter 7   Answer Sheet

1. _____
2. _____
3. _____
4. _____
5. _____
6. _____
7. _____
8. _____
9. _____
10. _____
11. _____
12. _____
13. _____
14. _____
15. _____
16. _____
17. _____
18. _____
19. _____

20. _____
21. _____
22. _____
23. _____
24. _____
25. _____
26. _____
27. _____
28. _____
29. _____
30. _____
31. _____
32. _____
33. _____
34. _____
35. _____
36. _____
37. _____
38. _____

39. _____
40. _____
41. _____
42. _____
43. _____
44. _____
45. _____
46. _____
47. _____
48. _____
49. _____
50. _____
51. _____
52. _____
53. _____
54. _____
55. _____
56. _____
57. _____

58. _____
59. _____
60. _____
61. _____
62. _____
63. _____
64. _____
65. _____
66. _____
67. _____
68. _____
69. _____
70. _____
71. _____
72. _____
73. _____
74. _____
75. _____

Chapter 8   Answer Sheet

1. _____
2. _____
3. _____
4. _____
5. _____
6. _____
7. _____
8. _____
9. _____
10. _____
11. _____
12. _____
13. _____
14. _____
15. _____
16. _____
17. _____
18. _____
19. _____

20. _____
21. _____
22. _____
23. _____
24. _____
25. _____
26. _____
27. _____
28. _____
29. _____
30. _____
31. _____
32. _____
33. _____
34. _____
35. _____
36. _____
37. _____
38. _____

39. _____
40. _____
41. _____
42. _____
43. _____
44. _____
45. _____
46. _____
47. _____
48. _____
49. _____
50. _____
51. _____
52. _____
53. _____
54. _____
55. _____
56. _____
57. _____

58. _____
59. _____
60. _____
61. _____
62. _____
63. _____
64. _____
65. _____
66. _____
67. _____
68. _____
69. _____
70. _____
71. _____
72. _____
73. _____
74. _____
75. _____

Chapter 9   Answer Sheet

1. _____
2. _____
3. _____
4. _____
5. _____
6. _____
7. _____
8. _____
9. _____
10. _____
11. _____
12. _____
13. _____
14. _____
15. _____
16. _____
17. _____
18. _____
19. _____

20. _____
21. _____
22. _____
23. _____
24. _____
25. _____
26. _____
27. _____
28. _____
29. _____
30. _____
31. _____
32. _____
33. _____
34. _____
35. _____
36. _____
37. _____
38. _____

39. _____
40. _____
41. _____
42. _____
43. _____
44. _____
45. _____
46. _____
47. _____
48. _____
49. _____
50. _____
51. _____
52. _____
53. _____
54. _____
55. _____
56. _____
57. _____

58. _____
59. _____
60. _____
61. _____
62. _____
63. _____
64. _____
65. _____
66. _____
67. _____
68. _____
69. _____
70. _____
71. _____
72. _____
73. _____
74. _____
75. _____

Chapter 10   Answer Sheet

1. _____

2. _____

3. _____

4. _____

5. _____

6. _____

7. _____

8. _____

9. _____

10. _____

11. _____

12. _____

13. _____

14. _____

15. _____

16. _____

17. _____

18. _____

19. _____

20. _____

21. _____

22. _____

23. _____

24. _____

25. _____

26. _____

27. _____

28. _____

29. _____

30. _____

31. _____

32. _____

33. _____

34. _____

35. _____

36. _____

37. _____

38. _____

39. _____

40. _____

41. _____

42. _____

43. _____

44. _____

45. _____

46. _____

47. _____

48. _____

49. _____

50. _____

51. _____

52. _____

53. _____

54. _____

55. _____

56. _____

57. _____

58. _____

59. _____

60. _____

61. _____

62. _____

63. _____

64. _____

65. _____

66. _____

67. _____

68. _____

69. _____

70. _____

71. _____

72. _____

73. _____

74. _____

75. _____

Chapter 11   Answer Sheet

1. _____
2. _____
3. _____
4. _____
5. _____
6. _____
7. _____
8. _____
9. _____
10. _____
11. _____
12. _____
13. _____
14. _____
15. _____
16. _____
17. _____
18. _____
19. _____

20. _____
21. _____
22. _____
23. _____
24. _____
25. _____
26. _____
27. _____
28. _____
29. _____
30. _____
31. _____
32. _____
33. _____
34. _____
35. _____
36. _____
37. _____
38. _____

39. _____
40. _____
41. _____
42. _____
43. _____
44. _____
45. _____
46. _____
47. _____
48. _____
49. _____
50. _____
51. _____
52. _____
53. _____
54. _____
55. _____
56. _____
57. _____

58. _____
59. _____
60. _____
61. _____
62. _____
63. _____
64. _____
65. _____
66. _____
67. _____
68. _____
69. _____
70. _____
71. _____
72. _____
73. _____
74. _____
75. _____

Chapter 12   Answer Sheet

1. _____
2. _____
3. _____
4. _____
5. _____
6. _____
7. _____
8. _____
9. _____
10. _____
11. _____
12. _____
13. _____
14. _____
15. _____
16. _____
17. _____
18. _____
19. _____

20. _____
21. _____
22. _____
23. _____
24. _____
25. _____
26. _____
27. _____
28. _____
29. _____
30. _____
31. _____
32. _____
33. _____
34. _____
35. _____
36. _____
37. _____
38. _____

39. _____
40. _____
41. _____
42. _____
43. _____
44. _____
45. _____
46. _____
47. _____
48. _____
49. _____
50. _____
51. _____
52. _____
53. _____
54. _____
55. _____
56. _____
57. _____

58. _____
59. _____
60. _____
61. _____
62. _____
63. _____
64. _____
65. _____
66. _____
67. _____
68. _____
69. _____
70. _____
71. _____
72. _____
73. _____
74. _____
75. _____

Chapter 13   Answer Sheet

1. _____
2. _____
3. _____
4. _____
5. _____
6. _____
7. _____
8. _____
9. _____
10. _____
11. _____
12. _____
13. _____
14. _____
15. _____
16. _____
17. _____
18. _____
19. _____

20. _____
21. _____
22. _____
23. _____
24. _____
25. _____
26. _____
27. _____
28. _____
29. _____
30. _____
31. _____
32. _____
33. _____
34. _____
35. _____
36. _____
37. _____
38. _____

39. _____
40. _____
41. _____
42. _____
43. _____
44. _____
45. _____
46. _____
47. _____
48. _____
49. _____
50. _____
51. _____
52. _____
53. _____
54. _____
55. _____
56. _____
57. _____

58. _____
59. _____
60. _____
61. _____
62. _____
63. _____
64. _____
65. _____
66. _____
67. _____
68. _____
69. _____
70. _____
71. _____
72. _____
73. _____
74. _____
75. _____